Patient Management in
Obstetrics and Gynecology

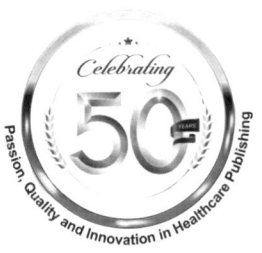

Patient Management in
Obstetrics and Gynecology

Editor

Rashida Begum
FCPS MS MSc PhD
Chief Consultant
Infertility Care and Research Center
Dhaka, Bangladesh

Foreword
TA Chowdhury

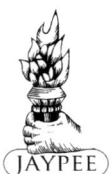

JAYPEE BROTHERS MEDICAL PUBLISHERS
The Health Sciences Publisher
New Delhi | London | Panama

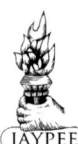 **Jaypee Brothers Medical Publishers (P) Ltd.**

Headquarters
Jaypee Brothers Medical Publishers (P) Ltd
4838/24, Ansari Road, Daryaganj
New Delhi 110 002, India
Phone: +91-11-43574357
Fax: +91-11-43574314
E-mail: jaypee@jaypeebrothers.com

Overseas Offices

J.P. Medical Ltd
83, Victoria Street, London
SW1H 0HW (UK)
Phone: +44 20 3170 8910
Fax: +44 (0)20 3008 6180
E-mail: info@jpmedpub.com

Jaypee-Highlights Medical Publishers Inc
City of Knowledge, Bld. 235, 2nd Floor, Clayton
Panama City, Panama
Phone: +1 507-301-0496
Fax: +1 507-301-0499
E-mail: cservice@jphmedical.com

Jaypee Brothers Medical Publishers (P) Ltd
17/1-B, Babar Road, Block-B, Shaymali
Mohammadpur, Dhaka-1207
Bangladesh
Mobile: +08801912003485
E-mail: jaypeedhaka@gmail.com

Jaypee Brothers Medical Publishers (P) Ltd
Bhotahity, Kathmandu
Nepal
Phone: +977-9741283608
E-mail: kathmandu@jaypeebrothers.com

Website: www.jaypeebrothers.com
Website: www.jaypeedigital.com

© 2019, Jaypee Brothers Medical Publishers

The views and opinions expressed in this book are solely those of the original contributor(s)/author(s) and do not necessarily represent those of editor(s) of the book.

All rights reserved. No part of this publication may be reproduced, stored or transmitted in any form or by any means, electronic, mechanical, photocopying, recording or otherwise, without the prior permission in writing of the publishers.

All brand names and product names used in this book are trade names, service marks, trademarks or registered trademarks of their respective owners. The publisher is not associated with any product or vendor mentioned in this book.

Medical knowledge and practice change constantly. This book is designed to provide accurate, authoritative information about the subject matter in question. However, readers are advised to check the most current information available on procedures included and check information from the manufacturer of each product to be administered, to verify the recommended dose, formula, method and duration of administration, adverse effects and contraindications. It is the responsibility of the practitioner to take all appropriate safety precautions. Neither the publisher nor the author(s)/editor(s) assume any liability for any injury and/or damage to persons or property arising from or related to use of material in this book.

This book is sold on the understanding that the publisher is not engaged in providing professional medical services. If such advice or services are required, the services of a competent medical professional should be sought.

Every effort has been made where necessary to contact holders of copyright to obtain permission to reproduce copyright material. If any have been inadvertently overlooked, the publisher will be pleased to make the necessary arrangements at the first opportunity. The **CD/DVD-ROM** (if any) provided in the sealed envelope with this book is complimentary and free of cost. **Not meant for sale.**

Inquiries for bulk sales may be solicited at: jaypee@jaypeebrothers.com

Patient Management in Obstetrics and Gynecology

First Edition: **2019**

ISBN: 978-93-5270-538-2

Printed at: Samrat Offset Pvt. Ltd.

Dedicated to

My parents, my siblings
my husband, my teachers
my daughters, and my patients
who gave me the scope of learning.

CONTRIBUTORS

Farhat Hossain MBBS FCPS
Professor and Head
Department of Obstetrics and Gynecology
Sir Salimullah Medical College
Dhaka, Bangladesh

Firoza Begum MBBS FCPS
Professor and Head, Fetomaternal Medicine Unit
Department of Obstetrics and Gynecology
Bangabandhu Sheikh Mujib Medical
University (BSMMU)
Dhaka, Bangladesh

Hosne Ara Baby MBBS FCPS
Fertility Specialist
Former Professor
Shahabuddin Medical College, Dhaka
Consultant
Infertility Care and Research Center
Dhaka, Bangladesh

Muna Shalima Jahan MBBS FCPS FAIMER Fellow
Associate Professor
Department of Obstetrics and Gynecology
Sir Salimullah Medical College
Dhaka, Bangladesh

Nurun Nahar Khanam MBBS FCPS MS Med LMCC
Associate Professor
Department of Obstetrics and Gynecology
Bangabandhu Sheikh Mujib Medical
University (BSMMU)
Dhaka, Bangladesh

Rashida Begum FCPS MS MSc PhD
Chief Consultant
Infertility Care and Research Center
Dhaka, Bangladesh

Rehana Parveen MBBS FCPS
Professor
Department of Gynecological Oncology
National Institute of Cancer Research
and Hospital
Dhaka, Bangladesh

Saria Tasnim MBBS FCPS Masters in Medical Education Diploma in Community Epidemiology
Professor and Head
Department of Obstetrics and Gynecology
Dhaka Community Medical College
Former Executive Director
Institute of Child and Mother Health
Dhaka, Bangladesh

Sayeba Akhter MBBS FCPS (BD) FICMCH (IN) DRH (UK) FCPS (PAK) FRCOG (UK) FICOG (IN)
Professor
Department of Obstetrics and Gynecology
MAMM's Institute of Fistula and
Women's Health (MIFWOH)
Dhaka, Bangladesh

FOREWORD

It is a matter of great pleasure for me to write a foreword for *Patient Management in Obstetrics and Gynecology* by Professor Rashida Begum and her collaborators. Unlike other similar textbooks, she has tried to focus on the way the patients generally present and then proceeds to discuss the possible etiology, pathology and management. This may prove to be a more interesting and effective way of learning in clinical medicine.

She has not tried to make the book comprehensive by including all possible topics, but has tried to focus on more important problems with which the patients present in the day to practice. Another useful addition was citing typical case scenarios to illustrate how the patients generally present and to relate this to the pathological features and management.

One important feature of the book that impressed me is the step-by-step details with which the management of the cases has been described. This, I presume will be useful not only to students, but to the obstetric practitioners in general who will be able to use the book as an up-to-date reference manual.

I hope this book will have wide acceptance among our students and obstetric practitioners.

TA Chowdhury
FRCS FRCOG FCPS (Bang) FCPS (Pak) PhD
Professor
Department of Obstetrics and Gynecology
Chief Consultant
Bangladesh Institute of Research and
Rehabilitation for Diabetes, Endocrine
and Metabolic Disorders (BIRDEM)
Dhaka, Bangladesh

PREFACE

Finally, I have completed it. I started the journey in 2011 when I observed that students in their fellowship examination could not correlate the clinical situation with their knowledge. Because there was a wide gap between their study and real situation as they did not get the chance of handling enough cases. According to Sir William Osler, "To study the phenomena of disease without books is to sail an uncharted sea, while to study books without patients is not to go to sea at all". So, there is no other alternative but to learn from patients. Patients are the greatest source of learning and they are the best teachers. However, all the cases may not be available in any institution. So, the concept of simulation emerged.

Simulation can be done either by human beings or by paper-pencil. Paper-pencil simulation has wide space to cover every aspect of the problem of the patient. Objective of introducing this book is to teach the students with paper-pencil simulation so that they can imagine the real situation.

This is a problem book, a variety of textbook. Problem books are textbooks usually at advanced undergraduate or postgraduate level, in which the material is organized as a series of problems, each with a complete solution given. Problem books are distinct from workbooks in that the problems are designed as a primary means of teaching, not merely for practice on material learned elsewhere.

In this book, I tried to teach the students about a particular disease in such a way that he/she can learn about so many different presentations of a particular disease. First of all, I started with a scenario of problems, then discussed about history taking. Next scenario was made by findings from history and examination. Those findings are usually the signs and symptoms of the disease. As all aspects could not be covered by the scenario and answer of the questions, other explanatory things are mentioned as related information.

This book is mainly planned for postgraduate students, but it is hoped that general gynecologists will also be benefited from this book.

It takes time to organize the whole spectrum of disease in a chapter. So, I could not cover all the topics. The book contains 21 chapters of both Obstetrics and Gynecology. To enrich the content of the topic, few chapters were written by gynecologists of respective specialty. Besides that, all chapters were reviewed by other experts of this field. Some chapters were also checked by postgraduate students to have their opinion.

I pay my humble respect and gratefulness to my seniors and juniors whose continuous encouragement and support helped me to prepare this book.

As first edition, this book may not be adequate enough and may not fulfill the desire of readers. I would invite constructive criticism from valued readers of this book so that errors and omission can be corrected in the next edition.

I acknowledge the contributors and reviewers for their efforts to enrich this book.

Lastly, I am grateful to M/s Jaypee Brothers Medical Publishers (P) Ltd, New Delhi, India, for taking the burden of publishing this book.

Rashida Begum

ACKNOWLEDGMENTS

I would like to acknowledge all my colleagues and well-wishers for their heartfully support to my endeavor, especially Professors Anowara Begum, Samina Chowdhury, Bayes Bhuiyan, Kohinoor Begum, Drs Maruf Siddiqui, Nusrat Mahmud, Jannatul Ferdous Jonaki, Afroza Kutubi, Mariya Ehsan, Nazia Ehsan, Shahina Begum Shanta, Farzana Khan, Farhana Sharmin, Nasrin Farhana, Nahid Parveen, and Tahera Begum.

CONTENTS

1. **Placenta Previa**   1
   Rashida Begum

2. **Abruptio Placenta**   14
   Rashida Begum

3. **Third Stage Complications**   24
   Rashida Begum

4. **Premature Birth**   39
   Rashida Begum

5. **Preterm Premature Rupture Membrane**   53
   Hosne Ara Baby, Rashida Begum

6. **Labor Dystocia**   61
   Rashida Begum

7. **Gestational Diabetes Mellitus**   78
   Rashida Begum

8. **Rhesus Isoimmunization**   89
   Nurun Nahar Khanam, Rashida Begum

9. **Pregnancy-induced Hypertension**   104
   Rashida Begum

10. **Ectopic Pregnancy**   128
    Rashida Begum

11. **Gestational Trophoblastic Diseases**   142
    Farhat Hossain, Rashida Begum

12. **Ovarian Masses**   162
    Rashida Begum, Rehana Parveen

13. **Ovarian Malignancy**   176
    Rehana Parveen, Rashida Begum, Farhat Hossain

14. Cervical Cancer   201
Farhat Hossain, Rashida Begum

15. Precancerous Disease of Cervix and its Prevention   221
Farhat Hossain

16. Endometriosis   238
Rashida Begum

17. Infertility   253
Rashida Begum

18. Abnormal Uterine Bleeding   286
Saria Tasnim, Rashida Begum

19. Postmenopausal Bleeding   298
Saria Tasnim, Farhat Hossain

20. Recurrent Pregnancy Loss   303
Rashida Begum, Firoza Begum

21. Genitourinary Fistula   318
Muna Shalima Jahan, Rashida Begum, Sayeba Akhter

Index   *339*

CHAPTER 1

Placenta Previa

Rashida Begum

INTRODUCTION

Bleeding during late pregnancy antepartum hemorrhage (APH) is a high-risk pregnancy. It is an emergency situation, which still is an important cause of maternal death in developing countries. APH occurs in 2–5% of all pregnancies. Placenta previa is one sort of APH, which complicates 0.3–0.5% of all pregnancies (Iyasu, 1993). In developing countries due to pre-existing anemia, poor transport condition and inadequate medical facilities placenta previa continues to be responsible for many maternal deaths. Though the death rate in developed countries is not significant.

> **Case scenario:** Mrs Hazera Khatun aged 35 years, a multiparous woman, has come to your hospital with history of amenorrhea for 32 weeks with sign symptoms of pregnancy and per vaginal (PV) bleeding for 1 hour. This is her first visit to you.
>
> How will you proceed for diagnosis?

Detailed History is to be Taken First

About bleeding
- When did PV bleeding start?
- How much bleeding occurred?
- Was there any clotted blood?
- Is it her first episode of bleeding?

To be sure about gestational age menstrual history is to be taken
- Whether the cycle was regular or not
- What was the length of the cycle?
- When was the last menstrual period?

About other associated factors
- Whether there is any pain in the abdomen?
- Whether there is any history of fall or trauma?
- Is she hypertensive?
- Is her parent hypertensive?

About fetal condition
- Whether fetal movement is present and adequate?

Obstetric history is to be taken
- Parity of the patient and number of previous conceptions
- Mode of previous deliveries
- History of any menstrual regulation (MR), dilatation and curettage (D&C) or manual removal of placenta

Examination

A quick general examination is needed to assess the effect of blood loss. *Abdominal examination* is to be done to assess fetal condition. Inspection of vulva and introitus is to be done to assess the amount of vaginal bleeding.

Note: Per vaginal examination is not done until and unless there is any sign of labor.

> On enquiry, you elicited that the patient has no complaints of abdominal pain. She started bleeding suddenly. This is her first episode of bleeding. It is not associated with any trauma. Amount of bleeding is like menstrual bleeding. On physical examination you found her pulse, blood pressure normal. Abdomen is soft nontender, fetal movement is present, fetal heart sound is audible and normal, and there is slight PV bleeding.
>
> On the basis of history and physical findings what might be your diagnosis?

Antepartum hemorrhage and most likely placenta previa.

Note: Any painless bleeding during late pregnancy should be considered as placenta previa until and unless proved otherwise.

RELATED INFORMATION

Antepartum Hemorrhage

Any bleeding from or into genital tract after 28 weeks of gestation, but before the onset of labor is called APH.

It is of four types:
1. Placenta previa
2. Abruptio placenta (1 and 2 are placental cause and comprise 70% of APH)
3. Indeterminant
4. Local cervicovaginal cause:
   – Vasa previa
   – Rupture of marginal sinus
   – Vulvo-vaginal and cervical varicosities
   – Cervical erosion, ectopy, injury, neoplasia
   – Vaginal neoplasia, infection, laceration.

Placenta Previa and Abruptio Placenta (Table 1.1)

When placenta lies in lower uterine segment then it is called *placenta previa* and when there is bleeding from the site of normally situated placenta then it is called *abruptio placenta*. *Painless bleeding* is characteristic of placenta previa.

Other *features of placenta previa* are:
- Bleeding is recurrent
- Malpresentation is common
- Fetus is usually alive
- Incidence is more in multiparous women.

So sudden onset, painless, causeless recurrent PV bleeding are diagnostic features of placenta previa.

Types of Placenta Previa

Placenta previa is of four types **(Fig. 1.1)**.

Type I (lateral): Placenta just reaches to lower uterine segment.

Type II (marginal): Placenta reaches to the level of internal os, but does not cover it.

Type III (incomplete central): Placenta completely covers the internal os when is closed, but does not cover entirely when os is fully dilated.

Type IV (central): Placenta completely covers the internal os even when os is fully dilated.

> What investigation would you like to do to confirm your diagnosis?

Ultrasonogram (USG).

Table 1.1 Differentiating points of placenta previa and abruptio placenta

Variables	Placenta previa	Abruptio placenta
Clinical features		
• Pattern and nature of bleeding	i. Painless, causeless and recurrent bleeding ii. Bleeding is always revealed iii. Usually bright red in color	i. Usually painful bleeding and followed by some precipitating factors such as preeclampsia or trauma ii. Bleeding is either revealed or concealed or mixed iii. Usually dark in color but may be bright
• General condition and pallor	Proportionate to visible blood loss	Out of proportionate to the visible blood loss in concealed or mixed variety
• Per abdominal examination: – Height of the uterus – Consistency of the uterus – Fetal heart sound – Presentation	 – Usually corresponds with gestational age – Soft and relaxed – Usually present – Malpresentation is common due to presence of placenta in lower segment. Head remains high up	 – May be disproportionately enlarged due to accumulation of blood in concealed type – May be tense, tender and rigid – Usually absent particularly in concealed type – There is no relation with presentation
Ultrasonography	Placenta lies in lower segment	Placenta lies in upper segment
Per vaginal examination, if performed	Placenta can be felt in lower segment	Placenta cannot be felt

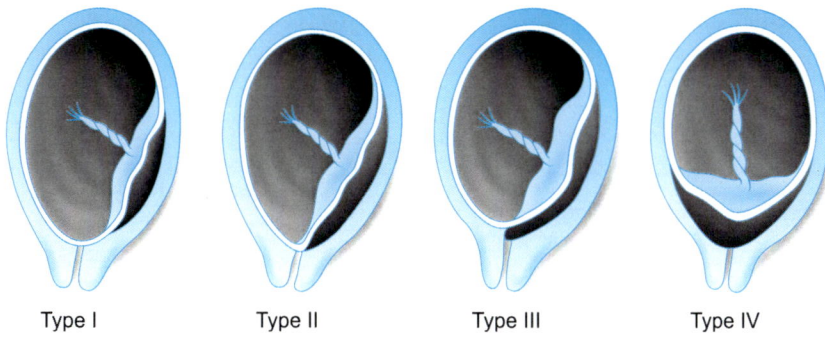

Fig. 1.1 Types of placenta previa

RELATED INFORMATION

Diagnostic Tools

Ultrasonogram

In modern obstetric practice USG is the single most important diagnostic aid. Both abdominal and transvaginal USG are safe, convenient and have reasonable accuracy. Though maternal obesity, over distension of the bladder, local myometrial contractions and acoustic shadowing from fetal parts can decrease the accuracy of transabdominal ultrasound. So it has been suggested that transvaginal ultrasonography (TVS) is more instructive than conventional transabdominal examination in cases of suspected placenta previa. Different studies have demonstrated the accuracy of transvaginal sonography for the diagnosis of placenta previa, and found superior to transabdominal sonography for this indication (Smith et al. 1997; Leerentveld et al. 1990). False-positive and negative rates are 2–25% for the diagnosis of placenta previa using transabdominal sonography.

There are potential advantages of TVS in this situation such as *imaging is better* and woman does not need full bladder. But insertion of ultrasound probe may provoke bleeding, so it is advocated that probe should be inserted no more than 3 cm into the vagina and should not therefore come into contact with cervix or lower segment.

The earlier, a scan is performed the higher the likelihood detecting low-lying placenta. About 26% pregnant women have low-lying placenta by USG at 18 weeks (16–22 week) but only 5% of them remain as low-lying placenta at 32 weeks of gestation and 1.9% remain as previa at term (Ruparelia and Chapman, 1985). This apparent shifting is due to the formation of lower segment and upward enlargement of the upper uterine segment as pregnancy advances from second to third trimester. At 20 weeks of gestation the length of lower segment is less than 1 cm. With progressive enlargement of the uterus the lower uterine segment enlarges and measures more than 5 cm at the end of the pregnancy. So there is relative shifting of placenta from below upwards and more than 90% of placenta previa move away from the cervical os by term. But a second trimester low-lying placenta, which is posterior or centrally located over the os is more likely to persist as previa at term.

So *routine rescanning is necessary* in women under following condition:
- Central or posterior located low placenta at second trimester
- History of previous cesarean section
- Continued bleeding
- With persistent malpresentation.

Now a days USG is available in almost all health services centers. Placental localization can be diagnosed radiologically, but USG replaced this method and radiology is obsolete nowadays. USG can differentiate placenta previa and abruptio placenta by detecting placental localization.

Magnetic Resonance Imaging (MRI)

The MRI can diagnose most accurately the placental localization and degree of adhesion in morbid adherent placenta. So it is valuable for the patients, who have history of previous cesarean section, who are more prone to have placenta previa and morbid adhesion. Considering the high expense of MRI it is not used to diagnose the localization of placenta.

> *Do you like to do PV examination to diagnose placenta previa?*

No. PV examination is not a diagnostic aid of placenta previa.

RELATED INFORMATION

The diagnosis of placenta previa *should not be made by digital vaginal examination* as 1 out of 16 examinations produce a major hemorrhage, and 1 out of every 25 examinations results in hypovolemic shock and accuracy of diagnosis is only 69%. But double setup examination or vaginal examination in the operating theater with full preparation of cesarean delivery and with crossmatched blood is still may be considered when:
- USG is not available and diagnosis is not confirmed in a woman with APH beyond 37 weeks gestation
- Type I or II anterior placenta previa is suspected in a woman with ongoing, but not life-threatening bleeding in active labor.

The procedure is *absolutely contraindicated* in situations where cesarean section is indicated such as:
- Profuse hemorrhage
- Fetal malposition and malpresentation
- Fetal distress
- Definite sonographically diagnosed major placenta previa.

> *Suppose you decided to do PV examination under general anesthesia with everything ready for cesarian section. What will be your approach for P/V examination?*

Approach of PV

- The head is to be pressed with left hand and introduce right hand for PV
- Gentleness should be applied
- Fornices are thoroughly checked for any intervening tissue between examining finger and fetal head
- Fingers are to be introduced through the cervix with great caution if soft tissue mass felt through fornix

- If placenta felt over the internal os (central placenta previa) further advancement of examination is to be postponed to avoid brisk hemorrhage
- If no placenta felt over the os, the finger is to be passed inside the lower segment and proceeded upwards palpating circumferentially as much as up to 7.5 cm from the os, to assess the presence of placenta and type of PP.

> *Why placenta gets implanted in lower uterine segment and what are the risk factors for development of placenta previa?*

Following theories are thought to be responsible for placental implantation in lower segment.
- *Defective migration*: In 5–28% cases *blastocyst gets implanted in lower uterine segment*, which with progressive enlargement of uterus shifted to upwards and only 0.5% left as placenta previa at term. This apparent migration is affected by:
  - *Previous scar in the uterus*: Previous lower uterine cesarean section. There is a strong positive correlation between the incidence of placenta previa and the number of previous cesarean section (McShane et al. 1985; Clark et al. 1985; Taylor et al. 1994; Gilliam et al. 2002). The mechanism of causation of previa by previous scar is poorly understood, but it may be due to reduced differential growth of the lower segment resulting in less upward shift in placental position as pregnancy advances (Dashe et al. 2002; Laughon et al. 2005).
  - Fibrosis due to previous injury by curettage.
- *Unsuitable upper segment for implantation*: In *multiparous* women due to repeated pregnancy upper segment placental site endometrium may be permanently damaged making it unsuitable for implantation. So embryo gets implanted in lower segment. Risk is 1 in 20 women who have had 6 or more pregnancies.

  Multiple induced abortions and curettage have a similar effect in increasing the incidence of placenta previa in multiparous women. Fibroid in upper segment may also favor implantation in lower segment.

- *Increased number of placenta or abnormally big placenta*:
  - In multiovular *multiple pregnancy* due to increased number of placenta there is less space for implantation and development of placenta in upper segment. So one may implants in lower segment or may gradually extends to lower segment with increment of size of placenta. Chance of developing placenta previa in multiple pregnancy is double.
  - *Increased surface area* leads to lower segment extension.
  - *Cigarette smoking* increased the risk of placenta previa due to relatively larger placenta, which probably occurs secondary to carbon monoxide related hypoxemia. Pregnant women who smoked 20 or more cigarettes per day are more than twice risky for developing placenta previa in relation to nonsmokers.
  - Placenta of *anemic* women and women *living at high altitude* grow larger to compensate decreased function of the placenta, which eventually develop placenta previa.
  - *Elderly women over 30 years* of age are three times risky to develop placenta previa than in women under 20 years of age. Changes in endometrial vascularization due to increased age causes compensatory enlargement of placenta and placenta previa.

> Suppose patient's PV bleeding is continuing and she has not any other complaint
> How will you stop her bleeding?

As amount of bleeding is small, patient is stable, baby is not matured and she has got no other complaints *nothing is to be done. Bleeding will stop spontaneously* due to thrombosis of open sinuses, placental infarction and due to mechanical pressure by presenting part. If needed intravenous (IV) fluid is to be given to maintain hemodynamics and blood loss is to be replaced by blood transfusion only.

Note: Artificial rupture membrane can stop bleeding. Due to rupture of the membrane presenting part comes close contact with placenta and compresses it. So due to pressure effect bleeding stops. But, which is not indicated in this case.

RELATED INFORMATION

The mean gestational age of first episode of bleeding is 29.6 weeks. About one-third of patients with placenta previa have their first episode of bleeding before 30 weeks, one-third from 30 to 35 weeks and one-third after 36 weeks (Crenshaw et al. 1973). First episode of bleeding is usually sudden and dramatic, but not so high to cause maternal catastrophes and completely stops a few hours after its onset. As lower segment dilates progressively with advancement of pregnancy then inelastic placenta separates from the wall of the lower segment. As a result uteroplacental blood vessels open up and causes bleeding, which is self-limiting by thrombosis of vessels. The separation of placenta is painless, so bleeding is not associated with pain.

> Patient is neither in labor nor she is a full term. After 2 days her PV bleeding completely stopped.
> Now what are you thinking about her obstetric management?

As fetus is not matured here and PV bleeding stopped patient is to be managed conservatively (expectant management). Pregnancy is to be continued till 37 completed weeks to attain fetal maturity.

Note: Rh anti-D immunoglobulin is to be given to all Rh-negative mother after first episode of bleeding to prevent Rh isoimmunization.

> Ultrasonography shows type II anterior placenta previa. You decided to continue the pregnancy up to term.
> In this circumstance what do you want to do?

Patient should be kept hospitalized for expectant treatment. Blood should be always kept ready at hand. In placenta previa there is recurrent episode of bleeding. *Subsequent bleeding is usually heavier.* So patient should be kept hospitalized till confinement.

But considering the cost of hospital stay type I and type II anterior placenta previa patient can be advised for domiciliary treatment to minimize the hospital stay if patient is:
- Aware about her situation and potential complications

- Able to come for weekly follow-up until delivery including serial hemoglobin levels and repeat sonography
- Able to attend the hospital immediately at any emergency situation.

What management patient needs during expectant treatment?

Treatment

- Absolute bedrest for at least 5–7 days after cessation of bleeding
- Sedative can be given at bedtime to relieve anxiety
- Correction of anemia by iron or blood transfusion, which is needed to keep the hemoglobin (HB) at upper level.

Monitoring and Investigations

- After 5–7 days of cessation of bleeding a gentle per speculum test is to be made to exclude cervical lesion
- Periodic enquiry about vaginal bleeding
- Regular assessment of fetal well-being by asking about kick count and by auscultating FHS
- Hemoglobin estimation (HB level should be kept at upper limit).

Precautions

- Anti-D immunoglobulin is to be given if patient is rhesus (Rh) negative
- Blood should be kept ready at hand
- Blood can be drawn from the patient and stored for autologous transfusion.

RELATED INFORMATION ABOUT TRANSFUSION

For management of a hemodynamically unstable patient, severity of bleeding should be assessed first. Pulse, blood pressure does not give the reflection of actual picture as those may remain within normal limit despite considerable amount of blood loss because of the unusual tolerance for the bleeding of the hypervolemic pregnant woman.

According to Gutiérrez et al. severity of bleeding can be classified into 4 groups (**Table 1.2**).

Class I or mild bleeding: Patients have lost <15% of their intravascular volume and show no change in vital signs or urine output.

Class II or moderate bleeding: Patients have lost between 15% and 30% of their volume and exhibit tachycardia, hypotension, pallor, cold and clammy extremities, changed mental status such as apathy or agitation.

Class III and class IV or severe bleeding case: Patients have lost 30% to more than 40% of their volume. Patient is in shock with decrease or nonrecordable blood pressure. Oliguria or anuria is present.

Management of Severe Bleeding

In severe bleeding with fetus in uterus patient is seating over a volcano. Quick and efficient

Table 1.2 Classification of severity of bleeding

Parameters	Class			
	I	II	III	IV
Blood loss	<750 mL (<15%)	750–1,500 mL 15–30%	1,500–2,000 30–40%	>2,000 >40%
Pulse rate/minute	<100	100–120	120–140	>140
Blood pressure	Normal	Decreased	Decreased	Decreased
Respiratory rate/minute	14–20	20–30	30–40	>40
Urine output (mL/h)	>30	20–30	5–15	Negligible
Central nervous system (CNS) symptom	Normal	Anxious	Confused	Lethargic
Gutiérrez et al. 2004.				

management plan including life support measure and *immediate operative intervention* is the only and right way to avoid maternal death.

Management includes the following:
- Intensive observation and monitoring:
  - The patient of APH with severe bleeding should never be left alone
  - Frequent monitoring of vital signs
  - Strict maintenance of intake output chart
  - Recording of amount of vaginal bleeding.
- *Administration of intravenous fluid*: One or two large wide-bored cannulas (18G) should be inserted for the administration of a balanced electrolyte solution such as Ringer's lactate. If patient is in shock two IV channels may be needed. About 1 L of crystalloid solution result in approximately 250 mL of intravascular volume expansion.
- Transfusion of blood and blood product in the form of:
  - *Whole blood*: Anticoagulant in the form of calcium gluconate is to be given after transfusion of 3 units of whole blood.
  - *Packed red cell (PRC)*: In case of massive transfusion there may be platelet depletion secondary to replacement with platelet poor blood. So after transfusion of 4 units of PRC clotting mechanism should be evaluated, particularly platelet count.
  - *Platelet*: It should be given if the count is <50,000/mm^3.
  - *Fresh frozen plasma*: If the patient is deficient in clotting factors as demonstrated by alterations in prothrombin time or partial thromboplastin time 1 unit of fresh frozen plasma should be administered for every 4 units of PRC.
- *Assessment of renal function and intravascular status*: Continuous catheterization (Foley catheter) is mandatory in moderate-to-severe bleeding cases. Severe bleeding is usually associated with shock, acute tubular and cortical necrosis, oliguria and anuria. Aggressive therapy by hydration, injection furosemide or mannitol is necessary for decreased urine output. Maintenance of a urine output of 30 mL/h should be ensured.
- Assessment of fetus.
- Delivery by cesarean section.

Management of Patients with Moderate Bleeding

Management of placenta previa with moderate bleeding depends upon gestational age of the fetus and stabilization of patient's condition.

If pregnancy is 34 weeks or more delivery by cesarean section should be performed along with resuscitation of the patient by fluid and blood transfusion.

If pregnancy is less than 34 weeks patient should be kept under intensive monitoring in labor ward with adequate fluid and blood transfusion. Steroid should be administered to induce lung maturation. If patients' condition remains unstable within 24–48 hours observation she should be delivered in spite of fetal immaturity.

If patient's condition becomes stable and remains stable for 24–48 hours she becomes a candidate for expectant management. But if there is rupture membrane or fetal distress then in spite of stable maternal condition pregnancy is to be terminated.

Management of Patients with Mild Bleeding

If fetus is at 37 completed weeks, pregnancy is to be terminated. If fetus is immature, expectant treatment is to be given till 37 completed weeks.

> What are the complications of transfusion of blood and blood products and how it can be minimized?

Complications

Complications of blood and blood product transfusion are the following:
- Transfusion reaction
- *Transmission of infection*: Hepatitis B and C, human immunodeficiency virus (HIV)
- Volume overload
- Bacterial contamination particularly with platelet transfusion.

Routine screening of donor's blood, cleaning of skin before blood collection and meticulous judgment for transfusion with strict maintenance of intake output chart can prevent the transfusion related complications.

Autologous transfusion also can minimize infection and transfusion reaction. It is safe, but is limited by the mother's hemoglobin concentration and by the potential effects on the fetus and on uterine activity of sudden changes in intravascular volume. So autologous transfusion for routine vaginal delivery and routine cesarean section is discouraged. It is difficult to predict, which patients will require transfusion. Also special arrangements and procedures are necessary for the collection of the blood, which poses a burden on the obstetrician and blood bank.

> Suppose Mrs Hazera reached at 37 weeks of gestation. She has type II anterior placenta previa. Fetal lie is longitudinal, presentation is cephalic. Fetal heart rate is 145/minute. As there is risk of bleeding and fetus gets matured you want to terminate the pregnancy.
> For termination what do you want to do?

For termination of pregnancy, there are two options, i.e. induction of labor and elective cesarean section. As there is no malpresentation, cephalopelvic disproportion is not predicted, placenta is type II anterior and there is no bleeding, there is no indication for elective cesarean section. So *labor can be induced*. But before induction PV examination is to be done to assess cervical ripening and adequacy of pelvis. In placenta previa PV examination may provoke bleeding. So PV examination will be done in operating theater, keeping everything ready for cesarean section. After assessing Bishop's score **(Table 1.3)** and adequacy of pelvis if quick vaginal delivery is predicted then *artificial rupture membrane (ARM) is to be done*. Oxytocin will be added for augmentation of labor. If Bishop's is not favorable and pelvis seems contracted cesarean section will be done.

RELATED INFORMATION

Table 1.3 Bishop's score

Score	0	1	2	3
Dilatation (cm)	0	1–2	3–4	5–6
Effacement (%)	0–40	40–60	60–80	80+
Station	–3	–2	–1 to 0	+1 to +2
Consistency	Firm	Medium	Soft	
Position	Posterior	Mid	Anterior	
Unfavorable score: 0–5				
Favorable score: 6–13				

Adequacy of Pelvis

Adequate pelvis shows following features:
- Sacral promontory could not be reached
- Ischial spine is everted
- Side walls are parallel
- Subpubic angle is obtuse and accommodates two fingers
- Intertuberous space accommodates knuckle of four fingers.

> You performed ARM successfully. How will you manage subsequently?

The ARM induces labor by synthesizing endogenous prostaglandins. If there is no initiation of uterine contraction or there is ineffective contraction oxytocin is to be added for augmentation. After addition of oxytocin if contraction remained ineffective cesarean section is to be done. On the other hand if pain has started and is increasing progressively and labor progresses reasonably then vaginal delivery is to be awaited.

> Suppose during expectant treatment, patient restarted bleeding, which is heavy in amount. You found patient's pulse became thready. You started blood transfusion, but per vaginal bleeding is continuing and outweighs the transfusion. Patient only passed another 2 weeks (34 weeks). 37 weeks is still far away.
> How will you manage the patient?

Although fetus is premature, patient started PV bleeding again, which is continuous and heavy in amount, so there is chance of maternal deterioration. On the other hand, extrauterine survivability of fetus at 34 weeks is good. In this situation, there is no indication of expectant treatment. *Pregnancy must be terminated*. A large wide bored (18G) IV line is to be established and blood transfusion must be started immediately. As bleeding is heavy and patient is not in labor cesarean section is to be done. In brisk hemorrhage there is no indication for induction of labor.
- When gestational age is less than 34 weeks injection glucocorticoids 12 mg intramuscular (IM) 12 hourly is to be given for fetal lung maturity. Two doses are recommended, but when there is no time at hand a single dose even at operation table is helpful.

Placenta Previa

> Suppose bleeding is moderate in amount and she is 34 weeks. At this time she also complaints of lower abdominal pain, which is rhythmic and progressively increasing.
> How will you manage her?

Rhythmic and progressively increasing pain is sign of labor. When patient goes in spontaneous labor then chance of vaginal delivery is more. Then after pelvic assessment (keeping everything ready for cesarean section in OT) ARM is to be done for augmentation of labor. ARM also helps to stop bleeding. If bleeding ceases or stops within 10 minutes then labor is to be continued for vaginal delivery. If bleeding continued cesarean section is to be done.

> Suppose Mrs Hazera has come to you at 35 weeks of pregnancy with history of PV bleeding 2 days ago. But now she has no PV bleeding at all. On examination you found that uterine contraction is absent. Fetal heart sound is not audible and fetal movement is also absent. USG shows dead fetus with type III placenta previa.
> What management do you plan for her? Explain.

Although there is no bleeding pregnancy is to be terminated as fetus is dead here. But in spite of dead fetus cesarean section is to be done as in type III placenta previa, placenta covers internal os. So along with cervical dilatation there will be brisk hemorrhage.

For this reason in type III and type IV placenta previa cesarean section is mandatory whether fetus is alive or dead.

RELATED INFORMATION

- In type I and type II anterior, vaginal delivery safely can be tried.
- In type II posterior, if fetus is alive, cesarean section is preferable because during descent presenting part *compresses the placenta and cord*, which causes uteroplacental insufficiency and leads to fetal distress and even death. In addition placental mass *reduces the anteroposterior diameter of the pelvis*, which prevents engagement and descent of the presenting part.

- In type II posterior, if fetus is *dead* vaginal delivery can be tried as there is no question of fetal distress here.
- In type III and type IV placenta previa for safety of the mother cesarean section is mandatory whether fetus is alive or dead.

> Suppose Mrs Hazera has breech presentation and type II anterior placenta previa.
> Will you go for vaginal delivery?

No. In placenta previa with any form of malpresentation, cesarean section is preferable.

> Suppose Mrs Hazera has come to you at 39 weeks of gestation with slight PV bleeding. She is not in labor. Ultrasonographically it is diagnosed as placenta previa type II anterior.
> Will you wait up-to expected date of delivery (EDD)? Explain.

No. Fetus is mature here. As there is chance of unpredictable bleeding at any time, pregnancy is to be terminated.

> What are the conditions where expectant treatment is contraindicated?

- When pregnancy is at 37 completed weeks
- With brisk hemorrhage
- With congenital anomaly
- With active labor
- With dead fetus
- Premature rupture of membranes (PROM) at ≥34 weeks of gestation.

> So who are the candidates for expectant treatment?

- Mother is in good health status (hemoglobin should be kept more than 12 mg%)
- Duration of pregnancy is less than 37 weeks
- Active vaginal bleeding is absent
- Fetal well-being is assured.

> As placenta lies in the lower segment, you predict difficulties during lower uterine cesarean section?
> What difficulties may arise during cesarean section?

Following are the difficulties may arise during cesarean section:
- Excessive bleeding, when placenta is anteriorly placed
- Difficulty in entering into amniotic cavity, when placenta is anteriorly placed
- There may be difficulty in delivering the baby in case of malpresentation
- There may be extension of uterine incision due to friability of the tissue causes excessive hemorrhage
- There may be morbid adhesion and removal of which gives rise to excessive bleeding and may need hysterectomy.

RELATED INFORMATION

Cesarean section in placenta previa could be a difficult one and should be performed by an experienced operator. A planned elective operation is preferable to an emergency operation as perinatal mortality and morbidity is higher with latter.

Approach for Cesarean Section

In cases of anterior placenta previa lower segment may be very vascular with engorged veins crossing over the site of incision. In that case veins may be ligated before giving incision on the lower segment. Usually transverse incision is given, but in prematurity with oblique or transverse lie where lower segment is poorly developed approach with transverse incision is very difficult and classical incision may needed. Fetus can be reached *either by* rapidly cutting through the placenta *or by* separating the placenta and approaching the membranes at the edge of the placenta by going above, below or to the side. The former approach may be quicker, but could result in serious fetal hemorrhage.

> Suppose during operation you found that there is profuse bleeding from placental site.
> How will you control it?

Due to less contractile power of lower segment bleeding is usually more in placenta previa.
- If there are large sinuses in placental bed, it can be controlled by giving mattress suture.
- Uterotonics such as oxytocin drip, injection ergometrine even direct intramyometrial injection of prostaglandin may be useful in such cases.
- If there is continuous oozing from the placental bed, uterine wound may be closed over a tight pack, which is to be removed vaginally 48 hours later. Alternatively balloon tamponade can be placed, which is to be removed after 48 hours.
- If packing or balloon tamponade cannot control bleeding bilateral internal artery ligation may control bleeding.
- If all measures fail to control bleeding hysterectomy is the last option for life-saving purpose.

> **Case scenario:** Mrs Nadira, a third gravid woman mother of two healthy children presents with history of two previous cesarean section and placenta previa. During her cesarean section you found that placenta is firmly adherent to lower segment. There is no sign of separation and there is no bleeding. Condition of the baby is good.
> What will you do?

This is due to morbid adhesion. As this is her third pregnancy preservation of fertility is not mandatory. So after proper counseling about subsequent risk of keeping the uterus as it is, hysterectomy is to be done. Total hysterectomy is preferable, but if not possible supracervical hysterectomy can be done.

Note: As there is no bleeding placenta can be kept *in situ* with preservation of uterus. Placenta will be autolysed in due course of time. But there is chance of partial separation and *bleeding* during autolysis, chance of infection and trophoblastic disease. Sometimes intrauterine infection could potentially be life-threatening. During autolysis there is discharge from the uterus, which in presence of placenta *in vivo* raise anxiety and tension to mother. Considering these things hysterectomy is better option for those who do not need to preserve it for future fertility.

> If this is patient's first pregnancy, then what should be done?

In this case, attempt is to be taken to conserve the fertility potential by preserving uterus. Preservation of uterus also reduces morbidity associated with hysterectomy. In this case placenta will be left *in situ* with no attempt of removal. Adjunctive procedure such as embolization of the internal iliac vessels or injection methotrexate can be given (Arulkumaran et al. 1986; Butt et al. 2002; Kayem et al. 2004; Weinstein et al. 2005). It can be left without further intervention. Placental tissue will regress gradually. In these cases subsequent hemorrhage may occur and may need hysterectomy. Intrauterine infection also sometimes may takes place, which may be life-threatening.

If total placenta is not adherent, then there is sign of separation. In that case easily removable part of placental tissue is to be removed. Adherent part is to be left out for resolution. Placenta may separate spontaneously and deliver vaginally.

> If anterior placenta involved the bladder and it is not approachable without injuring the bladder.
> What to do?

- If it is prediagnosed by ultrasonography (USG)
  - Careful preoperative planning should be done along with urologist
  - Placement of ureteric stent can prevent ureteric injury
  - Vertical uterine incision in upper segment is to be given
  - Placenta should be kept undisturbed.
- If it is diagnosed during operation again vertical incision and conservative approach can be adopted.

> How morbid adhesion can be diagnosed before hand?

By ultrasonography (USG) and magnetic resonance imaging (MRI)

Ultrasonography

Several studies have documented the efficacy of sonography in the diagnosis of placenta accreta (Comstock 2005; Comstock et al. 2004; Finberg and Williams 1992). Sonographic features suggestive of placenta accreta are:

- Irregularly shaped placental lacunae within the placenta give the placenta a 'moth-eaten' or 'Swiss cheese' appearance
- Thinning of the myometrium overlying the placenta
- Loss of the retroplacental 'clear space'
- Protrusion of the placenta into the bladder
- Increased vascularity of the uterine serosa-bladder interface and on Doppler ultrasonography, turbulent blood flow through the lacunae.

Magnetic Resonance Imaging

Several articles have described the use of MRI in the diagnosis of placenta accreta (Thorp 1998; Palacios et al. 2005; Levine 1997). Others show no more sensitive than USG for diagnosing placenta accreta (Comstock 2005; Levine 1997). In addition its high cost and limited availability limits its usefulness. For these reasons sonography considered as the primary imaging modality for diagnosing accreta. However, when there is a posterior placenta accreta, USG may be less adequate and MRI may be superior to USG for this specific indication (Comstock 2005; Levine 1997).

> It was not diagnosed beforehand and you approached lower segment incision. During separation of peritoneum, bladder opened up and there was profuse hemorrhage.
> What should be done?

Case is to be managed along with urologist. Depending upon the situation to save life of the patient along with hysterectomy partial resection of bladder may require.

> Is there any role of cervical cerclage?

According to some authors cervical cerclage has better outcome indicated by prolongation of pregnancy, greater birth weight, less neonatal complications and decreased cost of hospitalization (Arias, 1988). It may limits the development of lower uterine segment and avoids the partial detachment of the placenta from the lower uterine segment, which most probably is the cause of bleeding. But other did not find any difference between cerclage and conservative approach (Cobo et al. 1998). In view of the lack of convincing data to support cerclage in these women, cerclage should not be performed for treatment of placenta previa.

> What complications may arise in a case of placenta previa?

Maternal Complications

- Varying degrees of shock due to hemorrhage
- Premature labor either spontaneous or induced
- Early rupture of membranes
- Slow dilatation of cervix due to pressure of placenta in lower segment and *malpresentation, which is common in placenta previa*
- Intrapartum hemorrhage
- Increased incidence of operative interference due to malpresentation and for continuous bleeding
- Postpartum hemorrhage due to:
  - Imperfect retraction of the lower segment
  - Lower segment is thinner so there is chance of morbid adhesion of placenta in lower segment
  - Trauma to the cervix and lower segment because of extreme softness and vascularity.
- Retained placenta (due to morbid adhesion in thin lower segment)
- Sepsis due to:
  - Increased operative interference
  - Anemia and devitalized state of the patient.

Fetal Complications

- Low birth weight:
  - *Prematurity*: Due to premature labor either spontaneous or induced
  - *Intrauterine growth restriction (IUGR)*: Repeated small bouts of hemorrhage causes placental insufficiency, which leads to fetal growth retardation.
- Asphyxia due to:
  - Early separation of the placenta
  - Compression of placenta
  - Compression of cords.
- Intrauterine death due to severe degree of placental separation and massive hemorrhage
- Birth injuries due to increased operative interference.

General Consideration for Management

Any patient with bleeding in late pregnancy should be managed in the hospital with facility of cesarean section, blood transfusion and neonatal services. Initial management is same for all bleeding cases and include:

- Rapid assessment of maternal hemodynamic status and amount of blood loss
- Fetal assessment
- All patient should have a wide bored (18G) intravenous (IV) line and depending upon the amount of blood loss fluid replacement should be started
- If patient is hemodynamically unstable fluid and blood replacement should be the aim of initial management
- Subsequent management options include either immediate delivery or expectant management depending upon the patient's condition and fetal maturity
- A massive hemorrhage threatening maternal life requires termination of the pregnancy irrespective of gestational age of the fetus
- A mild-to-moderate bleeding episode at ≥37 weeks also should be managed by termination of pregnancy
- If the fetus is preterm and bleeding is not life-threatening—a more conservative approach is appropriate
- Cesarean section should be performed by skilled personnel.

BIBLIOGRAPHY

Arias F. Cervical cerclage for the temporary treatment of patients with placenta previa. Obstet Gynecol. 1988;71(4):545-8.

Arulkumaran S, Ng CS, Ingemarsson I, et al. Medical treatment of placenta accreta with methotrexate. Acta Obstet Gynecol Scand. 1986;65(3):285-6.

Butt K, Gagnon A, Delisle MF. Failure of methotrexate and internal iliac balloon catheterization to manage placenta percreta. Obstet Gynecol. 2002;99(6): 981-2.

Clark SL, Koonings PP, Phelan JP. Placenta previa/accrete and prior cesarean section. Obstet Gynecol. 1985;66(1):89-92.

Cobo E, Conde-Agudelo A, Delgado J, et al. Cervical cerclage: an alternative for the management of placenta previa? Am J Obstet Gynecol. 1998; 179(1):122-5.

Comstock CH, Love JJ Jr, Bronsteen RA, et al. Sonographic detection of placenta accreta in the second and third trimesters of pregnancy. Am J Obstet Gynecol. 2004;190(4):1135-40.

Comstock CH. Antenatal diagnosis of placenta accreta: a review. Ultrasound Obstet Gynecol. 2005;26(1): 89-96.

Crenshaw C, Jones DE, Parker RT. Placenta previa: a survey of twenty years experience with improved perinatal survival by expectant therapy and cesarean delivery. Obstet Gynecol Surv. 1973;28(7):461-70.

Dashe JS, McIntire DD, Ramus RM, et al. Persistence of placenta previa according to gestational age at ultrasound detection. Obstet Gynecol. 2002;99(5 pt 1): 692-7.

Finberg HJ, Williams JW. Placenta accreta: prospective sonographic diagnosis in patients with placenta previa and prior cesarean section. J Ultrasound Med. 1992;11(7):333-43.

Gilliam M, Rosenberg D, Davis F. The likelihood of placenta previa with greater number of cesarean deliveries and higher parity. Obstet Gynecol. 2002;99(6):976-80.

Gutiérrez G, Reines HD, Wulf-Gutierrez ME. Clinical review: hemorrhagic shock. Crit Care. 2004;8(5): 373-81.

Iyasu S, Saftlas AK, Rowley DL, et al. The epidemiology of placenta previa in the United States, 1979 through 1987. Am J Obstet Gynecol .1993;168(5):1424-9.

Kayem G, Davy C, Goffinet F, et al. Conservative versus extirpative management in cases of placenta accreta. Obstet Gynecol. 2004;104(3):531-6.

Laughon SK, Wolfe HM, Visco AG. Prior cesarean and the risk for placenta previa on second-trimester ultrasonography. Obstet Gynecol. 2005;105(5 Pt 1): 962-5.

Leerentveld RA, Gilberts EC, Arnold MJ, et al. Accuracy and safety of transvaginal sonographic placental localization. Obstet Gynecol. 1990;76(5 Pt 1):759-62.

Levine D, Hulka CA, Ludmir J, et al. Placenta accreta: evaluation with color Doppler US, power Doppler US, and MR imaging. Radiology. 1997;205(3):773-6.

McShane PM, Heys PS, Epstein MF. Maternal and perinatal mortality resulting from placenta previa. Obstet Gynecol. 1985; 65(2):176-82.

Palacios Jaraquemada JM, Bruno CH. Magnetic resonance imaging in 300 cases of placenta accreta: surgical correlation of new findings. Acta Obstet Gynecol Scand. 2005;84(8):716-24.

Ruparelia BA, Chapman MG. Early low-lying placenta- ultrasonic assessment, progress and outcome. Eur J Obstet Gynecol Reprod Biol. 1985;20(4):209-13.

Smith RS, Lauria MR, Comstock CH, et al. Transvaginal ultrasonography for all placentas that appear to be low-lying or over the internal cervical os. Ultrasound Obstet Gynecol. 1997;9(1):22-4.

Taylor VM, Kramer MD, Vaughan TL, et al. Placenta previa and prior cesarean delivery: how strong is the association? Obstet Gynecol. 1994;84(1): 55-7.

Thorp JM Jr, Wells SR, Wiest HH, et al. First-trimester diagnosis of placenta previa percreta by magnetic resonance imaging. Am J Obstet Gynecol. 1998; 178(5):616-8.

Weinstein A, Chandra P, Schiavello H, et al. Conservative management of placenta previa percreta in a Jehovah's Witness. Obstet Gynecol. 2005;105(5 Pt 2): 1247-50.

CHAPTER 2

Abruptio Placenta

Rashida Begum

INTRODUCTION

Abruptio placenta or accidental hemorrhage is an obstetric emergency. It occurs due to premature separation of normally situated placenta before birth of the baby. Approximately 30% of cases of third trimester bleeding are due to placental separation. If it occurs before 28th weeks of pregnancy, it cannot be distinguished from other causes of abortion. About 50% of separation occurs before the onset of labor. It occurs in 1% of all pregnancies worldwide.

> **Case scenario:** Alyea a second gravid woman is carrying for 38 weeks. She is a non-booked case. Suddenly she developed per vaginal (PV) bleeding and lower abdominal pain. With these complaints she has come to you.
> How will you proceed for diagnosis?

Detailed History is to be Taken

About bleeding
- When did per vaginal bleeding start?
- How much bleeding occurred?
- Was there any clotted blood?
- Is it her first episode of bleeding?

To be sure about gestational age menstrual history is to be taken
- Whether the cycle was regular or not
- What was the length of the cycle?
- When was the last menstrual period?

About pain
- When did pain start?
- Did it start before or after onset of bleeding?
- Is it rhythmic and progressively increasing or continuous?
- Did she use any painkiller? If so did she get relieved?

About other associated factors
- Whether there is any history of fall or trauma?
- Is she hypertensive?
- Is her parents hypertensive?

About fetal condition
- Whether fetal movement is present and adequate?

Obstetric history
- Whether there was any complication in previous pregnancy?
- What was the mode of previous delivery?

Examination

A quick 'both general and obstetrical examination' is to be performed.

> On enquiry you found that this is her first episode of bleeding. Bleeding started first then she developed lower abdominal pain. Bleeding is slight and fresh. Pain is severe and continuous. There is no history of trauma. She does not know about her parents or her own blood pressure status. She did not take any drug for these complaints. She had no complaints in previous pregnancy and delivery was normal. Her cycle was regular and last menstrual period (LMP) was 35 weeks back. She has not been feeling fetal movement for last 4–5 hours. After physical examination you found that she is pale, her pulse is 110/m, blood pressure (BP) is 90/50 mm Hg. Uterus is enlarged, tense and tender. Fetal heart sound is not audible. Cervix is soft, partially effaced and os is closed.
> What is your clinical diagnosis?

Most likely diagnosis is *abruptio placenta*.

> Why did you think so? (what are the diagnostic points)?

- Pervaginal bleeding in last trimester of pregnancy is due to antepartum hemorrhage either due to placenta previa or due to abruptio placenta
- Bleeding in placenta previa is painless, causeless and recurrent, and is not associated with tenderness of abdomen
- Patient is pale and is in a state of shock, which does not correspond with amount of blood loss, which goes in favor of concealed type of bleeding in abruptio placenta where general condition, pallor and shock is out of proportion of visible blood loss
- Uterine size is disproportionately enlarged and feeling is tense, tender and rigid
- Fetal movement and fetal heart sound is usually present in placenta previa; dead fetus is invariable in concealed abruptio placenta.

All these go in favor of abruptio placenta.

> What are the conditions with which confusion may arise? (DD)

- *Ruptured uterus*: May simulate concealed hemorrhage, since both have similar features such as continuous pain, shock, some revealed bleeding, tender and distended abdomen. But ruptured uterus must be associated with labor pain, whereas abruptio placenta may or may not. Prolonged labor pain particularly second stage of labor, multiparity, history of previous cesarean section (CS) are associated with ruptured uterus. On the other hand, high blood pressure, proteinuria, history of trauma, hydramnios are associated with abruptio placenta.
- *Acute appendicitis*: There will be pain and tenderness, and abdominal rigidity due to establishment of peritonitis. But there will be no predisposing factors of abruptio placenta and there will no sign of internal hemorrhage particularly pallor and sweating.
- *Ovarian torsion*: There will be no vaginal bleeding and sign of internal hemorrhage.
- *Placenta previa with labor pain*: May confused with revealed type of abruptio placenta. Ultrasonography (USG) and feeling of placenta at PV examination can differentiate these.
- *Acute hydramnios*: May be considered, but there will be no vaginal bleeding and no shock. USG can differentiate these.
- *Retroperitoneal hematoma* in the broad ligament may simulate concealed hemorrhage of abruptio placenta. In this situation, uterus is pushed to one side and itself is not tender or hard in consistency, though site of hematoma is acutely painful.
- *Hemorrhagic shock (hemorrhage from other site like rupture of splenic aneurism)*: Although, very rare situation may happen and confused with abruptio placenta.

> How will you confirm the diagnosis?

Ultrasonography can confirm the location of placenta. If it is normally situated and there is retroplacental hematoma (blood clot behind the placenta), then it confirms the placental abruption. But in this patient it is clinically so evident and patient needs urgent management, so ultrasonography is not essential for diagnosis.

RELATED INFORMATION

Abruptio placenta is one form of antepartum hemorrhage, where the bleeding occurs due to premature separation of normally situated placenta before birth of the baby.

Hemorrhage may be:
- *Revealed (80%)*: When blood is visible externally, it is called revealed. This is the most common type of bleeding in abruptio placenta. After separation of placenta, blood trickles down between the membranes and decidua to vaginal canal and becomes visible.
- *Concealed*: When the blood is not visible outside is called concealed. So absence of vaginal bleeding does not exclude a diagnosis of abruptio placenta. This is the dangerous type, but rare. Blood is collected behind the separated placenta or between membrane and placenta, and cannot come out due to pressure

of the presenting part of fetus. Absence of uterine contraction also plays an important role for the blood to remain concealed. Sometimes blood may percolate into the amniotic sac after rupturing the membrane.
- *Mixed*: When some part of the blood becomes visible and part becomes collected inside is called mixed. This is also common.
- Concealed and mixed (20%).

Symptoms

Symptoms may include:
- *Vaginal bleeding*: 80%
- *Abdominal or back pain and uterine tenderness*: 70%
- *Fetal distress*: 60%
- *Abnormal uterine contractions (Hypertonic)*: 35%
- *Premature labor*: 25%
- *Fetal death*: 15%.

There are differences in symptoms depending upon concealed and revealed type of bleeding.

Revealed Type

In revealed type there is continuous slight-to-severe bleeding, abdominal pain and discomfort. General condition is proportionate to visible blood loss. Shock is usually absent. Pallor is related to visible blood loss. Uterine size is proportionate to gestational age and feeling is soft with localized tenderness or rhythmic contraction may present. Fetal part can be felt easily and fetal heart sound (FHS) may or may not be present.

Concealed and Mixed Type

In concealed and mixed type there is continuous slight dark or fresh bleeding or no bleeding and intense abdominal pain. General condition, pallor and shock are out of proportion of visible blood loss. Uterine size is disproportionately enlarged and feeling is tense, tender and rigid. Fetal parts cannot be felt easily and FHS is usually absent.

Causes of Separation of Placenta

The exact cause of abruptio placenta is still unknown. It is thought that there is degenerative change of small arteries supplying the intervillous space, resulting in thrombosis; decidual degeneration and rupture of vessels causing retroplacental hematoma and placental separation. Due to continued arterial pumping, there is further separation of placenta from decidual attachment.

Though the exact cause is not known, there are certain associations and risk factors. These are:
- *Hypertension in pregnancy:* Among eclampsia, pre-eclampsia, chronic hypertension and chronic renal disease, the most common associated condition is hypertension in pregnancy. Pritchard et al. found that 45% of their patients with abruptio had elevated blood pressure (Pritchard et al 1970). Spasm of placental site blood vessels causes capillary anoxia. After cessation of spasm the damaged capillaries are unable to cope with the vascular engorgement that follows and get ruptured, and bleeding takes place.
- *Trauma:*
  a. Forceful external cephalic version.
  b. Road traffic accident.
  c. Needle puncture during amniocentesis.
- *Polyhydramnios and sudden decompression of the uterus:* In case of polyhydramnios, due to overdistension of the uterus, placenta may get detached and after ruptured membrane due to sudden release of fluid, uterus becomes contracted and placenta get detached (Ananth et al, 2004).
- *Multiple gestations:* Due to overdistension, placental abruption may occur (Salihu et al 2005).
- *Uterine fibroid:* Placenta fails to encroach adequately.
- *Uterine malformation:* Placentation over septum fails to encroach adequately.
- *Circumvallate placenta.*
- *Inherited thrombophilia* has association with placental abruption (Facchinetti et al 2003; Prochazca et al 2003) due to Factor V Leiden (FVL) mutation, *prothrombin* mutation and hyperhomocysteinemia.
- *Antiphospholipid antibody syndrome.*
- *Presence of lupus anticoagulant.*
- *Smoking:* Causes placental infraction due to vasoconstrictor effect of nicotine leads to abruption (Ananth 1999; Naeye 1980).

- *Cocaine abuse.*
- *Multiparity:* There is association between high parity and abruptio placenta, but the strongest association of abruption is with a previous history of abruption.
- *History of previous abruptio placenta:* The risk of recurrence is approximately 17% for patients with one abruption and as high as 25% for patients who have had more than one episode.

Controversies

Short umbilical cord itself is not responsible for placental detachment. This is only likely to operate as a cause if the patient is in labor with the presenting part advancing. If inferior vena cava is obstructed (*supine hypotension syndrome*) by the pressure of gravid uterus in supine position, occasional placental abruption may occur due to congestion and rupture of placental veins, but do not appear to be significant etiological factor. Role of *folic acid deficiency has not been confirmed*.

Placental abruption can be classified based on extent of separation (partial versus complete) and the location of separation (marginal versus central) into:

Class 0—asymptomatic: The diagnosis in this patient is made retrospectively by finding an organized blood clot or a depressed area on a delivered placenta. Volume of retroplacental clot never exceeds 500 mL (Sher 1978). With this small degree of abruption, fetuses are usually not at risk and favorable perinatal outcome is expected.

Class 1—mild 48% cases with mild symptom
- No vaginal bleeding to mild vaginal bleeding
- Uterine tenderness slight may be irritable
- Maternal blood pressure and heart rate are within normal limit
- No coagulopathy
- No fetal distress.

Class 2—moderate 27% cases with moderate symptoms:
- No vaginal bleeding to moderate vaginal bleeding; the retroplacental clot volume in these patients is usually 150-500 mL with one fourth of them having a clot larger than 500 mL
- Moderate-to-severe uterine tenderness; uterus may be tonically contracted
- Maternal hypotension and tachycardia present
- Fetal distress with high perinatal mortality, if delivered vaginally
- Hypofibrinogenemia (50-250 mg/dL).

Class 3—severe 24% cases with severe symptoms:
- No vaginal bleeding to heavy vaginal bleeding. Pritchard and Brekken demonstrated that when abruptio placenta is severe enough to kill the fetus then average blood loss is about 2,500 mL (Pritchard and Brekken, 1967).
- Uterus tonically contracted with severe tenderness.
- Maternal shock is obvious.
- Hypofibrinogenemia (less than 150 mg/dL).
- Coagulopathy.
- *Fetal death:* Indicates the severity of the disease. It is associated with large retroplacental hematoma and placental detachment more than 50%. Approximately 30% patients show evidence of coagulopathy and 10% may develop acute renal failure.
- *Maternal death:* Almost all maternal mortality is associated with 'class 3' abruptio placenta.

Diagnosis of Placental Location

Diagnosis of placental location is done by USG. Retroplacental hematoma may be recognized in 2-25% of all abruptio placenta. The sonographic identification depends on degree of hematoma formation and operators expertise. So normal sonographic findings do not exclude the condition. Magnetic resonance imaging (MRI) is diagnostically effective and can accurately depict placental abruption, in comparison to ultrasonogram. MRI is indicated if sonographic finding is negative in presence of bleeding in late pregnancy, where positive findings of abruptio placenta would change patient management.

Consequences of Placental Abruption

Both mother and fetus are at considerable risk in abruptio placenta. Fate of placental separation are as detailed below.

Maternal

- *Hypovolemic shock.*
- *Acute renal failure:* Due to persistent blood loss.

- *Uteroplacental apoplexy (Couvelaire uterus, associated with severe concealed bleeding):* In concealed accidental hemorrhage, there is formation of retroplacental hematoma, which gradually increases in size and creates pressure and further separates placenta. At a time, total placenta except margin becomes separated producing large hematoma due to absence outlet of blood. Uterus is distended to a size greater than would apply to the period of gestation. Large retroplacental clot may have tracked beyond the placental margin and may even burst into the amniotic sac. Blood enters into the muscle bundles of uterine wall and heavily infiltrated with extravasated blood and edema fluid. It extends between the layers of the broad ligament. Uterus shows ecchymoses on its serous surface, which may be fissured and from which blood may be oozing. This gives a characteristic port wine color to the uterus called *Couvelaire uterus* (**Fig. 2.1**). There is usually a blood clotting defect due to hypofibrinogenemia. The peritoneal cavity usually contains blood-stained fluid and occasionally the uterus may rupture due to damage of uterine wall though the condition is rare. The uterine muscle fibers may necrose in patchy areas, *which recovers completely after delivery* without any residual uterine structural weakness.
- *Disseminated intravascular coagulation (DIC) and coagulation failure (associated with severe concealed bleeding):* The basic pathology of DIC in abruptio placenta is formation of *retroplacental hematoma*, which may build-up sufficient pressure to rupture the basal plate and establish a communication between intradecidual space of the hematoma and maternal circulation of the placenta:
  a. Due to formation of large clot behind the uterus coagulation factors depleted due to *consumption of huge clotting factors* within the large clot. That is why, it is also called consumption coagulopathy.
  b. Moreover, there is autoextraction of tissue substances including *thromboplastin* from the decidua, damaged placenta and retained blood clot directly into the maternal circulation, causes *production of microthrombi throughout the maternal circulation,* consumes further clotting factors resulting in coagulopathy. These microthrombi use up the available supplies of circulating fibrinogen, which the liver cannot replace fast enough.
  c. Once the coagulation procedure starts, plasminogen activators released from damaged tissue to convert plasminogen to plasmin, which causes lysis of fibrinogen and fibrin to keep the vessels patent.
  d. So blood coagulation and fibrinolysis work side by side to maintain hemostasis and patency of the microvessels.
  e. Due to both *consumption and break down of fibrinogen,* hypofibrinogenemia develop and bleeding ensues.
  f. In late pregnancy, normal circulating level of fibrinogen is raised to about 450 mg%, when it falls below 100 mg% uncontrolled hemorrhage occurs. Though, the activation of fibrinolytic system is less pronounced in abruptio placenta, as quick delivery allows less time to absorb activator substances, but it is more pronounced in amniotic fluid embolism, retained dead fetus and septicemia.
- *Postpartum hemorrhage (PPH):* It may occur due to atonicity of the uterus and coagulopathy. Atonicity may be due to damaged muscle bundle in Couvelaire uterus and due to inhibition of myometrial contraction by increased fibrin degraded product (FDP).
- *Death* due to any isolated or combined effects.

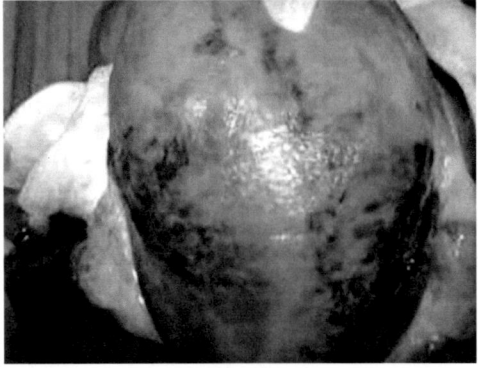

Fig. 2.1 Port wine colored couvelaire uterus
(For color version, see Plate 1)

Fetal

- Fetal ante-and intrapartum anoxia and distress.
- Growth retardation.
- Central nervous system (CNS) anomalies.
- Death as a result of anoxia due to placental separation or due to prematurity.

> *Diagnosis, abruptio placenta is confirmed. Fetus is dead. Patient is in shock, but external bleeding is not severe. So most of the bleeding is concealed. Patient is not in labor. Presentation is cephalic.*
> *How will you manage the case?*

Management depends on:
- Severity of abruption
- General condition of mother that is effect of blood loss
- Condition of labor
- Condition of fetus
- Complications such as coagulation abnormality.

Here the case is with severe symptom. Immediately just after quick assessment patient is to be resuscitated with close observation.

General Management for Resuscitation

- Intravenous (IV) channel is to be opened with wide bored (18 g) cannula.
- Blood is to be sent for grouping, crossmatching and coagulation profile such as bleeding time (BT), clotting time (CT), fibrinogen level, FDP, prothrombin time (PT), activated partial thromboplastin time (APTT) and platelet count. Transfusion is to be started as soon as possible.
- In the meantime infusion of Ringer's lactate solution and plasma expander is to be started before the blood becomes available.
- Foley's catheter is to be inserted to measure urine output.

Definitive Treatment

Here patient is not in labor and fetus is dead with cephalic presentation. As there is risk of coagulopathy and fetus is not concerned, induction of labor and vaginal delivery is preferred and safe:

- Along with resuscitation, labor is to be induced by artificial rupture of membrane (ARM). Labor usually initiates with ARM. ARM not only induces labor, but it increases the uterine tone and allowing the separated placenta to be compressed between the fetal bulk and the uterine wall, as a result bleeding ceases.
- Oxytocin drip is to be started to augment labor. Progress is to be watched. Labor progress is usually good, most of the time labor starts spontaneously. High doses of oxytocin may be required, because monitoring of uterine activity is unreliable as it remains tonically contracted. The best index of progress in labor is cervical change.
- If there is:
  - Delay in progress
  - Deterioration of maternal condition and
  - Continued bleeding.

  Cesarean section is to be done.

RELATED INFORMATION

Role of Cesarean Section in Abruptio Placenta

Unless there is a malpresentation other than breech, every effort should be made to deliver the patient with abruptio placenta with dead fetus vaginally. Cesarean section (CS) should be avoided unless there is clear indication for the procedure. Disseminated intravascular coagulation (DIC) is a strong contraindication for surgical intervention. So surgical intervention should be avoided if at all possible in presence of predicted hemostatic defect. If malpresentation is detected, pregnancy should be terminated by cesarean section with the exception of extreme small baby weighing less than 800 mg, which may be delivered vaginally even if there is transverse lie. Problem arises in clinical evaluation of fetal presentation and size due to rigid uterus in severe abruption. Therefore, ultrasonogram should be done in every case to determine fetal presentation, where there is any doubt. A failure to properly evaluate the fetal presentation may result in uterine rupture following oxytocin drip.

Indications

Indications of cesarean section are:
- Unfavorable cervix
- Delay in progress of labor
- Deterioration of patient's condition
- Malpresentation, except extreme premature small baby and breech presentation
- History of two or more previous cesarean section.

> Suppose patient's labor has started, but progress is not satisfactory. So you decided to do CS. During CS you found that uterus is dark port wine colored (almost black) and looks like a gangrenous uterus. It looks so unhealthy that seems better to remove it. This baby is dead and she has got no other children.
> In this situation what do you want to do?

This is the picture of Couvelaire uterus, which occurs commonly in severe form of concealed type of bleeding. *Couvelaire uterus is not an indication of hysterectomy.*

Uterus is to be kept as it is and the pathology will revert in due course of time. This occurs due to massive intravasation of blood into the uterine musculature up to the serous coat.

> Suppose Aleya has come with abruptio placenta with severe bleeding and shock. Fetus is dead, bleeding is continuing and cervix is tubular and firm.
> How will you manage her?

After initial management of resuscitation (as mentioned earlier) for definitive treatment, CS is to be done. No matter whether fetus is dead or alive. As maternal condition is poor and cervix is unfavorable for quick termination CS is to be done.

> Suppose she has same features, but she is in labor. Her cervix is 100% effaced and os is 6 cm dilated.
> What will you do for her?

After initial management for resuscitation (as mentioned earlier) for definitive treatment, ARM is to be done to augment labor. Bleeding usually stops after ARM. Progress of labor is to be observed:
- If bleeding stops and labor progresses smoothly, vaginal delivery is to be done
- To cut short second stage, ventouse or forceps can be applied
- If bleeding does not stop or labor does not progress, CS is to be done.

> Suppose Aleya has come at 30 weeks of gestation with slight abdominal pain. Uterus is soft in palpation. Ultrasonographically it is found that there is a slight collection of blood behind the placenta. Fetal movement and fetal heart sound is satisfactory.
> What will you do for this case?

This is 'class 0' abruptio placenta. Expectant treatment is suitable for this patient, as there is no symptom except mild pain:
- Patient should be observed for 24–48 hours to ensure that further separation is not occurring.
- Continuous fetal and maternal monitoring should be maintained. Changing in fetal status is sign of further separation.
- Pregnancy is to be continued till 37 completed weeks with regular follow-up and close monitoring.
- Conservative management is to be abandoned if the bleeding is recurrent and fetal condition deteriorates.

> Suppose patient has come with abruptio placenta at 35 weeks of gestation with mild bleeding. Uterus is soft, but irritable. Pulse is 90/m in, BP is 110/70 mm Hg. Fetal heart sound is audible. She is not in labor.
> How will you manage her?

Immediately after preliminary management, CS is to be done, as further separation of placenta is unpredictable. Any time excessive bleeding may occur due to further separation, which may jeopardies the fetus. So pregnancy is to be terminated by CS for quick delivery.

RELATED INFORMATION

In case of placental abruption with alive fetus, some authority advocate to classify the case into two groups. *If the uterus is rigid,* the abruption is probably large and chance of fetal distress or demise during labor is more than 90%. Patient should be delivered by CS provided there is no bleeding diathesis. *If the uterus is soft,* the pregnancy can be terminated by induction of labor. Because in this case, the abruption is not greater than 25% and chance of coagulopathy is extremely low and prospect of vaginal delivery with favorable outcome is excellent. But, if uterus becomes hypertonic, fetal heart rate (FHR) becomes nonreassuring it indicates further extension of abruption and immediate CS is to be done. In large majority cases of abruptio placenta should have vaginal delivery, if there is *no*

- Uterine rigidity
- Fetal distress
- Malpresentation
- Other indications for CS
- Continuous bleeding.

> Suppose patient has come with abruptio placenta at 33 weeks of gestation with moderate bleeding and alive fetus. Her pulse is 110/m in, BP is 90/50 mm Hg.
> How will you manage her?

As there is moderate bleeding, patient is to be resuscitated as mentioned earlier. CS is to be done, but before CS corticosteroids is to be given to mother for fetal lung maturity. At least one dose of injection corticosteroids even in operating (OT) table is helpful. Though fetus is premature, there is no scope of conservative treatment in abruptio placenta with moderate bleeding.

> After vaginal delivery in a case of abruptio placenta you found that there is profuse postpartum bleeding. Uterus is well-contracted and there is no tear or laceration.
> What might be the cause of bleeding?

Disseminated intravascular coagulation.

> How will you confirm it?

Coagulation profile such as fibrinogen, PT, partial thromboplastin time (PTT), platelet count, D-dimer and FDP are to be done. FDP and D-dimer will be more than normal and others will decrease. But it takes time to do the tests. So bedside coagulation test can be done to observe clot formation. In DIC, blood will not clot.

> How will you manage the case?

Aim of treatment is:
- To maintain hemodynamics and correction of coagulopathy.
- To prevent further blood loss.

For maintenance of hemodynamics and correction of coagulopathy: Blood and blood products is to be transfused in the form of:
 - Fresh whole blood
 - Packed red blood cells
 - Fresh frozen plasma
 - Cryoprecipitate packs
 - Platelets.

Fresh whole blood and fresh frozen plasma are commonly available and used.

For prevention of further blood loos: It takes time to correct coagulopathy by blood and blood products transfusion. So immediately intrauterine balloon tamponade can be used to prevent bleeding.

If not controlled:
 - Pelvic arterial embolization
 - Internal iliac arteries ligation can be done, even then in uncontrolled cases.

Hysterectomy may be needed even in presence of some degree coagulopathy.

> Suppose patient developed DIC and still she is undelivered. Fetus is dead. Bleeding is continuing. Her cervix is unfavorable.
> How will you deliver her?

In abruptio placenta with dead fetus always vaginal route of delivery is preferred. But here vaginal delivery will take time as cervix is not favorable. Moreover, bleeding is continuing.

So keeping the practical problem of uncontrolled hemorrhage in mind with all support of intensive care, with proper counseling of attendants and with double risk bond:
- Cesarean section is to be done to expedite delivery; vertical incision is ideal for such a case
- Adequate amount of blood and blood products should be transfused and kept at hand

- Patient and attendants should be counseled about emergency hysterectomy; but before taking the decision of hysterectomy uterine artery and hypogastric artery ligation is to be done to stop bleeding.

RELATED INFORMATION ABOUT DISSEMINATED INTRAVASCULAR COAGULATION

Obstetrical Causes of DIC

In disseminated intravascular coagulation (DIC), blood coagulation cascades starts as a sequale of some other conditions. DIC is never a primary disorder. Usually coagulation cascades starts due to endothelial injury, due to release of thromboplastin and phospholipids.

Obstetric Conditions

- Which causes endothelial injury?
  - Preeclampsia and eclampsia
  - Septicemia due to:
    - Septic abortion
    - Chorioamnionitis
    - Pyelonephritis.
  - Hypovolemia
- Which releases thromboplastin?
  - Amniotic fluid embolism
  - Intrauterine death of the fetus (dead fetus syndrome)
  - Abruptio placenta
  - Hydatidiform mole
  - Cesarean section
  - Intra-amniotic hypertonic saline infusion
  - Shock.
- Which releases phospholipids?
  - Fetomaternal bleeding
  - Incompatible blood transfusion
  - Hemolysis.

Basic Principles of Management

- Immediate management of triggering factors are utmost important to prevent the development of DIC and to arrest the consequences of DIC
- Prompt replacement of blood volume and coagulation factors.

> What is the role of heparin in the treatment of DIC?

Function of heparin is to prevent coagulation. So, if it can be given at consumption phase, then progression of the disease procedure is halted. But, if it is given in bleeding phase, then it will rather cause harm by preventing clotting. In acute cases, turnover of phases is very quick and it is very difficult to pinpoint the phase. So, it is better to avoid the use of heparin in acute cases. But in prolonged retention of intrauterine death (IUD), heparin can be used with normal coagulation profile to prevent development of DIC or with sign of consumption to prevent progression of DIC.

General Consideration for Management of Abruptio Placenta

Initial management is same for all bleeding cases and include:
- Rapid assessment of maternal hemodynamic status and amount of blood loss.
- Fetal assessment.
- All patients should have a wide bored (18 G) IV line and depending upon the amount of blood loss fluid replacement should be started.
- When abruptio placenta is severe enough to kill the fetus, it is assumed that about 2,500 mL blood lost in the retroplacental space (Pritchard and Brekken, 1967). So aggressive management is needed in this situation to avoid progressive organ perfusion damage.
- Normal hematocrit, hemoglobin, pulse and BP with fetal death due to abruptio placenta is sometimes misleading and transfusion must not be withheld in spite of normal vital signs.
- Blood pressure may be normal in spite of profuse blood loss if the patient is previously hypertensive and due to intense reactive vasoconstriction blood count may be within normal range in severe abruptio placenta.
- The aim of transfusion is to keep the hematocrit of at least 30% or more and urine output 30 mL/h, which is an indicator of effective intravascular volume maintenance.

- The most common cause of death in abruptio placenta is acute tubular necrosis and bilateral cortical necrosis, which can be avoided by maintaining the urinary output at 30 mL/h or more.
- Central venous pressure catheter should be inserted in severe abruption anticipating the need for large amount of intravenous fluid.

BIBLIOGRAPHY

Ananth CV, Oyelese Y, Srinivas N, et al. Preterm premature rupture of membranes, intrauterine infections and oligohydramnios: risk factors for placental abruptio. Obstet Gynecol. 2004;104(1):71-7.

Ananth C, Smulian JC, Vintzileos AM. "Incidence of placental abruptio in relation to cigarette smoking and hypertensive disorders during pregnancy: a meta-analysis of observational studies". Obstet Gynecol. 1999;93(4):622-8.

Facchinetti F, Marozio L, Grandone E, et al. Thrombophilic mutations are a main risk factor for placental abruptio. Haematologica. 2003;88(7):785-8.

Naeye RL. Abruptio placenta and placenta previa: frequency, perinatal mortality, and cigarette smoking. Obstet Gynecol. 1980;55(6):701-4.

Pritchard JA, Brekken AL. Clinical and laboratory studies on severe abruptio placentae. Am J Obstet Gynecol. 1967;97(5):681-700.

Pritchard JA, Mason R, Corely M, et al. Genesis of severe placental abruptio. Am J Obstet Gynecol. 1970;108(1):22-7.

Prochazca H, Happach C, Marsal K, et al. Factor V Leiden in pregnancies complicated by placental abruptio. BJOG. 2003;110(5):462-6.

Salihu HM, Bekan B, Aliyu MH, et al. Perinatal mortality associated with abruptio placenta in singletons and multiples. Am J Obstet Gynecol. 2005;193(1): 198-203.

Sher G. A rational basis for the management of abruptio placenta. J Reprod Med. 1978;21(3):123-9.

CHAPTER 3

Third Stage Complications

Rashida Begum

INTRODUCTION

Postpartum Hemorrhage

Postpartum hemorrhage (PPH) is the most common complication of third stage of labor and the most common cause of maternal death all over the world. All pregnant women are at risk of PPH and its sequelae when they carry pregnancy beyond 20 weeks. Although, death due to PPH has declined significantly in the developed world, it remains a leading cause of maternal death in developing countries. In Bangladesh, PPH is the number one cause of maternal death till today.

> **Case scenario:** *Asma, a 32-year-old primiparous lady gave birth a full term baby per vaginally at home 3 hours ago. She presents with heavy per vaginal (PV) bleeding. How will you proceed for management?*

Bleeding after delivery of the baby is called PPH. There is no diagnostic dilemma of PPH. So quick history taking, immediate examination and treatment are to be started simultaneously. Management of PPH depends on severity of bleeding. Severity is classified according to amount of bleeding. It is called minor when blood loss is between 500 and 1000 mL, major when blood loss is more than 1000 mL. Again major can be classified as moderate (1000–2000 mL) and severe (>2000 mL) (ACOG, 1997). Severe, heavy or massive hemorrhage can be determined by patients' vital signs like rapid and increased pulse rate and low blood pressure. Patients with massive hemorrhage need aggressive management to restore circulation and perfusion to vital organs. In case of massive hemorrhage, line of management will include:

- Communication with others
- Resuscitation to restore volume and oxygen carrying capacity
- Monitoring
- Attempt of arresting the bleeding: Mechanical and pharmacological measures are to be taken sequentially till stoppage of bleeding.

History taking, examination and treatment should be done simultaneously, as time is essence for PPH management:
- Shout for help
- Question about duration of labor
- Any difficulties of labor
- Query about delivery of placenta, whether complete or incomplete
- Examination of pulse, blood pressure (BP), respiration
- Designation of nurse or junior doctor to record vital signs, urine output, fluid and drugs administered
- Opening up of intravenous (IV) channel with 18G cannula
- Taking blood for grouping and crossmatching and making arrangement for blood
- Administration of oxygen by mask
- Infusion of normal saline or Ringer's lactate solution liberally to increase volume and raise blood pressure till arrival of blood. Total 3.5 liters of fluid, 2 liters crystalloid (Hartman's solution) and 1.5 liters colloid can be transfused till arrival of blood. Patient needs to be kept warm.
- Uterotonics:
  - Injection oxytocin 10 unit IV and 10 unit IM is to be given. Oxytocin infusion 40 unit in 500 mL Hartmann's solution 125 mL/h is to be started, unless there is any need for fluid restriction

- Injection ergometrine 0.5 mg IM or IV, maximum dose is 1.25 mg (contraindicated if there is high BP)
- Tablet misoprostol (prostaglandin E_1) 800 µg per rectally is to be given if uterus dose not contract and bleeding continues. The low cost and its heat stability makes it specially appealing for use in the developing countries
- Palpation of uterus to assess uterine contraction, if found laxed uterine massage is to be given to initiate uterine contraction
- Assessment of blood loss by observing wet cloths, clots in the vagina and free blood flow
- Catheterization is to be done and patient must be in continuous catheterization to empty the bladder, which helps in maintaining uterine contraction and to assess urine output
- After perineal toileting and maintaining asepsis, vaginal wall and cervix are to be inspected to exclude injury
- Assessment of any retained bits of placenta
- In absence of injury and retained placenta bleeding is due to atonicity of uterus, which needs immediate bimanual massage and compression.

Bimanual massage decreases bleeding from atonic uterus. Care should be taken to minimize the trauma in the lower genital tract during bimanual compression. The vaginal hand is to be placed in the anterior fornix and the abdominal hand over the posterior aspect of the fundus. The uterus is raised from the pelvis and compressed between the two hands. Due to compression clots expel out and bleeding ceases. Massaging is needed for sustained uterine contraction.

- Blood transfusion is to be started as soon as it is available
- Broad spectrum antibiotics is to be given.

Note:
- Prostaglandin F2α (PGF2α) carboprost can be used as second line if it is available at a dose of 0.25 mg IM injection stat and repeated at 15 minutes interval to a maximum 8 doses (contraindicated in asthma). Carboprost has been shown to be 80-90% effective in stopping PPH in cases refractory to oxytocin and ergometrine.
- A single dose of long-acting oxytocin derivatives carbetocin 100 µg IV can be given alternative to oxytocin drip, which is as effective as oxytocin infusion.

> After history taking and examination, you elicited that she had an easy delivery within a reasonable period. Patient is in a state of shock that is pulse is thready, feeble and 120/minute, BP 75/40 mm Hg, sweating present, respiration is hurried. There were large clots in the vagina, which was removed, cloths were soaked completely, no vaginal and cervical tear found. Uterus was laxed. You started blood transfusion, BP is increasing gradually. Uterotonics are going on, bimanual compression is applied. But bleeding is not controlled.
>
> What other measures can be taken for management of this patient?

If bimanual compression cannot stop bleeding, condom tamponed is to be introduced. Inflated condom can apply pressure over open sinuses and stops bleeding in atonic uterus. As balloon tamponade is the least invasive, cheaper and the most rapidly approachable, should be introduced when bleeding is not controlled by other means.

Note: Other temporary measures until substantive care is available are bimanual uterine compression, external aortic compression and non-pneumatic anti-shock garments. If resources are available, uterine artery embolization should be considered in case of persistent uterine bleeding.

RELATED INFORMATION

Resuscitation

Patient of severe hemorrhage remains in a state of shock. She must be resuscitated to maintain intravascular volume and to increase oxygen-carrying capacity. So that patient can maintain optimum blood pressure to supply vital organs and prevent from renal shutdown. Otherwise long hypotension and deoxygenation causes renal failure.

Component of resuscitation
- High concentration oxygen 10-15 L/minute via face-mask should be administered.
- Intravenous fluid infusion and blood transfusion:
  - Fluid:
    - *Crystalloid*: Up to 2 L
    - *Colloid*: Up to 1-2 L, until blood arrives.

About 4–5 L of crystalloid is needed to replace 1 L of blood loss, as most of the infused fluid shifted to the interstitial space. This shift along with oxytocin causes peripheral edema. If cause of bleeding can be arrested, in a healthy pregnant woman up to 1,500 mL blood loss can usually be managed by infusion of crystalloid alone. Blood and blood products are needed when blood loss is >1500 mL. Crystalloid is preferable to colloid as colloid may be responsible for more complication and mortality (Choi et al. 1999; Roberts et al. 2004)

- *Blood and blood products*: Crossmatched blood should be given, but in emergency situation uncrossmatched 'O negative blood' can be given:
  - *Whole blood*: To replace volume.
  - *Fresh frozen plasma (FFP)*: If fibrinogen, thrombin time, blood film and D-dimer results are abnormal and needle prick oozing present, FFP is to be given.
  - *Platelet concentrate:* It is to be used if bleeding continues and platelet count is less than $50 \times 10^9/L$.
  - *Cryoprecipitate:* It can be used when bleeding continues and abnormal coagulation test results are not corrected in-spite of transfusion of FFP.
  - *Cryoprecipitate and platelet:* Both need to be transfused before surgical intervention.

Criteria for fully resuscitated patient

Clinical improvement (must observed)
- Systolic blood pressure must be 100 mm Hg or more
- Pulse must be less than 100 beats per minute (bpm)
- Respiration must be less than 20 per minute
- Temperature must be less than 100°F
- Urine output must be 30 mL or more per hour.

Others
- Hemoglobin (Hb) must be > 8 g/dL
- Platelet count must be $> 75 \times 10^7/L$
- Prothrombin < 1.5 × mean control
- Activated prothrombin times < 1.5 × mean control
- Fibrinogen > 1.0 g/L.

Monitoring

Frequent monitoring is the cornerstone of management of a hemorrhagic case:
- Continuous pulse, BP recording and respiratory rate using oximeter, electrocardiogram and automated BP recording if available; otherwise manual recording of pulse, BP and respiration every 15 minutes
- Temperature recording every 15 minutes
- Monitoring of urine output hourly
- Frequent auscultation of lung field to assess fluid overload
- Consider central venous line, if volume cannot be maintained by peripheral line
- Consider arterial line, which may aid in monitoring BP and allowing easy access for blood work
- Consider transfer to intensive care unit, once bleeding is controlled, but general condition is not improved
- Full blood count and coagulation screening including fibrinogen is to be done
- Documentation of intake and output chart maintaining chart of fluid, blood and blood products.

Arresting of Hemorrhage

After failure by uterotonics before going for surgical ligation of arteries intrauterine compression of placental sinuses by roller gauze packing was considered as an important management. But uterine packing fell into disfavor, as pressure may not be evenly distributed and bleeding may continued, which will be concealed due to presence of roller gauze. That might further deteriorate the patient's condition. Moreover, there is increased risk of infection. So uterine packing is no longer recommended. Uterine packing is replaced by intrauterine balloon tamponade. Various type of hydrostatic balloon catheter supersede uterine packing for control of atonic PPH. Foley catheter (Ikechebelu et al. 2005), Bakri balloon (Bakri et al. 2001), Sengstaken-Blackmore esophageal catheter (Chan et al. 1997; Condous et al. 2003) the urological Rusch balloon (Keriakos et al. 2006) and Sayeba's condom tamponade **(Fig. 3.1)** (Akhter et al. 2003) are different types of balloon tamponade can control PPH successfully. Among all

Third Stage Complications

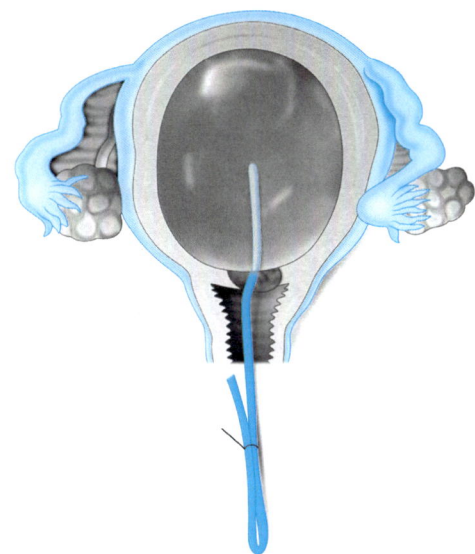

Fig. 3.1 Sayeba's condom tamponade

Sayeba's condom tamponade is the cheapest, easily available and easy to use.

How to Use Condom Tamponade?

- Maintaining aseptic precautions, a sterile rubber catheter is to be inserted within the condom and catheter is tied near the mouth of the condom by a silk.
- Indwelling Foley's catheter is to be introduced to keep the bladder empty.
- Maintaining lithotomy position of the patient, the condom is to be inserted within the uterine cavity.
- Inner end of the catheter will be within the condom.
- A saline set is fixed with outer end of the catheter and the condom is to be inflated with running normal saline till development of resistance of fluid flow.
- Bleeding is observed and further inflation will be stopped when bleeding is reduced considerably along with development of resistance of flow. Then outer end of the catheter is folded and tied with silk.
- Oxytocin drip is to be continued for at least 6 hours after the procedure to keep the uterus contracted.
- The inflated condom is kept tight in position by vaginal pack or another inflated condom placed in the vagina.
- The condom tamponade needs to be kept for 24–48 hours and then will be deflated gradually over 10–15 minutes and then removed.
- Prophylactic IV triple antibiotic, amoxicillin (500 mg every 6 hours) + metronidazole (500 mg every 8 hours) + gentamicin (80 mg every 8 hours) is to be given for 7 days.

Out of 23 patients bleeding stopped totally within 15 minutes of introduction of condom tamponade in all cases (Akhter et al. 2003).

> You are observing patient's condition. Bleeding is still continuing. Uterotonics are going on with maximum dose. Blood transfusion is going on. Bimanul compression and condom tamponade were applied. But PV bleeding outweighs the transfusion.
> What measure you can be taken for arresting bleeding?

Surgical Management

Surgical management is necessary if the uterus does not remain contracted and bleeding persists despite all efforts. Laparotomy is to be done for ligating the vessels.

Surgical approaches include the following:
- Adequate resuscitation of the patient
- Proper counseling and consent
- Laparotomy under general anesthesia
  - *Bilateral uterine and ovarian artery ligation:* Almost 90% of uterine blood flow comes from uterine arteries. So bilateral uterine artery ligation, which is relatively simple procedure can be highly effective in controlling bleeding. As portion of uterine supply comes from ovarian vessels, ovarian arteries ligation along with uterine arteries ligation becomes more effective. Menstrual flow and fertility is not affected due to bilateral uterine artery ligation
  - B Lynch suture if above measure fail
  - Internal iliac arteries ligation if others fail
  - Finally peripartum hysterectomy may be needed for life saving purpose.

Note: Selective arterial embolization is very effective and can be done on rare occasion where there is intractable hemorrhage, surgical options have been exhausted and fertility is desired. It is also effective in case of unmanageable hematoma (Pelage et al. 1998). Return of menstruation and fertility is not affected after uterine artery embolization (Chauleur et al. 2008). Drawback is that it needs stable condition of the patient and 24 hours availability of radiological expertise. Complications are hematoma formation at insertion site, infection, ischemia, contrast related adverse effect and on rare occasion uterine necrosis due to severe ischemia.

RELATED INFORMATION

Postpartum hemorrhage is defined as blood loss of more than 500 mL following vaginal delivery or more than 1,000 mL following cesarean delivery or any amount, which effects woman's health status or threatens hemodynamic stability of the woman such as falling of BP, tachycardia (Baskett, 1999).

The PPH can be minor (500–1,000 mL) or major (more than 1,000 mL). Major could be divided to moderate (1,000–2,000 mL) or severe (more than 2,000 mL) **(Table 3.1)**.

The effect of blood loss varies from woman to woman. As there is 30–50% increment of blood volume in a normal singleton pregnancy, a healthy woman can tolerate much blood loss than a woman who has pre-existing anemia, an underlying other volume contracted conditions like dehydration and pre-eclampsia. When bleeding occurs within 24 hours of delivery then it is called early or *primary PPH*, and when it occurs after 24 hours of delivery till 6 weeks postnatally then it is called *secondary PPH* (Alexander et al. 2002). PPH is the primary cause of maternal death in many parts of the world.

According to World Health Organization (WHO) statistics 25% of maternal deaths are due to PPH, accounting for more than 100,000 maternal deaths per year (Abouzahr, 1998).

Causes of Postpartum Hemorrhage

For easy remembering sources have suggested using the 4 *T's*' as a mnemonic, i.e. tone, tissue, trauma and thrombosis.

Atonicity of Uterus (Tone)

Atonicity of the uterus is the most common and dangerous cause of postpartum hemorrhage. It leads to rapid and massive hemorrhage and hypovolemic shock. Uterine smooth muscles arranged in a crisscross manner and vessels that supply the placental site traverse a weave of myometrial fibers and open sinuses lies between these interlacing muscle fibers. So after separation of placenta these muscle fibers of uterus contract and retract firmly, and occlude these supplying vessels and open sinuses by compression and kinking. Retraction is the unique characteristic of the uterine muscle to maintain its shortened length following each successive contraction. That is why it is called 'living ligatures' or 'physiological sutures' of the uterus (Baskett, 1999). But in certain situations, uterus remains atonic as it lost its contractile and retractile power and lead to massive hemorrhage.

Causes of Atonicity

- Overdistension of the uterus due to:
  a. Polyhydramnios
  b. Multiple pregnancies
  c. Fetal macrosomia

Table 3.1 Clinical findings in obstetric hemorrhage (ACOG, 1997)

Blood volume loss	Blood pressure (systolic)	Symptoms and signs	Degree of shock
500–1,000 mL (10–15%)	Normal	Palpitations, tachycardia, dizziness	Compensated
1,000–1,500 mL (15–25%)	Slight fall (80–100 mm Hg)	Weakness, tachycardia, sweating	Mild
1,500–2,000 mL (25–35%)	Moderate fall (70–80 mm Hg)	Restlessness, pallor, oliguria	Moderate
2,000–3,000 mL (35–50%)	Marked fall (50–70 mm Hg)	Collapse, air hunger, anuria	Severe

d. Congenital abnormality like hydrocephalus
  e. Failure to deliver the placenta or distension with blood before or after placental delivery.
- Poor contractile capacity of uterus due to:
  a. Uterine fatigability due to prolonged and obstructed labor or rapid forceful labor, especially if stimulated
  b. Inco-ordinate uterine action and inhibition of contraction due to use of some drugs like nitrates, nonsteroidal anti-inflammatory drugs, magnesium sulfate, halogenated anesthetic agents, beta-sympathomimetics and nifedipine
  c. Uterine structural abnormality, e.g. septate or subseptate uterus, placental implantation in the lower uterine segment
  d. Bacterial toxins, e.g. chorioamnionitis, endomyometritis, septicemia
  e. Hypoxia due to hypoperfusion due to severe anemia or Couvelaire uterus in abruptio placenta and hypothermia due to massive resuscitation or prolonged uterine exteriorization
  f. Mechanical barrier, e.g. fibroid uterus leads to ineffective contraction.
- Mismanagement of third stage of labor:
  a. Premature attempt to deliver the placenta before its separation
  b. Kneading and fiddling of the uterus
  c. Pulling the cords
  d. Manual removal of placenta during cesarean section.
     A, b and c these three cause irregular uterine contraction and partial placental separation leading to hemorrhage.

Note: Recent data suggest that grand multiparity is not an independent risk factor for PPH.

Retained Placenta (Tissue)

Due to inefficient uterine contraction and retraction or due to morbid adhesion placenta may retained in the uterus. Partial detachment opens the sinuses and interfere further uterine contraction leads to hemorrhage. Retention of a portion of the placenta is more in a placenta succenturiate or having an accessory lobe. Retained placenta is more common in extreme preterm pregnancies, especially in gestational age <24 weeks. Placenta accreta and its variants also fail to separate and causes retention. In this condition, the placenta is abnormally adherent due to invasion beyond the normal cleavage plane. When entire placenta is abnormally attached with deep invasion is called placenta increta or percreta. There may not be severe bleeding as sinuses are not open. But bleeding may occur if aggressive efforts are made to remove the placenta. The condition is serious when placenta implants over uterine scar due to C/S and other causes, especially if associated with placenta previa. So all patients with placenta previa should be taken seriously as there is risk of severe PPH, including the possible need for transfusion and hysterectomy. Retained blood clots also may cause uterine distension and prevent effective contraction.

Injury to Genital Tract (Trauma)

- Genital tract trauma may occur either spontaneously or following any operative delivery.
- Blood loss is almost twice in cesarean delivery than vaginal delivery.
- Trauma may occur in vagina, cervix and even in the body of the uterus following prolonged labor with manipulation.
- Trauma to the lower vagina, posterior fourchette, periurethral and clitoral region may occur either spontaneously or because of episiotomy.
- There may be complete perineal tear.
- Vaginal sidewall laceration is also most commonly associated with forceps delivery. It may also occur spontaneously, especially if a fetal hand presents with the head. Lacerations may occur during manipulations for any reason.
- Cervical tear and laceration is most commonly associated with forceps delivery specially when applied in incompletely dilated cervix. Spontaneous cervical laceration also may occur if mother cannot resist bearing down effort before full dilatation of the cervix. Very rarely, the cervix is purposefully incised at the 2 and/or 10 o'clock positions to facilitate delivery of an entrapped fetal head during a breech delivery (Dührssen incision).

- Rupture uterus: (*see* page 75).
  - Most common cause of rupture uterus is obstructed labor. It may also occur secondary to external or internal version. The highest risk is probably associated with internal version and extraction of a second twin. Scar rupture may occur spontaneously or after starting of labor pain. Trauma also may occur during manual removal of placenta or with instrumentation.
- Broad ligament hematoma: Occurs due to
  - Slippage of any vessels from lower uterine cesarean section wound
  - Extension of cervical or vaginal vault laceration
  - Spontaneous rupture of paravaginal venous plexus.
- Valval hematoma: Occurs due to:
  - Improper hemostasis during repair of vaginal, perineal and episiotomy wound resulting from missing suturing the apex of the wound and failure to obliterate dead space of the wound
  - Rupture of paravaginal venous plexus either spontaneously or following instrumental delivery.

Coagulation Defect (Thrombosis)

Pre-existing coagulation disorder is not very common. Acquired abnormalities are more commonly problematic. Disseminated intravascular coagulation (DIC) related to abruptio placenta, HELLP syndrome, intrauterine fetal death, amniotic fluid embolism, fatty liver in pregnancy and sepsis may cause PPH.

Other Causes

Uterine Inversion

> *Suppose Mrs Asma came with profuse PV bleeding. Her pulse is 100/minute, BP is 90/50 mm Hg. You found the uterus laxed and placenta is partially separated. No injury in cervix and vagina. During examination you applied gentle traction to bring out the placenta, but it did not come out.*
>
> *How will you manage the case?*

- Shout for help (resuscitation and monitoring as mentioned earlier)
- Opening up of IV channel with 18 G cannula
- Taking blood for grouping and crossmatching and making arrangement for blood
- Infusion of normal saline or Ringer's lactate solution liberally to increase volume and raise blood pressure till arrival of blood
- Uterine massage is to be given
- Uterotonics like injection oxytocin 10 unit IV and 10 unit IM is to be given and 20 unit in 500 mL drip is to be started. Injection ergometrine and tablet misoprostol are not recommended as those may cause firm contraction and further retention of placenta
- Blood transfusion is to be started as soon as it is available
- Patient must be in continuous catheterization to assess urine output
- After giving uterotonics bleeding supposed to be controlled and placenta supposed to be come out, which are to be assessed
- If after 15–20 minutes placenta still does not come out an attempt is now made to deliver it with cord traction and uterine counter traction. Care must be taken about uterine inversion. If still placenta does not come out or cord avulsed manual removal under general anesthesia is to be arranged with the following procedure:
  - Under general anesthesia with surgical preparation and all aseptic precaution, patient is to be drapped and placed in lithotomy position
  - Broad spectrum antibiotics are to be given
  - Maintaining asepsis one hand is to be introduced into the uterus in cone-shaped manner following the cord, which is made taught by other hand; margin of the placenta is to be felt
  - Uterus needs to be kept steady by other hand. Counter pressure is to be applied and needs to follow the movement of fingers of inside hand
  - After reaching the placental margin the fingers are insinuated between the placenta and the uterine wall with the back of hand. The placenta is gradually separated by slicing movement of hand from outwards to inwards till separation of whole placenta

- When placenta is totally separated, traction is given by abdominal hand by keeping the uterine hand inside to check that nothing is left behind
- Oxytocin drip is to be continued and injection ergometrine 0.25 mg is to be given and uterine hand is to be removed gradually. Uterine massage is to be given by abdominal hand to keep the uterus contracted
- Cervix and vagina are to be checked for any injury
- Placenta and membranes are need to be checked for completeness
- Tonicity of the uterus and PV bleeding are to checked for few hours.

> *Suppose during separation you found that there is no cleavage and finger cannot be introduced, but significant portion of placenta felt detached inside the cavity.*
> *What will you do?*

This may be the case of morbid adhesion to a part of placenta:
- If it is firmly attached, then attempt should not be taken to separate this portion
- Only the detached portion needs to bring down and attached portion should be kept as it is
- After removing the detached portion, uterine content will cleared off significantly and uterine contraction is possible. Though the retained portion may interfere uterine contraction, uterotonics may overcome it
- If uterotonics fails to stop bleeding, intrauterine condom tamponade can be applied
- The left over portion of the placenta will autolyze automatically
- Broad-spectrum antibiotics are to be continued for 7 days to prevent infection
- Role of methotrexate is debatable (Kayem et al. 2004). So one has to wait for spontaneous autolysis

> *If there is difficulty in introducing the hand due to hour glass contracture. What to do?*

- Injection hyoscine butylbromide and nitrous oxide (NO) can relax the ring for easy entrance of hand.

> *What are the complications of manual removal of placenta?*

- Hemorrhage due to incomplete removal
- Shock
- Injury to the uterus
- Infection
- Inversion
- Subinvolution
- Thrombophlebitis
- Embolism.

Note: For tear of cervix and vagina, meticulous repair should be done. In case of uterine perforation or rupture, laparotomy needs for repair.

> *Suppose Mrs Asma bleeds profusely after delivery of the baby and placenta as a whole. You examined and found no tear and uterus is firmly contracted. She has given history of severe pain in the abdomen, hardening of abdomen and bleeding before delivery.*
> *How will you manage her?*

This may be due to DIC, consequence of abruptio placenta. Bedside coagulation test is to be done to observe clotting. If blood fails to clot it is due to DIC.

Prompt replacement of blood volume is to be done by fresh blood transfusion and coagulation factors. It is vary important part of management.

Following tests are to be done:
- Platelet count
- Fibrinogen
- FDP
- PT
- D-dimer

Usually elevated D-dimer, very low fibrinogen and prolonged thrombin time is characteristic. As there is markedly depressed fibrinogen level, fresh frozen plasma and cryoprecipitate may be useful. Injection of low-molecular weight heparin can be given to prevent coagulation.

So if it can be given at consumption phase then progression of the disease procedure is halted. But if it is given in bleeding phase, then it will rather cause harm by preventing clotting. In acute cases, turnover of phases is very quick and it is very difficult to pinpoint the phase. So it is better to avoid the use of heparin in acute cases. *The use of heparin and antifibrinolytic therapy is* not recommended in women with DIC of obstetric origin.

> **Case scenario:** Mrs Ayesha delivered a baby by cesarean section at night. Next morning nurse called you due to restlessness of the patient. You examined her and found she is anxious, pale, restless due to severe pain in the abdomen and in a state of shock. PV bleeding is average. Abdomen is tender in left iliac region with a swelling above the inguinal ligament pushing the uterus to right side. Vaginal examination revealed bulging of the fornices towards vagina and a boggy swelling felt through the fornices.
>
> How will you manage her?

- Immediately patient should be resuscitated (as mentioned before)
- Blood should be sent for complete blood count (CBC), HB%, fibrinogen, FDP, D-Dimer and blood should be transfused as quickly as possible
- Ultrasonogram (USG) to identify intra-abdominal fluid or lump
- Arrangement for reopening the abdomen to explore the cavity.

> You could arrange USG and it did not find any free fluid in the abdominal cavity. An irregular lump is identified at left border of uterus, extending from lower part of body of uterus to fundus. Uterine cavity contains a small amount of fluid.
>
> After resuscitation what should be your next plan of action?

This is most likely broad ligament hematoma. So laparotomy should be done immediately to explore the hematoma and to ligate the bleeding points.

RELATED INFORMATION

Management of Genital Tract Trauma

Genital tract trauma is the most likely cause if bleeding persists or is present despite a well-contracted uterus. Cervical tear, cervical laceration and vaginal laceration are common. Beside those rarely concealed bleeding may occur forming hematomas in different sites. Vaginal sidewall hematoma, episiotomy wound hematoma and broad ligament hematoma formations may occur.

Injury and Laceration to Cervix and Vagina

Injuries are to be repaired preferably under general anesthesia (GA) with good light and positioning (lithotomy). Lacerations, which are small and non-bleeding, need not to be sutured. Any laceration with significant bleeding must be sutured. By an absorbable, continuous interlocking stitch tear should be repaired. Ensure that the stitch begins above the apex of the tear. If the apex cannot be visualized, place the stitch as high as possible and then apply gentle traction to bring the apex into view. Cervix must be checked for bleeding after approximation of torn edges. To control bleeding from laceration, vaginal pack may be applied.

Repair of Complete Perineal Tear

Significant amount of bleeding may occur from complete perineal tear. With maintaining proper aseptic condition and under general anesthesia (GA) tear should be repaired immediately after delivery of the placenta.

Traumatic Pelvic Hematomas

Collection of blood anywhere between pelvic peritoneum and the perineal skin is called pelvic hematoma. Traumatic hematomas are rare and may occur in isolation or along with other lacerations.

They are usually:
- Vulvar and paravaginal hematomas.
- Broad ligament and retroperitoneal hematomas.

Vulval hematoma is a localized swelling having intense pain. Vulva becomes dusky and purple in color and tender to touch. Broad ligament hematomas may be palpated as lump adjacent to the uterus. Due to significant concealed hemorrhage patient may go into shock. All these situations should be managed as massive revealed hemorrhage like resuscitation followed by specific management.

Lower genital tract or vulval hematomas are usually managed by incision and drainage, although expectant management is acceptable if the lesion is not enlarging. All bleeding vessels should be tied off. To control bleeding from oozing vaginal packing can be done, which should be removed after 24–36 hours. An indwelling Foley catheter is to be kept to prevent retention, which might occur due to severe pain and tissue distortion.

If the patient remains stable and hematoma is not expanding, both broad ligament and retroperitoneal hematomas can be managed expectantly. Ultrasound is good enough to assess the size and progress of these hematomas. Computed tomography (CT) scanning, and magnetic resonance imaging (MRI) can be used if needed. If it occurs after cesarean section laparotomy or if it occurs as an extension of vaginal vault laceration laparoscopy can be done for exploration. Hematomas need to be evacuated and all bleeding vessels are to be ligated. Skilled personnel should be involved to manage large retroperitoneal hematomas. Anterior leaf of the broad ligament is incised and the blood clot is scooped out and visible bleeding vessels are to be secured and ligated. Random blind suture should not be placed to prevent ureteric injury. If bleeding is not controlled, anterior division of internal iliac artery may be ligated. If facilities available and hematomas are not big enough and do not need to be evacuated, selective arterial embolization may be the treatment of choice. It is also applicable in cervical and vaginal vault lacerations that continue to bleed or are associated with hematomas.

> **Case scenario:** Mrs Amena, a fourth gravid woman is carrying for 31 weeks. She is a high-risk pregnancy, as she is carrying triplet pregnancy. As uterus is overdistended there is a risk of atonicity of the uterus and PPH.
>
> What precaution you need to be taken?

Antenatal Precautions

- As pregnancy is triplet there is big placental surface area due to three placenta. Triplet usually cannot be uniovular. Even in uniovular multiple pregnancies placental size is bigger than singleton pregnancy. Antenatally iron supplementation is to be given to keep the HB nearly 12 g%. If oral iron cannot increase the HB percentage parenteral iron therapy is to be given. Even then if HB percentage is below 10 g% blood transfusion is to be given so that patient can cope with any amount of postpartum blood loss.
- Delivery must be conducted in any institution with facilities of blood banking, surgery and neonatal care.
- Cross-matched blood donor should be kept ready.

Intranatal Precautions

Active management of third stage of labor:
- Injection oxytocin a dose of 10 IU is administered intramuscularly with the delivery of anterior shoulder of the baby. In addition, 10–20 IU is placed in 500–1,000 mL of crystalloid and run quickly
- Assessment of size and tone of the uterus
- A continuous and downward controlled cord traction (CCT) and counter traction is given when uterus is well-contracted
- Early cord clamping, not recommended by World Health Organization (WHO)
- Oxytocin drip is to be continued for 24 hours.

Note: Preventive measure should be taken for any case who has risk factors for developing PPH.

RELATED INFORMATION

Risk Factors for Postpartum Hemorrhage and how to Minimize?

- Certain factors, which are responsible for uterine atonicity are predictive risk factors must be taken into consideration. Plans of management must be modified according to present risk factors. Patients should be counseled about place of delivery and risk and safety of both the mother and the baby.
- Management should be started from antenatal period to keep the HB level at upper limit (more than 11 g/dL) so that patient can cope with PPH to some extent.

- All women who have previous cesarean section, must have ultrasound to determine the placental localization.
- If facilities available, MRI can be done to determine whether the placenta is accreta or percreta.
- Women with accreta or percreta should be managed by multidisciplinary approach. Consultant obstetrician, anesthetist, pediatrician and urologist should be in the team. Patient must be managed in a facility where blood and blood products are available.
- Blood donor with crossmatching should be kept ready.
- Active management (use of uterotonics, early clamping of the umbilical cord and CCT and counter traction) should be applied. A Cochrane review of five trials found that active management of third stage of labor was associated with reduced risk of PPH, prolonged third stage and reduced blood loss (Prendiville et al. 2000). Though nausea, vomiting and raised BP are the unpleasant effects of uterotonics, it reduces the risk of PPH by 60% and need for therapeutic oxytocin by about 50% (Cotter et al. 2001). For prophylaxis injection ergometrine along with injection oxytocin is not recommended, as it increases the risk of unpleasant side effects five times than oxytocin alone with similar efficacy in prevention of PPH.
- Misoprostol 600 µg orally is not as effective as injection oxytocin 10 IU intravenously in preventing PPH (You and Zahn, 2006). Due to adverse effects, which are dose related misoprostol is not recommended for routine use for prevention of PPH. A review of 32 trials concluded that conventional uterotonics are preferable to prostaglandins for routine prophylaxis of PPH. They recommended the use of prostaglandins in treatment rather than prevention of PPH (Gulmezoglu et al. 2007). But in rural areas where oxytocin injection is not available or skilled birth attendants are not available tablet misoprostol 600 µg orally or per rectally can be given by community healthcare providers, which reduces the risk of hemorrhage.
- In cases where there is chance of atonicity of uterus long-acting oxytocin derivative carbetocin can be used. A single dose (100 µg) of carbetocin is as effective as oxytocin infusion (Boucher et al. 1998; Dansereau et al. 1999). If carbetocin is not available oxytocin drip is to be continued for 24 hours.

Note: WHO recommendation for certain facts:
- Controlled cord traction is not recommended where skill, birth attendants are not available.
- For all births cord should be clamped within 1-3 minutes of birth. Early cord clamping within <1 minute is not recommended until and unless baby is asphyxiated and needs resuscitation.
- Oxytocin (10 IU, IV/IM) is the recommended uterotonic drug for the prevention of PPH.
- Ergometrine/methylergometrine or the fixed drug combination of oxytocin and ergometrine, or oral misoprostol (600 µg) is recommended, where oxytocin is not available.
- Tab misoprostol 600 µg orally can be given by community health workers, where skill birth attendants are not present.
- Women who have received prophylactic oxytocin do not need sustained uterine massage. So it is not recommended.
- For early identification of uterine atony postpartum abdominal uterine tone assessment is recommended for all women.
- Oxytocin (IV or IM) is the recommended uterotonic drug for the prevention of PPH in cesarean section.
- Controlled cord traction is the recommended method for removal of the placenta in cesarean section. Manual removal of placenta is not recommended during cesarean section.

Case scenario: *Mrs Anuradha Mondol delivered a baby by cesarean section 10 days back. Her wound healed completely and her lochial discharge was normal. But suddenly she developed severe PV bleeding.*

How will you manage her?

Per vaginal bleeding 10 days after cesarean section is usually due to:
1. Either separation of slough from the wound due to infection and exposing the vessels.
2. Retention of bits of placenta:

Keeping these two things in mind resuscitation, history taking, examination and ordering investigation should be done simultaneously:
- To assess the amount of blood loss
- To find out the specific cause to take appropriate measure to correct it.
    a. Immediately an IV channel with 18 G cannula is to be established
    b. Infusion of crystalloid is to be started to maintain volume
    c. Crossmatched blood should be arranged and transfused as soon as it arrives
    d. Uterotonics are to be given to minimize atonicity if there is any. Injection ergometrine 0.5 mg intramuscularly
    e. History is to be taken regarding:
        - History of any temperature
        - Foul smelling discharge
        - Pain in the abdomen.
    f. *Examination*: Pulse, BP, temperature needs to be assessed
        - *Per abdominal (PA)*: Any tenderness or rigidity
        - *Per vaginal*:
            - Observation of amount of bleeding
            - Before going to bimanual examination high vaginal and intracervical swab is to be taken for culture and sensitivity
            - Assessing presence of any retained product of conception.
    g. Starting of IV broad spectrum antibiotics; injection ceftriaxone, metronidazole and gentamicin are to be started after taking high vaginal and intracervical swab for culture and sensitivity.
    h. Ultrasonogram is to be done to see any product of conception
    i. If detected exploration of the uterus is to be done under general anesthesia (GA) with maintaining caution
    j. If USG is not available and bleeding continues in spite of using uterotonics exploration of the uterus is to be done under GA.

> You have started antibiotics, given uterotonics, transfused two units of blood, USG did not find any retained bits of placenta and even after exploration you did not find any retained bits of placenta. Uterus remained contracted and PV bleeding controlled, but patient's condition is not improving. Abdomen is tender and a bit distended.
> What might be the case and how will you manage?

This may be due to separation of slough from cesarean section wound and opening up of vessels. So laparotomy is to be done for exploration, toileting and ligature of bleeding vessels. Whole uterine wound may need to be sutured. If specific bleeding points cannot be identified or suturing of uterine wound cannot control bleeding, bilateral internal iliac artery ligation may be needed. Even then if bleeding cannot be controlled, hysterectomy may be the last resort of management.

Note: In secondary PPH, bleeding usually occurs between 8th and 14th day of delivery. Causes are:
- Retained bits of cotyledon or membranes
- Infection and separation of slough from cesarean section wound or deep cervicovaginal laceration
- Endometritis and subinvolution.

> **Case scenario:** Mrs Alyea a 25-years-old lady came to the hospital with history of vaginal delivery at home, severe PV bleeding and hanging of the placenta, severe lower abdominal pain with bearing down sensation. Dai tried to deliver the placenta. She was fourth gravid and during third pregnancy she had history of morbid adhesion of placenta. She is in a state of shock. On abdominal examination there was a depression in the center of the uterus or in other words fundus could not be palpated. On vaginal examination you found that no cervix could be felt, rather there is a reddish purple, colored mass on which placenta is firmly attached partly and partly is hanging.
> What might be the case? How will you manage her?

This is a case of acute inversion of uterus with retention of placenta due to morbid adhesion. As dai tried to remove the placenta in presence of morbid adhesion uterus became upside down:
- *General treatment*: Immediately patient should be resuscitated as other severe hemorrhagic patients except uterotonics (fluid, blood, antibiotics and catheterization).
- *Specific treatment*:

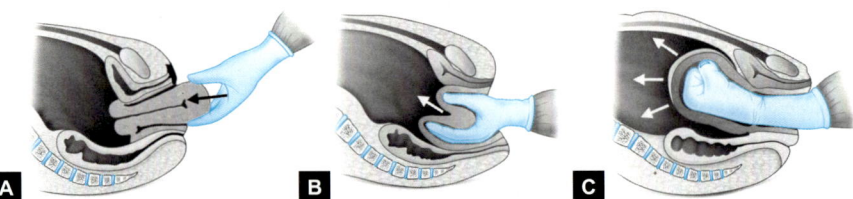

Figs 3.2A to C (A) Complete inversion; (B) Manual reposition; (C) Reposition completed

- Once inversion is recognized, all oxytocic agents should be withheld until correction has been established
- Manual correction of inversion **(Figs 3.2A to C)** is to be done through the vagina, known as the Johnson maneuver, consists of pushing the inverted fundus through the cervical ring with pressure directed toward the umbilicus. Reposition should be started from that part that is inverted last (Kochenour, 1991).
- It is commonly suggested that removal of the placenta before correction will result in increased blood loss and worsening hemodynamics (Momani, 1989; Kochenour, 1991).
- Procedure is to be done under GA so that uterus remains relaxed, which will facilitate reposition and constriction ring also will be relaxed.
- Magnesium sulfate or terbutaline or nitroglycerin can be used for uterine muscle relaxation.
- After complete reposition hand should be kept *in situ* and injection ergometrine 0.5 mg IM and oxytocin 40 unit in 1,000 mL fluid is to be started to initiate uterine contraction. Once uterus is contracted placenta is to be removed manually. Oxytocin drip should be continued till 24 hours.
- Alternatively hydrostatic pressure by O'Sullivan method can be applied. Warmed fluid is hung above the level of the patient and allowed to flow, into the vagina through a tube. The pressure of the water, held in place by the clinician's hands, results in correction of the inversion.
- Surgical correction is needed when all attempts of manual reduction of the inversion are failed. It can be done by adopting one of the two methods, Huntington and Haultain procedures.
- Laparotomy is needed for Huntington procedure. Cup of the uterus formed by the inversion is located and clamps are placed in the cup of the inversion below the cervical ring. Gentle upward traction is applied. Repeated clamping and traction continues until the inversion is corrected.
- Haultain procedure also is done through laparotomy. An incision is made in the posterior portion of the inversion ring to increase the size of the ring and allow repositioning of the uterus.

RELATED INFORMATION

Uterine Inversion

Uterine inversion is a rare, but a life-threatening complication in third stage of labor in which uterus is turned inside out partially or completely. It is not clear that's why uterine inversion occurs.

Some factors are associated with uterine inversion are:
- *Iatrogenic:* Due to mismanagement of third stage of labor.
  - This occurs due to strong traction on the umbilical cord before placental separation, particularly when the placenta is in a fundal location.
  - Excessive fundal pressure or Crede's expression in a laxed uterus.
  - Inappropriate technique of manual removal of placenta.
- *Spontaneous*: It includes the following.
  - Localized atony of the placental site over the fundus associated with sharp rise in

intrauterine pressure such as coughing, sneezing or bearing down effort
- Relaxed uterus, lower uterine segment and cervix
- Placenta accreta particularly in fundal attachment
- Short umbilical cord
- Congenital weakness or anomalies of the uterus
- Primiparity and rapid emptying of the uterus after prolonged distention as possible predisposing factors (Salomon, 1990; Zahn, 1990).

Types of Inversion

Uterine inversion is classified into:
- By the degree of inversion:
  - *First degree*: There is dimpling of the fundus, which still remains above the level of internal os
  - *Second degree*: The fundus passes through cervix, but lies inside the vagina
  - Third degree:
    - Complete inversion when the endometrium with or without the attached placenta is visible outside the vulva fundus extends beyond the external os (Salomon, 1990).
    - A prolapsed inversion when inverted uterine fundus extends beyond the vaginal introitus (Lewin, 1989).
- By the time of onset:
  - *Acute inversion*: Occurs before cervical ring contraction
  - *Subacute inversion*: Occurs after the cervical ring contraction
  - *Chronic inversion*: Occurs after 4 weeks of delivery.

Complications of Massive Postpartum Hemorrhage

- Renal failure
- Irreversible shock
- Sheehan's syndrome
- Death.

BIBLIOGRAPHY

Abouzahr C. Antepartum and postpartum hemorrhage. In: Murray CJ, Lopez AD (Eds). Health Dimensions of Sex and Reproduction. Boston: Harvard University Press; 1998.pp.172-4.

Akhter S, Begum MR, Kabir Z, et al. Use of a condom to control massive postpartum hemorrhage. Med General Med. 2003;5(3):38.

Alexander J, Thomas PW, Sanghera J. Treatments for secondary postpartum hemorrhage. Cochrane Database Syst Rev. 2002;(1):CD002867.

ACOG educational bulletin. Hemorrhagic shock. Number 235, April 1997 (replaces no. 82, December 1984). American College of Obstetricians and Gynecologists. Int J Gynaecol Obstet. 1997;57(2): 279-26.

ACOG educational bulletin. Hemorrhagic shock. Number 235, April 1997 (replaces no. 82, December 1984). American College of Obstetricians and Gynecologists. Int J Gynaecol Obstet. 1997;57(2):219-26.

Bakri YN, Amri A, Abdul Jabbar F. Tamponade-balloon for obstetrical bleeding. Int J Gynaecol Obstet. 2001;74(2):139-42.

Baskett TF. Complications of the third stage of labour. Essential Management of Obstetrical Emergencies. 3rd edition. Bristol, England: Clinical Press; 1999. pp.196-201.

Boucher M, Horbay GL, Griffin P, et al. Double-blind, randomized comparison of the effect of carbetocin and oxytocin on intraoperative blood loss and urine tone of patients undergoing cesarean sections. J Perinatol. 1998;18:202-7.

Chan C, Razvi K, Tham KF, et al. The use of a Sengstaken-Blakemore tube to control post-partum hemorrhage. Int J Gynecol Obstet. 1997;58(2):251-2.

Chauleur C, Fanget C, Tourne G, et al. Serious primary post-partum hemorrhage, arterial embolization and future fertility: a retrospective study of 46 cases. Hum Reprod. 2008;23(7):1553-9.

Choi PT, Yip G, Quinonez LG, et al. Crystalloids vs. colloids in fluid resuscitation: a systematic review. Crit Care Med. 1999;27(1):200-10.

Condous GS, Arulkumaran S, Symonds I, et al. The "tamponade test" in the management of massive postpartum hemorrhage. Obstet Gynecol. 2003; 101(14):767–72.

Cotter AM, Ness A, Tolosa JE. Prophylactic oxytocin for the third stage of labor. Cochrane Database Syst Rev. 2001;(4):CD001808.

Dansereau J, Joshi AK, Helewa ME, et al. Double-blind comparison of carbetocin versus oxytocin in prevention of uterine atony after cesarean section. Am J Obstet Gynecol. 1999;180:670-6.

Gulmezoglu AM, Forna F, Villar J, et al. Prostaglandins for prevention of postpartum hemorrhage. Cochrane Database Syst Rev. 2007;(3):CD000494.

Ikechebelu JI, Obi RA, Joe-Ikechebelu NN. The control of postpartum hemorrhage with intrauterine Foley catheter. J Obstet Gynecol. 2005;25(1):70-2.

Kayem G, Davy C, Goffinet F, et al. Conservative versus extirpative management in cases of placenta accreta. Obstet Gynecol. 2004;104(3):531-6.

Keriakos R, Mukhopadhyay A. The use of the Rusch balloon for management of severe postpartum hemorrhage. J Obstet Gynecol. 2006;26(4):335-8.

Kochenour NK. Intrapartum obstetric emergencies. Crit Care Clin. 1991;7(4):851-64.

Lewin JS, Bryan PJ. MR imaging of uterine inversion. J Comput Assist Tomogr. 1989;13(2):357-9.

Momani AW, Hassan A. Treatment of puerperal uterine inversion by the hydrostatic method; reports of five cases. Eur J Obstet Gynecol Reprod Biol. 1989;32(3):281-5.

Pelage JP, Le Dref O, Mateo J, et al. Life-threatening primary postpartum hemorrhage: treatment with emergency selective arterial embolization. Radiology. 1998;208(2):359-62.

Prendiville WJP, Elbourne D, McDonald SJ. Withdrawn: Active versus expected management in the third stage of labor. Cochrane Database Syst Rev. 2000;(3):CD000007.

Roberts I, Alderson P, Bunn F, Chinnock P, Ker K, Schierhout G. Colloids versus crystalloids for fluid resuscitation in critically ill patients. [Cochrane Database Syst Rev. 2004;18(4):CD000567].

Salomon CG, Patel SK. Computed tomography of chronic nonpuerperal uterine inversion. J Comput Assist Tomogr. 1990;14(6):1024-6.

You WB, Zahn CM. Postpartum hemorrhage: abnormally adherent placenta, uterine inversion, and puerperal hematomas. Clin Obstet Gynecol. 2006;49(1):184-97.

Zahn CM, Yeomans ER. Postpartum hemorrhage: placenta accreta, uterine inversion, and puerperal hematomas. Clin Obstet Gynecol. 1990;33(3): 422-31.

CHAPTER 4

Premature Birth

Rashida Begum

INTRODUCTION

Premature birth is defined as birth of the baby before 37 completed weeks before the organs become mature enough for extrauterine survival. It may be due to spontaneous or induced preterm labor. Premature infants are at greater risk for short- and long-term complications, including disabilities, and impediments in growth and development both mentally and physically. Approximately 12.9 million preterm births take place annually worldwide (Martin et al. 2010). It is an important cause of low birth weight and the major cause of death of infants worldwide. Management and prevention of spontaneous preterm labor is very challenging for obstetrician.

> **Case scenario:** Mrs Rabeya, a 30-year-old lady has come with history of pregnancy for 30 weeks and lower abdominal pain for 5 hours.
>
> How will you proceed for diagnosis?

Detailed History is to be Taken First

- About pain:
  - Is it rhythmic in nature?
  - Is it progressively increasing in intensity and frequency?
    - Rhythmically progressive increasing pain is characteristics of labor pain.
  - Did she take any pain killer? If so, did it reduce the pain?
    - Labor pain does not subside by any painkiller.
- About gestational age:
  - When was her last menstrual period (LMP)?
  - Was her cycle regular? Chance of miscalculation of date is less in regular cycle.
  - Did she take any contraceptive before this pregnancy?
    - Oral contraceptive pill (OCP) causes post pill amenorrhea. So chance of miscalculation of date is more in case of pregnancy after withdrawal of OCP.
  - Date of positive pregnancy test: It will give clue of gestational age.
  - Any ultrasound done in early weeks: More informative about gestational age.
- Past obstetric history:
  - History of previous abortions: Recurrent abortions are risk factors for premature labor.
  - History of previous premature labor: Risk of premature labor, 7 times more, who has history of previous premature labor.
  - Number of live children.
- History of any medical and obstetrical diseases:
  - Diabetes
  - Hypertension
  - Pregnancy-induced hypertension
  - Antepartum hemorrhage
  - Fever due to any cause
  - Infection in urinary tract and genital tract: Genitourinary tract infection is responsible for 20–40% of all cases of preterm birth
  - Query about fetal movement.
- History of any trauma: Fall or blow in the abdomen may initiate labor pain

Patient is to be examined thoroughly to evaluate.

- Pulse
- Blood pressure (BP)

- Temperature, anemia
- Per abdominal examination to assess:
  - Gestational age of the fetus by assessing height of the uterus
  - Fetal heart activity
  - Fetal movement
  - Pattern of contraction and its association with pain, if there is any. Number of contraction per 10 minutes and duration of each contraction.
- Per vaginal examination:
  - Cervical effacement
  - Cervical dilatation
  - Any show.

> After history taking and performing examination, you elicited that her pregnancy is for 30 weeks according to her LMP and ultrasound done at 7 weeks of pregnancy. Her pulse, temperature, BP is within normal limit. She has got no medical or obstetrical complications. Per abdominal examination revealed corresponding uterine height. Fetal movement and heart sound is normal. Uterine contraction is 3–10 minutes, which is associated with pain and persists for 20 seconds. Per vaginal examination revealed short cervix 50% effaced and 2.5 cm dilated, slight show is present. She is first gravid, so no significant past history is present.
> What is your diagnosis?

This is a case of premature labor. This is an early preterm labor as dilatation is less than 3 cm.

> How you will evaluate the case for management?

When cervix is 80% effaced or more, but dilatation is less than 3 cm then it is called early preterm labor. Dilatation 3 cm or more is advanced preterm labor. If labor is in early stage 60–65% of women respond to tocolysis and pregnancy can be continued till term or near term.

Test to be done for Assessment

Following tests are to be done for assessment:
- Complete blood count (CBC) and C-reactive protein (CRP) to assess any sign of infection. Elevated white blood cell (WBC) count and CRP will raise the suspicion of intra-amniotic infection. Upper limit of CRP during pregnancy is 0.9 mg/dL with no variation due to gestational age (Watts et al. 1991).
- *Blood sugar*: 2 hours postprandial.
- Transabdominal ultrasonography is to be done to assess the fetal condition, whether there is any congenital anomaly, which may be an initiator of labor pain. Fetal weight is to be measured. Localization of placenta, placental size and any retroplacental bleeding is to be sought for.
- Color Doppler USG to see placental circulation to evaluate placental insufficiency, which may cause intrauterine growth restriction (IUGR), fetal stress and might initiate labor.
- Urine routine, microscopic and culture and sensitivity (C/S)
- High vaginal swab, intracervical swab culture and sensitivity.

Note:
- *Fetal fibronectin (FFN) test:* Presence of FFN in the vaginal secretion is a predictor of premature labor. It is a glycoprotein acts as glue between the fetal membranes and decidua. Any interruption due to uterine contraction or infection releases the fibronectin in cervicovaginal secretion. Value less than 50 ng/mL is negative and ≥ 50 ng/mL is positive. It is a valuable test for predicting preterm birth in both symptomatic and asymptomatic women (Faron et al, 1998) but fallacy is that speculum or digital examination, endovaginal ultrasound examination even sexual intercourse interferes with the accuracy of the test. Here digital examination was done. So 24–48 hours interval is to be given in these situations to get the accurate result.
- *Transvaginal ultrasound (TVS) to measure cervical length:* Though cervical length can be measured by TVS, digital examination also can assess at a time. Cervical effacement 50% corresponds with 0.50 cm cervical length, 75% corresponds with 0.25 cm and 100% is paper-thin.
- Amniocentesis for amniotic fluid C/S and test for fetal lung maturity can be done after initial management.

RELATED INFORMATION

Preterm labor is defined as onset of labor after the age of viability (20–28 weeks depending upon definition of different societies), but before 37 completed weeks. There should be documented uterine contractions at least 1/10 minutes, ruptured membranes, or cervical change like cervical length <1 cm or cervical dilatation of more than 2 cm. Uterine contraction without cervical change is known as threatened preterm labor.

Causes of Premature Birth

The exact cause of preterm birth is remained undetermined. In 50% cases, the cause of preterm births is never determined.

Primarily four factors are responsible for premature birth:
1. Activation of myometrium due to any cause resulting premature contraction and premature labor.
2. Premature rupture of the membrane due to premature activation of membrane for any reason leads to premature labor.
3. Premature ripening of the cervix due to cervical incompetence or other causes leads to premature rupture of membrane and labor.
4. Iatrogenic preterm delivery for fetal and maternal indications.

Following conditions are responsible for pre-term activation of common pathways of labor:
1. Complications during present pregnancy are:
   A. Maternal:
      a. *Obstetrical complications:*
         - Pregnancy-induced hypertension
         - Antepartum hemorrhage
         - Gestational diabetes mellitus
         - Polyhydramnios
         - Premature rupture of the membrane.
      b. *Uterine defect:*
         - Cervical insufficiency
         - Maldevelopment of the uterus (bicornuate, didelphus, septate and subseptate uterus).
      c. *Medical and surgical illness:*
         - High fever
         - Acute pyelonephritis
         - Recurrent urinary tract infection (UTI)
         - Acute appendicitis
         - Toxoplasmosis
         - Diarrhea
         - Chronic renal disease
         - Hypertension
         - Hepatitis
         - Diabetes mellitus
         - Decompensated heart lesion
         - Severe anemia.
      d. *Genital tract infection:*
         - Bacterial vaginosis
         - Group B streptococcus (GBS)
         - Bacteroids
         - Chlamydia
         - Mycoplasma
   B. Fetal:
      - Multiple pregnancy
      - Congenital malformation
      - Intrauterine fetal death.
   C. Placental: Abnormalities in morphology, implantation and function of the placenta is associated with preterm birth.
      - Placental insufficiency
      - Abnormal placentation: Lack of physiological changes of spiral arteries causing small placenta having extensive infarction, fibrosis and calcification.
      - Anatomic abnormalities of placenta: Battledore placenta, circumvallate placenta and marginal insertion of the umbilical cord are associated with preterm birth.
2. Iatrogenic: When labor is induced due to maternal and obstetrical complications.
3. Maternal other predisposing factors:
   - Low and high body mass index (BMI)
   - Maternal stress
   - Smoking
   - History of recurrent pregnancy loss
   - History of previous premature labor
   - Pregnancy following assisted reproductive technology
   - Low social class.
4. Idiopathic.

Pathogenesis

1. **Premature activation of myometrium:** (Predominant causes endocrine factors and bleeding)
   A. *Maternal and fetal stress:* Both maternal and fetal stress causes premature acti-

vation of myometrium. Under normal condition the uterus is under the effect of multiple inhibitors of uterine contraction. Progesterone, relaxin, nitric oxide and prostacyclin are the factors responsible to keep the uterus quiescent. As pregnancy advances myometrium becomes more responsive to estrogen and increases the synthesis of gap junctions, oxytocin and prostaglandin receptors and gets prepared for contraction. In certain situations where these phenomenon come in advance causes premature activation of myometrium and uterine contraction.

Maternal stress: It causes release of corticotropin releasing hormone (CRH) from maternal hypothalamus. Maternal CRH releases ACTH from pituitary, which in turn increases the synthesis of cortisol from maternal adrenal gland. This cortisol though inhibits maternal hypothalamic CRH, stimulates placental CRH production. Placenta is a major source of CRH during pregnancy. Placental CRH increases the production of fetal ACTH, which leads to production of fetal cortisol and dehydroepiandrosterone (DHEA). The fetal cortisol stimulates the production of placental CRH and a vicious circle established to produce more fetal DHEA. This DHEA eventually transformed into estriol having properties of multiple activities such as:

- Increment of myometrial gap junctions, density of prostaglandin and oxytocin receptors.
- Increase release of oxytocin from hypothalamus and prostaglandins from decidua. Prostaglandin cause cervical ripening and stimulates myometrial contraction and initiates onset of labor.

Fetal stress: It is due to sickness either by maternal disease such as pre-eclampsia, eclampsia, diabetes, anemia or by fetal congenital anomaly, metabolic and infectious disease. In these situations labor starts with the fetal production of CRH as a response to stress.

B. *Abnormal placentation:* Abnormal placental implantation decreases uteroplacental blood flow, which in turn causes fetal stress that in turn causes production of CRH for initiation of contraction.
C. *Bleeding in choriodecidual interface:* Separation of placenta and abruptio placenta causing bleeding in choriodecidual interface, thrombin release and activation of labor pain.
D. *Overdistention of the uterus:* Overdistention of the uterus induce myometrial contractility by possible early activation of CRH and mechanical force might activates protein kinase and increased expression of guanine nucleotide binding protein (G proteins).
E. *Uterine abnormalities:* Septate and bicornuate uterus is responsible for preterm labor. Most possible mechanism is initiation of myometrial activity.

2. **Premature activation of membranes:** (Predominant cause is infection)
Premature activation of the membrane causes premature rupture of the membrane (PROM). PROM may occur due to:
A. Reduction of membrane strength
B. Increased intrauterine pressure or both.

A. Reduction of membrane strength: The amniotic membranes are a connective tissue structure and their tensile strength depends on the synthesis, degradation and quality of their collagen.
Causes of decreased tensile strength are:
  i. *Abnormal collagen structure:*
     - Connective tissue disorder
     - Tobacco smoking
     - Copper deficiency
     - Ascorbic acid deficiency.
   Degradation of collagen occurs due to sequential activity of several matrix metalloproteinases.
  ii. *Infection:* Infection by ascending organism or colonial organism may cause alteration in the tensile strength of the fetal membranes. Microorganisms produce proteolytic enzymes that can weaken the fetal membranes (Mc Gregor and Frence, 1977).

Another mechanism is host inflammatory response includes the production of cytokines that stimulates the production of prostaglandins by amnion and chorion. Prostaglandins stimulate uterine contractility and cause increased collagen degradation. In addition corticoids produced in response to stress may facilitate rupture of the membrane.

 iii. *Genetic:* Genetic factors may responsible for reduced tensile strength for some races and which might explain the higher incidence of PROM in African American population.

B. Increased intrauterine pressure: The possibility of PROM by increased intrauterine pressure is less as patient can tolerate intrauterine pressure, secondary to polyhydramnios or to uterine contraction for long time without rupture:

3. **Premature ripening of the cervix in cervical insufficiency:** Predominant cause is anatomic or functional abnormalities of the cervix. Cervical insufficiency may be congenital or acquired.
   - *Congenital:*
     - Defect in embryologic development of mullerian duct
     - Defect in collagen composition in Ehlers Danlos syndrome and Marfan's syndrome.
   - *Acquired:*
     - Forceful mechanical cervical dilatation
     - Cervical trauma during childbirth
     - Cervical conization or loop electrocautery excision procedure (LEEP) for the treatment of cervical intraepithelial neoplasia.

4. **Iatrogenic preterm delivery:** Due to maternal and fetal complications. One third of preterm births are due to maternal and fetal indications.

Mrs Rabeya's CBC is normal, CRP is negative, blood sugar is normal, ultrasonography shows gestational age is 30 weeks and normal fetus, liquor is adequate, placental size and localization is normal. According to menstrual history and early ultrasonogram, she is a case of 30 weeks pregnancy.

How will you manage the case?

Management depends upon the status of labor and maternal, and fetal condition. Here, it is a case of early preterm labor and there is no maternal infection or any fetal problem. So, pregnancy can be continued with follow-up.

Line of Management

Patient must be hospitalized.

A. *Use of tocolysis*
   Most of the women in their early preterm labor respond well to oral tocolysis:
   - *Drug and dose:* Nifedipine 30 mg stat followed by 20 mg every 6 hours is to be given to control uterine contraction. Drug should be continued till complete subsidence of contraction, but in some cases continuous administration is necessary to prevent further contraction.
   - *Mode of action:* It blocks uterine contraction by blocking calcium (Ca) channel (King et al. 2003). The drug is tolerable and only headache can occur in some cases and has no fetal effects.

B. *Steroids:* It is to be given to accelerate fetal lung maturity and to prevent neonatal respiratory distress syndrome.
   - *Drug and dose:* Injection betamethasone 12 mg intramuscularly in two consecutive doses, 24 hours apart is to be given. Though effect of glucocorticoids on the fetal lungs does not last more than 1 week, no booster or repeat dose is indicated, if woman continue pregnancy more than 7 days to avoid significant fetal and neonatal side effects.
   Alternatively injection dexamethasone 6 mg IM/IV every 12 hours for four doses can be given. In Bangladesh betamethasone is not available and dexamethasone is the drug of choice.

C. *Antibiotics:* To prevent infection, prophylactic antibiotics are to be given. If there is any growth in the HVS specific antibiotics are to be given after getting the result of culture and sensitivity.

D. *Expectant management:* Once the contraction subsides the woman can be managed on an outpatient basis provided FFN is negative. The woman should stop working and limit her activities at home and should have weekly antenatal check up.

If FNF is positive, the risk of preterm delivery is substantial. So pregnancy is to be continued with bed rest in hospital. FNF testing is to be repeated every 2–3 weeks and if become negative then outpatient treatment can be allowed.

> What other tocolytic drugs can be used to stop uterine contraction?

A number of tocolytic drugs are available for controlling premature uterine contraction.

Magnesium Sulfate

Mechanism of action: Calcium channel blocker and prevent myometrial contraction by preventing activity of calcium.

Dose and duration: About 4 g IV bolus over 20 minutes, followed by 1 g/hour maintenance dose for 24 hours or until delivery whichever occurred first (Crowther et al. 2003).

Side effects: Most frequent maternal side effects are flushing, nausea, vomiting, headache, pulmonary congestion, respiratory depression, hypothermia and neuromuscular toxicity. Fetal side effects are intraventricular hemorrhage and central nervous system (CNS) depression when high dose is needed to control contraction. A RCT shown 32% neonatal adverse effect with magnesium sulfate in comparison to 19% with placebo (Mittendorff et al. 2002).

Efficacy: According to Cochrane systematic review it is an ineffective tocolytic agent (Crowther et al. 2002; Cox et al. 1990).

Recommendation: Considering its poor efficacy and adverse effect to mother and fetus, it is recommended to abandoning magnesium sulfate as tocolytic therapy.

Beta-adrenergic Agents

Beta-adrenergic agents are β receptor blocker, which stop uterine contraction by inhibiting β receptors. The intravenous beta-adrenergic has the powerful tocolytic effect in established preterm labor. Commonly two forms are available for use:
1. Terbutaline.
2. Ritodrine.

Terbutaline
Dose and duration: About 5 mg of terbutaline is dissolved in 500 mL of Ringer's lactate solution and started at 5 μg/minute. It is to be increased by 5 μg/minute every 10–20 minutes until a dose adequate to stop contraction or till development of any side effects. Maximum dose is 30 μg/minute.

Side effects: Pulmonary edema, increased glucose level, lowering serum potassium level and tachyphylaxis in asthmatic patients who already are taking beta-adrenergic agents.

Contraindications of use: Include the following:
- Cardiac disease
- Hyperthyroidism
- Sickle-cell disease
- Uncontrolled insulin-dependent diabetes
- Chorioamnionitis
- Eclampsia and severe pre-eclampsia.

Retordine
Dose and duration: 100 μg/minute and increased by 50 μg/minute until the contractions stop or toxicity develops. Maximum dose is 350 μg/minute.

Side effect and contraindications are same as terbutaline.

Indomethacin

Dose and duration: 25–30 mg orally is starting dose followed by 25 mg orally every 4–6 hours and continued for 3 days.

Side effects: Mostly fetal side effects and these are premature closer of ductus arteriosus, necrotizing enterocolitis and grade III and IV intraventricular hemorrhage, pulmonary hypertension, persistent open ductus and reduced urinary output. Effects are rapidly reversible after discontinuing the drug.

The sensitivity of the fetal ductus increased with gestational age and that is why this drug is not used after 32 weeks of gestation.

Nitroglycerine

Nitroglycerine is a powerful smooth muscle relaxant and can prevent uterine contraction rapidly.

Dose and duration: 100 µg IV bolus followed by a continuous infusion at a rate of 1 µg/kg/minute.

Side effects: Hypotension and headache. This drug is not commonly used.

Diazoxide

Diazoxide inhibits smooth muscle activity, hence uterine contractility.

Dose and duration: It can be given in bolus doses or as infusion. Bolus is given as 50–100 mg IV every 5 minutes till the contractions stop. Infusion is given as one ample dissolved in 250 mL normal saline and administered within 30 minutes. Contraction usually stops within 15 minutes and duration of action varies from patient to patient. In many cases one single dose stops uterine contraction indefinitely. Second dose, if needed can be used, but not beyond that.

Side effects: Most commonly maternal side effects and these are hypotension, tachycardia, hyperglycemia and decreased uteroplacental circulation secondary to hypotension. Fetal side effects are hyperglycemia secondary to maternal hyperglycemia and fetal distress secondary to reduced uteroplacental circulation. To avoid hypotension, administration of 500–1,000 mL Ringer's lactate or normal saline is desirable to expand maternal intravascular volume before diazoxide therapy. This drug is also not commonly used.

> *Suppose Mrs Rabeya's per vaginal findings at admission is short cervix with 80% effacement and cervix is 4 cm dilated instead of 50% effacement and 2.5 cm dilatation. How will you manage her?*

This is an advanced stage of preterm labor. In certain situations of advanced preterm labor such as infection and in placental insufficiency premature labor is protective mechanism for fetus. So, steps are to be taken to assess whether patient need to be delivered or patient might get benefit from prolongation of pregnancy by giving tocolysis and steroids.

As there is no signs of amnionitis prolongation of pregnancy can be tried with tocolysis and steroid. But, cervical dilatation is 4 cm here, which is an indicator of inevitable delivery, because more than 50% of patients deliver within 48 hours despite aggressive tocolysis if cervical dilatation is 4 cm or more. (Amon et al. 2000). So at least to administer the doses of steroids labor is to be delayed by applying tocolysis.

Note: Tocolysis and steroid is to be given as described before. Patient is to be monitored every 2 hours to avoid the consequence of high-dose tocolysis. If maternal pulse is >120/m, blood pressure is <100/60 mm Hg oxygen saturation is 95% and temperature raised treatment is to be discontinued.

> *Suppose with advanced labor Mrs Rabeya has foul smelling discharge, both maternal and fetal heart rate is increased, temperature is raised to 100.6°F, C-reactive protein is 5 mg/dL, leucocyte count is 15000/mm^3.*
> *How will you manage her? Would you like to use tocolysis to halt the labor process?*

No these are clearly the signs of amnionitis. So labor is to be allowed and measures are to be taken for quick delivery.

Broad-spectrum intravenous antibiotics are to be started in the form of ceftriaxone 2 g 12 hourly and clindamycin 900 mg 8 hourly and continued till the patient remains afebrile for 24 hours.

In some cases of amnionitis, there may be abnormal uterine action without further progress in cervical dilatation and descent of the head. If such occurs cesarean section is to be done.

RELATED INFORMATION

Role of cervical length measurement in predicting preterm labor.

Cervical length measurement using the three-dimensional endovaginal, ultrasound is precise and can be predictor of premature labor (Bega et al. 2000). The cervical length slowly decreases from a mean of 4 cm at 16 weeks to 3 cm at 40 weeks:

- Cervical length up to 2.5 cm is not risky for preterm delivery
- If cervical length is less than 2.5 cm, but >1.5 cm risk of preterm delivery is about 35%. If labor is threatened FNF and CRP should be done

- If CRP positive, it indicates intrauterine infection and pregnancy is to be terminated.
- If CRP negative, FNF positive patient is to be treated by tocolysis and steroids for 48-72 hours to get the benefit of steroids
- If CRP and FNF are negative chance of delivery within 2-3 weeks is minimum and patient can be managed on outpatient basis, so long FNF is negative with weekly FNF testing.
- If cervical length is 1.5 cm or less the risk of preterm delivery is substantial and 50% will deliver before 32 weeks and 90% will deliver before 34 weeks of gestation (Hassan et al. 2001). All patients with cervical length 1.5 or less should be managed in the hospital. If FNF is negative delivery might occur within 2-3 weeks of testing. In these cases CRP detection is indicated. If CRP present it indicates intrauterine infection, where termination is indicated. If CRP is negative pregnancy is to be continued with tocolytic agents, steroids and antibiotics.
- If cervical length is 1.5 cm or less and FNF is positive chance of delivery is within 1-2 weeks of testing. Steroid is to be given. Tocolysis will not be effective and it only can be given to get the time for effect of steroids.

> **Case scenario:** Mrs Saleha a second gravid woman is carrying for 28 weeks. On examination and routine investigation she is found apparently normal. But her first pregnancy was a premature delivery on 30 weeks gestation and baby died in NICU on 4th postnatal day. She had no history of any cervical operations. Labor was sudden without any significant labor pain. This time she is worried about this pregnancy.
>
> How will you manage her?

This might be a case of cervical incompetency or insufficiency due to inherent weakness of the cervix.

Diagnosis is to be made by assessing cervical length and funneling of the cervix by ultrasonography. If cervical length is less than 2.5 cm and there is significant funneling, it indicates cervical insufficiency.

Cervical cerclage operation is to be done on the basis of cervical shortening and history of previous premature labor.

If cervical length is >2.5 cm then only on the ground of previous one premature labor cervical cerclage operation is not indicated.

RELATED INFORMATION

What is Cervical Insufficiency?

Inability of the cervix to retain a pregnancy in the absence of uterine contractions is known as cervical incompetence or cervical insufficiency. It causes painless dilatation of the cervix.

Predisposing and Risk Factors for Preterm Labor

- Congenital abnormality of the connective tissue (Marfan's syndrome, Ehlers-Danlos syndrome)
- Anatomical abnormalities of the uterus (Bicornual or septate uterus)
- Deep cervical laceration from previous childbirth or D&C
- Cervical treatment for abnormal cytology (Freezing, conization, LEEP and trachelorrhaphy)
- Short cervix <1 cm found in initial prenatal visit
- History of previous short labor
- History of two or more second trimester loss
- In 50% cases associated with intra-amniotic infection/inflammation (Romero et al. 1992).

Pathophysiology of Cervical Insufficiency

Cervix constitutes both muscular tissue and connective tissue with preponderance of connective tissue (90%) and capacity to retain the product of conception depends on the content of the connective tissue. Due to this connective tissue component cervix can withstand increased intrauterine pressure. During pregnancy, due to influence of estrogen and prostaglandins cervical connective tissue undergoes significant changes. Due to synthesis of collagenases, hyaluronic acid and infiltration of inflammatory cells such as neutrophil and macrophages, there is degradation of collagen, disruption of collagen structure, increased synthesis of proinflammatory cytokines and increased accumulation of water. As a result cervix becomes soft, easy to stretch, becomes short progressively and starts to dilate in response to uterine contractions. Gradually intrauterine pressure threshold decreased due to cervical ripening.

In certain situations, where significant amount of cervical tissue lost as a consequence of a surgical procedure or who have an abnormal composition of connective tissue, cervical threshold for intrauterine pressure decreased. As a result cervical canal opens up even without uterine contraction.

Presentations

- Painless dilatation of the cervix
- Pelvic or rectal pressure
- No uterine contraction
- Increased mucus (mucoid and curdy white) vaginal discharge: This is an important information as the cervical mucus comes out due to opening up of cervical canal.
- Digital or speculum examination reveals a cervix dilated 2 cm or more, effacement greater than or equal to 80% and bag of waters visible through the external os or protruding into the vagina (in acute cases).

Diagnosis

- *By history:* In most of the cases diagnosis is made on a historical basis and called historical diagnosis:
  - History of painless cervical dilatation
  - History of ruptured membrane without contraction
  - History of congenital abnormality, cervical laceration and trauma.
- *By ultrasonogram:* It is called sonographic diagnosis. Findings are:
  - Shortening of the cervical length
  - Funneling of the cervical canal ('Y' shaped and finally 'U' shaped instead of T)
  - Protruding of amniotic sac into cervical canal.

  Note: Serial sonographic surveillance is needed, when there is history of second trimester pregnancy loss or preterm birth.
- *Prepregnancy techniques:*
  - Hysterography
  - Cervical resistance indices
  - Insertion of cervical dilator.

Case scenario: Mrs Rahela is a primigravid woman has come to you at 32 weeks of pregnancy with the complaints of thick curdy white vaginal discharge for 2 days. On speculum examination you found that cervix is dilated about 2–2.5 cm and membrane is protruding through the external cervical os.

How will you manage the case?

This is an acute presentation of cervical insufficiency. Cervical cerclage (*Rescue cerclage*) operation in an emergency basis is to be done. Curdy white discharge is indicator of opening of cervical canal.

As in 50% cases, it is associated with intra-amniotic infection it is to be excluded first before cerclage operation. Cerclage operation is contraindicated in case of intra-amniotic infection.

So, CRP and WBC count are to be done. If WBC is $\geq 14,000/mm^3$ and CRP >3 mg/dL, it indicates infection and cervical cerclage will not help.

Note: Cervical cerclage is also not applicable when cervical dilatation is >4 cm.

RELATED INFORMATION

Cervical Cerclage

Cervical cerclage is a suture around the cervix, which is commonly performed as prophylactic intervention in cervical insufficiency. Cerclage may provide a degree of structural support to a weak cervix, maintains the cervical length and endocervical mucus plug. There are a lots of controversies about indications, timing and type of cerclage operation.

Indications of Cerclage

History Indicated Cerclage

Cervical cerclage is given based on previous obstetric and gynecological history, which are the risk factors for cervical insufficiency and previous preterm birth. It is given as prophylactic measure in asymptomatic women electively at 12–14 weeks of gestation. Followings are the conditions for history indicated cerclage.

- History of two or more previous preterm birth or second trimester loss.
- One or two losses with other risk factor like short cervix ≤2.5 cm.

Note:
Following conditions individually are not an indication of cervical cerclage
- Previous painless dilatation of the cervix
- History of one or two losses without short cervix
- History of previous premature ruptured membrane
- Risk factors such as cervical surgery, cervical trauma
- Multiple pregnancy
- Uterine anomaly

Ultrasound Indicated Cerclage

Cerclage is given prophylactically in an asymptomatic woman on the basis of ultrasonographically diagnosed risk factors between 14–24 weeks of gestation. Risk factors are a) short cervix ≤2.5 cm along with history of previous preterm birth or midtrimester loss b) funneling with short cervix.

Note:
- Short cervix alone is not an indication for cerclage
- Funneling alone is not an indication for cerclage.

Rescue Cerclage

When cerclage is given as an emergency basis by senior obstetrician in case of premature dilatation of the cervix >4 cm with exposed fetal membrane in the vagina. Dilatation of cervix can be diagnosed by ultrasonography or speculum examination in women with symptoms such as vaginal discharge, bleeding and sensation of pressure. Study shows that following rescue cerclage average prolongation of pregnancy was 7 weeks 1 day and average neonatal survival was more than 70% (Cockwell and Smith, 2005). It should be individualized with assessing risk benefit ratio.

Success of rescue cerclage depends on the following conditions:
- Proper placement of the patient and proper exposure
- Good light
- Good anesthesia, regional is preferable, general anesthesia increases intra-abdominal pressure
- Avoidance of contact of the exposed membranes with chemical irritants.

Types of Cerclage Operation

McDonald Suture (Transvaginal)

The procedure is done transvaginally and a purse-string suture is given at the level of cervicovaginal junction without mobilization of the bladder (McDonald, 1957) **(Figs 4.1A to C)**.

Shirodkar Suture (High Transvaginal)

It is also done vaginally and a purse-string suture is given at a higher level than McDonald suture above the level of cardinal ligament after mobilization of the bladder (Shirodkar, 1955).

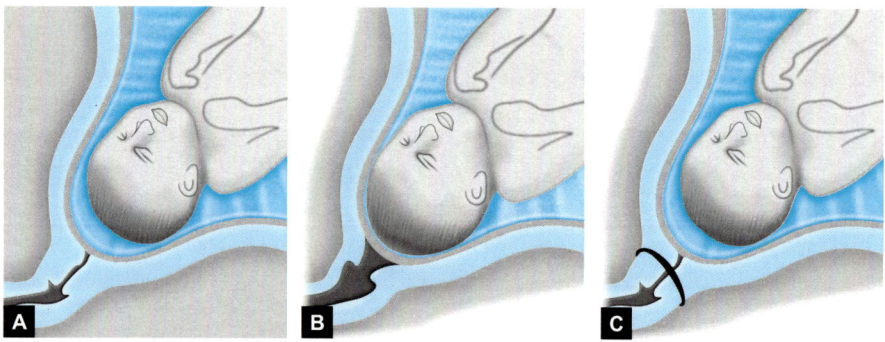

Figs 4.1A to C (A) Competent cervix; (B) Incompetent cervix and; (C) McDonald suture

Occlusion Cerclage

Occlusion of the external os by placing continuous non-absorbable suture in an intention to retain the cervical mucus plug (Secher et al. 2007).

Espinosa-flores Operation

It is done as rescue cerclage where membrane is visualized. In this operation after displacing the bag of water (BOW) by inflated balloon (30 mL) of Foley catheter anterior and posterior lips are grasped with a ring forceps. Cardinal ligament is exposed and suture is given by Mersaline band at this level from posterior to anterior then anterior to posterior in other side of the cervix. The two ends tied over the posterior aspect of the cervix. It is simple and effective, and can be used for both prophylactic and rescue cerclage.

Wurm Operation

It is also done as rescue operation where cervix is dilated and BOW is visible, cervical effacement is >80% and cervical dilatation is 3 cm or more. In this operation BOW is displaced inside by using Foley catheter balloon (30 mL), the lips of cervix are grasped with the ring forceps. Two 'U' suture are placed by prolene, one is vertically from 2 to 12 o'clock position and other is transversely from 3 to 9 o'clock position through whole thickness of the cervix.

Transabdominal Cerclage

Suture is given via laparotomy or laparoscopy at the level of cervicoisthmic junction. Laparotomy is preferable. It is usually done in following cases:
- Severe trauma to the cervix like.
  - Deep lacerations following a difficult vaginal delivery
  - Extensive conization
  - Repeated LEEP for treatment of carcinoma cervix (Davis et al. 2000; Zaveri et al. 2002).
- Repeated second trimester loss
- Failed vaginal cerclage.

Timing of Cerclage

- It can be given at prepregnancy period where in anticipated future pregnancy
- During pregnancy between 12 and 14 weeks of gestation, when uterus come out of the pelvic cavity.

Contraindications of Cerclage Operation

- Active premature labor
- Clinical evidence of chorioamnionitis
- Vaginal bleeding
- PPROM
- Fetal compromise
- Fetal anomaly
- Fetal death.

Precaution to be Taken before and after Cerclage Operation

- Ultrasonogram to see fetal viability and to exclude fetal anomaly whenever applicable.
- In suspected cases amniocentesis to exclude both aneuploidy and intra-amniotic infection. Amniocentesis does not increase the risk of preterm delivery.
- Routine perioperative antibiotic therapy is not recommended, it depends on clinicians choice. But in case of positive culture of vaginal swab antibiotic therapy is to be given.
- Prophylactic tocolysis is not recommended as there is no evidence to support the use of this. A retrospective study shows no difference in premature labor before 35 weeks with or without prophylactic tocolysis (Visintine et al. 2008).
- Routine bed rest and avoidance of coitus is not recommended as there is no evidence of risk of preterm delivery, if those are allowed or not. Decision should be individualized according to clinical manifestation.
- Progesterone supplement has not any effect on premature labor before 35 weeks of gestation (Owen et al. 2009). So routine use of progesterone is not recommended to prevent premature labor.

Patients should be informed about potential risk of cerclage operation.
- Maternal pyrexia may develop, but chance of chorioamnionitis is least.
- It is not associated with induction of labor, preterm delivery or cesarean section.

- There is a small chance of bladder damage, cervical trauma, membrane rupture and bleeding during surgery.
- Suture must be removed immediately, if labor starts as there is risk of cervical laceration and trauma.
- Removal of Shirodker suture may need anesthesia.
- Elective transvaginal cerclage can be done as a day case basis.
- Those who need rescue cerclage or cerclage for short cervix have risk of PPROM, preterm delivery or infection may benefit from hospital stay at least for 24 hours.
- Abdominal cerclage by laparotomy needs to stay at hospital at least for 48 hours.

Time of Removal of Cerclage Suture

- At any time, if patient starts pain and bleeding to minimize potential trauma to the cervix and to allow quick expulsion to stop bleeding.
- If vaginal delivery planned, suture should be removed between 36 and 37 weeks of gestation as any time labor may start and there is potential risk of cervical injury.
- In case of elective cesarean section suture is to be removed at that time.
- All women with transabdominal suture require cesarean section and suture may be left in place following delivery.
- In emergency situation, where cesarean section is not applicable, abdominal suture is to be removed by colpotomy.

> **Case scenario:** Mrs Ayesa has undergone Shirodker suture due to historical indication during 30 weeks of pregnancy. After two weeks at 32 weeks pregnancy she suddenly developed PPROM. There is no sign of maternal infection and fetus is normal.
> How will you manage her?

Cerclage is to be removed but a latency period can be taken for 48 hours as there is no sign of infection and fetal condition is good to get the benefit of steroid. A course of prophylactic steroid is to be given for lung maturation.

> Suppose along with PPROM you found that she has tachycardia, her CRP is >4.5 mg/dL and WBC is 15,000/c mm.
> How will you manage her?

There is increased risk of maternal and neonatal sepsis, if suture removal is delayed. So, it should be removed without delay.

> Suppose she developed PPROM at 34 weeks and 5 days. She has no sign of infection and fetus is in good condition.
> How will you manage her?

Here fetus reached to a stage where extrauterine survival rate is good. Delayed suture removal is unlikely to be advantageous in this situation. So suture should be removed without delay and no need of giving prophylactic steroids. Labor is to be allowed with prophylactic antibiotic coverage.

> **Case scenario:** Mrs Rumana has history of three consecutive pregnancy losses between 18–30 weeks. Every time delivery occurred within very short time of starting pain. She again gets pregnant and has come to you for advice. Now her pregnancy is 8 weeks. She is nondiabetic, no-PCOS and has no other medical disorder. All three labors were spontaneous, sudden and with short period of labor pain.
> How will you manage her?

This might be a case of cervical insufficiency. To test cervical insufficiency it is ideal to test cervical length as early as 18 weeks of pregnancy. FNF test is not useful before 22 weeks of pregnancy. So, at the 8 weeks of pregnancy no need of testing anything for cervical insufficiency. But she had history of 3 mid- and last-trimester loss. So she must be treated for prevention.

Preventive Measures

Following preventive measures are to be taken:
1. **Modification of working pattern:**
   - Works standing up on feet most of the time are to be avoided
   - Vibrating works and which need to move around are to be avoided
   - Strenuous activities should be avoided
   - Complete bed rest should be discouraged.
2. **Coitus should be prohibited:** Though one study showed no association between coitus and preterm labor (Sayle et al. 2001), one very old study found significant amniotic fluid infection with intact membranes in women who had coitus one or more per week than

those who did not have coitus. Amniotic fluid infection might initiate preterm labor (Naeye and Ross, 1982).
3. **Administration of progesterone:** Use of progesterone is controversial. There is lots of debate about benefit of progesterone to prevent premature labor. In general it is said that progesterone is effective to prevent preterm birth in women who have history of previous spontaneous preterm birth. It increases cervical tone, make the cervical mucus thick and keep the uterus quiescent. By its anti-inflammatory properties it may alters progesterone receptor expression and the onset of preterm labor.

   Types and Dose
   a. *Vaginal progesterone*:
      - Natural progesterone, 200 mg twice daily from 18 weeks to delivery (Borna and Sahabi, 2008; Dodd et al. 2008).
      - Micronized progesterone, 200 mg daily from 20 weeks till 34 weeks (Fonseca et al. 2007).

      Note: The first randomized clinical trial to examine the effects of vaginal progesterone on the prevention of PTB in women with a short cervix was reported by Fonseca et al. in women with a short cervix (defined as ≤15 mm by transvaginal ultrasound) between 20 and 25 weeks of gestation were allocated to receive either vaginal progesterone (200 mg of micronized progesterone) or placebo (safflower oil) till 34 weeks. The primary outcome of the trial was the frequency of spontaneous PTB at <34 weeks of gestation. Overall PTB rate was 19.2% in comparison to 34.4% in placebo group. He again analyzed the reduction rate of PTB by cervical length. And found that vaginal progesterone reduce the rate of spontaneous preterm delivery at <34 weeks of gestation by 15% when cervical length is 1–5 mm, 25% with a cervical length of 6–10 mm and 75% in patients with a cervical length between 11 and 15 mm (Fonseca et al. 2007).
   b. 17 hydroxy progesterone: Synthetic progesterone 250 mg IM weekly from 16–20 weeks to 36 weeks (Rouse et al. 2007; Meis et al. 2003; Dodd et al. 2005; Dodd et al. 2008).
4. **Cervical cerclage:** Cerclage is to be given between 12 and 14 weeks of gestation.

Complications of Preterm Birth

- Prematurity
- Low birth weight
- Sever birth asphyxia
- ARDS
- Intraventricular hemorrhage
- Death
- Infection
- Necrotizing enterocolitis
- Developmental anomaly: Skeletal compression deformities, amniotic band syndrome, pulmonary hypoplasia, intestinal obstruction, diaphragmatic hernia, clubfoot, scoliosis and hip dislocation
- Cerebral palsy.

Premature preterm rupture membrane (PPROM) is described in Chapter 5 (Preterm Premature Rupture Membrane).

BIBLIOGRAPHY

Amon E, Midkiff C, Winn H, et al. Tocolysis with advanced cervical dilatation. Obstet Gynecol. 2000;95(3):358-62.

Bega G, Lev-Toaff A, Kuhlman K, et al. Three-dimensional multiplanar transvaginal ultrasound of the cervix in pregnancy. Ultrasound Obstet Gynecol. 2000;16(4):351-8.

Borna S, Sahabi N. Progesterone for maintenance tocolytic therapy after threatened preterm labor: a randomised controlled trial. Aust N Z J Obstet Gynaecol. 2008;48(1):58-63.

Cox SM, Sherman ML, Leveno KJ. Randomized investigation of magnesium sulfate for prevention of preterm birth. Am J Obstet Gynecol. 1990;163(3):767-72.

Cockwell HA, Smith GN. Cervical incompetence and the role of emergency cerclage. J Obstet Gynaecol Can. 2005;27(2):123-9.

Crowther CA, Hiller JE, Doyle LW. Magnesium sulphate for preventing preterm birth in threatened preterm labor. Cochrane Database Syst Rev. 2002;(4):CD001060.

Crowther CA, Hiller JE, Doyle LW, et al. Effect of magnesium sulfate given for neuroprotection before preterm birth: a randomized controlled trial. JAMA. 2003;290(20):2669-76.

Davis G, Berghella V, Talucci M, et al. Patients with a prior failed transvaginal cerclage: a comparison of obstetric outcomes with either transabdominal or transvaginal cerclage. Am J Obstet Gynecol. 2000;183(4):836-9.

Dodd JM, Crowther CA, Cincotta R, et al. Progesterone supplementation for preventing preterm birth: a systematic review and meta-analysis. Acta Obstet Gynecol Scand. 2005;84(6):526-33.

Dodd JM, Flenady VJ, Cincotta R, et al. Progesterone for the prevention of preterm birth: a systematic review. Obstet Gynecol. 2008;112(1):127-34.

Fonseca EB, Celik E, Parra M, et al. Progesterone and the risk of preterm birth among women with a short cervix. N Engl J Med. 2007;357(5):462-9.

Hassan SS, Romero R, Maymon E, et al. Does cervical cerclage prevent preterm delivery in patients with a short cervix? Am J Obstet Gynecol. 2001;184(7):1325-31.

King JF, Flenady V, Papatsoni S, et al. Calcium channel blockers for inhibiting preterm labor; a systematic review of the evidence and a protocol for administration of nifedipine. Aust N Z J Obstet Gynaecol. 2003;43(3):192-8.

Martin JA, Hamilton BE, Sutton PD, et al. Births: final data for 2007. Natl Vital Stat Rep. 2010;58(24):1-85.

McDonald IA. Suture of the cervix for inevitable miscarriage. J Obstet Gynaecol Br Emp. 1957;64(3):346-50.

Meis PJ, Klebanoff M, Thom E, et al. Prevention of recurrent preterm delivery by 17 alpha-hydroxyprogesterone caproate. N Engl J Med. 2003;348(24):2379-85.

Mittendorf R, Dambrosia J, Pryde PG, et al. Association between the use of antenatal magnesium sulfate in preterm labor and adverse health outcomes in infants. Am J Obstet Gynecol. 2002;186(6):1111-8.

Naeye RL, Ross SM. Amniotic fluid infection syndrome. Clin Obstet Gynaecol. 1982;9(3):593-607.

Owen J, Hankins G, Iams JD, et al. Multicenter randomized trial of cerclage for preterm birth prevention in high-risk women with shortened mid-trimester cervical length. Am J Obstet Gynecol. 2009;201(4):375.

Romero R, Gonzalez R, Sepulveda W, et al. Infection and labor. VII. Microbial invasion of the amniotic cavity in patients suspected cervical incompetence: prevalence and clinical significance. Am J Obstet Gynecol. 1992;167(4):1086-91.

Rouse DJ, Caritis SN, Peaceman AM, et al. A trial of 17 alpha-hydroxyprogesterone caproate to prevent prematurity in twins. N Engl J Med. 2007;357(5):454-61.

Sayle AE, Savitz DA, Throp JM JR, et al. Sexual activity during late pregnancy and risk of preterm delivery. Obstet Gynecol. 2001;97(2):283-9.

Secher NJ, McCormack CD, Weber T, et al. Cervical occlusion in women with cervical insufficiency: protocol for a randomised, controlled trial with cerclage, with and without cervical occlusion. BJOG. 2007;114(5):649.

Shirodkar VN. A new method of operative treatment for habitual abortion in the second trimester of pregnancy. Antiseptic. 1955;52:299-300.

Visintine J, Airoldi J, Berghella V. Indomethacin administration at the time of ultrasound-indicated cerclage: is there an association with a reduction in spontaneous preterm birth? Am J Obstet Gynecol. 2008;198:643.

Watts DH, Krohn MA, Wener MH, et al. C-reactive protein in normal pregnancy. Obstet Gynecol. 1991;77(2):176-80.

Zaveri V, Aghajafari F, Amankwah K, et al. Abdominal versus vaginal cerclage after a failed transvaginal cerclage: a systematic review. Am J Obstet Gynecol. 2002;187(4):868-72.

CHAPTER 5

Preterm Premature Rupture Membrane

Hosne Ara Baby, Rashida Begum

INTRODUCTION

Spontaneous rupture of amniotic membrane before the onset of labor is called premature or prelabor rupture of membranes (PROM). It is called preterm PROM if it occurs before 37 weeks of pregnancy. The incidence of PROM is 6–19% of term pregnancies (NICE, 2008), and that of PPROM is 2% of all pregnancies (RCOG, 2006). Among preterm deliveries PPROM is responsible for 30% cases. It increases the risk of prematurity and leads to a number of other perinatal and neonatal complications. There is 1–2% risk of fetal death.

> **Case scenario:** Mrs Salma aged 27 years admitted in your hospital at 31 weeks of pregnancy with complaints of watery discharge per vaginal (PV).
> How will you proceed to diagnose the case?

History Taking

First of all *detailed history is to be taken* regarding following points:
- *Type of discharge:* Sudden gush, intermittent leaking, continuous leaking, drop by drop or occasional leaking.
  Sudden gush, continuous leaking or intermittent leaking of variable amount of watery, clear odorless discharge indicates PROM. Occasional wetting of underclothes, small and whitish foul-smelled discharge with associated itching indicates vaginal infection.
- *Amount of discharge:* Profuse or scanty, whether the underclothing soaked or not. It will indicate the volume of liquor amni drainage.
- *Color of discharge:* Clear and watery discharge indicates amniotic fluid or normal vaginal secretion, whitish curd-like discharge indicates monilial infection, frothy discharge indicates trichomonas infection and blood-stained discharge indicates early labor.
- *Odor of discharge:* Odorless or foul smelled or urinary smelled.
- *Associated symptoms:* Vaginal bleeding, itching per vagina, lower abdominal pain or tenderness, fever and urinary problem. Small blood-stained discharge with associated lower abdominal pain indicates premature labor pain. Associated bleeding indicates abruptio placenta.
- *History of recent intercourse.*
- *Menstrual cycle and last menstrual period* to confirm gestational age.
- *Presence of any risk factors of PROM* including previous obstetrical history.

Examination

Then thorough *examination* is to be done.
- *General examination:* Anemia, temperature, pulse and blood pressure (BP) are to be checked.
- *Pre abdominal (PA) examination:* Uterine height, tenderness, contractions, liquor volume, fetal size, lie, presentation and fetal heart rate (FHR) are to be assessed.
- Then a sterile *speculum examination* is to be done to observe the following things:
  - Whether fluid is seen coming through the cervical os spontaneously or on coughing or by fundal pressure or if there is pool of fluid seen collected in the posterior fornix
  - Whether there are any signs of labor, e.g. cervical effacement and or dilatation

- Whether there is prolapse of cord or any other fetal parts
- Whether there are any signs of vaginitis, e.g. redness, whitish discharge and its characteristics, etc.

> On enquiry you elicited that there was sudden gush of clear odorless watery discharge per vaginally and then there was intermittent leaking, which soaked her underclothing. On PA examination, height of the uterus seemed 30 weeks of pregnancy size and there was no contraction, tenderness or irritability of the uterus. Fetal movement and heart sound is normal. Per speculum examination shows fluid is escaping through the cervical os. Cervix is tubular with closed external os.
>
> What is your diagnosis?

This is a case of preterm PROM.

> Can we do digital vaginal examination instead of per speculum examination?

It is better to avoid digital cervical examination in case of PPROM unless the patient is in active labor and imminent delivery is anticipated. Because such examinations have been shown to decrease the latent period and increase the chance of ascending infections thereby increasing the fetal and maternal morbidity and mortality. (Alexander et al. 2000; Schutte et al. 1983; Lewis et al. 1992). Morover, the difference between speculum and digital examination in assessing cervical effacement and dilatation is not clinically significant (Munson et al. 1985).

> What investigations do you like to do to confirm the diagnosis?

For this patient no investigation is needed to confirm the diagnosis as fluid is seen coming through the cervical os, so diagnosis is obvious.

> In cases where clinical examination is not conclusive, how can you confirm PROM?

The following tests can be done to confirm the diagnosis of PROM:
- *Nitrazine paper test:* The alkaline amniotic fluid causes the yellow nitrazine paper turn into blue (fallacy-contaminated substances such as blood, semen). Alkaline antiseptics and bacterial vaginosis may produce false-positive result.
- *Fern test:* Ferning due to presence of protein and chloride in amniotic fluid indicates PROM. So fluid from the posterior fornix or vaginal sidewall is collected and allowed to dry on a slide to observe the ferning under low power microscope. Vaginal blood can obscure the presence of fern and cervical mucus can give false-positive result if swab is collected from cervical os.

The sensitivity of nitrazine paper test and fern tests in diagnosis of PROM is about 90% (Davidson, 1991).
- *Ultrasonography* (*USG*): By assessing decreased liquor volume indirect diagnosis can be made by ultrasonogram.
- *Dye test by indigo carmine:* Transabdominal USG-guided instillation of indigo carmine dye '1 mL' is mixed in '9 mL' of sterile saline. If membranes are ruptured, the blue dye should pass onto a vaginal tampon within 30 minutes of instillation. This test is indicated when both the physical findings and USG results are inconclusive. Methylene blue should not be used, as it causes hyperbilirubinemia and hemolytic anemia in infants (Naylor et al. 2001).
- *Microscopic examination of vaginal fluid:* To examine lanugo hair and fetal epithelial cells staining with nile blue sulfate.
- *Fetal fibronectin immunoenzyme testing:* Fetal fibronectin is a large-molecular-weight glycoprotein present in large amount in amniotic fluid. It can be detected in the endocervix or vagina in 93.85% of women with PROM. This test is highly accurate and is not affected by blood, but meconium may interfere (Lockwood et al. 1991). It may be useful confirmatory test in doubtful cases.
- *Alpha-fetoprotein (AFP):* Detection of AFP by monoclonal antibody test in the vaginal secretion is an accurate test for PROM, as it is present in amniotic fluid, but absent in urine and vaginal secretions. Sensitivity and specificity of this test is 98% and 100% respectively (Rochelson et al. 1987).

But it is unreliable at term and accuracy is affected by maternal blood contamination.

- *Immunoassay test [placental alpha-microglobulin-1 (PAMG-1) Test (AmniSure Assay)]*: Detection of trace amount of PAMG-1, a protein expressed by the decidua and found in the amniotic fluid has sensitivity of 99% at any gestational age (Lee et al. 2007).

RELATED INFORMATION

Pathophysiology

Fetal membranes consist of amnion (composed of five layers) and chorion (composed of three layers). These membranes are thin but tough, having no blood vessels and nerves but rich in collagen, which gives them strength and elasticity. Regulatory inhibitor control the collagenolytic enzymes from breaking down the collagen throughout pregnancy. During labor the collagenolytic enzyme increases and phospholipids (precursor of prostaglandins) decreases causing the membrane to rupture. PROM may occur as a result of reduction in membranes strength or increase in intra-amniotic pressure or both. In infection, bacterial proteases and collagenases along with inflammatory response of neutrophils decrease the collagen content of the membrane. Bacterial proteases also activate the prostaglandin cascade. Reactive oxygen species (ROS) may also cause damage of the membranes. Overproduction of relaxin also increases collagenase activity.

Risk Factors of PROM

- Racial variation and blacks are at increased risk than white.
- Lower social class and, low body mass index (BMI <19 kg/m^2)
- Micronutritional deficiencies, ZINC, Vit C, E and copper deficiency.
- Reduced immunity.
- Smoking
- Sexually transmitted disease (STDs), bacterial vaginosis and other lower genital tract infection, and urinary tract infection (UTI).
- Previous preterm delivery or PROM
- Vaginal bleeding
- Overdistension of uterus due to multiple pregnancies.
- Cerclage operation, amniocentesis
- Choriodecidual infection
- Decreased collagen content of the membranes
- Cervical incompetence
- Malpresentation
- Trauma: For example, accidental trauma over the abdomen, external cephalic version.

> What will you do for subsequent management of the patient?

Following investigations are needed to assess maternal and fetal well-being and to exclude associated complications:
- To see fetal well-being:
  - *Ultrasonography to see*:
    - Volume of liquor
    - Estimated fetal weight
    - Confirmation of gestational age
    - Placental localization and exclusion of any abruption
    - Fetal presentation
    - Fetal anomaly
    - Fetal well-being: Biophysical profile.
  - *Non-stress test*
  - *Assessment of fetal lung maturity*:
    - Amniotic fluid from the vaginal pool tested for phosphatidylglycerol: It and collection of amniotic fluid are under the heading assessment of fetal lung maturity. Both will be shifted to right. Presence of PG indicates probable fetal lung maturity
    - Collection of amniotic fluid by amniocentesis and tested for lecithin/sphingomyelin (L/S) ratio. L/S ratio (1:8–2:1) indicates probable lung maturity. Difficult to collect fluid by amniocentesis in cases of decreased liquor volume.
- To diagnose infectious status:
  - High vaginal swab (HVS), endocervical swab and anal swab for culture and sensitivity (C/S). Women with chlamydia and gonorrhoea are seven times more likely to develop PROM (Ekwo et al. 1993). Intrapartum group B *Streptococcus (GBS)* prophylaxis should be given if GBS present in vaginal and anal swab.

- Following tests are to be done
  - Total and differential count of white blood cell (WBC)
  - C-reactive protein (CRP).
  - Gram staining and culture of amniotic fluid (collected by amniocentesis) to detect subclinical infection.

> On evaluation you found that liquor volume is reduced, weight of the baby is 1.5 kg, L/S ratio is >2 and no organism is isolated from Gram staining and C/S. WBC and CRP are normal.
> How will you treat this case?

The woman is at 31 weeks of pregnancy. At this gestational age, delivery is associated with severe neonatal morbidity and mortality and benefit of continuation of pregnancy outweigh the risk of chorioamnionitis. As fetus is not mature and there is no contraindication of continuation of pregnancy such as fetal distress, signs of chorioamnionitis, abruptio placenta and labor expectant or conservative management is the better option for this woman.

> How long do you want to continue the pregnancy?

The specific gestational age of reduced neonatal morbidity in PPROM is 34 weeks (Neerhof et al. 1999). After 34 weeks continuation of pregnancy is associated with increased risk of chorioamnionitis and fetal acidosis without any improvement in neonatal morbidity (Naef et al. 1998; Lieman et al. 2005). So pregnancy is to be continued up to 34 weeks.

Note: Pregnancy can be terminated earlier than 34 weeks even before if lung maturity is confirmed by amniocentesis.

> What management do you like to do during continuation of pregnancy?

Pregnancy is to be continued with the following management:

A. *Hospitalization:* Patient should be hospitalized in a specialized center with neonatal intensive care unit (NICU) facility to manage the premature baby properly.
B. *Bed rest with bathroom privileges.* Sterile vulval pad should be used.
C. *Prophylactic antibiotics* is to be given:
   - *Injection ampicillin*: 2 g IV 6 hourly for 48 hour followed by amoxicillin 250 mg 8 hourly for 5 days
   Or
   - *Injection erythromycin*: 250 mg 6 hourly for 48 hours followed by 333 mg 8 hourly for 5 days
   Or combination of both ampicillin and erythromycin.
   Routine prophylactic antibiotics to patient with PPROM reduce maternal and fetal morbidity, and prolong the latent period. Use of antibiotics reduces the incidence of chorioamnionitis, postpartum endometritis, neonatal sepsis, neonatal pneumonia and intraventricular hemorrhage and subsequent pelvic infection of mother. (Mercer et al. 1995; Egarter et al. 1996).
D. *Corticosteroid:* Consequences of PROM like respiratory distress syndrome, intraventricular hemorrhage and necrotizing enterocolitis can be minimized by administration of antenatal corticosteroids (Harding et al. 2001). Recommended dose of corticosteroids; intramuscular betamethasone, 12 mg every 24 hour for 2 days or intramuscular dexamethasone 6 mg 12 hourly for 2 days. (National Institute of Health (NIH) Consensus statement, 1994)
E. Daily monitoring of the patient.

The woman should be observed for chorioamnionitis, labor pain and fetal distress in the following way:
   a. Enquiry about:
      - *Rise of temperature:* Increased temperature indicates chorioamnionitis
      - *Fetal movement:* Reduced movement indicates fetal distress
      - *Lower abdominal pain (constant or rhythmic):* Rhythmic progressively increasing pain is suggestive of labor pain
      - *Blood-stained discharge per vagina:* Show of labor
      - *Foul smelling discharge per vagina:* Sign of infection (chorioamnionitis).
   b. Physical examination:
      - *Temperature:* High in chorioamnionitis

- *Maternal pulse rate:* High in chorioamnionitis
- *Uterine tenderness:* Tender in chorioamnionitis
- *Uterine contraction:* Present in labor
- *Monitoring of fetal heart rate:* To detect fetal distress
- *Inspection of the vulval pad:* For amount, color and smell of discharge, whether it is clear or blood-stained or meconium-stained or foul smelling
- *In case of suspected labor pain, cervical effacement and dilatation are to be noted by sterile speculum examination.*

c. Investigations:
- *Daily USG:* For biophysical profile (BPP) and amniotic fluid index (AFI)
- *Nonstress test.*

Note: Laboratory tests such as serial full blood count, CRP, weekly vaginal culture and amniotic fluid culture can facilitate diagnosis of intra-amniotic infection. Due to low sensitivity of these tests Royal College of Obstetricians and Gynaecologists do not recommend to do these tests (RCOG Guideline 2006). So weekly high vaginal swab, full blood count and C-reactive protein testing are not needed to detect intrauterine infection (RCOG Guidelines 2010).

> With those above measures do you think pregnancy can be continued till 34 weeks?

No. Even with these above measures many patient will deliver within 1 week of preterm PROM (Schucker and Mercer, 1996).

> After 1 week Mrs Salma develops fever, lower abdominal pain, abdominal tenderness. Her pulse is also increased and discharge is a bit fowl smelled.
> Will you continue the pregnancy?

No. These are the features of chorioamnionitis. Pregnancy must be terminated.

> Suppose there is no sign of chorioamnionitis. Patient develops rhythmic contraction of the uterus.
> Do you like to use tocolysis to prevent labor?

No. Right at this moment there is no role of tocolysis. It is usually given to give time to corticosteroid therapy. Here patient has already received corticosteroid beforehand. So no need of tocolysis. Besides that tocolytic therapy is not recommended in PPROM, as this treatment does not significantly increase the interval between rupture of membranes and delivery or improve neonatal morbidity (How et al. 1998; Levy and Warsof, 1985; Dunlop et al. 1986; Jazayeri et al. 2003).

RELATED INFORMATION

Clinical Indicators of Chorioamnionitis

- Maternal fever and lower abdominal pain
- Maternal tachycardia
- Fetal tachycardia
- Abdominal tenderness
- Foul smelling vaginal discharge
- Nonreactive FHR (nonstress test) and abnormal BPP.

Clinical Indicators of Labor Pain

- Rhythmic lower abdominal pain
- Uterine contraction
- Presence of show
- Cervical effacement and dilatation.

Clinical Indicators of Fetal Distress

- Decreased fetal movement
- Fetal heart rate abnormality
- Abnormal nonstress tests: Variable deceleration; late deceleration accompanying with variable deceleration indicates placental abruption
- Abnormal BPP.

Role of Therapeutic Tocolysis if Patient Starts Labor Pain at the Onset of Rupture Membrane or During Conservative Management

There is no clear evidence that therapeutic tocolysis improve the outcome of premature labor. In addition tocolysis could have adverse effect such as delaying delivery from an infected environment.

But it should be considered if patient needs time for completing the course of corticosteroid and or her transfer to a better facility.

> *Suppose during expectant treatment, your patient responded very well and except drainage of a little fluid she has no other additional complaints.*
> *When and how will you deliver the baby?*

Baby should be delivered at 34 completed weeks of pregnancy, as baby is competent enough for independent extrauterine survival at this gestational age. Moreover, continuation beyond this gestational age bears risk for both mother and fetus.

The PPROM is not a contraindication of vaginal delivery. So if the lie is longitudinal and fetal condition is good, labor can be induced by misoprostol or oxytocin with meticulous monitoring of the labor.

> *If there is sign of chorioamnionitis, then how will you deliver the baby?*

It will depend upon fetal condition and condition of the cervix. Only chorioamnionitis is not the indication of cesarean section. Rather chance of postpartum infection is more after cesarean section. So if fetal condition is good and cervix is favorable, labor can be induced by misoprostol or oxytocin with meticulous monitoring of the labor.

RELATED INFORMATION

Management Based on Gestational Age

34–36 Weeks

Labor should be induced if PPROM occurs at 34–36 weeks of gestation. Conservative management at this gestation is associated with chorioamnionitis and fetal acidosis without improving major or minor neonatal morbidity (Naef et al. 1998; Lieman et al. 2005). After 34 weeks only appropriate antibiotics for GBS prophylaxis is to be given. Corticosteroids are not indicated at this gestational age.

32–33 Weeks

For patients with preterm PROM at 32 or 33 weeks gestation with documented pulmonary maturity, induction of labor is performed in a place where neonatal services are available (Ehrenberg and Mercer, 2001). Prolonging pregnancy after pulmonary maturity unnecessarily increases the likelihood of maternal infection, umbilical cord compression, prolonged hospitalization and neonatal infection (Mercer, 2003). A course of corticosteroids and intravenous antibiotics are to be administered and delivery is to be considered 48 hours later. Alternatively a careful assessment of fetal well-being, intra-amniotic condition is to be done to continue the pregnancy to 34 weeks. A careful assessment about leucocyte count (<16000 with neutrophil <90%), fetal fibronectin (FNF) (<50 ng/mL), CRP (<3 mg/dL), cervical length (>15 mm), cervical effacement (<80%) and cervical dilatation (<5 cm) should be considered before conservative treatment.

Patients with amnionitis should be treated by broad-spectrum antibiotics and all patients should receive appropriate intrapartum GBS prophylaxis, if indicated.

24–31 Weeks

Delivery before 32 weeks' gestation is associated with severe neonatal morbidity and mortality. Attempt is to be taken to prolong the pregnancy until 34 weeks' gestation if patient is free from infection. Despite these efforts, many patients deliver within 1 week of preterm PROM (Schucker and Mercer, 1996). Chorioamnionitis, abruptio placenta and nonreassuring fetal testing are contraindications for conservative treatment. A course of corticosteroids and intravenous broad spectrum antibiotics are to be given. Fetal well-being is to be assessed by fetal monitoring or USG.

To continue pregnancy safely daily fetal monitoring is essential as umbilical cord compression is about 32–76% at this period (Smith et al. 1987). So patient should be transferred to a facility where fetus can be monitored properly. Close observation is needed during conservative treatment to diagnose amnionitis earlier by maternal tachycardia, rise of temperature 100.4°F, uterine tenderness and leukocytosis.

- Leukocyte count may increase after corticosteroid in PROM. So WBC is not a good predictor of intrauterine infection.

- Evidence suggests that prolonged latency may increase the risk of intra-amniotic infection (Gopalani et al. 2005).
- The CRP should be less than 3 mg/dL. It is a better predictor of infection. Level 3–4 mg/dL indicates acute chorioamnionitis.
- Delivery should be considered if there is infection.
- The route of delivery will depend on the cervical and fetal condition. Birth weight <1,000 g should be delivered by cesarean section to prevent intraventricular hemorrhage. Delivery through underdeveloped lower segment is more dangerous than vaginal delivery. So in thick and tough lower segment, vertical incision is to be considered.

Before 24 Weeks

- It is very difficult to manage and continue the pregnancy when PROM occurred before 24 weeks.
- Perinatal mortality rate is very high (60–90%) as baby is too premature. Almost all deliver within one week when preterm PROM occurs before 24 weeks' gestation (Schutte et al. 1983). Depending upon the time of membrane rupture and amount of liquor amnii many infants suffer from numerous long-term problems including chronic lung disease, developmental and neurologic abnormalities, hydrocephalus, cerebral palsy and Potter's syndrome, which results in pressure deformities of the limbs and face and pulmonary hypoplasia.
- Almost 50% mother will have chorioamnionitis.
- No plan of management has been shown to improve the outcome of pregnancies if it is less than 24 weeks.
- So considering the above mentioned things induction of labor and delivery is to be considered to avoid maternal morbidity.

Complications of Preterm Premature Rupture of Membrane

Maternal

- Chorioamnionitis
- Abruptio placenta
- Increased operative intervention
- Postpartum hemorrhage
- Puerperal sepsis
- Psychological problem.

Fetal

- Prematurity
- Low birth weight
- Sever birth asphyxia
- Cord compression
- Oligohydramnios and malpresentation
- Intrauterine fetal death (IUFD)
- *Developmental anomaly:* Skeletal compression deformities, amniotic band syndrome, pulmonary hypoplasia, intestinal obstruction, diaphragmatic hernia, clubfoot, scoliosis and hip dislocation
- Intraventricular hemorrhage
- Necrotizing enterocolitis
- Fetal infection and neonatal infection.
- Acute respiratory distress syndrome (ARDS)
- Cerebral palsy.

BIBLIOGRAPHY

Alexander JM, Mercer BM, Miodovnik M, et al. The impact of digital cervical examination on expectantly managed preterm rupture of membranes. Am J Obstet Gynecol. 2000;183(4):1003-7.

Davidson KM. Detection of premature rupture of membranes. Clin Obstet Gynecol. 1991;34(4):715-22.

Dunlop PDM, Crowley PA, Lamont RF, Hawkins DF. Preterm ruptured membranes, no contractions. J Obstet Gynecol. 1986;7:92-6.

Ehernberg HM, Mercer BM. Antibiotics and the management of preterm premature rupture of the fetal membranes. Clin Perinatol. 2001;28(4):807-18.

Ekwo EE, Gosselink CA, Woolson R, et al. Risks for premature rupture of amniotic membranes. Int J Epidemiol. 1993;22(3):495-503.

Gopalani S, Krohn M, Meyn L, et al. Contemporary management of preterm premature rupture of membranes: determinants of latency and neonatal outcome. Obstet Gynecol. 2005;60:16-7.

Harding JE, Pang J, Knight DB, et al. Do antenatal corticosteroids help in the setting of preterm rupture of membranes? Am J Obstet Gynecol. 2001; 184(2):131-9.

How HY, Cook CR, Cook VD, et al. Preterm premature rupture of membranes: aggressive tocolysis versus expectant management. J Mater Fetal Med. 1998; 7(1):8-12.

Jazayeri A, Jazayeri MK, Sutkin G, et al. Tocolysis does not improve neonatal outcome in patient with preterm premature rupture of membranes. Am J Perinatol. 2003;20:189-93.

Lee SE, Park JS, Norwitz ER, et al. Measurement of placental alpha-microglobulin-1 in cervicovaginal discharge to diagnose rupture of membranes. Obstet Gynecol. 2007;109(3):634-40.

Levy D, Warsof SL. Oral ritodrine and preterm premature rupture of membranes. Obstet Gynecol. 1985;66:621-3.

Lewis DF, Major CA, Towers CV, et al. Effects of digital vaginal examinations on latency period in preterm premature rupture of membranes. Obstet Gynecol. 1992;80(4):630-4.

Lieman JM, Brumfield CG, Carlo W, et al. Preterm premature rupture of membranes: is there an optimal gestational age for delivery? Obstet Gynecol. 2005;105(1):12-7.

Lockwood CJ, Senyei, Dische MR, et al. Fetal fibronectin in the cervical and vaginal secretions as predictor of preterm delivery. N Engl J Med. 1991;325(10):669-74.

Mercer BM, Arheart KL. Antimicrobial therapy in expectant management of preterm premature rupture of the membranes. Lancet. 1995;346:1271-9.

Mercer BM. Preterm premature rupture of the membranes. Obstet Gynecol. 2003;101(1):178-93.

Munson LA, Graham A, Koos BJ, et al. Is there a need for digital examination in patients with spontaneous rupture of the membranes? Am J Obstet Gynecol. 1985;153(5):562-3.

Naef RW, Allbert JR, Ross EL, et al. Premature rupture of membranes at 34 to 37 weeks' gestation: aggressive versus conservative management. Am J Obstet Gynecol. 1998;178(1 pt 1):126-30.

Naylor CS, Gregory K, Hobel C. Premature rupture of the membranes: an evidence-based approach to clinical care. Am J Perinatol. 2001;18(7):397-413.

Neerhof MG, Cravello C, Haney EI, et al. Timing of labor induction after premature rupture of membranes between 32 and 36 weeks' gestation. Am J Obstet Gynecol. 1999;180:349-52.

NICE. Induction of labor, NICE Clinical Guideline (July 2008). www.nice.org.uk/CG070.

NIH Consensus. Effect of corticosteroids for fetal maturation on perinatal outcomes. NIH Consens Statement. 1994;12(2):1-24.

Rochelson BL, Rodke G, White R, et al. A rapid colorimetric AFP monoclonal antibody test for the diagnosis of preterm rupture of the membranes. Obstet Gynecol. 1987;69(2):163-6.

Royal College of Obstetricians & Gynecologists. Green-top Guidelines No. 44: Preterm Prelabor Rupture of Membranes. London: RCOG; 2006. www.rcog.org.uk/globalassets/documents/guidelines/gtg_44.pdf

Schucker JL, Mercer BM. Midtrimester premature rupture of the membranes. Semin Perinatol. 1996;20(5):389-400.

Schutte MF, Treffers PE, Kloosterman GJ, et al. Management of premature rupture of membranes: the risk of vaginal examination to the infant. Am J Obstet Gynecol. 1983;146(4):395-400.

Smith CV, Greenspoon J, Phelan JP, et al. Clinical utility of the nonstress test in the conservative management of women with preterm spontaneous premature rupture of the membranes. J Reprod Med. 1987;32(1):1-4.

Tanya M Medina, D Ashley Hill. Preterm Premature Rupture of Membranes: Diagnosis and Management. American Family Physician. 2006;73:659-66.

CHAPTER 6

Labor Dystocia

Rashida Begum

INTRODUCTION

Labor dystocia is an abnormal or difficult labor or abnormally slow progress of labor. Approximately one fifth of human labors have dystocia (Zhu et al. 2006). Dystocia may arise due to inefficient and incoordinate uterine activity, abnormal fetal lie or presentation, absolute or relative cephalopelvic disproportion or rarely due to fetal congenital anomaly such as sacrococcygeal teratoma and hydrocephalus. Dystocia often ended with assisted deliveries such as forceps, ventouse and cesarean section. It is the most common current indication for primary cesarean section. Both maternal and fetal mortality and morbidity rates increased with abnormal labor.

> **Case scenario:** Mrs Zohra a 25-year-old woman has come to you with the complaints of amenorrhea for 38 weeks and lower abdominal pain for 16 hours.
> How will you proceed to diagnose the case?

For diagnosis:
- Detailed history is to be taken
- Examination is to be performed
- If necessary some investigations are to be done.

History

Following points are to be elicited:
- Exact duration of pregnancy by knowing last menstrual period (LMP), and ultrasonogram of early weeks
- Character of pain—whether it is rhythmic with progressively increasing frequency and intensity associated with hardening of uterus, which is characteristics of labor pain
- *Exclusion of false labor pain:* Whether subsided with drug or not
- Exact duration of pain
- Antenatal care in this pregnancy
- History of any trauma
- Visit to any health workers with pain, history of taking any drugs
- Whether membrane is ruptured, if so for how long?
- Fetal movement
- Number of previous pregnancies
- Number of previous deliveries
- Mode of previous deliveries
- Any problem during previous pregnancies and labor
- About immunization.

Examination

- General condition—pulse, blood pressure (BP), respiratory rate, anemia, edema, dehydration are to be noted whether there is any sign of exhaustion due to labor pain
- Per abdominal examination—to note uterine contraction number per 10 minutes, duration of each contraction per second, fetal heart rate
- Presentation, engagement
- Per vaginal examination—to assess whether she is in labor or not:
  - Cervical effacement and dilatation
  - Presence of show
  - Formation of bag of water, rupture of the membrane.
- If in labor, stage and progress of the labor:
  - Amount of cervical dilatation
  - Assessment of presenting part to identify malpresentation and malposition
  - Descent of the presenting part

- Adequacy of pelvis
- Color of liquor, if membrane is ruptured.

Investigations

- Hemoglobin (Hb) percentage
- Blood for grouping and Rhesus (Rh) typing
- Blood sugar
- Bedside urine for ketone bodies

(First three, if done beforehand not needed now).

> You completed history taking and physical examination and explored that she is a primigravid woman, without antenatal care (ANC), pain started 16 hours ago, which was rhythmic and progressively increasing both in frequency and intensity, but remained static for last 8 hours. Per abdominal examination revealed uterine contraction 3/10 minutes, which was persisted for 20 seconds. Fetal heart rate (FHR) 135/minute. Per vaginal (PV) examination revealed cervix is 100% effaced and 4 cm dilated. Presentation cephalic, station minus 1, membrane is intact, pelvis is adequate.
>
> On the basis of these findings what is your diagnosis?

This is a case of prolonged labor or labor dystocia in active phase of labor. When total duration of first and second stage of labor exceeds 16 hours then it is called prolonged labor. Here patient is in early first stage of labor in-spite of passing 16 hours. So it can be diagnosed as prolonged labor.

> What is your decision for management of the patient?

Here patient is in active labor but uterine contraction is not effective. So to expedite the labor, it is to be augmented. As labor is prolonged there may be fetal compromise. Here pelvis is adequate so vaginal delivery can be allowed. But further management will depend on the fetal condition. To assess the fetal condition two parameters are to be assessed, fetal heart sound and color of liquor. Here heart sound is normal. To assess color of liquor:

- Artificial rupture of the membrane is to be done, which also augment the labor pain.

Note: As station is –1 there is chance of cord prolapse so it is to be observed till settlement of head in the pelvis. There will be no gap between presenting part and pelvis.

- If liquor is stained it indicates fetal distress. So labor is to be terminated by doing cesarean section (CS).
- If liquor is clear oxytocin drip is to be added and labor will be followed up. After establishment of effective uterine contraction PV examination is to be done at 2 hours interval and progress of labor will be assessed. In good progress cervix will be dilated at least 1 cm/hour and descent of presenting part is at least 1 cm/hour. If progress is satisfactory labor will be continued for vaginal delivery. If progress is not satisfactory CS is to be done.

Note: During any intervention such as artificial rupture of membrane (ARM) or administration of oxytocin labor should be monitored at 2 hours interval rather than 4 hours.

- Proper hydration is to be maintained by infusion of fluid
- Antibiotics is to be given to prevent infection
- Analgesics is to be given after establishment of good uterine contraction.

> Suppose after ARM and oxytocin drip, effective pain has started and after 4 hours, it is found that cervix is full dilated and station is zero. But after full dilatation of the cervix, patient passed 2 hours and delivery did not take place. Uterine contraction is adequate. FHR is normal. Liquor is slightly stained. Station is still zero with formation of a small capute. Mother is a bit exhausted.
>
> What do you want to do?

Here labor became arrested in second stage. There is possibility of *deep transverse arrest*. There are four modalities of treatment of deep transverse arrest:

1. Application of ventouse
2. Cesarean section, if station is high and there is features of obstructed labor.
3. Manual rotation and application of forceps
4. Rotation by forceps and delivery—by Kielland forceps

Note: Last two options used previously, which is obsolete in modern obstetric practice. As liquor is stained, mother is exhausted and there is formation of capute, considering all these cesarean section would be logical option.

RELATED INFORMATION

During normal labor cervical dilatation follows a sigmoid shaped with distinct three parts (Friedman 1978):
1. First part of curve corresponds to latent phase where there is little progression of cervical dilatation.
2. The active phase of labor where there is fast progression in cervical dilatation corresponds to middle part of the curve.
3. The deceleration phase where the cervical dilatation slows again and corresponds to final part of the curve. The descent of the fetus through birth passage follows a hyperbolic curve with little change during latent and active phase of labor, followed by rapid progress starting at the deceleration phase.

Both latent and active phases correspond to first stage of labor and deceleration phase corresponds to second stage of labor.

Stages of Labor

Normal duration of labor, rate of cervical dilatation, descent of fetal head and lack of progress in labor are detailed below:
A. *First Stage of Labor:* It extends from onset of labor pain to full dilatation of the cervix. It has two phases (a) Latent phase and (b) active phase
- Latent phase: Latent phase extends from starting of onset of labor to 4 cm dilatation of cervix.
  - The mean duration of latent phase is 8.6 hours in nulliparous and 5.3 hours in multiparous.
  - In primiparous cervical effacement takes place at this stage. Dilatation and descent of fetal part is minimum or nil both in primi and multiparous women.

Lack of progress in latent phase
- Lack of progress is declared, if duration exceeds 8 hours in both nulliparous and multiparous women.
- Most common cause in nulliparous patients is an unripe cervix at the onset of labor. In multiparous the most common cause is misinterpretation of false labor as latent phase of labor.

- *Active phase:* Active phase of labor is characterized by regular and frequent uterine contraction, 3/10 minutes with duration of 40 seconds accompanied by cervical changes (dilatation and effacement). Active phase of labor starts from 4 cm cervical dilation and ends to 10 cm or full dilatation of the cervix.
  - Duration of active phase is 5.5-7.7 hours for nulliparous (Zhang et al. 2002) and 5.7 hours in multiparous women (Albers et al. 1996).
  - Cervical dilatation is 1 cm/hour in nulliparous and 1.5 cm/hour in multiparous women.

Lack of progress in active phase of labor
- Lack of progress declared when there is little or no change (less than 1 cm/hour) in cervical dilatation for 2 hours during active phase of labor.
- Labor is considered to be prolonged when the duration is more than 12 hours.

Causes of lack of progress or dystocia in active phase
Usually there may be defect in power, passage and passenger:
- Defect in power (contraction)
  - Uterine inertia where uterus becomes inert and there is no effective contraction in active phase-most common cause
  - Incoordinate uterine contraction
  - Injudicious use of sedatives and analgesics before establishing active labor causing abnormal uterine action.
- Defect in birth passage
  - Contracted pelvis causing cephalopelvic disproportion (CPD)
  - Cervical dystocia: Cervix is failed to dilate in spite of effective uterine contraction
  - Impacted pelvic tumor.
- Defect in passenger (fetal cause)
  - Big baby
  - Malposition (asynclitism, extended head)
    - In multiparous women most frequent malposition is occiput posterior (OP) 40.7% and then occiput transverse (OT) 25.4%
    - In nulliparous patients 60% is OT and 26.3% is OP
  - Malpresentation

- Hydrocephalus, encephalocele, cystic hygroma, fetal goiter, hydrops and other abnormalities that increases the size of the fetus.
B. *Second Stage of Labor:* Extends from full dilatation of the cervix to delivery of the baby. Second stage of labor is the phase of expulsion of baby. Descent of the presenting part into the maternal pelvis usually starts at the end of the active phase of labor:
  - Normal rate of descent is 3.3 cm/hour in nulliparous women and 6.6 cm/hour in multiparous women.
  - Normal duration of second stage is 2 hours in nulliparous and 1 hour in multiparous according to National Institute for Health and Clinical Excellence guideline (NICE, 2007).

Lack of progress or arrest in second stage of labor

Arrest is declared when there is less than 1 cm/hour or no descent of the presenting part into the birth canal after complete dilatation of the cervix.

Second stage is considered to be prolonged or arrested when:
- It lasted more than 2 hours in nulliparous women and more than 1 hour in multiparous women [NICE clinical guide line, 2007]
- According to Ottawa's Hospital clinical practice guideline 2006, second stage dystocia (Spraque et al. 2006).
  - Nulliparous without epidural:
    - Nearly 2 hours active pushing without imminent delivery
    - Total length of second stage >3 hours and birth is not imminent
  - Nulliparous with epidural:
    - Nearly 2 hours active pushing without imminent delivery
    - Total length of second stage >4 hours and birth is not imminent.
  - Multiparous without epidural:
    - Nearly 1 hour active pushing without imminent delivery
    - Total length of second stage >2 hours and birth is not imminent.
  - Multiparous with epidural:
    - Nearly 1 hour active pushing without imminent delivery
    - Total length of second stage >3 hours and birth is not imminent.

Causes of lack of progress or dystocia or arrest in second stage
- *Defect in power:*
  - Uterine inertia
  - Inability to bear down due to epidural analgesia or exhaustion
  - Constriction ring
- *Defect in birth passage:*
  - Contracted pelvis or (CPD)
  - Undue resistance of the pelvic floor or perineum
  - Soft tissue pelvic tumor.
- *Defect in passenger (fetal cause):* Same as active phase.

Malpositions and Labor Dystocia

Posterior position of vertex is called malposition. In vertex presentation where occiput is placed posteriorly over the sacroiliac joint or directly over the sacrum is called OP position. At the onset of labor about 10% of all vertex is OP, though it is much less during second stage of labor. Due to dextrorotation of the uterus and presence of the sigmoid colon in the left side, right OP position is five times more common than left OP position.

Causes

Most common causes are android and anthropoid pelvis of the mother and marked deflexion of the head of the fetus.

Diagnosis

The OP position can be predicted by observing the flat abdomen below the umbilicus. Head remains high, not engaged and maximum intensity of FHS heard on the flank. Sometimes it is difficult to locate FHS in left occipitoposterior (LOP). In direct OP the FHS is heard in the midline.

On PV examination the anterior fontanelle is felt more easily because of deflexion of the head. Posterior fontanelle is felt near the sacroiliac joint.

In late labor due to capute formation fontanelle cannot be felt and make the diagnosis difficult.

Ultrasonography can diagnose the attitude of the head and its relation to the pelvic walls.

Fate of OP Position

- *Normal vaginal delivery (90%):* In favorable condition where uterine contraction is effective, pelvis is adequate, liquor is adequate and fetal size is average occiput moves *anteriorly* 3/8th of a circle to lie behind symphysis pubis. Then deliver by same mechanism of occipito anterior position (in occipito anterior position head moves one eighth of a circle to lie behind symphysis pubis).
- *Deep transverse arrest (incomplete rotation):* In unfavorable situation where head is much deflexed, uterine contraction is not effective, pelvis is not adequate or fetal size is bigger the occiput cannot rotate completely. It rotates through 1/8th of a circle anteriorly and the sagittal suture comes to lie in the bispinous diameter. Thereafter further rotation does not occur and head arrest in this position is called deep transverse arrest (Management discussed before).
- *Oblique arrest (nonrotation):* When both sinciput and occiput touch the pelvic floor simultaneously due to moderate deflexion of the head, occiput cannot rotate. Further mechanism is unlikely and head becomes arrested at the same oblique position called oblique posterior arrest. CS should be done in oblique posterior arrest.
- *Persistent occipitoposterior position (malrotation):* In extreme deflexion the sinciput touches the pelvic floor first resulting in anterior rotation of the sinciput to 1/8th of a circle and putting the occiput to the sacral hollow. This condition is called occipito-sacral or persistent occipito-posterior position.

In favorable situation where uterine contraction is effective, pelvis is adequate and fetal size is average spontaneous delivery may occur as 'face to pubes' 26% in nulliparous and 57% in multiparous women (Ponkey et al. 2003). In unfavorable situation delivery does not occur and it is called occipito-sacral arrest. CS is to be done in occipito-sacral arrest.

Both deep transverse and occiput sacral arrest are associated with increased maternal morbidity and neonatal morbidity and mortality.

Malpresentation and Labor Dystocia

Cesarean section is the ideal option for labor dystocia with any malpresentation.

> How will you assess and monitor progress of labor in dystocia?

Assessment and monitoring of progress of labor is to be done by assessing different components:
- Leopold maneuvers (all grips) to assess fetal lie, position, presentation and engagement.
- Uterine contraction:
  - By clinical palpation (most commonly used)
  - By external monitor (tocodynamometer, measures duration of contraction and interval between them but not strength)
  - Quantitative measurement by intrauterine pressure catheter used to (IUPC) measures duration, interval and strength of contraction. For this test membrane must be ruptured.

  It is rarely used in obstetrical practice. Uterine work can be expressed as Montevideo Units (MVUs). Three contractions in 10 minutes produce approximately 100–200 MVUs. Adequate uterine activity when contraction pattern generates >200 MVUs. Strong contractions every 2 minutes generate more than 300 MVUs.
- Vaginal examination:
  a. To see cervical condition and descent of head. There are six ways to determine progress (Simkin and Ancheta, 2000)
     i. Cervix moves from posterior to an anterior position (position).
     ii. Cervix ripens or softens (consistency).
     iii. Cervix effaces (opening up of cervical canal from above downwards or oblitering cervical canal).
     iv. Cervix dilates.
     v. Fetal head rotates.
     vi. Fetus descends.
  b. Clinical pelvimetry to assess pelvis:
     i. An attempt should first be made to feel the tip of the sacral promontory.

In doing so, one is trying to establish the length of the diagonal conjugate. If it is easily tipped, it should alert one to the possibility of a contracted pelvis.
  ii. The curvature of the sacrum is assessed to see if it is flat or well curved. A well curved sacrum allows for internal rotation of the fetal head.
  iii. The pelvic side walls are next assessed to see, if they are parallel or convergent.
  iv. The ischial spines should next be palpated to see if they are prominent and sticking in.
  v. Then the subpubic angle is assessed to see if it is acute or obtuse. If it accommodates two fingers it is obtuse.
  vi. Having removed the fingers, the intertuberous diameter is assessed to see, if it accommodates more than four knuckles.

Features of an adequate (gynecoid) pelvis include a wide diagonal conjugate, a well-curved sacrum, parallel side walls, ischial spines are not prominent, a wide subpubic angle and lastly a wide intertuberous diameter.

- Assessing fetal conditions by:
  - The FHR auscultation
  - External monitoring
  - Internal monitoring, if external monitoring is inadequate or closer surveillance is needed.
    Advantage of internal monitoring is that it can prevent unnecessary cesarean section for fetal distress. Disadvantages are:
    a. Risk of infection of mother and fetus
    b. Restricts maternal movement
    c. Reduction of movement can cause more pain
    d. Membrane must be ruptured.
  - Observing liquor color after ruptured membrane.
- Assessing maternal condition by pulse, BP, hydration status and ketone bodies.

RELATED INFORMATION ABOUT UTERINE FUNCTION

- *Pattern of contraction:* Normally uterine contraction generated by pace maker placed at two cornu of the uterus, propagates towards lower uterine segment with decreasing duration and intensity as it moves away from pacemaker.
- *Polarity of uterus:* When upper segment contracts lower segment relaxes.

Characteristics of Normal Uterine Contraction

- Comes at regular interval
- Interval gradually shortens
- Intensity gradually increases
- Feeling of pain in the back and abdomen
- Associated with cervical dilatation
- Pain is not relieved by sedation
- Adequate contraction, e.g. 1 in 3 minutes lasting for 45 seconds with good relaxation in between
- Basal tone 5–20 mm Hg with a peak pressure around 60 mm Hg.

Abnormal Uterine Action

Any deviation from normal pattern of uterine contraction affecting the normal course of labor is designated as abnormal uterine contraction. Overall incidence of labor abnormality is 25% in nulliparous and 10% in multiparous.

Types of Abnormal Uterine Action

A. *With normal polarity of uterus:*
   a. Hypertonic dysfunction (Hypertonic uterine inertia):
      - *Precipitate labor*: When delivery takes place after an unusually rapid labor within <2 hours
      - *Tonic contraction and retraction and formation of Bandl's ring*: Where there is obstruction.
   b. Hypotonic dysfunction (Hypotonic uterine inertia)

B. *With abnormal polarity of uterus (incoordinate uterine action)*:

Characteristics of incoordinate uterine action
- Usually occurs in active phase of labor
- New pacemakers appear all over the uterus
- Fundal dominance is lacking and pacemakers do not work in rhythm
- The myometrium contracts spasmodically and irregularly
- The contraction force neither dilates the cervix nor pushes the fetus down
- Inadequate or no relaxation in between contractions.
- Uterine tonus is elevated above 20 mm Hg
- Pain is present before, during and after contractions.

Types of Incoordinate Uterine Action

- Spastic lower segment
- Colicky uterus
- Constriction ring
- Generalized tonic contraction
- Cervical dystocia.

> How will you diagnose and manage a case of hypotonic uterine action?

Hypotonic uterine action is also called uterine inertia where the uterine contraction is inefficient:
- It may be *primary* where poor uterine contractions from the start of labor
- It may be *secondary* where uterine contractions become weaker after a period of good uterine contraction.

Diagnosis
- Labor is prolonged at various stages such as prolonged latent phase, active phase and second stage of labor.
- Uterine contractions are weak, infrequent and have short duration. This can be detected by
  a. Clinical Palpation
  b. External monitor (tocodynamometer):
     – Apart from prolonged labor mother and fetus are usually not seriously affected specially when membrane is intact.

Management
- General measure
- Proper diagnosis of true labor
- Exclusion of CPD and risk factors for use of oxytocin such as grand multiparity, scarred uterus, malpresentations (except breech) and fetal distress
- Oxytocin stimulation to increase the strength, frequency and duration of uterine contraction
- ARM for further augmentation
- Monitoring the progress of labor
- If labor is prolonged and/or fetal distress in first stage cesarean section is to be done.
- If labor is prolonged and/or fetal distress in second stage ventouse (in absence of fetal distress) forceps (in presence of fetal distress) is to be done.

> How will you diagnose and manage tonic uterine contraction?

- In primaparous, labor comes to a stand still—a state of exhaustion after intense and frequent contraction and retraction
- In multiparous, contraction and retraction continues
- Patient is anxious looking
- Features of exhaustion and ketoacidosis are present
- Upper segment is tender and hard
- Lower segment is distended and tender
- Bladder is distended
- Development of circular groove between upper and lower segment called Bandl's ring.

Management
- Correction of dehydration and ketoacidosis by rapid IV fluid (Ringer's lactate) infusion
- Adequate pain relieve medication
- Parenteral antibiotics
- Exclude rupture uterus
- Deliver by cesarean section.

Note: As uterus is in a state of hypertonicity, mother becomes exhausted and fetus is in jeopardy due to placental insufficiency resulting from tonic contraction of the uterus, there is no role of oxytocin and ARM in hypertonic uterine action.

> How will you diagnose and manage spastic lower segment?

- Unbearable pain (patient is in a state of agony)
- Increased uterine contraction with poor relaxation in between
- Fundal dominance is lacking (reverse polarity)
- Lower segment contractions are stronger
- Uterine tenderness present
- Palpation of fetal parts is difficult
- Bladder is distended often with retention of urine
- Premature bearing down effect
- Dehydration and ketoacidosis present
- Fetal distress in the form of fetal tachycardia
- On PV exam:
  - Cervix is thick loose edematous hanging like a curtain; not well applied to the presenting part
  - Inappropriate dilatation of the cervix
  - Absence of membrane and meconium stained liquor may be there.

Management

General management of dehydration, ketoacidosis, pain killer and parenteral antibiotics followed by cesarean section

Note: No role of oxytocin and ARM for the same reason, which discussed above.

> What is constriction ring (Schroeder's ring)? How it can be managed?

Constriction ring is a variety of in coordinate uterine action where localized myometrial contraction forms a ring of circular muscle fibers of the uterus.

Characteristics

- It may appear in all stages of labor
- It is situated at the junction of upper and lower segment usually around the constricted part of the fetus such as neck in cephalic presentation.
- Maternal condition is not usually affected
- Fetal distress may occur

- Caused by:
  - Injudicious administration of oxytocin
  - Premature rupture of membranes
  - Premature attempt of instrumental delivery.
- Uterus never ruptures
- Difficult to diagnose as ring is not palpable on PA exam
- Can be diagnosed during:
  - Cesarean section
  - Forceps delivery
  - Manual removal of placenta (Hour glass contracture).
- Ring is usually passes of by deepening plane of anesthesia.

Management

- Delivery by cesarean section
- If ring does not pass off it may have to cut vertically to deliver the baby.

> What are the difference between constriction ring and Bandl's ring? (Table 6.1)

> What is cervical dystocia? How it can be managed?

Failure of progressive cervical dilatation in spite of adequate uterine contraction is called cervical dystocia.

It may be *primary* when it happens in first birth due to rigid cervix, insufficient uterine contraction and malposition and malpresentation

It may be *secondary* due to excessive scarring or rigidity of cervix from previous operation or any growth in the cervix.

Management

General management according to patient's general condition:

Delivery
- If malposition, malpresentation or any growth of cervix is present CS is preferred.
- If there is no complication and a thin rim of cervix is left behind—it is pushed up manually during contraction and traction is given by ventouse.

Table 6.1 Difference between constriction ring and Bandl's ring

Constriction ring	Bandl's ring
• Result of localized incoordinate uterine action	• It is the end result of tonic uterine contraction and retraction
• Undue irritability of uterus	• Following obstructed labor
• Usually at the junction of upper and lower uterine segment	• Always at the junction of upper and lower uterine segment
• Upper segment contracts and retracts with relaxation in between	• Upper segment tonically contracted
• Lower uterine segment thick and loose	• Lower uterine segment thinned out
• Ring cannot be felt abdominally	• Ring can be felt abdominally
• Maternal exhaustion is usually absent but may occur at late stage	• Maternal exhaustion is early appearance
• Fetal distress is also late feature	• Fetal anoxia and even death are usually early
• Chance of uterine rupture is absent	• In multigravida rupture uterus is common

- *If cervix is thinned out, but only half dilated*: Duhrssen's incision is given at 2 o'clock and 10 o'clock position followed by forceps or ventouse extraction.

What are the characteristics of generalized tonic contraction (uterine tetany)? How it can be managed?

Characteristics

- The whole uterus undergoes tonic muscular spasm
- Pronounced retraction occurs involving uterus up to internal os
- There is no differentiation of active upper segment and passive lower segment
- Fetus is held inside the uterus
- Usually there is no risk of rupture
- Usually occurs due to:
  - CPD
  - Obstruction
  - Injudicious use of oxytocin
- Labor is prolonged having severe and continuous pain
- Uterus is tense, tender and smaller
- Fetal parts are not palpable and heart sound is not audible
- On PV exam vagina is dry and hot with jammed head with a big capute.

Management

- General management:
  - Correction of dehydration and ketoacidosis
  - Antibiotic
  - Adequate pain relieve.
- Tocolytic agent, e.g. terbutalin, or MgSO$_4$ and oxytocin infusion is to be stopped if it is due to abuse of oxytocin
- Cesarean section.

What is the role of amniotomy in labor dystocia?

In labor dystocia amniotomy is the treatment of choice both in first stage and second stage, if membrane is intact till that time. After establishment of diagnosis of labor pain amniotomy can be done as active management of labor to overcome labor dystocia. Also it can be done in diagnosed labor dystocia where cause is inefficient uterine contraction.

It helps by:
- Accelerating labor
- Allowing early detection of meconium
- Allowing for placement of internal monitors.

The value of amniotomy have been argued by proponents and opponents for many years. Although, some has reported that amniotomy does not enhance labor progress (Garite et al. 1993), a large randomized trail shows early amniotomy shortens duration of labor by 2 hours without lowering the rate of CS (Fraser et al. 1993). The United Kingdom (UK) amniotomy group shows statistically significant reduction of duration of labor in the amniotomy group (8.43 hours) in comparison to control group (9.35 hours). But there was no difference in CS or operative vaginal delivery rate (The UK amniotomy group, 1994).

While Cochrane review in 2000 shows reduction of first stage by 1–2 hours with no effect in second stage of labor with an increasing trend to CS rate (Fraser et al. 2000), in 2013 it shows no evidence of shortening of the length of first stage of labor and a possible increase in CS (Smyth et al. 2013). Routine amniotomy was not recommended by them as part of standard labor management and care. As no study shows any adverse effect on fetal heart rate, neonatal outcome or postpartum hemorrhage, so amniotomy may be practiced in reduction of duration of first stage in labor dystocia.

Risks of Amniotomy

Risks of amniotomy are:
1. Risk of infection
2. Lost of buffer mechanism during labor due to fluid loss
3. Risk of abnormal fetal heart tracing.

> What is the role of oxytocin in labor dystocia?

If labor dystocia is due to inadequate uterine activity, oxytocin is to be administered with a starting dose 0.5–1.0 mU/minute with an increment of 1–2 mU/minute every 20–30 minutes up to 12 mU/minute. Sometimes, higher dose may be needed, which reduces both cesarean and operative vaginal delivery rate. Higher dose at 20 minutes interval significantly reduces CS rate (Satin et al. 1992; Satin et al. 1994). Oxytocin significantly increases cervical dilatation in comparison to amniotomy or expectant management (Blanch et al. 1998). Combined oxytocin and amniotomy is more effective than either oxytocin or amniotomy alone (Nachum et al. 2010). Oxytocin augmentation also may be needed in second stage of labor due to ineffective uterine contraction. Careful monitoring is needed to avoid hyperstimulation of the uterus and to prevent uterine rupture. Direct FHR monitoring is needed during second stage of labor because fetus becomes progressively acidotic during the second stage (Modanlou et al. 1973).

> What is active management of labor?

Intervention of spontaneous labor in nulliparous women with singleton fetus in an intention to keep the labor to fewer than 12 hours and operative rates to a minimum. Components of active labor are:
- Early diagnosis of the labor following strict criteria
- Early amniotomy
- High dose oxytocin augmentation with a starting rate of 6 mU/minutes and increased by 6 mU/minutes every 15 minutes to a maximum of 40 mU/minutes. The goal is no more than 7 uterine contractions per 15 minutes
- Frequent vaginal examination
- Personal, psychological support for the women
- One-on-one nursing care.

> **Case scenario:** Mrs Lutfa aged 34 years has come to you with her labor pain for 10 hours. She is a mother of three children, all were home deliveries. First two were uneventful, but third delivery was with prolonged duration of second stage. Baby's cry was delayed after delivery. She is a non-booked case, but immunized by tetanus (TT) vaccine. This time she is amenorrhoic for 39 weeks and developed labor pain, which was typical in nature and started 10 hours earlier. Her membrane was ruptured 6 hours ago. Dai tried for delivery, but failed. Head is seen in introitus for 4 hours. On general examination: patient is anxious, exhausted, dehydrated, pulse 100/minute, BP 110/75 mm Hg. On PA examination—uterus is tonically contracted, fetal heart is rapid 178/minute, bladder is distended. On PV examination—vagina is hot and dry, presentation is cephalic, station is zero, membrane ruptured, liquor is deeply stained. There is a big capute with ++ moulding.
>
> On the basis of above history and findings what is your diagnosis?

Obstructed Labor (Dystocia in Second Stage of Labor)

By the definition when in spite of effective uterine contraction fetus is failed to deliver or progressive descent of the presenting part is arrested due to mechanical obstruction is called obstructed labor.

> What are the points in favor?

Suggestive Past History

- *Multiparity:* In multiparous women due to subluxation of sacrum due to repeated pregnancy and delivery anteroposterior diameter of pelvis reduced, so obstruction occurs.

Labor Dystocia

- Difficult and delayed last delivery indicates that there was mild obstruction in last delivery.
- Delayed crying of baby may be due to effect of prolonged second stage of labor.

Present Situation

- This time total duration is prolonged with second stage prolongation.
- Head is seen in introitus for 4 hours, this indicates that she entered into second stage 4 hours back or even more.
- Mother is exhausted and dehydrated and pulse is raised. All are signs of effects of prolonged labor.
- Tonically uterine contraction indicates exhausted uterus, which occurs in obstructed labor.
- Fetal tachycardia indicates distress due to prolonged second stage.
- Bladder is distended due to failure to evacuate due to impacted fetal head in pelvis.
- Hot and dry vagina are sign of prolonged and obstructed labor
- Though head is seen in the introitus, it is not actual head, it is capute. Station zero indicates that actual head is above the ischial spine. Due to obstruction it could not descent.
- Deeply stained liquor is due to fetal distress due to prolonged obstructed labor.
- Capute and moulding are the signs of obstructed labor.

> What might be the cause here?

Cephalopelvic Disproportion

- Due to subluxation of sacrum (causes secondary contracted pelvis, occurs in multiparous women)
- Due to big baby
- Due to both subluxation and big baby.

> What are the factors those can cause obstruction?

Maternal Factors

- Contracted pelvis and CPD are the most common causes:
  - True or primary contracted pelvis
  - Secondary contracted pelvis.
- Soft tissue obstruction due to:
  - Cervical or broad ligament fibroid
  - Impacted ovarian tumor
  - Non-gravid horn of bicornuate uterus below the presenting part.

Fetal Factors

- Big baby
- Transverse lie (shoulder presentation)
- Brow presentation
- Congenital anomaly of the baby (Hydrocephalus, encephalocele, cystic hygroma, fetal goiter and hydrops fetalis)
- Compound presentation
- Locked twin.

> How will you manage this case?

General Management

- Dehydration is to be corrected by infusion of fluid at least 1,000 mL at running drip then at 25 drops/minute
- Blood is to be sent for grouping and cross matching as there is chance of excessive blood loss from atonic uterus and from injury. One pint of blood is to be kept ready at hand.
- A vaginal swab is to be sent for culture and sensitivity test before starting antibiotics. Patient was handled by *dai*. So there is chance of introduction of infection.
- Antibiotic: Broad spectrum antibiotics are to be given covering gram positive and negative bactericidals. Ceftriaxone, metronidazole and gentamycin combination is to be given.
- Catheterization is to be done.

Obstetric or Specific Management

This is a case of obstructed labor with alive fetus. So CS is to be done to deliver the baby. As baby is distressed neonatologist should be present during delivery to manage the baby. Baby may be severely asphyxiated and need neonatal intensive care unit (NICU) services.

> What are the effects of prolonged and obstructed labor in mother and fetus?

- Prolonged latent phase of first stage of labor may be worrisome to the patient, but may not cause any adverse effect to mother and fetus
- It may be associated with increased incidence of CS, chorioamnionities and postpartum bleeding
- It may associated with low Apgar score and admission to the NICU.

Prolonged active phase of first stage and second stage of labor have adverse effect to mother and fetus. Prolonged second stage of labor is associated with significant maternal and fetal morbidity independent of the need for operative intervention.

Effects on Mother

- *Exhaustion:* Due to constant agonizing pain
- *Dehydration:* Due to increased muscular activity without adequate fluid intake
- *Metabolic acidosis:* Due to accumulation of lactic acid and ketones. Powerful uterine contractions compress uterine blood vessels, causing transient hypoxic episodes. The myometrium responds by producing adenosine triphosphate (ATP) anaerobically. More pyruvate converts into lactic acid rather than entering the Krebs cycle for oxidative metabolism resulting in acidosis.
- *Genital sepsis:* Due to prolonged ruptured membrane and repeated PV examination and malhandling by health professionals.
- *Rupture uterus:* In neglected cases rupture of the uterus may occur particularly in multiparous women where uterus becomes weak due to replacement of muscular tissue by fibrous tissue in repeated pregnancy.
- *Injuries* to cervix, vagina, perineum may occur due to mal-handling and manipulation.
- *Postpartum hemorrhage* and shock due to injuries, atonic uterus and combined effect.
- *Subinvolution*

All these lead to increased maternal morbidity and mortality.

Rupture uterus, sepsis and postpartum hemorrhage (PPH) are the main causes of death in obstructed labor.

Remote

a. Vesicovaginal, ureterovaginal and rectovaginal fistula:
   - Base of the bladder and urethra are trapped in between presenting part and symphysis pubis and undergo pressure necrosis due to impediment of blood circulation to maternal parts. The devitalized tissue becomes infected and later on slough off resulting in the development of vesicovaginal fistula (VVF) (most common fistula). Other fistulas also occur due to pressure necrosis. Rectovaginal fistulas are less common, presumably because of the absence of a maternal bony surface in close proximity posteriorly.
   - In case of instrumental delivery due to direct injury.
b. Asherman syndrome
c. Amenorrhea
d. Infertility
e. Vaginal stenosis
f. Chronic pelvic pain
g. Osteitis pubis and
h. Foot drop.

Effects on the Fetus

- Asphyxia:
  - Due to impaired uteroplacental circulation caused by repeated uterine contraction.
  - Due to cord prolapse in shoulder presentation (if delivery takes place immediately otherwise fetus invariably dies).
- *Acidosis:* Due to fetal hypoxia and maternal acidosis.
- *Intracranial hemorrhage* due to excessive moulding causing tentorial tear or due to traumatic delivery.
- *Intrauterine infection* particularly after rupture of the membrane.
- *Increased operative delivery.*

All these lead to increased perinatal mortality and neonatal morbidity.

> What are the risks of cesarean section in such a case?

- Hemorrhage
- Shock

Labor Dystocia

- Extension of lower segment incision
- Injury to bladder, ureter
- PPH
- Sepsis
- Wound dehiscence
- Subinvolution.

> *Suppose with the same feature fetal heart sound is not audible. What will be your management?*

Here presentation is cephalic and presenting part lies just above the ischial spine. So craniotomy is possible and craniotomy will be done.

Note: Craniotomy is applicable for vertex, brow, face and after-coming head of breech.

> *What precaution do you need to take before craniotomy?*

- Patient's dehydration must be corrected by, intravenous (IV) fluid infusion
- Catheterization must be done
- Blood must be kept ready at hand
- Antibiotic is to be started.

> *What precaution should be taken after craniotomy?*

- Uterus is to be explored to check whether there is any injury. Rupture uterus is very common after destructive operation in obstructed labor
- Cervix and vaginal canal are to be checked for injury
- Foley's self-retaining catheter is to be kept for at least 10 days to prevent the development of VVF.

> *What are the complications of craniotomy?*

- Postpartal shock
- Injury to uterus, cervix, vagina and perineum
- Injury to bladder and rectum
- PPH due to atonicity or injury.

> *In obstructed labor, if fetus is alive with good Apgar score at CS and vaginal tissue is pink indicating optimum circulation.*
>
> *Would you like to retain the catheter for prevention of fistulas?*

Alive fetus with good Apgar score and healthy vaginal wall (no sign of ischemia) indicates obstruction of short period. In such case as there is no ischemic change of vaginal tissue fistula formation is unlikely. So retention of catheter is not necessary in such a case.

> *Suppose in the above mentioned case presentation is shoulder due to transverse lie rather than cephalic.*
>
> *How will you deliver the fetus?*
> *a. When it is alive?*
> *b. When it is dead?*

In this case, CS is to be done irrespective of fetal condition because:
- In dead fetus destructive operation such as evisceration should not be done in multiparous women due to risk of uterine rupture.
- In alive fetus there is no role of internal podalic version in multiparous women with features of obstructed labor due to risk of uterine rupture.

Note: Transverse lie with obstructed labor should be delivered by CS irrespective of fetal condition and parity of mother.
- In modern obstetric practice advances in anesthesia, blood banking and pre- and postsurgical care have made the CS much safer than manipulated vaginal delivery in obstructed labor.
- Even in primiparous and second gravid women though uterine integrity is stronger than that in multiparous women chances of uterine rupture is there.

So considering future reproductive potential and safety of the mother, CS is safer than manipulated vaginal delivery.

> *Why rupture is more common in multiparous women and less in primiparous?*

Primiparous

- In primigravid women uterine contractility is diminished in obstructed labor. The uterus stops contracting because of myometrial acidification, which results from local myometrial energy depletion, anaerobic metabolism and systemic ketosis. So uterus becomes fatigue

and there is no contraction and no chance of rupture (Neilson, 2003).
- No loss of muscular tissue in primiparous women, which retains the strength of the uterus.

Multiparous

- In parous women the myometrium might becomes tolerant to the effects of acidification by an unknown mechanism and does not stop contracting. Due to continued contractions in the presence of myometrial energy depletion lower segment continues to thin and hypoxia are likely to lead to myometrial edema and necrosis contributing to uterine rupture (Neilson, 2003).
- Due to replacement of muscular tissue by fibrous tissue in previous pregnancies strength of uterus reduced.

> Why VVF is more common in primiparous women?

In primigravid women due to fatigability of the uterus resulting from tissue acidosis contractility diminishes. The presenting part retains within pelvis till definitive management, causing ischemia, infection and necrosis of tissue leads to fistula formation. Whereas in parous women, contractility may be maintained with the risk of uterine rupture. Fetal head usually becomes loosen after dehiscence of the uterus, releases the pressure of head to vaginal wall and minimizes the chance of ischemia of vaginal tissue.

> How prolonged and obstructed labor can be prevented?

- By identifying labor dystocia in time by using partogram
- Timely appropriate management of dystocia in active phase of labor
- By active management of labor.

> **Case scenario:** Mrs Jobaida Khatun, aged 38 years, a multiparous woman has come to the hospital with the complaints of amenorrhea with signs and symptoms of pregnancy for 9 months and lower abdominal pain for 24 hours. Her abdomen is distended. The patient is restless and her general condition is very poor.
>
> How will you proceed for diagnosis?

As patient's general condition is very poor a quick assessment should be the first attempted for proper management:
- Her pulse and BP is to be checked quickly
- Abdomen is to be examined as it is distended
- Fetal heart is to be ausculted to assess fetal condition
- Inspection of vulva to see whether there is any PV bleeding
- Observation of general look.

> On examination, it is found that patient is distressed, sweating is present, pulse: 120/minute, BP: 80/40 mm Hg, patient is pale. On PA examination it is found that abdomen is tender, irregular fetal parts can be felt easily, fetal heart sound is absent. On inspection PV bleeding is present.
>
> What should be your next action?

- Immediately an IV channel is to be opened
- Before going to other examination or investigations opening up of an IV channel is mandatory as patient is in a state of shock
- Immediately blood is to be sent for grouping and cross matching
- Running IV fluid dextrose in normal saline (DNS), Hartman solution or plasma expander is to be started
- Blood transfusion is to be started as soon as it is available.
- As patient is in a state of shock she should be catheterized to assess urine output
- Detailed history is to be taken afterwards
- Finally PV examination is to be done.

> What points do you need to ask during history taking?

- Whether she is a booked case or not?
- When was her LMP? Calculate estimated date of delivery (EDD)
- About parity
- Mode of previous deliveries
- Complication during past pregnancy and labor
- When pain has started?
- Character of pain. Rhythmic progressively increasing pain indicates labor pain
- Rupture of the membrane
- Whether there is any intervention and application of any drug?
- From when abdomen begins to be distended?

> On further enquiry, it was elicited that her LMP was 39 weeks 3 days back that is gestational age is 39 weeks 3 days. She is para 4, all were normal vaginal delivery without any complications during pregnancy and labor. Pain has started 18 hours earlier with increasing frequency and intensity. Membrane was raptured 12 hours ago. Traditional birth attendance (TBA) tried for vaginal delivery but she did not use any drug. There is history of agonizing pain 3 hours ago. Afterwards rhythmic contraction stopped and abdomen was gradually distended. On PV examination it is found that vagina is hot and dry. Bleeding (+). Presentation vertex. Capute (+++). Moulding (++).
>
> On the basis of the above findings what is your likely diagnosis? Explain points in favor.

Ruptured Uterus

- There is a history of prolonged (18 hours) obstructed labor.
- Hot and dry vagina is a sign of prolonged labor
- Capute and moulding are the signs of obstruction
- History of agonizing pain and then subsidence of rhythmic uterine contraction is characteristics of ruptured uterus
- Ruptured uterus is more common in multiparous women
- Distinctly palpable fetal parts indicate that fetus is within the abdominal cavity, which, occurs in ruptured uterus
- Features of shock and pallor are due to internal hemorrhage. Presenting part remains tight within the birth passage, so there is no heavy PV bleeding.

> With all these data gathered it can be diagnosed as a case of ruptured uterus.
> What immediate management needed?

- Inject pethidine 100 mg intramuscularly (IM) is to be given to relieve pain
- Broad-spectrum antibiotics ceftriaxone, gentamycin and metronidazole is to be started to prevent sepsis. Patient was handled by *dai* and membrane is ruptured for long time. So there is chance of development of sepsis.

> Will you go for any investigation for confirmation the diagnosis?

No. History and clinical examination is enough for diagnosis of ruptured uterus. No need to do any investigation for confirmation.

> Fetus is dead here. Now how will you deliver the fetus?

Laparotomy is to be done to deliver the fetus and to repair or remove the ruptured uterus.

> You are going to do surgery. You know patient's general condition is very poor. There is risk of general anesthesia in a patient with poor general condition. So what precautions do you need to take before going for operation?

The patient is a case of prolonged and obstructed labor with ruptured uterus. In obstructed labor patient becomes dehydrated and develops metabolic acidosis. In addition this patient has internal hemorrhage and she is in a state of shock. *So first of all she should be resuscitated by liberal transfusion of blood and fluid. After resuscitation surgery is to be done.*

Criteria of Resuscitated Patient

- Pulse should be less than 100/minute.
- Systolic BP should be >100 mm Hg.
- Temperature should be <100°F.
- Urine output should be at least 30 mL/hour.

Note: In practice it is not feasible to wait till falling of pulse <100. So after settling BP, surgery is to be done.

> After opening the abdomen and removing the fetus, placenta and blood clots you found that uterus is ruptured completely in its anterolateral aspect involving both upper and lower segment.
> Now what is decision about further management?

Subtotal hysterectomy is to be done.

> Why subtotal hysterectomy?

The patient is multiparous and rupture is extensive and complete. So removal of uterus is ideal treatment. But in a parturient woman where cervix is fully dilated it is difficult to do total hysterectomy. So subtotal hysterectomy is ideal option here. After hysterectomy abdominal toileting is to be done by normal saline. A drain tube is to be kept in abdominal cavity before closing the abdomen.

Suppose tear is small and clean cut. Then what do you like to do in such a multiparous woman?

If tear is small and clean cut then repair is possible. So in a multiparous woman repair with bilateral tubal ligation will have to be done.

Suppose a patient who has got no children and rupture is small and clean cut. Then what do you like to do?

As patient has got no children only repair is to be done. So that she can have future pregnancy.

Suppose patient has got no children and rupture is irregular and extensive. Then what do you like to do?

Though patient has got no children *subtotal hysterectomy* is to be done, as repair is not possible in extensive rupture. Moreover, it will leave a damaged uterus, which will be more prone to rupture in future pregnancy.

What are the causes of rupture of the uterus?

- Obstructed labor most common cause in developing countries.
- Grand multiparity.
- Scar rupture of previous lower segment cesarean section (LSCS) or hysterotomy.
- Previous damage and weakening of the uterine walls following dilatation and curettage and manual removal of placenta.
- Injudicious administration of oxytocin and prostaglandins for induction and augmentation of labor.
- Forcible external cephalic version.
- Internal podalic version in obstructed labor.
- Destructive operation.
- Manual removal of placenta.
- Application of forceps or breech extraction through incompletely dilated cervix.

Ruptured uterus is an avoidable condition. Still it is one of the important causes of maternal mortality in developing countries like ours. We should try to overcome this situation.
What do you think about the prevention of such happening?

- At risk mothers are likely to rupture should be identified during antenatal check-up. So every pregnant mother must have access to health care delivery system.
- All high-risk patients should have mandatory hospital delivery. High-risk patients are:
  - Grand multiparity
  - Previous history of CS
  - Malpresentation such as shoulder and brow presentation, deep transverse arrest
  - Contracted pelvis
  - Hydrocephalus
- In the hospital during labor meticulous management should be done
- Proper selection of cases for external and internal podalic versions
- Judicious use of drugs such as oxytocin and prostaglandins
- Destructive operations and manual removal of morbid adherent placenta should be done by expert personnel.

What postoperative cares are needed for this patient?

- Continuous catheterization for 10 days to prevent the development of VVF
- Blood transfusion, if Hb% is less for better wound healing.

What postoperative complications might occur in such a case?

Same mentioned in obstructed labor.

Labor dystocia is an obstetric emergency that needs meticulous judgment for management. It is the most common cause of primary CS. Dystocia at active stage and second stage of labor is associated with both maternal and fetal risks. So labor should be monitored by using partogram to identify dystocia at earlier stage and manage accordingly.

BIBLIOGRAPHY

Albers LL, Schiff M, Gorwoda JG. The length of active labor in normal pregnancies. Obstet Gynecol. 1996;87:355-59.

A UK Amniotomy Group multicentre randomized trial of amniotomy in spontaneous first labor at term. Br J Obstet Gynaecol. 1994;101:307-9.

Blanch G, Lavender T, Walkinshaw S, Alfirevic Z. Dysfunctional labor: a randomised trial. Br J Obstet Gynaecol. 1998;105(1):117-20.

Fraser WD, Marcoux S, Moutquin JM, Christen A. Effect of early amniotomy on the risk of dystocia in nulliparous women. The Canadian Early Amniotomy Study Group. N Engl J Med. 1993;328: 1145-9.

Fraser WD, Turcot L, Krauss I, Brisson-Carrol G. Amniotomy for shortening spontaneous labor. The Cochrane Database of Systematic Reviews. 2000, Issue 1.

Friedman EA. Labor: clinical evaluation and management, 2nd edition. New York. Appleton-Century-Crofts, 1978.

Garite TJ, Porto M, Carlson NJ, et al. The influence of elective amniotomy on fetal heart rate patterns and the course of labor in term patients; a randomized study. Am J Obstet Gynecol. 1993;168: 1827-31.

Modanlou H, Yeh SY, Hon EH, et al. Fetal and neonatal biochemistry and Apgar scores. Am J Obstet Gynecol. 1973;117(7):942-51.

Nachum Z, Garmi G, Kadam Y, Zafran N, Shalev E, Salim R. Comparison between amniotomy, oxytocin or both for augmentation of labor in prolonged latent phase: a randomized controlled trial. Reproductive Biology and Endocrinology. 2010;8:136. doi:10.1186/1477-7827-8-136.

National Institute for Health and Care Excellence (NICE 2007). Intrapartum care: care of healthy women and their babies during childbirth. (Clinical Guideline 55.) 2007.

Neilson JP, Lavender T, Quenby S, et al. Obstructed labor. Br Med Bull. 2003;67:191-204.

Ponkey SE, Cohen AP, Heffner LJ, et al. Persistent fetal occiput posterior position: obstetric outcomes. Obstet Gynecol. 2003;101:915-20.

Rouse DJ, Owen J, Hauth JC. Active-phase labor arrest: oxytocin augmentation for at least 4 hours. Obstet Gynecol. 1999;93(3):323-8.

Satin AJ, Leveno KJ, Sherman ML, et al. High-dose oxytocin: 20-versus 40-minute dosage interval. Obstet Gynecol. 1994;83(2):234-8.

Satin AJ, Leveno KJ, Sherman ML, et al. High- versus low-dose oxytocin for labor stimulation. Obstet Gynecol. 1992;80(1):111-6.

Simkin P, Ancheta R. The Labor Progress Handbook: Early Interventions to Prevent and Treat Dystocia [Paperback]. 3rd edition. Wiley-Blackwell. 2000.

Smyth RMD, Markham C, Dowswell T. Amniotomy for shortening spontaneous labour. Cochrane Review. 2013.

Sprague AE, Oppenheimer L, McCabe L, et al. The Ottawa Hospital's Clinical Practice Guideline for the Second Stage of Labor. J Obstet Gynaecol Can. 2006;28(9):769-79.

Zhang J, Troendle JF, Yancey MK. Reassessing the labor curve in nulliparous women. Am J Obstet Gynecol. 2002;187(4):824-8.

Zhu BP, Grigorescu V, Le T, et al. Labor dystocia and its association with interpregnancy interval. Am J Obstet Gynecol. 2006; 195(1):121-8.

CHAPTER 7

Gestational Diabetes Mellitus

Rashida Begum

INTRODUCTION

Gestational diabetes mellitus (GDM) is currently defined as any degree of glucose intolerance with onset or first recognition during current pregnancy (American Diabetes Association, 2006; ACOG practice bulletin, 2001; Metzger et al. 1998; Metzger et al. 2007). Pregnancy induces progressive changes in maternal carbohydrate metabolic process. As pregnancy advances insulin resistance and diabetogenic stress due to placental contrainsulin hormones necessitate compensatory increase in insulin secretion. When this compensatory mechanism fails due to pancreatic β cells inadequacy gestational diabetes develops. The GDM affects 1–2% of all pregnancies. In majority of patients it is mild and can be adequately controlled with diet alone, but a minority will require antidiabetogenic agents such as glyburide or insulin.

> **Case scenario:** *Mrs Fatema Begum a 33-year-old primigravida has come to you with the complaints of amenorrhea for 9 weeks with sign and symptom of pregnancy. You confirmed diagnosis by ultrasonography. On history taking you elicited that her father is diabetic. Her weight is 70 kg. Other physical examination findings are normal.*
>
> *What are the risk factors present here? For which 'with routine booking investigations' what additional investigation you need to do?*

Patient's father is diabetic and she is obese. So she is a potential candidate for gestational diabetes mellitus. For which one-step glucose tolerance test is to be done. Test is to be done 2 hours after ingestion of 75 g glucose in nonfasting state. If plasma glucose (PG) level lies between 7.8–11 mmol then it is glucose intolerance. If value is more than 11 mmol then it is diabetes.

> *Her PG was 7.5 mmol after 75 g glucose ingestion. Does she need any further glucose testing?*

Yes. She has got risk factors for GDM. So she needs to be tested around 16 weeks then again between 24 and 28 weeks, and around 32nd to 34th weeks and also in later weeks if necessary, particularly when rapid weight gain occurs or fetal macrosomia is suspected (Franks et al. 2006).

> *How will you interpret the tests?*

Interpretation is shown in **Table 7.1** in next page.

RELATED INFORMATION

Reason of Testing During Pregnancy

In pregnancy along with other bodily changes carbohydrate metabolism is also altered leads to glucose intolerance. About 3–5% of all pregnant women show some degree of glucose intolerance and about 90% of these women have gestational diabetes due to diabetogenic effect of pregnancy. Though majority reverse to normal after delivery of the baby, almost 50% of them develop type 2 DM later in their life. There is ethnic variation and Asian women are more prone to develop glucose intolerance than other ethnic groups. To prevent the adverse effects of GDM on mother and fetus early diagnosis and appropriate management is essential. Classification of glucose intolerance after 75 g glucose is shown in **Table 7.1**.

Table 7.1 Classification of glucose intolerance by 75 g 2-hour oral glucose tolerance test (OGTT)

Diagnosis	Fasting plasma glucose (FPG) mg/dL (mmol)	2-hour plasma glucose (PG) mg/dL (mmol)
Normal glucose tolerance (NGT)	<100 (<5.5)	<140 (<7.8)
Impaired fasting glucose (IFG)	100–125 (5.55–6.94)	
Impaired glucose tolerance (IGT)		140–199 (7.78–11.05)
Diabetes mellitus (DM)	≥126 (≥7)	≥200 (≥11.11)

Why Glucose Intolerance Occurs in Pregnancy?

With the advancement of pregnancy following changes occur:
- *Increased insulin resistance due to:*
  - Increased production of human placental lactogen, which acts as contra-insulin factor.
  - Increased production of other contra-insulin factors like cortisol, estriol, and progesterone.
  - Increased catabolism of insulin by placental and renal insulinage (Arias et al. 2008).
- *Increased blood glucose level because:*
  - During pregnancy mother utilizes fat for her calories and saves glucose for her baby.
  - As a result of these physiological changes the normal blood sugar pattern in pregnant woman is fasting—65 ± 9 mg/dL (3.6 mmol), nonfasting—80 ± 10 mg/dL (4.44 mmol), postprandial—140 ± 10 (7.78 mmol) mg/dL (Cousins et al. 1980).

How GDM can be Diagnosed?

In pregnancy all potential candidates should be screened to diagnose GDM. There are a number of screening procedures and diagnostic criteria in different countries like American Diabetes Association (ADA), World Health Organization (WHO), Canadian Diabetes Association (CDA), National Diabetes Data Group (NDDG) and Australian criteria.

Types of Screening

Basically two types of screening are adopted by different populations:
1. *Selective screening:* Where only high risk peoples are screened.
2. *Universal screening:* Where all pregnant women are screened. In selective screening some cases may be missed but universal screening can diagnose more cases of GDM (Dorendra et al. 2006). As a result maternal and neonatal prognosis improves. Therefore, universal screening appears to be the most reliable and desired method of diagnosis of GDM (Shamsuddin et al. 2001).

ADA screening: The ADA recommends two steps screening.

Step 1: A 50 g glucose challenge test (GCT) is used for screening without regard to the time of last meal or time of the day (Swami et al. 2008).

Step 2: If 1 hour GCT value is more than 140 mg/dL, 100 g oral glucose tolerance test (OGTT) is recommended and plasma glucose is estimated at 0, 1, 2 and 3 hours. GDM is diagnosed if any two values meet or exceed fasting plasma glucose (FPG) >95 mg/dL (>5.28 mmol), 1 hour postprandial glucose (PG) >180 mg/dL (>10 mmol), 2 hour PG >155 mg/dL (>8.61 mmol) and 3 hour PG >140 mg/dL (>7.78 mmol). But drawback of this method is that, the glycemic control cut-off was originally validated against the future risk of mother only and on the fetal outcome (Divakar et al. 2008). Other problems are the number of blood samples requirement is more, 1 for screening and 4 for 3 hour OGTT to confirm the diagnosis. Moreover, patients have to visit the antenatal clinic at least on two occasions for diagnosis leading to their inconvenience.

WHO procedure: To standardize the diagnosis of GDM the World Health Organization (WHO) recommends using a 2 hours OGTT with a threshold plasma glucose concentration of greater than 140 mg/dL (7.78 mmol) at 2 hours, similar to that of impaired glucose tolerance (IGT) in nonpregnant state (Beischer et al. 1991). The

WHO procedure also was not based on maternal and fetal outcome, but probably the criteria was recommended for its easy adaptability in clinical practice. The WHO criteria of 2-hour plasma glucose ≥140 mg/dL (7.78 mmol) identifying a large number of cases may have greater potential for prevention of GDM (Metzger et al. 1998).

A single test procedure for diagnosis of GDM: All the diagnostic criteria require the women to be fasting.

- For successful implementation of universal screening the procedure should not impose any restriction.
- So a single test 2 hours after 75 g glucose in a nonfasting state irrespective of last meal can make the diagnostic procedure simple, feasible and economical.
- It serves as both screening and diagnostic procedure, causes least disturbance to a pregnant woman's routine activities and avoids the inconvenience of fasting in a pregnant woman.

No significant difference in plasma glucose (PG) level was observed in 75 g glucose testing between fasting and nonfasting state, irrespective of last meal timing (Anjalakshi et al. 2009). So rationality of performing this test in nonfasting state is that, glucose concentration are affected little by the time since last meal in a normal glucose tolerant woman. But meal timing affects in a woman with GDM (Seshiah et al. 2004). The nonfasting 2-hour post 75 g glucose correctly identified subjects with GDM (Pettitt et al. 1994) and strongly predict adverse outcome for the mother and her baby (Pettitt et al. 1991). Thus, the single test procedure performed irrespective of the last meal timing seems to be a more rational and patient-friendly approach.

Risk Factors for Development of GDM

Any woman can develop gestational diabetes, but some women are at greater risk. Risk factors for gestational diabetes include:

- *Age greater than 35:* Women older than age 35 are more likely to develop gestational diabetes.
- *Family or personal history:* It includes:
  - Family history of type 2 diabetes mellitus, parent or siblings
  - History of diabetes in previous pregnancy
  - History of unexplained stillbirth
  - History of previous overweight baby (>4 kg).
- *Excess weight:* Overweight women (>90 kg) are more prone to develop GDM.
- *PCOS:* Patients of polycystic ovarian syndrome (PCOS) are prone to develop GDM.
- *Non-white race:* For reasons that are not clear, women who are black, Hispanic, American, Indian or Asian are more likely to develop gestational diabetes.

High-risk GDM

Both mother and fetus are affected by GDM, which is a complication of pregnancy. From fetal point of view adverse affects are sometimes severe and fatal. Some GDM patients are at higher risk for complications than others. High-risk GDM patients are those who have the:

- History of fetal macrosomia, stillbirth and neonatal death in previous pregnancy
- Maternal weight gain, obesity and hypertension
- Development of polyhydramnios, oligohydramnios and preeclampsia
- Inadequate metabolic control by diet alone.

Women at high risk should be identified as soon as the diagnosis is made, because they need meticulous management to prevent such complications. They need antepartum fetal surveillance testing and may require delivery before their expected date.

> You did screening test for the patient at booking visit.
> Is it necessary to do screening at this earliest period?

Yes. Testing at earlier has many advantages. It has been suggested that women at high risk should be screened as soon as pregnancy is confirmed (American Diabetes Association, 2003). Because increasing maternal carbohydrate intolerance in pregnant woman without GDM is associated with adverse maternal and fetal outcome (American Diabetes Association, 2002). By following the usual recommendation for screening between 24–28 weeks of gestation many early onset of GDM and prepregnant unidentified diabetes mellitus (DM) can be missed, which may adversely affect fetal outcome. Seshiah et al. detected 16.3% glucose intolerance within 16 weeks of pregnancy (Seshiah et al. 2007). Other two studies reported about 40-66% of women with GDM can be detected early during pregnancy (Super et al. 1991; Nahum et al. 2002). Nahum et al. suggested that the ideal period to screen for GDM is around 16 weeks of gestation and even earlier in high-risk groups with a history of fetal wastage (Nahum et al. 2002). The GDM diagnosis may not be missed by screening around 24-28 weeks of gestation, but a substantial number of pregnant women who develop GDM in the earlier weeks of gestation are likely to have delayed diagnosis and may not receive appropriate medical care. So it is safe to screen for GDM during early weeks of pregnancy as by early detection of glucose intolerance during pregnancy and adequate care to the antenatal women a good fetal outcome can be achieved similar to that of normal glucose tolerance (NGT) pregnant women (Seshiah et al. 2006; Seshiah et al. 2008). If a woman is found to have normal glucose tolerance test in the first trimester, she should be tested for GDM around 24th to 28th weeks and around 32nd to 34th weeks and also in later weeks if necessary, particularly when rapid weight gain occurs or fetal macrosomia is suspected (Franks et al. 2006).

> *Suppose Fatema's PG level was normal throughout pregnancy.*
> *What precaution is needed during delivery?*

As PG was normal throughout pregnancy, no extra caution is needed for her.

> *During follow-up at 22 weeks you found that her PG level 2 hours after 75 g glucose was 198 mg/dL (11 mmol).*
> *How will you manage her?*

Her glucose tolerance is impaired here. She should be managed by medical nutrition therapy and is to be followed up by monitoring FPG and 2-hour postprandial PG. Aim is to bring down the FPG to ≤90 mg/dL (≤5 mmol) and 2-hour postprandial glucose level to ≤120.6 mg/dL (≤6.7 mmol).

Approximately 30-40 kcal/kg and an increment of 300 kcal/day above the basal requirement are needed in second and third trimester. For majority of women the optional total daily caloric intake will be between 2,000 and 2,500 kcal/day.

RELATED INFORMATION

To prevent maternal and fetal complications treatment at appropriate time is necessary. Early detection of glucose intolerance during pregnancy and instillation of treatment at earliest state can prevent the complications and a good fetal outcome can be achieved.

Aim of Management

So, aim of management is to:
- Maintain euglycemia
- Prevent obstetrical complications
- Fix optimal time and appropriate mode of delivery.

Combined management by obstetrician, endocrinologist, nutritionist and neonatologist is necessary for better outcome. Management include:
- Counseling of the patient.
- Treatment of blood glucose control.
  - Medical nutrition therapy
  - Drug therapy (oral hypoglycemic agent and insulin).
- Management during labor.
- Neonatal management.

Counseling of the Patient

It is important to counsel the patient with impaired glucose tolerance (IGT) and GDM about the condition and its management, so that they can acquire a clear understanding of the characteristics and demands be emphasized on: (a) the importance of exercise and diet control, (b) importance of blood glucose control, (c) self-monitoring of blood glucose and (d) identification and treatment of hypoglycemia.

Treatment of Blood Glucose Control

The fundamental objective of the care of every pregnant diabetic is control of blood glucose to a desirable level for good fetal outcome. The aim is to maintain the fasting glucose level between 80-90 mg/dL (4.44-5 mmol) and 2 hours postprandial glucose level between 110-129 mg/dL (6.11-7.17 mmol).

Medical Nutrition Therapy

Dieting is an important step for blood glucose control. But pregnancy needs extra calories for growth and development of fetus. So GDM patients need strict maintenance of diet to maintain adequate calories without affecting blood glucose level to have a healthy baby. The concept of dietary management of the GDM or any other diabetic pregnant woman is that a healthy diet for them is not different from a healthy diet for any other nondiabetic pregnant woman. Patients should know that carbohydrate containing food increase blood glucose levels above normal limits and that persistently abnormal elevation of the blood glucose levels are harmful both for mother and fetus. So to prevent abnormal glucose levels a food plan should be made to maintain adequate calories without affecting blood glucose levels. Patient needs to understand the quantity or servings of carbohydrate present in her meals and snacks, and the effect of different types of carbohydrate on her blood glucose levels.

The meal pattern should provide adequate calories and nutrients to meet the needs of pregnancy. The expected weight gain during pregnancy is 300-400 g/week and total weight gain is 10-12 kg by term. So the meal plan aims to provide sufficient calories to sustain adequate nutrition for the mother and fetus, and to avoid excess weight gain and postprandial hyperglycemia. Calculation of daily caloric intake is based on body weight, age, physical activities and gestational age. Approximately 30-40 kcal/kg and an increment of 300 kcal/day above the basal requirement are needed in 2nd and 3rd trimester. For majority of women with GDM the optional total daily caloric intake will be between 2,000 and 2,500 cal/day. The total caloric intake is split into three meals and one to three snacks depending on the patient's habit. In a nondiabetic woman the peaking of the plasma glucose is high after breakfast due to 'Dawn phenomenon' and the insulin secretion also matches the glycemic excursion that occurs with the meal (Polonsky et al. 1988). But GDM mothers have deficiency in first phase insulin secretion leads to increased postprandial glucose level after heavy breakfast. To avoid the postprandial plasma glucose peaking with breakfast, it can be split into two halves and consuming these portions with a 2 hours gap. By this, the undue peak in plasma glucose levels after ingestion of the total quantity of breakfast at one time is avoided.

The total daily caloric allowance should be distributed among the different food groups in such a way that approximately 40-50% of the calories come from complex carbohydrate. The carbohydrate component of the diet should be distributed as 10-15% at breakfast, 20-30% at lunch and 30-40% at dinner. Approximately 30-40% from fat and the rest from protein. Postprandial elevations of blood sugar are due almost exclusively to the carbohydrate content of the diet. So carbohydrate should be taken as small frequent meal. Growthwer et al. showed the benefit of medical nutrition therapy (MNT) in a series of 1,000 pregnant women in comparison to routine care. Serious complications were 1% in MNT and 4% in routine care. Macrosomia rate was 10% in MNT and 21% in routine care. There was no perinatal death in MNT group whereas five perinatal deaths were in routine care (Crowther et al. 2005). Benefits of MNT are:

- Decreases hospital admission
- Decrease in insulin use
- Improved likelihood of normal fetal and placental growth
- Reduced risk of perinatal complications specially when diagnosed and treated early.

> With MNT, her PG level did not fall to desired level. What should be your next step of action?

Along with MNT she will be advised to take oral hypoglycemic agent in the form of Glibenclamide 2.5 mg once or twice daily, which needs to be adjusted by estimating her PG routinely.

RELATED INFORMATION

Oral hypoglycemic agents can be used to control blood glucose where nutritional therapy is failed. Two important agents are used.

Glibenclamide

Glibenclamide (Glyburide) is safe therapy for many GDM women. This drug decreases the insulin resistance and improves insulin secretion.

Placental transfer of glibenclamide is negligible. Langer et al. concluded that glyburide is as effective as insulin in maintaining the desired glycemic levels and resulted in a comparable outcome (Langer et al. 2000). Only 4% of women in the glyburide group were not adequately controlled and required insulin. The usual starting dose of glyburide is 2.5 mg once or twice daily. A randomized clinical trial comparing the effect of insulin and glyburide showed equally good glycemic control and similar perinatal outcome (Anjalakshi et al. 2007). The total daily dose may be increased up to 20 mg if necessary. The peak plasma level occurs 2–4 hours after administration and duration of action is 10–12 hours. Women with fasting hyperglycemia, but normal postprandial blood glucose may do well with a single dose of glyburide at bedtime. Glyburide is a sulfonylurea and its primary mechanism of action is stimulation of the release of insulin from the storage granules of pancreatic beta cells. Secondarily it decreases insulin resistance. It is nonteratogenic and is classified as a category B drug. The main side effect of glyburide is hypoglycemia.

Metformin

Though use of metformin in pregnancy is controversial, studies shows that it can prevent the development of GDM in high risk for developing that. There were no adverse effects to fetus and mother (Glueck et al. 2002; Begum et al. 2009). Metformin trial in gestational diabetes found that in women with GDM, metformin was not associated with increased perinatal complications as compared with insulin (Glueck et al. 2004). Usual dose is 500–1,500 mg daily in divided doses. Metformin appears to suppress hepatic glucose uptake and decreases intestinal absorption of glucose. It is also a category B drug and it does not cause hypoglycemia. More studies needed before recommendation for routine use in pregnancy.

> Suppose at 22 weeks of gestation you found her 2-hour PG 216 mg/dL (12 mmol). Predicting that only MNT may not work, you also have started oral hypoglycemic agent (Glibenclamide) and tried to adjust with 2.5 mg twice daily. But after 2 weeks of treatment her FPG and 2-hour postprandial PG were 108 mg/dL (6 mmol) and 145.1 mg/dL (8.06 mmol) respectively.
> What should be your next action?

As PG is not controlled to a desired level [FPG of ≤90 mg/dL (≤5 mmol) and 2-hour postprandial glucose level of ≤120.6 mg/dL (≤6.7)] with MNT and oral hypoglycemic agent insulin therapy is to be stared. The aim is to maintain the postprandial peak plasma glucose level of 120.6 mg/dL (6.7 mmol).

> Suppose at 24 weeks you found her PG level 2 hours after 75 g glucose is 197 mg/dL (10.94 mmol).
> Do you like to start with oral hypoglycemic agent?

No. Here PG level is high and needs to control efficiently. For which insulin therapy is needed. But MNT is to be advised along with insulin therapy.

RELATED INFORMATION

Human insulin is the insulin of choice for the first time. Most patients require a mixture of intermediate (NPH) and regular (short-acting) insulin twice daily. It is preferable to start with premix insulin (mixture of NPH and regular insulin) of any brand. Usually women with GDM do not require >20 unit insulin per day for glycemic control (Schmidt et al. 2001). Recommended dosing schedule is two-thirds of the total insulin dose is to be given in the morning and remainder before dinner. The morning dose should be two thirds NPH and one third short-acting insulin and the predinner dose should be equal parts NPH and short-acting insulin. However, dose schedule requires modification according to patent's body mass index (BMI), glucose level and lifestyle.

Insulin Analog

If postprandial glucose is still not under control, rapid-acting insulin analog is to be considered. Rapid-acting insulin analogs [aspart-(Novorapid), lispro (Humalog)] have been found to be safe and effective during pregnancy. Pregestational diabetic women during pregnancy may require high dose of insulin. A few may require multiple-daily injections usually given as short acting insulin before breakfast and lunch and intermediate acting insulin or premix before dinner. Insulin dose is always individualized and has to be adjusted according to need of the patient.

> During insulin therapy how will you monitor the patient?

For monitoring two things need to be tested.
1. Blood glucose.
2. HbA1c.

Measuring Blood Glucose Level

Once targeted blood glucose level is achieved woman with GDM require monitoring of both fasting and 2-hour post breakfast glucose once in a month till 28th weeks of gestation. After 28th weeks blood glucose monitoring should be done fortnightly or more frequently if needed. After 32 weeks blood glucose monitoring should be done once a week till delivery. In high risk pregnancies continuous glucose monitoring may be needed to know the glycemic fluctuations and to plan proper insulin dosage.

Meticulous monitoring is essential to achieve desired level of plasma glucose and to prevent postinsulin hypoglycemia. The success of treatment for a woman of GDM depends on glycemic control. Two hours postprandial blood glucose monitoring is preferable as the diagnosis of GDM is also based on two hour plasma glucose. GDM women have high post-breakfast plasma glucose level compared to post lunch and post dinner. So increased morning dose of short acting insulin is needed together with careful adjustment of meal timing and snacks to avoid hypoglycemia.

Measuring HbA1c

The A1c level is useful in monitoring the glucose control during pregnancy, but not for the day to day management. It serves as a prognostic value. In euglycemic state A1c value should be ≤6%. In early weeks of pregnancy A1c level is helpful to differentiate GDM from prepregnant diabetes. If A1c level is more than 6% it indicates that woman is pre-GDM (Balaji et al. 2007). Though treatment approach is not changed based on A1c level.

> GDM is a high-risk pregnancy.
> What measures need to take for fetus in intrauterine life?

The management of GDM, based on the fetal growth and developmental defect if there is any. USG is the key diagnostic tool to detect developmental defect as well as to monitor the fetal growth. Low-risk GDM patients who have glycemic control with diet alone and who do not develop any complications like polyhydramnios, pre-eclampsia or macrosomia need ultrasonogram around 24 weeks of gestation and thereafter as needed. High-risk GDM patients who are on insulin or oral antidiabetic agent should have antepartum fetal surveillance by ultrasonogram in every trimester. A fetal echo is a must at 24 weeks to rule out congenital defect. In last trimester biophysical profile is recommended twice in a week or weekly if fetus is at risk.

> Mrs Fatema is now at 34 weeks of gestation. Her blood sugar is under control and fetus is also fine with longitudinal lie and vertex presentation.
> How long you want to continue pregnancy and what will be mode of delivery?

As she is low-risk GDM and is not complicated, she will be allowed to term for spontaneous labor. Before allowing labor pelvis must be assessed to ensure pelvic adequacy.

RELATED INFORMATION

Low-risk or uncomplicated GDM patients may be allowed to develop spontaneous labor and to deliver at term. There is no need to deliver before term unless there is evidence of macrosomia, polyhydramnios, poor glycemic control or other obstetric complications such as, pre-eclampsia or intrauterine growth retardation. Once the uncomplicated GDM patient reaches 40 weeks labor should be induced if cervix is ripe. If cervix is not ripe and estimated fetal weight (EFW) is >4,000 g elective cesarean section is to be done. High-risk GDM patients should have their labor induced when they reach 38 weeks. Again CS is to be done if EFW is >4,000 g. Preterm pregnancy termination may be needed in GDM with complications such as pre-eclampsia, polyhydramnios, fetal compromise (less fetal movement) and uncontrolled diabetes. Glucocorticoid for 48 hours should be administered to accelerate lung maturity in preterm termination. Insulin requirement may be increased due to hyperglycemic effect of glucocorticoids. Spontaneous preterm labor is common in patient with GDM. Tocolysis in the form of magnesium sulfate or nifedipine can be used in preterm labor to delay delivery so that glucocorticoid therapy to accelerate lung maturity can be administered over 48 hours.

Management During Labor

Most insulin treated GDM do not need insulin during labor and after delivery. During labor it is essential to monitor blood glucose every 2-4 hours. Upward deviations from normal are corrected with small doses of regular insulin or low-dose IV insulin to maintain blood glucose between 100 and 120 mg/dL. If blood glucose is >120–140 mg/dL (>6.67–7.78 mmol), 4 unit insulin, if >140–180 mg/dL (>7.78–10 mmol) 6 unit insulin and if >180 mg/dL (>10 mmol) 8 unit insulin is to be given in a drip of normal saline at a rate of 16–20 drops/minute. Maternal capillary blood glucose is to be checked by glucometer every 1 hour and drip rate is to be adjusted. Dextrose infusion should be avoided. If it is given neutralizing dose of insulin is to be given. 1 unit insulin is needed to neutralize 2.5 g glucose. So to neutralize the glucose of 1,000 mL 5% dextrose saline 20 unit insulin is to be added with the drip. Drip rate is to be judged according to patient's requirement. Oral feeding is to be started as early as possible to avoid infusion of fluid. Monitoring should be done after delivery and 24 hours postpartum. Usually blood glucose level falls to baseline after delivery.

Neonatal Management

A neonatologist should be present during delivery as GDM is a high-risk pregnancy and there is chance of neonatal morbidity. Neonates are at risk of all complications similar to the infants born to mothers with overt diabetes (Carpenter et al. 2007). Neonates should be monitored closely after delivery for respiratory distress. Capillary blood glucose should be monitored at 1, 2 and 4 hours after birth and before starting of feeding. Cut-off value is 2.6 mmol. Early breastfeeding is strongly encouraged. If mother's blood glucose is not normalized insulin is advisable in lactating woman for good glycemic control.

> What are the complications of GDM?

The complications associated with GDM can affect both the mother and the fetus.

Mother

- *Type 2 DM:* Women who have had GDM are much more likely to develop type 2 DM later in life. A systematic review of 28 studies covering 28 years showed the cumulative incidence of type 2 DM to range from 2.6% to 70% of women who had GDM (Kim 2002).
- *Recurrent GDM:* In addition to developing type 2 DM later in life, women who have had GDM with one pregnancy are 30–69% more likely to develop GDM again in future pregnancies.
- *Obstetric complications:* Maternal polyhydramnios, hypertension and pre-eclampsia are often associated with GDM.

Fetus and the Neonate

- *Congenital malformations*: The risk of congenital malformations is slightly increased in infants of mothers with GDM compared to the general population. Diabetes strictly related to pregnancy has no increased risk of congenital malformations, but diabetes diagnosed during pregnancy, but pre-existing before pregnancy is associated with similar risk of congenital malformations to that of pre-existing diabetes. Thus, increased risk is of congenital malformations is associated with the presence of undiagnosed type 2 diabetes among women with GDM (Sheffield et al. 2002). There is a relationship between the risk of congenital malformations, maternal blood glucose levels and gestational age at which diabetes is diagnosed.
- *Macrosomia*: The complication that is perhaps the hallmark of GDM is macrosomia, defined as an infant weighing more than 4 kg. There is a positive correlation between maternal blood glucose levels and macrosomia. This relationship is probably due to fetal hyperinsulinism, secondary to maternal hyperglycemia. Maternal overweight and obesity is an additional risk factor for macrosomia (Ehrenberg et al. 2004). But appropriate treatment of GDM reduces the incidence of macrosomia (Horvath et al. 2010).

- *Perinatal death*: The increased risk of intrauterine fetal death and neonatal death associated with GDM when it is not well controlled and it is undiagnosed type 2 diabetes. Maternal obesity is often associated with GDM and is in itself an independent risk factor for perinatal complications, and macrosomia is the main factor linked to perinatal complications in GDM.
- *Birth injury*: Birth injuries and brachial plexus injuries are rarely associated with GDM and an increased risk of birth injuries due to untreated GDM has not been demonstrated. The absolute risk is low and mainly associated with macrosomia. Shoulder dystocia, a complication associated with macrosomia, is defined as impaction of the anterior shoulder of fetus behind the maternal pubic symphysis. This can lead to fetal injury and injury to mother.
- *Birth asphyxia*: May develop birth asphyxia, but it is not possible to establish a link between GDM and neonatal respiratory problems due to insufficient data.
- *Neonatal hypoglycemia*: Neonatal hypoglycemia occurs more often in pregnancies complicated by GDM, resulting in possible coma or even death if undetected. The risk of neonatal hypoglycemia is difficult to quantify in the absence of a consensual definition. However, the incidence of hypoglycemia requiring intravenous therapy is low.

> What is the long-term complication of GDM and how it can be prevented?

There is increased risk of development of type 2 DM in patients of GDM (Bartha et al. 2000) and incidence of type 2 DM is about 44% in patients who required insulin or OHA or onset of GDM before 24 weeks (Kjos and Buchanan, 1990). GDM may also recur in a future pregnancy and approximately 55% of patients who were obese or with macrosomic infants will have GDM in subsequent pregnancy (Philipson and Super, 1989). So it is important to perform a 75 g GTT at 6-8 weeks postpartum. If found normal, GTT is repeated after 6 months and every year to assess glucose tolerance. Patients should be informed that about 40–60% of them will have overt diabetics when they are in their fifth decades. Weight loss, dietary control and exercise will obviously help to prevent overt diabetes later in life (Grant et al. 1986). The GDM has a far reaching consequence in predisposing their offsprings to glucose intolerance. Debelea et al. found that more than 50% children who were born to women with GDM developed type 2 DM by the age 35 (Dabelea et al. 2000). The important aspect of GDM is that the intrauterine milieu whether one of nutritional deprivation or nutritional plenty, results in fetal pancreatic development and peripheral response to insulin that may lead to adult onset GDM and type 2 DM (Savona and Chircop, 2003). So the timely action in all pregnant women with glucose intolerance to achieve euglycemia may prevent transmitting glucose intolerance from one generation to another (Aerts, 2004).

Gestational diabetes mellitus (GDM) women are at increased risk of future type 2 diabetes mellitus and their children are also at risk of developing type 2 DM later in their life. Universal screening for GDM at early weeks of gestation can detect more cases at an early stage leading to early interventions and hence improves maternal and fetal outcome as early detection leads to early treatment and prevent complications and adverse effect to mother and fetus. A 2-hour 75 g postglucose ≥7.8 mmol/L serves both as screening and diagnostic criteria, which is a simple and economical one step procedure. Early detection and treatment of GDM can only prevent the all probable complications and the vicious cycle of transmitting glucose intolerance from generation to generation.

BIBLIOGRAPHY

Aerts L. Intergenerative transmission of DM. Abstract volume of the 36th Annual Meeting of the DPSG, Luso-Portugal, 2004.

American College of Obstetricians and Gynecologists Committee on Practice Bulletins Obstetrics ACOG Practice Bulletin. Clinical management guidelines for obstetrician gynecologists. September (2001). Replaces Technical Bulletin Number 200, December 1994. Gestational diabetes. Obstet Gynecol. 2001; 98(30):525-38.

American Diabetes Association. Diagnosis and classification of diabetes mellitus. Diabetes Care. 2006; (Suppl 1):S43-8.

American Diabetes Association. Gestational diabetes mellitus. American Diabetes Association. Diabetes Care. 2003; (suppl 1):5103-5.

American Diabetes Association. Gestational Diabetes Mellitus: American Diabetes Association-Clinical Practice Recommendations Diabetes Care. 2002; 25(1):S94-6.

Anjalakshi C, Balaji V, Balaji MS, et al. A prospective study comparing insulin and glibenclamide in gestational diabetes mellitus in Asian Indian women. Dia Res Clin Pract. 2007;76(3):474-5.

Anjalakshi C, Balaji V, Balaji MS, et al. A single test procedure to diagnose gestational diabetes mellitus. Acta Diabetol. 2009;46(1):51-4.

Arias F, Daftary SN, Bhide AG. Practical guide to high-risk pregnancy and delivery. A South Asian perspective. Elsevier. Diabetes and pregnancy; 2008.pp.440-64.

Balaji V, Madhuri BS, Ashalatha S, et al. A1c in gestational diabetes mellitus in Indian Asian women. Diabetes Care. 2007;30(7):1865-7.

Bartha JL, Martinez del fresno P, Comino delgado. Gestational diabetes mellitus diagnosed during early pregnancy. Am J Obstet Gynecol. 2000;182(2):346-50.

Begum MR, Khanam NN, Quadir E, et al. Prevention of GDM by continuing metformin therapy throughout pregnancy in women with polycystic ovary syndrome (PCOS). J Obstet Gynecol. 2009;35(2):282-6.

Beischer NA, Oats JN, Henry OA, et al. Incidence and severity of gestational diabetes mellitus according to country of birth in women living in Australia. Diabetes.1991;40(Suppl: 2):35-8.

Carpenter MW, Canick JA, Hogan JW, et al. Amniotic fluid insulin at 14-20 weeks' gestation: association with later maternal glucose intolerance and birth macrosomia. Diabetes Care. 2001;24(7): 1259-63.

Cousins L, Rigg L, Hollingsworth D, et al. The 24 hour excursion and diurnal rhythm of glucose, insulin and C-peptide in normal pregnancy. Am J Obstet Gynecol. 1980;136:483-488.

Crowther CA, Hiller JE, Moss JR, et al. Effect of treatment of gestational diabetes mellitus. N Engl J Med. 2005;352(24):2477-86.

Dabelea D, Knowler WC, Pettitt DJ. Effect of diabetes in pregnancy and offspring: follow-up research in the Pima Indians. J Matern Fetal Medicine. 2000;9:83-8.

Divakar H, Tyagi S, Hosmani P, Manyonda IT. Diagnostic criteria influence prevalence rates for gestational diabetes: implications for interventions in an Indian pregnant population. Perinatology. 2008.pp.155-61.

Dorendra Singh IBidhumukhi Devi Th, Ibeyaima Devi Kh, Premchand Singh Th. Scientific Presentation Volume of the First National Conference of the DIPSI, 2006; Chennai. 68.

Ehrenberg HM, Mercer BM, Catalano PM, et al. The influence of obesity and diabetes on the prevalence of macrosomia. Am J Obstet Gynecol. 2004;191:964-8.

Franks PW, Looker HC, Kobes S, et al. Gestational Glucose tolerance and risk of type 2 diabetes in Young Pima Indian Offspring. Diabetes. 2006;55(2): 460-5.

Glueck CJ, Goldenberg N, Pranikoff J, et al. Height, weight and motor-social development during the first 18 months of life in 126 infants born to 109 mothers with polycystic ovary syndrome who conceived on and continued metformin throughout pregnancy. Hum Reprod. 2004;19(6):1323-30.

Glueck CJ, Wang P, Kobayashi S, et al. Metformin therapy throughout pregnancy reduces the development of gestational diabetes in women with polycystic ovary syndrome. Fertil Steril. 2002;77:520-5.

Grant PT, Oats JN, Beischer N. The long term follow-up of women with gestational diabetes. Aust N Z J Obstet Gynecol. 1986;26:17-22.

Horvath K, Koch K, Jeitler K, et al. Effects of treatment in women with gestational diabetes mellitus: systematic review and meta-analysis. BMJ. 2010;340: c1395.

Kim C, Newton R, Knopp R. Gestational diabetes and the incidence of type 2 diabetes: a systematic review. Diabetes Care. 2002;25:1862-8.

Kjos SL, Buchanan. Gestational diabetes mellitus: the prevalence of glucose intolerance and diabetes mellitus in the first two months postpartum. AM J Obstet Gynecol. 1990;163:93-8.

Langer O, Cornway DL, Berkus MD, et al. A comparison of glyburide and insulin in GDM. N Engl J Med. 2000; 343(16):1134-8.

Metzger BE, Buchanan TA, Coustan DR, et al. Summary and recommendations of the Fifth International Workshop-Confer ence on Gestational Diabetes Mellitus. Diabetes Care. 2007;(Suppl 2):S: 251-60.

Metzger BE, Coustan DR. Summary and Recommendations of the Fourth International workshop-Conference on Gestational Diabetes Mellitus. Diabetes Care. 1998;B:161-7.

Metzger BE, Coustan DR. Summary and recommendations of the Fourth International Workshop-Conference on Gestational Diabetes Mellitus. The Organizing Committee. Diabetes Care. 1998; (Suppl 2):B:161-7.

Nahum GG, Wilson SB, Stanislaw H. Early pregnancy glucose screening for gestational diabetes mellitus. J Reprod Med. 2002;47(8):656-62.

Pettitt DJ, Bennett PH, Hanson RL, et al. Comparison of World Health Organization and National Diabetes Data Group procedures to detect abnormalities of glucose tolerance during pregnancy. Diabetes Care. 1994;17(11):1264-8.

Pettitt DJ, Bennett PH, Saad MF, et al. Abnormal glucose tolerance during pregnancy in Pima Indian women: Long term effects on the offspring. Diabetes. 1991;40(2):126-30.

Philipson EH, Super DN. Gestational diabetes mellitus: does it recur in subsequent pregnancy? AM J Obstet Gynecol. 1989;160:1324-31.

Polonsky KS, Given BD, Van Cauter E. Twenty four hour profiles and pulsatile patterns of insulin secretion in normal and obese subjects. J Clin Invest. 1988;81(2):442-8.

Savona Ventura C, Chircop, M. Birth weight influence on the Subsequent development of gestational diabetes mellitus. Acta Diabetol. 2003;40:101-4.

Schmidt MI, Duncan BB, Reichelt AJ, et al. For the Brazilian Gestational Diabetes Study Group. Gestational diabetes mellitus diagnosed with a 2-h 75-g oral glucose tolerance test and adverse pregnancy outcomes. Diabetes Care. 2001;24(7): 1151-5.

Seshiah V, Alexander C, Balaji V, et al. Glycemic control from early weeks of gestation and pregnancy outcome. Diabetes. 2006; Supp1:604.

Seshiah V, Balaji V, Balaji MS, et al. Gestational Diabetes Mellitus manifests in all trimesters of pregnancy. Dia Res Clin Pract. 2007;77(3):482-4.

Seshiah V, Balaji V, Madhuri S Balaji, et al. Gestational Diabetes Mellitus in India. JAPI. 2004;52:707-11.

Seshiah V, Cynthia A, Balaji V, et al. Detection and care of women with gestational diabetes mellitus from early weeks of pregnancy results in birth weight of newborn babies appropriate for gestational age. Dia Res Clin Pract. 2008;80(2):199-202.

Shamsuddin K, Mahdy ZA, Siti Rafiaah I, et al. Risk factor screening for abnormal glucose tolerance in pregnancy. Int J Gynecol Obstet. 2001;75: 27-32.

Sheffield JS, Butler-Koster EL, Casey BM, et al. Maternal diabetes mellitus and infant malformations. Obstet Gynecol. 2002;100:925-30.

Super DM, Edelberg SC, Philipson EH, et al. Diagnosis of gestational diabetes in early pregnancy. Diabetes Care. 1991;14(4):288-94.

Swami SR, Mehetre R, Shivane V, et al. Prevalence of Carbohydrate Intolerance of Varying Degrees in Pregnant Females in Western India (Maharashtra). A Hospital based Study. J Indian Med Association. 2008;106:712-5.

CHAPTER 8

Rhesus Isoimmunization

Nurun Nahar Khanam, Rashida Begum

INTRODUCTION

The rhesus (Rh) blood group is the most complex human blood group. In the year 1940 Landsteiner discovered some specific antigen system on the human erythrocytes. The same antigen also present in the Rhesus monkey, thus the antigen was named Rh antigen. The individual having the antigen called Rh positive and those who does not have is called Rh negative. The Rh factor is modified by two genes *RHD* and *RHCE*. The complete genetic makeup of the Rh blood group of an individual is its genotype. The Rh antigens are grouped in three pairs: Dd, Cc, and Ee. The major antigen in this group is RhD, particular concern. An Rh-negative mother carries an Rh positive fetus, serious complications may pursue due to production of antibody against the fetal Rh-antigen that enters the maternal circulation. An individual carrying D of both sets of antigen (DD) is called homozygous and when carrying D only in one set (Dd), it is called heterozygous. Heterozygous persons are always classified as Rh-positive because D is dominant to d. Rh-positive persons are either (DD) homozygous (45%) or (Dd) heterozygous positive (55%). If father is homozygous (DD) positive, all of his children will be heterozygous (Dd) Rh-positive but if he is heterozygous positive (Dd), his children will have a 50% chance of being heterozygous Rh-positive (Dd) and 50% will be Rh-negative (dd). Alloimmunization to antigens other than D, i.e. C and E is rare. So, C and E antigens usually cause immunization via blood transfusion, not as a consequence of fetal-maternal bleeding (Roman and Pernoll, 2007).

Case scenario: Mrs Beauty with Rh-negative blood group presents at her 28 weeks of pregnancy with history of previous two pregnancy loss.
How will you proceed to manage her?

When an Rh-negative woman presents with previous fetal loss, one has to keep in mind that the possibility of severe form of Rh isoimmunization. To manage this patient, we need to go through her history, perform examination and do some investigations.

Detailed History is to be Taken First

- History of previous blood transfusion
- Current pregnancy complaints should be noted. Any history of threatened abortion, antepartum hemorrhage (APH) or trauma should be noted.
- Whether she was under regular antenatal checkup or not in this pregnancy?
- Has she done Rh antibody titer? If yes, was the antibody present? If yes, what was the level at first trimester and what is the present level? Is the titer gradually increasing or suddenly increased. Sudden rise of titer indicates new fetomaternal hemorrhage. A titer of 1:4 is significant and indicates maternal sensitization (Gilbert, 2011).
- Does she suffer from diabetes mellitus or any other infection, which may results non-immune hydrops of her fetus?
- Was there any anomaly scan in the present pregnancy?
- Does she know about her husband's blood group?

Past Obstetric History

- How many times she did conceive?
- What were the fate of those pregnancies?
- History of abortion, menstrual regulation (MR), ectopic, pregnancy, molar pregnancy, preterm or term delivery
- History of any still birth or abnormal fetus
- What were the gestational age of previous pregnancies? This is important for management purpose because we have to start fetal surveillance at least 4 weeks prior to the gestational age of previous affected pregnancy loss.
- Was she under antenatal care (ANC) in last pregnancies?
- Did she receive any anti-D prophylaxis in previous pregnancies?

Clinical Examination

- Anemia should be looked for
- Blood pressure (BP) should be checked because there may be associated pre-eclampsia
- Edema should be checked
- Abdominal girth may be raised, if there is polyhydramnios
- By assessing BP, edema and abdominal girth it is to be assessed whether her current pregnancy is complicated with polyhydramnios or pre-eclampsia, as these conditions are associated with Rh-isoimmunization.

> On enquiry you elicited that her first pregnancy was aborted completely at 14 weeks of gestation. She did not consult with any doctor. Again she conceived spontaneously after 6 months of abortion and was not under antenatal check-up. At her 36 weeks of gestation labor pain started and delivered an edematous dead baby vaginally at home. At this current pregnancy this is the first time at 28 weeks she came to consult with the doctor. She does not know about her husband's blood group. On examination she found with normal parameters.
>
> What initial investigations will you suggest for her?

- Routine investigations for pregnancy such as HB%, urine R/E, blood sugar, hepatitis B surface antigen (HBsAg) should be checked.
- Blood group of husband, if Rh-positive, then genotyping is to be done to find out zygosity (DD or Dd).
- Estimation of Rh antibody titer. Critical level varies from center to center. A titer of 1:32 is always considered critical.
- Ultrasonography to see fetal condition.

> On preliminary investigation, you found her antibody titer is 1:32. Her husband's blood group is Rh-positive with Dd genotype. Ultrasound revealed nothing gross abnormality of the fetus.
>
> What is your diagnosis?
>
> What is the basis of your diagnosis?
>
> What will you do for further evaluation of the fetal condition?

Diagnosis

Possibly it is a case of Rh isoimmunization with previously affected pregnancy.

Basis of the Diagnosis

Her blood group is negative and husband's blood group is Rh-positive; she lost her first pregnancy by abortion and no anti-D was given at that time. She was not under antenatal check up during her second pregnancy, though there is no evidence of Rh-isoimmunization as she did not measure her antibody titer, but she told her second baby had hydropic changes. So, possibly that baby was affected by Rh-isoimmunization.

Evaluation of the Fetal Condition

Following investigations should be done for fetal evaluation.

Noninvasive

- Cell-free fetal DNA (cffDNA) from maternal plasma to identify fetal Rh typing and genotype. It can be found positive as early as 38th days of conception with 99.5% accuracy (Geifman-Holtzman et al. 2006). Advantage of this testing is that it can avoid routine antenatal anti-D prophylaxis (RAADP) in 40% Rh-negative women, who carries Rh-negative babies (Lee et al. 1999).
- Middle cerebral artery (MCA) peak systolic velocity (PSV) to detect fetal anemia.

- Non-stress test: Fetus affected by anemia shows following changes in electronic fetal monitoring:
  - A base line heart rate of 180 beats/minute or greater
  - Deceleration or loss of short-term variability with presence of sine wave long-term variability (sinusoidal pattern).

Invasive

- Amniocentesis to detect bilirubin concentration and fetal Rh typing
- Cordocentesis for precise measurement of the fetal hematocrit and hemoglobin concentration.

Both tests will be done to detect any affection of the baby and severity of affection if any.

> How frequently do you want to test her Rh antibody?

This patient does not need further antibody testing as predictive value of antibody is lost in previously immunized women.

RELATED INFORMATION

Monitoring of Rh-negative Women by Antibody Testing

Anti Rh antibody titers are done to determine the risk of fetal anemia. The frequency of testing depends on whether the mother is immunized or not immunized. If immunized, whether for the first time or subsequent time.

First test is to be done within 12th weeks of pregnancy:
1. If it is negative or mother is not immunized, it is to be repeated at 28th and 36th week in primigravida. In multigravida, the test is to be repeated at monthly intervals from 24th weeks onwards.
2. If test is positive or mother is immunized for the first time:
   - Test is to be done every 4 weeks, up to 36 weeks of gestation if titer remains under the critical level (1:32). Afterwards delivery should be planned by elective induction between 38 and 40 weeks of gestation. Nonaffected or mildly affected Rh-positive fetus is anticipated.
   - There is no further use of antibody titer for follow-up of first immunized mother if:
     - The titer is found to be at or above the critical level (1:32) on the initial evaluation
     - The titer reaches or exceeds the critical level (1:32) at any time during gestation
     - There is a significant rise in titer between two consecutive samples
   - In these circumstances further management will be based on fetal assessment using:
     a. The middle-cerebral artery peak systolic velocity (MCA PSV)
     b. The concentration of bilirubin in the amniotic fluid by amniocentesis.
3. Immunized women with previously affected pregnancy do not need antibody titer for follow-up of pregnancy because the ability to predict fetal anemia from maternal anti D titers is lost. Titers are no longer predictive for fetal outcome in women with prior affected pregnancies. They should be followed with:
   - Serial determinations of the MCA PSV
   - With concentration of bilirubin in the amniotic fluid.

> Mrs Beauty's first MCA PSV shows 1.5 multiples of the median. How frequently do you like to do MCA PSV and high-resolution ultrasonography for Beauty.

If any baby is affected by Rh-isoimmunization, chance of affection of Rh-positive baby in next pregnancy is about 90%. Moreover, subsequent affection occurs earlier than previous one. So, she should be monitored by MCA PSV Doppler ultrasonography and high-resolution real time ultrasonography every 1–2 weeks to detect fetal anemia and structural changes at earlier.

RELATED INFORMATION

Role of Ultrasonography in the Management of Sensitized Rh-negative Patients

Ultrasonography is the non-invasive assessment of fetal condition.

Doppler Ultrasound

Fetal anemia can be predicted by peak flow velocity in the fetal MCA. So MCA and PSV can be considered as an accurate noninvasive method for the diagnosis of fetal anemia (Mari et al. 1995). As fetal hemoglobin decreases the correlation between MCA PSV and fetal anemia becomes stronger (Mari et al. 2000). When fetus becomes anemic, cardiac output increased and blood viscosity drops, which causes an increased blood flow velocity in the cerebral artery (ACOG, 2006; Moise, 2008).

Advantages of MCA-PSV

Advantages of MCA-PSV are that fetal anemia can be detected at earlier when high-resolution ultrasound evaluation is still normal. It is a noninvasive procedure without risk to mother and fetus. Fetal anemia can be diagnosed by two methods PSV and amniotic fluid bilirubin. PSV has better predictive values than amniotic fluid bilirubin concentration (Nishie et al. 2003, Pereira et al. 2003). PSV can reduce the need for invasive diagnostic procedures like amniocentesis and cordocentesis by more than 70% (Zimmerman, 2002). PSV also can be used to fix the time for repeat fetal transfusion. If needed MCA Doppler studies can be started as early as 18 weeks' of gestation, but the test is not reliable after 35 weeks' of gestation (ACOG, 2006).

Disadvantage of MCA-PSV

Disadvantage is that a false positive rate for the diagnosis of fetal anemia is high about 12%.

High-resolution Real Time Ultrasonography

Fetal hemolytic disease causes fetal ascites, pericardial effusion, liver enlargement and placental swelling. As fetal structure can be clearly visualized by *High-resolution real time ultrasonography* fetal structural changes due to hemolysis can be detected at the earliest. Accuracy of ultrasound in detecting the signs of fetal hemolytic disease is better than invasive amniotic fluid bilirubin measurement (Frigoletto et al. 1986, Reece et al. 1989). Another advantage of assessment of fetal anemia by ultrasound is, it has no false positive result like MCA PSV and the amniotic fluid bilirubin as detection of ascites is proof of anemia.

But, disadvantage is that it can detect only advance degree of fetal anemia when hydrops develops with a hematocrit of less than 20% and intrauterine transfusion is necessary. In many patients, onset of hydrops is sudden, so serial ultrasound is needed to detect it.

> Suppose on ultrasonography, there is no features of fetal abnormality, but MCA PSV showed more than 1.5 MoM.
>
> What will be your next step to manage her?

The next step should be amniotic fluid analysis for the assessment of severity of anemia and to assess fetal pulmonary maturation as well.

> Patient has history of previous delivery of IUD. This time titer is also high. You did amniocentesis at initial visit at 28 weeks. Spectrophotometric reading falls into zone 2 of Lily's graph.
>
> When do you like to do next amniocentesis?

Next amniocentesis will be done after 1 week to see any changes of Lylie's graph.

RELATED INFORMATION

Amniocentesis in evaluation and management of fetus in Rh isoimmunization.

Amniocentesis is done to collect amniotic fluid:
- To detect fetal genotype, if father is heterozygous positive
- To measure bilirubin to determine whether fetus is affected or not:
  - When antibody titre rises more than 1:8
  - When MCA PSV value is >1.5 MoMs.
- To measure lecithin sphingomyelin ratio to assess fetal lung maturity.

It is done for determining the optimal time for intrauterine transfusion or for delivery of the fetus:
- Usually the first amniocentesis is performed at 20 weeks
- But, in women who start off with high titer, who have had a baby that was hydropic or died in uterus or whose ultrasound evaluation demonstrates early sign of fetal hydrops, the first amniocentesis may done at 16 weeks and

should be repeated according to Liley's graph, discussed below
- When there is no history of previously affected baby test is to be done at 30–32 weeks and second test should be repeated after 3–4 weeks.

Spectrophotometric analysis of amniotic fluid is done for bilirubin concentration. About 5–10 mL of amniotic fluid is required for spectrophotometric analysis. The result is recorded in Liley graph, which has been divided into 3 zones, upper (Zone 3), middle (Zone 2) and lower (Zone 1). The $\Delta OD450$ value is used for patient management (Fig. 8.1):

A. When $\Delta OD450$ value lies in lower zone or zone 1 (<0.09), there is no immediate danger of IUD and procedure should be repeated at 4 weeks interval.
   - If values remained in zone 1 at repeated test delivery at term will be allowed. Either non-affected or mildly affected baby is anticipated.
   - If at any time values go up to that of zone 2, patient is to be managed as zone 2 described below.
   - If at any time values go up to that of zone 3, patient is to be managed as zone 3 described below.

B. When $\Delta OD450$ value lies in middle zone or zone 2 (0.09–1.5) it indicates that fetus is affected in range of *mild to severe* form (*moderately affected*):
   - Repeat the test after 1 week. Management will depend upon the following results:
     - If values go down to the zone 1 patient is to be managed as zone 1 mentioned above
     - If values decreasing, but still in zone 2, repeat amniocentesis in 2 weeks. If repeat values unchanged and still in zone 2, repeat amniocentesis in 1 week. If the horizontal trend continues plan delivery, if lung is mature and cordocentesis, and fetal hematocrit assessment is indicated, if lung is not matured.
     - If values go up to zone 3, patient is to be managed as zone 3 described below.

C. When $\Delta OD450$ value lies in upper zone or zone 3 (>0.15) at first test or previously was in zone 1 or zone 2 and moved to zone 3, it indicates that fetus is *severely affected* and is in imminent danger of IUD.
   - If gestational age is between 34 and 37 weeks, lung maturity test is to be done. If it is positive, delivery is to be planned. If lung is not matured, corticosteroid is to be given to accelerate lung maturity and delivery is to be planned.

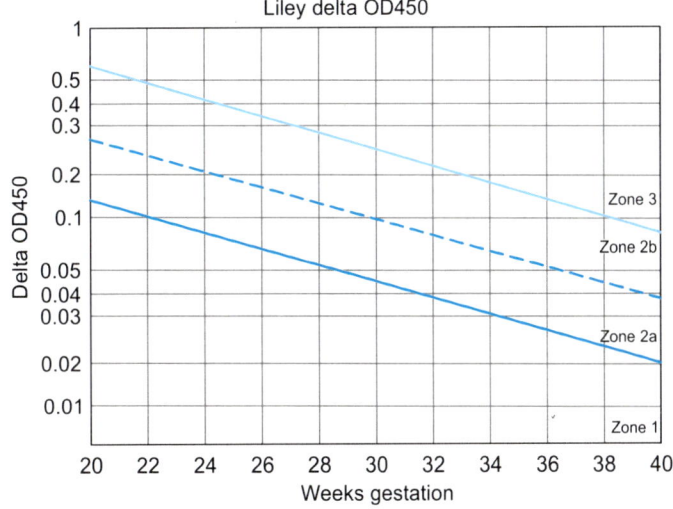

Fig. 8.1 Liley's curve

- If gestational age is <34 weeks, cordocentesis is to be done to measure fetal hematocrit:
  1. If hematocrit is <30%, intrauterine transfusion (IUT) is to be given to raise hematocrit up to 40–45%.
  2. Repeat cordocentesis and IUT is to be done at weekly interval till 34 weeks. Beyond 34 weeks of gestation, the risk of cordocentesis and IUT is higher than delivery, and neonatal exchange transfusion.
  3. If hematocrit is >30% fetus will be followed-up with repeat cordocentesis and USG till 34 weeks. Delivery is to be planned after lung maturity testing.

Limitation of Liley Curve

Limitation of Liley curve is that it starts at 26 weeks, gestation and extrapolation of the lines to earlier gestational ages is inaccurate. Some investigators (Queenan et al. 1993) have developed a curve for fetal assessment from 14 to 40 weeks, divided into 4 zones.

Complications of amniocentesis: Infections resulting chorioamnionitis leads to preterm labor and preterm delivery.

Caution

- Mild contractions may occur following the procedure, which usually subsides after 30–40 minutes. Patient should be instructed to report, if contractions continue or increased. Tocolysis therapy may be needed in that case.
- In multiple pregnancy fluid should be collected from each gestational sac.

False Interpretation

- Meconium causes a marked rise in bilirubin value. So, meconium stained specimen should not be used for patient management.
- Increased amount of fluid in polyhydramnios dilute the bilirubin content of amniotic fluid resulting in falsely low bilirubin values.
- Contamination of maternal blood will distort the measurement of bilirubin and should not be used for patient management. In gross contamination amniocentesis should be postponed for 1 week.

> After 4 weeks at 32 weeks of gestation, MCA Doppler studies shows >1.5 multiples of the median, ultrasound shows scalp edema and ascites of the fetus and spectrophotometric reading after amniocentesis falls into zone 3 of the Liley graph.
> What is your next plan to do?

This is the indication of severely affected fetus. At this moment fetal blood sampling or cordocentesis is necessary to determine the degree of anemia and need of intrauterine blood transfusion.

> You did cordocentesis and found hematocrit is 25% and HB is 9 g/dL.
> What is your next plan to do? How many times do you like to do it?

Intrauterine transfusion is to be given to raise the hematocrit to 40–45%. Intrauterine transfusion can be given every 1–4 weeks. For this patient cordocentesis will be done at weekly interval till 34 weeks. After that delivery will be planned with corticosteroid therapy as IUT is more risky than premature delivery and newborn exchange transfusion.

RELATED INFORMATION

Cordocentesis (Fetal Blood Sampling) in Management of Rh Isoimmunization

Cordocentesis is the puncture of umbilical vein:
- To collect blood to detect fetal blood type, hematocrit, DCT and total bilirubin level. HCT value <15% is associated with hydrops.
- To transfuse blood in severely affected fetus.

Indications of Cordocentesis

The main indications of cordocentesis are:
1. A combination of MCA PSV >1.5 MoMs above the mean and an amniotic fluid bilirubin values in the high-middle zone or zone 3.
2. Hydrops fetalis in ultrasonogram
   Blood sample is collected to determine the severity of the hemolytic process. A hematocrit

of less than 35% is an indication for intrauterine transfusion. Intrauterine transfusion also given through the same vein. Umbilical vein is identified by high-resolution ultrasonogram and color flow mapping.

Disadvantages

- It is an invasive procedure and the most common complication of umbilical vein blood sampling is bleeding, which is usually transient:
- Blood loss from cordocentesis may be severe and may cause fetal death
- May also cause fetomaternal bleeding
- Thrombosis of the umbilical vessels and severe vasospasm with secondary fetal bradycardia are procedural complications
- The risk of fetal death following cordocentesis is approximately 1.5% after 24 weeks and it may be as high as 5% before 24 weeks.

Intrauterine Transfusion

Since 1963, intrauterine transfusion (IUT) has been instrumental in saving hundreds of infants affected by hemolytic disease secondary to Rh-isoimmunization. Blood transfusion is given to replace fetal red blood cells (RBC) those are being destroyed by immune system of Rh-sensitized mother. Due to hemolysis fetus becomes anemic. So to keep the fetus healthy until it's maturity, intrauterine transfusion is given to replace the red blood cells. Outcome depends on the experience and skills of the performer, severity of the disease, fetal lie and position and maternal obesity.

Indications

Intrauterine blood transfusions are done when:
- Fetus is anemic, diagnosed by Doppler ultrasound of the middle cerebral artery, and fetal blood sampling.
- Fetus is moderately or severely affected diagnosed by amniocentesis (shows increased value of bilirubin in amniotic fluid).
- Hydrops fetalis diagnosed by Ultrasound.

In a severely affected fetus, transfusions are given every 1–4 weeks till fetal maturity, which is determined by assessing fetal lung maturity by amniocentesis.

Types of IUT

There are two type of IUT: (i) Intraperitoneal, (ii) Intravascular. In both methods, the procedure is carried out under visual control with real-time ultrasound. Umbilical cord vessel transfusion is the preferred method because it permits better absorption of blood and has a higher survival rate than does transfusion through the abdomen (Moise, 2008). Compatible blood ideally 'O' negative irradiated blood is transfused.

In intraperitoneal IUT, the blood is injected into the peritoneal cavity and transported by the lymphatic system into the fetal blood stream. In intravascular IUT blood is injected into the umbilical circulation.

The two types of IUT are not mutually exclusive. They complement each other and either one or both of them may be used depending on the circumstances. Although, the direct intravascular approach is the procedure of choice, but if the approach to umbilical cord is difficult, then intraperitoneal transfusion is done.

The overall survival rate of the fetuses is 80.1–84.8% for hydropic and 89.5% for non-hydropic fetuses.

Risk of IUT

Intrauterine transfusion has a potential for serious complications. The procedure related complication is 3.1%:
- Uterine infection
- Fetal infection
- Preterm labor
- Excessive bleeding and mixing of fetal and maternal blood
- Rupture of membrane
- Fetal death
- Perinatal death was 11% (Van Kamp et al. 2005).

> When and how fetal pulmonary maturity is considered?

The classical to the management of sensitized Rh-negative mother was early delivery depending on the severity of the fetal hemolytic process.

This has changed and at present most maternal-fetal medicine specialists perform the last transfusion at about 35–36 weeks and deliver at 37–38 weeks' gestation. If delivery before 35 weeks, then lung maturity test is necessary when delivery is the treatment of choice. The use of steroids to accelerate the maturity of fetal lung is recommended (Arias, et al. 1979 and Caritis, et al. 1977) by betamethasone 12 mg IM daily for 2 consecutive days or dexamethasone 6 mg every 12 hours for four doses is equally effective.

> Suppose you planned to deliver the baby by cesarean section.
> What precaution do you need to take during and after surgery.

Following precautions should be taken to reduce fetomaternal hemorrhage (FMH):
- Precautions during cesarean section is to prevent blood spilling into the peritoneal cavity and manual removal of placenta should not be done as a routine.
- Prophylactic ergometrine should preferably be withheld, as it may facilitate fetomaternal transfusion.
- Manual removal of placenta should be done gently (Roman and Pernoll, 2007).

After delivery, cord blood is to be collected to test the following to assess whether exchange transfusion is needed or not.
- Fetal blood grouping and Rh typing is need to know, which is already known in this case from blood sampling.
- HB%, HCT, reticulocyte count, Coombs test and bilirubin level.

> Does Mrs Beauty need anti-D immunoglobulin after delivery?

No, once mother is immunized, there is no use of anti-D prophylaxis. Antibody remains in the circulation rest of the life.

RELATED INFORMATION

Incidence of Rh-negative Blood Group

The incidence of Rh negativity in Indian subcontinent is 5–10%. Basque populations have the highest incidence of Rh negativity (30–35%). Caucasian populations have the higher incidence (15–16%). Blacks in the United States have a rate of 8% and African blacks are 4%. The incidence in Indian subcontinent is 5–10%.

In Rh-negative mothers, the overall risk of isoimmunization for an Rh positive ABO compatible infant is about 16%. Of these, 1.5–2% of reactions will occur antepartum, 7% within the 6 months of delivery and the remainder 7% early in the second pregnancy. ABO incompatibility between the Rh positive fetus and Rh negative mother provides some protection against Rh isoimmunization; the overall incidence is 1.5–2%. In mothers who receive prophylaxis with Rh immunoglobulin, the risk of isoimmunization is reduced to 0.2% (Roman and Pernoll, 2007).

> What is Rh incompatibility?

Presence of Rh-positive fetus in an Rh-negative mother is known as Rh incompatibility.

> What is Rh-isoimmunization?

The Rh-isoimmunization is the production of immune antibodies in an individual in response to foreign red cell antigen derived from another individual of the same species provided the first one lacks the antigen.

> Diagnosis of Rh-isoimmunization.

For the diagnosis of Rh-isoimmunization, we need to do following test:
- All Rh-negative pregnant women should screen for Rh-antibody at their first antenatal visit. The presence of anti-D antibodies in the serum is diagnostic of maternal Rh alloimmunization or isoimmunization.
- The possibility of Rh-isoimmunization before delivery is small (about 1%).
- If first test is negative, to identify the few Rh-negative women who will develop antepartum sensitization, the antibody screening should be repeated at 20, 24, and 28 week of gestation.

How does Rh-isoimmunization occur?

Rh antigens are lipoproteins that are confined to the red cell membrane. Isoimmunization may occur by 2 mechanisms:
1. Following incompatible blood transfusion.
2. Following FMH between a (Rh-negative) mother and an incompatible (Rh-positive) fetus. FMH may occur during pregnancy or at delivery. About 15–50% occur during third stage of labor and following cesarean section or manual removal of placenta. Though in 1–2% cases a continuous fetomaternal bleed occurs throughout normal pregnancies. With no apparent predisposing factors, fetal red cells have been detected in maternal blood in 6.7% of women at first trimester, 15.5% during the second trimester and 28.9% during the third trimester.

- When Rh-negative mother carries a Rh-positive fetus mother develops antibodies against fetal RBC after FMH.

What are the predisposing factors for FMH?

- Spontaneous, induced and threatened abortion
- Surgical dilation and curettage (D and C) or medical treatment (prostaglandin) of abortion
- Ectopic pregnancy
- Molar pregnancy
- Chorionic villus sampling
- Amniocentesis
- Cordocentesis
- Feto reduction
- Abdominal trauma by accident or external version
- Placenta praevia with bleeding
- Abruptio placenta
- Fetal death
- Multiple pregnancy
- Normal delivery
- Cesarean section
- Manual removal of placenta
- Lack of prenatal care.

Why all Rh-negative women do not develop isoimmunization?

Immunization is unlikely to occur unless at least 0.1 mL of fetal blood enters into the maternal circulation. About 17% of Rh negative women will become alloimmunized by a single delivery. Risk of sensitization depends largely upon following factors, so all Rh negative women do not develop Rh-isoimmunization:

1. Extent of maternal immune response:
   - Inborn inability to respond to the Rh-antigen stimulus
   - Immunologic nonresponder is found in 30% of Rh negative women
   - Variation in the strength of the Rh-antigenic stimulus, which depends on the Rh genotype of the fetal blood, e.g. *CDe/cde* genotype.
2. *Volume of transplacental hemorrhage*: Volume of fetal blood entering into the maternal circulation (0.1 mL is considered as critical sensitizing volume) (Konar, 2012). Although exact number of Rh-positive cells necessary to cause isoimmunization of the Rh-negative women is unknown, as little as 0.1 mL of Rh-positive cells can cause sensitization. When the number of fetal cells entering into the maternal circulation is more, possibility of maternal sensitization is more.
3. *Concurrent presence of ABO incompatibility*: ABO incompatibility is protective against the development of Rh sensitization. When the mother is type O and the father is type A, B or AB the incidence reduced dramatically to 1–2%. As mother's blood contains antibodies against the ABO blood group of fetus, fetal RBC those enter into maternal circulation are destroyed rapidly by maternal antibody before Rh sensitization. As a result ABO incompatibility does not take place.

How does first baby escape from affection?

For the first time mother is not immunized unless she has any history of taking Rh positive blood transfusion. An immune response is elicited during pregnancy (<1%) or at delivery (10–15%) in an Rh negative mother, who carries an Rh positive fetus. Even with delivery, this amount occurs in less than half of the cases. Initial maternal immune response to Rh sensitization is formation of high molecular weight immunoglobulin (Ig) M, which is too large to cross the placenta. Within 6 weeks to 6 months, IgG antibodies become detectable, which are capable of crossing the placenta and destroy fetal Rh positive cells. As this takes a long time, immunization in first pregnancy is unlikely. Thus first fetus usually remains unaffected (Roman and Pernoll, 2007).

Manifestations of Rh-isoimmunization

Although the mother will exhibit no symptoms of Rh incompatibility, Rh antibodies adversely affect fetal health. Maternal Rh antibodies cross the placenta, enter into fetal circulation and cause hemolysis of fetal RBC. As a consequence, large amounts of bilirubin are produced from the breakdown of fetal hemoglobin. However, *in utero*, heme and bilirubin are effectively removed by placenta and metabolized and excreted by the mother.

Antepartum Manifestations

- Some fetuses are mildly affected and may have little or no anemia but have only mild hyperbilirubinemia.
- Fetuses who are moderately affected may have a combination of anemia and hyperbilirubinemia/jaundice.
- In severely affected fetus a serious life-threatening condition occurs called erythroblastosis fetalis, which is characterized by severe hemolytic anemia and jaundice. Hydrops fetalis is the most severe form of erythroblastosis fetalis is characterized by generalized edema, ascites, hydrothorax, pericardial effusion, high output cardiac failure and extramedullary hematopoiesis.
- Intrauterine death (IUD): If left untreated, 20–30% of fetuses affected by erythroblastosis fetalis die in utero.

Postnatal Manifestations

- Newborns with hydrops fetalis are extremely pale due to severe anemia with hematocrits usually less than five.
- Neonatal death soon after delivery.
- *Icterus gravis neonatorum:* After delivery low levels of glucuronyl transferase in the infant can not conjugate large amounts of bilirubin and may result in elevated levels of serum bilirubin, severe jaundice and eventual tissue deposition. Tremendously high level of bilirubin develops kernicterus several days after delivery, which is a neurologic syndrome caused by deposition of bilirubin into central nervous system (CNS) tissues. It is characterized by loss of the Moro (i.e. startle) reflex, posturing, poor feeding, inactivity, a bulging fontanelle, a high-pitched shrill cry, and seizures. Long term sequelae are hypotonia, hearing loss, and mental retardation.
- Congenital anemia of the newborn.

> How does erythroblastosis fetalis develop?

If the Rh-negative mother conceived with Rh positive fetus, antibody formed in maternal circulation in response to Rh-antigen coming from the fetal blood, if there is fetomaternal transfusion. These antibodies can cross the placental barrier and enter into fetal circulation. The antibodies then attach to the antigen sites on the surface of fetal erythrocytes. Resulting in hemolysis of RBC and development of hemolytic anemia of the fetus. Fetal anemia stimulates extramedullary erythropoietic sites to produce high level of nucleated red cell elements. Immature erythrocytes (erythroblast) are present in the fetal blood because of poor maturation control. That is why it is called erythroblastosis fetalis. Hemolysis produces heme, which is converted to bilirubin; both of these substances are neurotoxic. However, *in utero*, heme and bilirubin are effectively removed by placenta and metabolized by the mother.

When red cell destruction far exceeds the production, severe anemia occurs, which leads to tissue anoxemia and metabolic acidosis. As a result of anoxemia and extensive erythropoiesis, there is damage to the liver leading to hypoproteinemia, which is responsible for generalized edema (hydrops fetalis) ascites pericardial effusion, hydrothorax and congestive heart failure. There is hepato and splenomegaly due to compensatory extramedullary hematopoiesis and accumulation of fluid because of congestive heart failure.

If untreated, 20–30% of fetus affected by erythroblastosis die in utero. Kernicterus and jaundice are not the components of erythroblastosis fetalis during intrauterine life as accumulation of bilirubin is prevented by its removal through placental circulation and metabolism in the maternal liver. But, after birth the newborn liver cannot effectively metabolize the large amount of pigment during the rapid hemolytic process, which leads to rapid increment of serum bilirubin and eventually deposition in tissue.

Affection of Mother

Though mother is not affected by Rh-isoimmunization, there is association of pre-eclampsia, polyhydramnios, big baby and related hazard, hypofibrinogenemia due to prolonged retention of IUD and postpartum hemorrhage due to big placenta. Big placenta is the effect of Rh-isoimmunization as placenta becomes hypertrophic to give more supply to severely anemic baby.

> Is it always necessary to do paternal genotype?

If father of baby is Rh-negative, the fetus will be negative and will not be affected and further tests are not necessary.

There are different school of thoughts for testing Rh-positive father's genotype. One school of thought is that if father is Rh-positive, genotype testing is necessary for antenatal management. Exception is previous birth of Rh-negative baby, which indicates that father is heterozygous positive. All babies of homozygous Rh-positive (DD) father will be heterozygous (Dd) Rh-positive. But, if father is heterozygous positive 50% babies will be Rh-negative (dd) and 50% babies will be heterozygous Rh-positive (Dd). So fetal Rh testing is mandatory to avoid unnecessary testing in the 50% fetuses that will be Rh negative. As all the babies of homozygous Rh-positive father are Rh-positive fetus, Rh testing will be unnecessary and can avoid invasive amniocentesis.

Another school of thought is that it is not necessary to determine Rh genotype of father because even in the best of the circumstances, the probability that the fetus will be Rh positive is substantial and the plan of management will be identical to that for the homozygous father. If the father is positive, it is necessary to design a strategy to diagnose immunization by antibody testing and to prevent immunization by routine antenatal anti-D prophylaxis.

> **Case scenario:** Razia is pregnant, her blood group is B negative. This is her first conception and she has no history of blood transfusion. You did Rh-antibody titer and found negative during first antennal visit at 12 weeks. What will be your subsequent steps to manage her?

If the Rh-antibody titer is negative during screening at first antenatal visit, it indicates that this mother is still non-immunized. To manage her following steps should be taken:
- Determination of Rh-phenotype of the baby's father. If father is Rh-negative, no further test is required. Patient will be followed as Rh positive pregnant women. If father is Rh positive then following tests are done.
- Antibody screening is repeated at 20, 24 and 28 weeks of gestation.
- If no evidence of alloimmunization, patient should receive anti-D immune globulin at 28 weeks.
- Pregnancy can be continued up to spontaneous on set of labor. There is no contra indication of vaginal delivery for Rh negative blood group.
- Precaution should be taken during delivery to minimize FMH.
- After delivery cord blood is to be tested for grouping and Rh typing, Hb%, HCT, Coombs test and reticulocyte count.
- Patient should receive anti-D immunoglobulin within 72 hours of delivery, if the baby is Rh-positive.

RELATED INFORMATION

Immunoprophylaxis

Routine Antenatal Anti-D Prophylaxis (RADDP)

- RADDP should be offered to all non-sensitized RhD negative women
- RADDP is not required in women who are RhD sensitized.

Administration of anti-D: According to recommendation of RCOG immunoprophylaxis should be given once at 28 weeks of pregnancy (1,500 IU/300 μg). It also can be given twice at 28 and 34 weeks of pregnancy at a dose of 500 IU or 100 μg. (RCOG, 2011). Antibody screening must be done at 28 weeks before administration of first dose.

Silent sensitization secondary to occult FMH occurs in 55–80% cases when there is no recognized sensitization feature present (Hughes et al. 1994). As gestational age advances frequency of silent FMH increases and maximum (45.4%) occurs in third trimester (Bowman et al. 1986). A few instances (<10%) silent FMH occur even before 28 weeks of pregnancy. So the rationale for RADDP is to protect against these unpredictable sensitizations and to prevent complications in subsequent pregnancies. In absence of RADDP approximately 1% Rh-negative women having Rh-positive baby is sensitized. (Lcc et al. 1999).

A few women have undetected level of anti-D 12 weeks after a single injection of 1,500 IU of anti-D Ig (Bowman and Pollock, 1987). Therefore, anti-D given at 28 weeks of gestation may not protect those women who progress at or beyond 40 weeks of gestation. So giving two doses at 28 and 34 weeks is more protective than a single dose at 28.

Antenatal Prophylaxis with Sensitizing Events before Delivery

According to RCOG guideline 2011, all non-sensitized Rh negative women should have Anti-D Ig prophylaxis after potentially sensitizing events of pregnancy even after routine antenatal anti-D prophylaxis (RCOG, 2011). Events are:
- Invasive prenatal diagnostic procedures such as amniocentesis CVS and cordocentesis
- Intrauterine procedure such as embryo reduction
- Antepartum hemorrhage
- External cephalic version
- Abdominal trauma
- Fetal death
  What is the dose for these cases?
  – A minimum dose of 250 IU is to be given up to 19 weeks of gestation
  – 500 IU is to be given at or after 20 weeks of gestation and additional anti D Ig should be given after quantifying the size of FMH
  – If there is history of recurrent episode of vaginal bleeding after 20 weeks of gestation, anti D Ig should be given at 6 weeks interval irrespective of the presence or absence of passive anti-D.

Prophylaxis Following Miscarriages, Ectopic Pregnancy, Molar Pregnancy and Termination of Pregnancy

Miscarriage
- Anti-D Ig should be given to all non-sensitized Rh-negative women:
  – After miscarriage at or after 12 weeks of gestation, either complete or incomplete miscarriage.
  – After surgical evacuation, irrespective of gestational age.
  – After medical evacuation of the uterus.
- Anti-D is not recommended for spontaneous miscarriage (no instrumentation and no medication) before 12 weeks of gestation.

Threatened miscarriage
- Anti-D Ig should be given to all non-sensitized Rh-negative women with a threatened miscarriage after 12 weeks of gestation.
- Before 12 weeks of gestation only when there is heavy and repeated bleeding and abdominal pain.
- If bleeding continues intermittently after 12 weeks of gestation, anti-D should be given at 6 weekly intervals.

Other conditions
- Irrespective of mode of treatment of ectopic pregnancy Anti-D Ig should be given to all non-sensitized Rh-negative women.
- In therapeutic termination of pregnancy Anti-D Ig should be given to all non-sensitized Rh-negative women irrespective of surgical or medical method and age of gestation.

Dose of anti-D Ig for above mentioned cases
- 250 IU up to 19 weeks of gestation
- 500 IU at or above 20 weeks of gestation.

Postnatal Prophylaxis

1,500 IU anti-D Ig must be given to all non-sensitized Rh negative women after delivery.

In the Event of Rh-D Positive Blood Transfusion

Anti-D Ig must be given to all nonsensitized Rh-negative women after inadvertent transfusion of Rh-D positive blood. The dose should be calculated on the basis of that 500 IU of anti-D Ig will suppress immunization by 4 mL of Rh-D positive RBC.

> What is the timing for administration of anti-D Ig.

For successful immunoprophylaxis anti-D Ig should be given as soon as possible after the potentially sensitizing event, but always within 72 hours. If it is not given before 72 hours still it should be given at any time within 10 days, as a dose given within 10 days may provide some protection.

> How does the size of FMH can be assessed? What is the significance of it?

Kleihauer Betke test is a method by which approximate amount of fetal blood entered into maternal circulation can be calculated. Test should be done within two hours of event. Acid elution technique is used to note the number of dark refractile fetal red blood cells. If there are 80 fetal erythrocytes in 50 low-power fields in maternal peripheral blood films, it represents a fetomaternal transfusion to the extent of 4 mL.

Significance

In 99% cases women have an FMH of less than 4 mL at delivery. Usually 500 IU anti-D Ig is needed to neutralize 4 mL of fetal blood. Additional dose is needed if FMH is higher. So to fix the appropriate dose of anti-D Ig, the test is done.

Following are the situations where larger FMH may occur:
- Traumatic delivery including cesarean section
- Manual removal of placenta
- Multiple pregnancies
- Unexplained hydrops fetalis
- Stillbirths and fetal death
- Abdominal trauma during third trimester.

> About 99% women have FMH of less than 4 mL. To neutralize this amount 500 IU anti-D Ig is appropriate.
>
> Why 1,500 IU is scheduled for postnatal prophylaxis?

Approximately 1% women have FMH more than 4 mL who need more than 500 IU anti-D Ig for complete protection. So, to quantify the amount routine Kleihauer test is needed. But, it is found that a standard postnatal dose of 1,000–1,500 IU does not require a routine Kleihauer test. So, where there is no facility to perform Kleihauer test 1,500 IU can be used to protect more than 99% women. However, 0.3% women have FMH is more than 15 mL and may not be protected by 1,500 IU anti-D Ig.

> What are the objectives of follow-up of Rh negative pregnant women?

1. Objective of follow-up of Rh-nonimmunized women is prevention of Rh alloimmunization.
2. Objective of follow-up of Rh-immunized women is early detection and adequate treatment of fetal anemia and to prevent serious fetal complications.

Summary of Management of Rh-isoimmunized Women

Positive antibody titer at early pregnancy indicates Rh-isoimmunization, possibly from the fetomaternal transfusion of previous pregnancy with Rh positive fetus. Here, the steps of management should be as follows:

- Determination of paternal Rh phenotype; if father is Rh-positive, it is necessary to determine whether he is homozygous or heterozygous for the *Rh D* gene.
- If father is heterozygous amniocentesis is done to determine fetal Rh factor.
- If fetus is Rh-negative, next step will be as that of Rh positive pregnancy.
- If fetus is Rh-positive and this pregnancy is the *first affected pregnancy*, maternal anti Rh antibody titers can be used to determine the risk of fetal anemia.
- Antibody titers done every 4 weeks. If titer remains under critical level up to 36 weeks, delivery should be done between 38 and 40 weeks.
- If titer is at or above the critical level (usually 32) or if there is a significant rise in titer (two-tube dilution) between two consecutive samples, even if the upper dilution does not reach the critical level, further assessment

will be based on Middle Cerebral Artery Peak Systolic Velocity (MCA PSV). If MCA PSV is less than 1.5 multiples of median (MoM) for the gestational age, which is within normal value, patients will be followed by MCA PSV 2 weekly. If MCA PSV is at or above 1.5, indicates severely affected fetus; the next step is amniocentesis.
- Amniocentesis is to be done to determine the concentration of bilirubin and fetal pulmonary maturation. If fetal pulmonary maturation is certain, pregnancy can be terminated. If not, bilirubin level will be assessed by spectrophotometric analysis of amniotic fluid and plotting the value in Lily's curve (**Fig. 8.1**). Management will be according to the values given in the following (**Flowchart 8.1**). Women with a *previous affected pregnancy* need to be followed with serial determinations of the MCA PSV and amniocentesis to determine the concentration of bilirubin in the amniotic fluid.
- Ultrasound assessment: To detect fetal hydrops.
- Fetal blood sampling (indication): A MCA PSV >1.5 MoM, amniotic fluid bilirubin values in the high middle zone or in zone 3, and fetal pulmonary maturation is not adequate or finding of fetal hydrops by USG.
- Intrauterine transfusion: If fetal hematocrit is <30; intrauterine blood transfusion is necessary. Hematocrit >30 needs followed-up by fetal blood sampling and ultrasound.
- Early delivery and glucocorticoids: If delivery before 36 weeks is necessary, the use of steroids to accelerate fetal lung maturation is recommended. The drug used is injection betamethasone 12 mg IM daily for 2 consecutive days or dexamethasone 6 mg every 12 hours for 4 doses (Moise K, 2008).

> If a nonpregnant patient having high antibody titer comes to you with history of two fetal losses and one healthy baby, she wants one more baby, what will be your advice?

If the patient wants to have pregnancy with same Rh-positive husband, there is every chance to loss

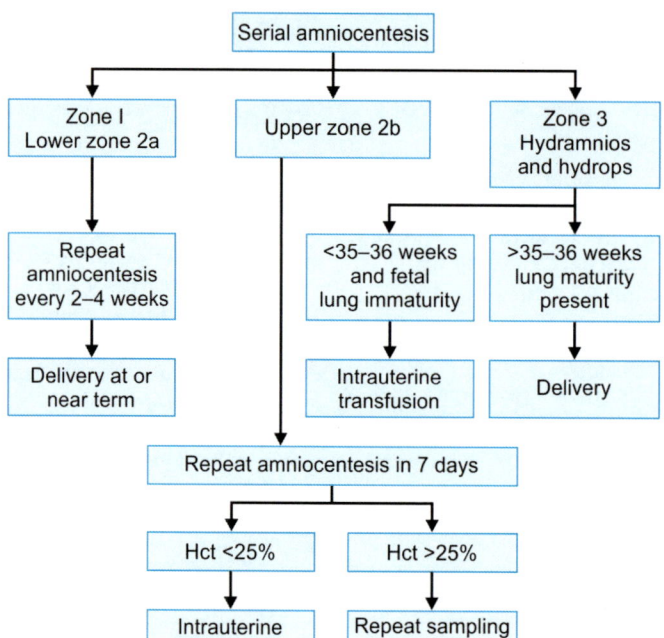

Flowchart 8.1 Suggested management after amniocentesis for ΔOD 450

her subsequent pregnancy even earlier than that of the previous one. This patient might have the following options:
- Wait for 2–3 years and when the antibody titer lower down, then try for pregnancy.
- There is another procedure, known as plasmapheresis, where several liters of maternal plasma is removed to reduce maternal anti-D; after then patient can try for pregnancy.

Due to lack of definite benefit, it is not commonly done.

BIBLIOGRAPHY

American College of Obstetricians and Gynecologists (ACOG). Management of alloimmunization during pregnancy, Clinical Management Guidelines for Obstetricians-Gynecologists, No. 75, Washington, DC, 2006, ACOG.

American college of obstetricians and gynecologists. ACOG Practice Bulletin No. 75: Management of alloimmunization during pregnancy. Obstet Gynecol. 2006;108(2):457-64.

Arias F, Pineda J, Johnson LW. Changes in human amniotic fluid lecithin/sphingomyelin ratio and dipalmitoyl lecithin associated with maternal betamethasone therapy. Am J Obstet Gynecol. 1979;133 (8):894-8.

Bowman JM, Pollock JM. Failure of intravenous Rh immunoglobulin prophylaxis: an analysis of the reasons for such failures. Transfuse Med Rev. 1987;1(2):101-12.

Caritis SN, Mueller-Heubac E, Eldestone DI. Effect of betamethasone on analysis of amniotic fluid in the rhesus- sensitized pregnancy. Am J Obstet Gynecol. 1977;127(5): 529-82.

Frigoletto FD, Greene MF, Benacerraf BR, et al. Ultrasonographic fetal surveillance in the management of the isoimmunized pregnancy. N Eng J Med. 1986;315(7):430-2.

Geifman-Holtzman O, Grotegut CA, Gaughan JP. Diagnostic accuracy of noninvasive fetal Rh genotyping from maternal blood–a meta-analysis. Am J Obstet Gynecol. 2006;195(4):1163-73.

Gilbert ES. Hemolytic Incompatibility. Manual of High Risk Pregnancy & Delivery 5th edition Mosby; Elsevier; 2011. p.406.

Hughes RG, Craig JI, Murphy WG, et al. Causes and clinical consequences of Rhesus (D) haemolytic disease of the newborn: a study of a Scottish population, 1985-1990. Br J Obstet Gynaecol. 1994;101(4):297-300.

Konar H. Pregnancy in a Rh negative woman. In: Keith Edmonds (Ed) DC. Dutta's Test Book of Obstetrics; 7th edition. Delhi: Jaypee Brothers Medical Publishers (P) Ltd. 2012.p.332.

Lee D, Contreras M, Robson SC, et al. Recommendations for the use of anti-D immunoglobulin for Rh prophylaxis. British Blood Transfusion Society and the Royal College of Obstetricians and Gynaecologists. Transfus Med. 1999;9(1):93-7.

Mari G, Adrignolo A, Abuhamad AZ, et al. Diagnosis of fetal anemia with Doppler ultrasound in the pregnancy complicated by maternal group immunization. Ultrasound Obstet Gynecol. 1995;5(6):400-5.

Mari G, Deter RL, Carpenter RL, et al. Noninvasive diagnosis by ultrasonography of fetal anemia due to maternal red cell alloimmunization. Collaborative Group for Doppler Assessment of the Blood velocity in Anemic Fetuses. N Engl J Med. 2000;342(1):9-14.

Moise K. Management of rhesus alloimmunization in pregnancy. Obstet Gynecol. 2008;112(1):164-76.

Nishie EN, Brizot ML, Liao AW, et al. A comparison between middle cerebral artery peak systolic velocity and amniotic fluid optical density at 450 nm in the prediction of fetal anemia. AM J Obstet Gynecol. 2003;188(1):214-9.

Pereira L, Jenkins TM, Berghella V. Conventional management of maternal red cell alloimmunization compared with management by Doppler assessment of middle cerebral artery peak systolic velocity. Am J Obstet Gynecol. 2003;189(4):1002-6.

Queenan JT, Tomai TP, Ural SH, et al. Deviation in amniotic fluid optical density at a wavelength of 450 nm in Rh-immunized pregnancies from 14 to 40 weeks' gestation: a proposal for clinical management. Am J Obstet Gynecol. 1993;168(5):1370-6.

Reece EA, Cole SW, Romero R, et al. Ultrasonography versus amniotic fluid spectral analysis: are they sensitive enough to predict neonatal complications associated with isoimmunization? Obstet Gynecol. 1989;74(3):357-60.

Roman AS, Pernoll ML. Late pregnancy complications. In: Decherney AH, Nathan L, Goodwin TM, Laufer N (Eds). Current Diagnosis and Treatment Obstetrics and Gynecology, 10th edition. New York: McGraw-Hill; 2007. p. 282-6.

Royal College of Obstetricians and Gynaecologists. Rhesus D prophylaxis, The use of anti-D immunoglobulin for (Green-top Guideline No 22). 2011.

Van Kamp IL, Klumper FJ, Oepkes D, et al. Complications of intrauterine intravascular transfusion for fetal anemia due to maternal red-cell alloimmunization. Am J Obstet Gynecol. 2005;192:171-7.

Zimmerman R, Carpenter RJ Jr, Durig P, et al. Longitudinal measurement of peak systolic velocity in the fetal middle cerebral artery for monitoring pregnancies complicated by red cell alloimmunisation: a prospective multicentre trial with intention-to-treat. BJOG. 2002;109(7):746-52.

CHAPTER 9

Pregnancy-induced Hypertension

Rashida Begum

INTRODUCTION

Pregnancy-induced hypertension (PIH) is the leading cause of maternal morbidity and mortality worldwide. The global incidence of pre-eclampsia has been estimated at 5–14% and in developing countries it is 4–18% (Villar, 2001; Khedun et al. 1997) with second most common obstetric cause of stillbirth and early neonatal deaths (Ngoc et al. 2006). Both mother and fetus are at increased risk of mortality and morbidity from complications of hypertension. It is a high-risk pregnancy, which needs meticulous care throughout pregnancy and afterwards.

> **Case scenario:** Maleka Khatun aged 21 years wife of a shopkeeper has come to the outpatient department for consultation. She is amenorrheic for 32 weeks. She went to a doctor and came to know that her blood pressure is 145/100 mm Hg. She noticed that her leg is swelling gradually. So, for better consultation she has come to you.
>
> How will you proceed to diagnose the case?

Detailed History

What other complaints does she have?
Is there any oliguria, nausea, vomiting, insomnia or epigastric pain, which are symptoms of severe form of pre-eclampsia (PE). As leg edema may be due to pre-eclampsia, it should be taken into consideration. Though incidence of pre-eclampsia is similar in patients with or without edema and for that reason edema is no longer considered as a diagnostic sign of pre-eclampsia.

To determine gestational age, menstrual history is to be taken
If the case is pre-eclampsia, gestational age determination is very important as termination of pregnancy is the definitive treatment of pre-eclampsia and decision of termination will be made by balancing the risk benefit ratio of maternal pathogenesis and fetal maturity:
- Whether menstrual cycle was regular or not?
- What was the length of the cycle?
- When was the last menstrual period?

About obstetric history and other associated factors
- Is it her first pregnancy? PIH is more common in nulliparous and in young age group.
- If not how was her previous pregnancy? Was there any similar complain?
- Whether she gained weight rapidly this time? Though excessive weight gain is no longer considered as sign of pre-eclampsia, sudden weight gain can be taken into consideration.
- Whether her parents are hypertensive or not? If one of them is hypertensive then there is chance of development of pre-eclampsia.
- Whether she was hypertensive before pregnancy?
- Whether she received any treatment from previous doctor?
- Whether fetal movement is adequate or not?

Next she should be examined thoroughly:
- General examination: Height, weight, pulse, blood pressure are to be recorded. Anemia and edema are to be looked for. Heart and lungs are to be examined.

- Obstetrical examination to assess gestational age and well-being. Fundal height, volume of liquor amni, uterine irritability are to be assessed. Fetal heart rate is to be counted.

> On enquiry you elicited that she is pregnant for the first time. Duration of gestation is about 32 weeks. She gained weight very rapidly. She does not know about her parents' status, whether they are hypertensive or not. She also does not know whether she was hypertensive or not before pregnancy.
>
> After performing physical examination you found that her BP is 145/100 mm Hg. Pulse is 80/m. Heart and lungs-NAD. Edema (++). Anemia mild. Uterus is 32 weeks size. Fetal movement is present. Fetal heart rate is 148/m.
>
> On the basis of history and physical findings what do you think about the case? Justify your answer.

This is a case of pre-eclampsia. Hypertension and edema in 33% cases are characteristic features of PE, which develops after 20th weeks of gestation. Incidence is more in primiparous women and in young age.

> How will you confirm the diagnosis?

Heat coagulation test of urine (dipstick urine test) should be done to detect the presence of albumin. Urinary albumin is present in PE. Hypertension and proteinuria are diagnostic features of PE.

RELATED INFORMATION

Hypertension in Pregnancy

- Raised blood pressure to the extent of 140/90 mm Hg or more on 2 or more occasions at least 4–6 hours apart after 20 weeks of gestation in a previously normotensive woman is called hypertension in pregnancy (ACOG 2002; Sibai 2002)
  Or
- Diastolic blood pressure ≥110 mm Hg on any one occasion
  Or
- Increment of systolic blood pressure 30 mm Hg and diastolic blood pressure 15 mm Hg from previous blood pressure.

Classification of Hypertension in Pregnancy [NHBPEP 2000]

1. *Gestational hypertension*: Hypertension, which is *not associated with proteinuria* and develop after 20th weeks of gestation, during labor or during puerperium in a previously normotensive woman is called gestational hypertension. Blood pressure (BP) returns to normal within less than 12 weeks postpartum.
2. *Chronic hypertension*: Hypertension, which present before 20th weeks of pregnancy or before pregnancy is called chronic hypertension. It occurs due to:
   - Essential hypertension
   - Chronic renal disease
   - Coarctation of aorta
   - Pheochromocytoma
   - Thyrotoxicosis
   - Systemic lupus erythematosus.
3. *Pre-eclampsia*: Hypertension associated with proteinuria after 20th weeks of gestation is called pre-eclampsia. *Edema is no longer considered as diagnostic criteria.*
4. *Eclampsia*: Pre-eclamptic cases when complicated with convulsion is called eclampsia.
5. *Chronic hypertension with superimposed pre-eclampsia*: It is a condition when proteinuria develops for the first time in pregnancy in a woman with known chronic hypertension.

Pregnancy-induced hypertension

Pregnancy-induced hypertension (PIH): The PIH is defined as the hypertension that develops as a direct result of the gravid state. It includes:
a. Gestational hypertension
b. Pre-eclampsia
c. Eclampsia.

Pre-eclampsia

Pre-eclampsia: It is a multisystem disorder characterized by raised blood pressure to the extent of 140/90 mm Hg or more at least two different occasions at 6 hours apart with *proteinuria* greater than 0.3 g/L in a 24 hour urine collection corresponds to 1+ by qualitative urine examination after 20th weeks gestation in a previously normotensive and nonproteinuric woman.

Pre-eclampsia is classified as mild or severe:
i. *Mild pre-eclampsia:* When systolic blood pressure is less than 160 mm Hg and diastolic blood pressure is less than 110 mm Hg with 0.3 g or more protein in 24-hour urine collection corresponds with 1+ or greater on a urine dipstick test and there is no additional symptoms then it is called mild pre-eclampsia (ACOG, 2002; NHBPEP, 2000).
ii. *Severe pre-eclampsia:* When systolic blood pressure is 160 mm Hg or higher and diastolic blood pressure is 110 mm Hg or higher associated with one or more of the following symptoms then it is called severe pre-eclampsia:
   - 24-hours urinary protein 5 g or more
   - Oliguria of less than 400 mL in 24 hour
   - Severe headache
   - Cerebral or visual disturbance
   - Pulmonary edema
   - Epigastric pain due to stretching of the Glisson's capsule of the liver
   - Impaired liver function
   - Thrombocytopenia due to microangiopathic hemolysis induced by spasm
   - Fetal growth restriction (ACOG 2002; NHBPEP 2000).

Severe pre-eclampsia may be complicated as:
a. **Impending eclampsia:** When severe pre-eclampsia associated with oliguria, epigastric pain, vomiting, headache (occipital or frontal), insomnia and blurring or dimness of vision then it is called impending eclampsia. These are the ominous symptoms, which may be evident either singly or in combination.
b. **HELLP syndrome:** It is a severe form of pre-eclampsia characterized by hemolysis, low platelet count ($<100,000/mm^3$) and elevated liver enzymes (LDH >600 U/L).

> What other investigations are needed for this patient?

Following baseline investigations are needed for diagnosis of severity of disease and to see progress in follow-up visit (NHBPEP 2000; ACOG 2001):
- Routine tests:
  - Complete blood count (CBC)
  - Hb%
  - Routine urine analysis
  - Blood grouping and Rh typing if not known before
  - Blood sugar 2 hours postprandial.
- Kidney function tests:
  - Blood urea
  - Creatinine
  - Serum uric acid
  - 24-hours urinary total protein
  - Protein/Creatinine ratio.
- Liver function tests:
  - Aspartate transaminase (AST)
  - Alanine transferase (ALT)
  - PT or activated partial thromboplastin time (APTT)
  - Platelet count.
- Hemolysis and coagulopathy related:
  - Indirect bilirubin
  - Lactate dehydrogenase (LDH)
  - Peripheral smear
  - Fibrin degradation product (FDP)
  - Fibrinogen
  - D-dimer.
- USG for fetal well-being and to assess fetal growth.

Note: Fibrinogen and D-dimer are to be done if there is coagulopathy.

RELATED INFORMATION

- Total urinary protein increased in PE. It will be more than 0.3 g/L in 24 hours. Value increases with severity of the disease. In mild PE, it is more than 0.3 g/L in 24 hours, but less than 5 g/24 hours. In severe PE, it is 5 g or higher in 24-hour urine specimen or 3+ or greater on two random urine samples collected at least 4 hours apart.
  Correlation of dipstick test with total urinary protein:
  Trace = 0.1 g/L; 1+ = 0.3 g/L; 2+ = 1 g/L; 3+ = 3 g/L; 4+ = 10 g/L; boiled egg = >10 g/L.
- Serum uric acid value is also increased in PE. It has got more prognostic value. With progression of the disease level increases. Value more than 4.5 mg/dL is pathognomic. Uric acid is secreted from distal tubules. Raised serum uric acid level indicates renal involvement and diminished renal blood flow.

- Liver function tests will be altered in PE. All values increases. When LDH level increased it indicates HELLP syndrome. AST ≥72 IU/L and LDH >600 IU/L is diagnostic for HELLP syndrome.
- Coagulation profile is also deteriorated. Platelet count is reduced in HELLP syndrome.

These tests have got both diagnostic and prognostic value. Response to the treatment or progression of the disease is to be assessed by observing the changes of these values.

Risk Factors for Developing Pre-eclampsia

There are certain risk factors for development of PE. Some risk factors contribute to poor placentation, whereas others contribute to increased placental mass and poor placental perfusion secondary to vascular abnormalities (ACOG, 1996).

According to ACOG, following are the risk factors for development of PE (ACOG, 2001).
- Pregnancy-associated factors:
  - Chromosomal abnormalities
  - Hydatidiform mole
  - Hydrops fetalis
  - Multifetal pregnancy
  - Oocyte donation and donor insemination
  - Structural congenital anomalies
  - Urinary tract infection.
- Maternal-specific factors:
  - Teenage and older than 35
  - Nulliparity
  - Family history of hypertension and pre-eclampsia
  - Obesity
  - Diabetes mellitus
  - Thyroid disorder
  - Chronic hypertension
  - Renal disease
  - Collagen vascular disease
  - Sudden weight gain
  - History of pre-eclampsia in previous pregnancy
  - Antiphospholipid syndrome
  - Black race
  - Stress.
- Paternal-specific factors:
  - First-time father
  - Previously fathered a pre-eclamptic pregnancy in another woman.

Etiology and Pathology of Pre-eclampsia

The exact cause of pre-eclampsia is not known. But it is definite that placenta is the initiation of the disease. That is why hyperplacentosis in multiple pregnancy, hydatidiform mole and diabetes mellitus aggravate the disease and removal of placenta or in other words termination of pregnancy cures the disease.

It is thought that decreased placental oxygenation due to some reasons cause release of a variety of vasoactive substances including thromboxane-A2, interleukin-1, tumor-necrosing factors. These substances cause maternal vascular endothelial injury, which plays a central role in the disorder, alterations in metabolism, inflammation and other possible reactions.

Reduced Placental Oxygenation

Reduced placental oxygenation is due to:
1. Abnormal endovascular trophoblast invasion early in pregnancy.

   In normal women during first trimester proliferative trophoblast invades the decidual segment of maternal spiral arteries, replacing endothelium in a process called pseudo-vascularization (Zhou et al. 1997; Redman and Sargent, 2005) and destroying the medial elastic and muscular tissue of the arterial wall and replaced by fibrinoid material by expressing a number of different classes of molecules (Zhou et al. 1993; Lim et al. 1997). In second trimester, a second wave of endovascular trophoblastic invasion extends down the lumen of the spiral arteries deeper in the myometrium. The endothelium and musculo-elastic architecture of the spiral arteries destroyed resulting in dilated, thin walled, funnel-shaped vessels for easy uteroplacental circulation.

   In a subset of patient for unknown reason, the first wave of endovascular trophoblastic invasion is incomplete and second wave does not occur, so retained the musculoelastic architecture of spiral arteries and reduced placental perfusion leads to placental hypoxia. There is lipid deposition, fibrinoid necrosis and macrophage and mononuclear cell infiltration in vessel wall resulting in acute

atherosis and may lead to vascular lumen obliteration, placental infarction and reduced uteroplacental circulation. This subset of patient develops pre-eclampsia. With increasing fetal and placental oxygen demand with advancing gestational age the clinical manifestation increased. That is why the condition is more common in third trimester.
2. Reduced placental oxygenation may be due to maternal vasculopathy such as chronic hypertension, renal disease and collagen vascular disease.
3. In other cases, it is due to hyperplacentosis in multiple pregnancy, diabetes mellitus and hydatidiform mole without evidence of characteristic features of abnormal placentation.

When PE occurs due to abnormal placentation, it is called placental pre-eclampsia and when placentation is normal, but PE occurs due to maternal pathological condition, it is called maternal pre-eclampsia (Redman and Sargent, 2005). In either case, decreased placental oxygenation triggers the placenta to release unknown factors in maternal circulation, which is capable of *damaging or altering the function of maternal endothelial cells.*

Results of Endothelial Damage

Several circulating markers of endothelial injury have been shown to be increased in women who develop pre-eclampsia. These are endothelin, circular fibronectin, plasminogen activator-1 with an altered prostacyclin/thromboxane (Friedman et al. 1995; Taylor et al. 1998). Following events take place in pre-eclamptic patients:
- Decreased production of prostacyclin I_2, which is a potent vasodilator and platelet aggregation inhibitor. As a result vasoconstriction and platelet aggregation is not inhibited.
- Increased production of thromboxane A2 (TXA2), which is a potent vasoconstrictor and platelet aggregation stimulator. As a result vasoconstriction and platelet aggregation aggravated.
  Normal ratio of prostacyclin and TXA2 is altered and contribute to the generalized vasoconstriction and hypertension that is central feature of the disorder.
- Elevated intravascular pressure combined with damaged vascular endothelium results in movement of fluid from the intravascular to the extravascular spaces leading to edema in the brain, retina, lungs, liver and subcutaneous tissue.
- Hypertension and glomerular endothelial damage lead to proteinuria. Severe hypoxia may lead to cortical damage, oliguria and renal failure.
- As a result of proteinuria there is decreased colloid osmotic pressure, contributes further loss of intravascular fluid.
- Reduced vascular compartment about 500 mL resulting hemoconcentration with rising hematocrit.
- Consumption of platelets and activation of the clotting cascade at the site of endothelial damage may leads to thrombocytopenia and disseminated intravascular coagulation (DIC). The process of DIC also appears to be initiated by the release of thromboplastin in the circulation from platelets as in Shwartzman reaction or from trophoblastic fragments. Microthrombi affect the arterioles of all the vital organs. Fibronectin, D-dimer and thrombin levels are elevated.
- Deposition of soluble fibrin monomers produced by coagulation cascade may precipitate in the microvasculature leading to microangiopathic hemolysis and elevated serum LDH.
- Cerebral vasoconstriction and capillary endothelial damage lead to edema and hypoxia resulting in convulsion. Extreme hypertension may cause intraventricular hemorrhage. Computed tomography (CT) scan reveals cerebral edema, capillary thrombosis, infarctions, intraventricular and parenchymal hemorrhage and necrosis.
- Hepatic edema and hypoxia may lead to hepatocellular injury and elevation of serum transaminase and lactate dehydrogenase. Hepatic edema and hemorrhage cause stretching of Glisson's capsule resulting in right upper quadrant or epigastric pain.

- Subendothelial hemorrhage and focal necrosis in the myocardium may affect the conducting system leading to heart failure. In severe PE the low CO and elevated PVR also causes heart failure, which leads to pulmonary edema.
- Intravascular fluid loss across damaged capillary endothelium in the lungs may result in pulmonary edema. Heart failure and aspiration also lead to pulmonary edema.
- Vasoconstriction and/or edema in the retina may lead to visual disturbances, retinal detachment or blindness.
- Movement of fluid from intravascular space into the subcutaneous tissue causes generalized edema.

Note: Net result is multiorgan damage and failure.

> Mrs Maleka's BP is 145/100 mm Hg. Pulse is 80/m. Heart and lungs-NAD. Edema (++). Anemia mild. Uterus is 34 weeks size. Fetal movement is present. Fetal heart rate is 148/m. You did heat coagulation test and found albumin ++.
>
> How will you manage the case?

This is a case of mild pre-eclampsia. It can be managed at home with advice. *Though there is no role of domiciliary treatment in established PE,* in developing countries like Bangladesh where number of PE is more, but hospital facility is not adequate, domiciliary treatment can be given after proper counseling. Patient and attendants must aware of the situation and must follow the instruction of the clinician. Patient should be taught about ominous signs of PE.

Baseline investigations are to be done to see the effects on the organs. For domiciliary treatment, all baseline values should be normal or slightly raised.

Note: Baseline investigations mentioned before.

Advice and Treatment

- *Rest:* Bed rest increases renal and uteroplacental circulation, which is beneficial both for mother and fetus. As renal flow increases it increases urinary output so help reduce blood pressure.
- *Sedative:* To cut down anxiety mild sedatives orally is to be given. Phenobarbitone 60 mg or diazepam 5 mg daily is helpful to reduce anxiety and tension so as to reduce blood pressure.
- *Antihypertensive:* Antihypertensive is not recommended at this level of blood pressure. But in case of domiciliary treatment either oral labetalol or methyldopa can be used to prevent the rise of blood pressure. Target is to keep the blood pressure systolic 140 mm Hg and diastolic 90 mm Hg.

> How will you follow-up the patient?

Patient will be advised for *weekly* check-up. At *each visit* she will be monitored by the following:

History

- Development of any new signs and symptoms of severe PE
- About fetal movement (kick count).

Examination

- Blood pressure
- Height of the uterus
- Weight of the mother
- Fetal heart sound.

Investigations

- Heat coagulation test, if presence of albumin is ++ or more 24-hours total protein is to be estimated
- Liver function test
- Kidney function test
- Coagulopathy and hemolysis-related tests
- USG for fetal biometry and biophysical profile *fortnightly*
- Umbilical and cerebral Doppler where facility is available.

> At follow-up you found that Maleka's blood pressure remained the same in spite of treatment rather she complaints of insomnia for two days.
>
> What will be your next decision?

Patient will be advised for immediate admission to the hospital. Either she is not following the instruction or is not responding to the treatment. So, she will be kept under vigilant supervision in the hospital.

In the hospital, patient will be monitored by maintaining a chart, which will record the following:
- Questioning about fetal movement (kick count) and development of new symptoms and ominous signs daily
- Blood pressure at least four times a day
- Fetal heart sound every 4 hourly
- State of edema daily
- Daily urine output
- Daily heat coagulation test
- Measurement of body weight every other day
- Liver function test, kidney function test and coagulation profile once in a week
- USG for fetal biometry and biophysical profile every fortnightly. More frequent testing, twice in a week may needed in less fetal movement (ACOG, 1996; ACOG, 2001)
- Umbilical and cerebral Doppler every week if facility is available.

How will you assess that the patient is responding to treatment?

- Blood pressure will fall; diastolic blood pressure should be kept between 90 and 95 mm Hg
- Subsidence of edema
- No abnormal weight gain
- Optimum urine output
- Diminishing proteinuria
- No development of new symptoms or no further progression of the disease.

After hospitalization she responded well to the treatment. How long will you continue such treatment?

The aim of the treatment is to:
- Prevent further progression of the disease and development of complications
- Gain fetal maturity so as to able to survive in extrauterine environment independently.

Definitive treatment of PE is termination of pregnancy: As such treatment will be continued by assessing the risk benefit balance of mother and fetus.

Thus, the duration of treatment depends on:
- Severity of pre-eclampsia
- Duration of gestation
- Response to treatment.

As patient is a case of mild PE, responded to treatment and becomes stable, pregnancy is to be continued till 37 completed weeks. After that period termination of pregnancy is safe to avoid complications of PE. Though with good response of treatment under strict follow-up pregnancy can be continued till EDD (40 weeks of gestation) to get benefit of spontaneous onset of labor and vaginal delivery.

Suppose she has passed her EDD and did not go into labor. What do you like to do?

In PE, even in mild cases with good control of the disease, one can wait till EDD, but should not wait beyond that as it is a high-risk pregnancy and anytime any complication may develop. So pregnancy is to be terminated.

She is young primipara with average height and she has got no medical or obstetrical complications. Pelvis seems adequate.
For termination what do you want to do?

For termination labor is to be induced.

What will be the mode of induction and how will you monitor the labor?

Both medical and surgical induction are applicable for PE. Depending upon the cervical condition following are the procedure of mode of induction:
A. If cervix is ripe then ARM is to be done:
- *If liquor is clear:* Oxytocin drip is to be added and increased gradually till effective contraction achieved.
  Labor is to be monitored by using partograph and observing the following parameters:
  - Uterine contraction
  - Cervical dilatation
  - Descent of the head
  - Fetal heart rate
  - Color of liquor
  - Blood pressure
  - Urinary protein
- If liquor is stained and there is no prediction of quick delivery
  Cesarean section is to be done as fetuses of PE are usually compromised due to reduced placental circulation.

B. If cervix is not ripe, prostaglandins is to be given for ripening of the cervix then ARM is to be done.

> Suppose Maleka did not follow the instruction during domiciliary treatment. During follow-up visit you found that her BP is 160/110 mm Hg, dipstick test shows +++ albumin.
> How will you manage her?

Due to progressive pathology she developed severe PE.

Patient is to be managed in the tertiary level hospital with vigilant monitoring and treatment as mentioned before. (Hospital follow-up mentioned under mild PE)

Hypertension is the main pathognomic feature of PE. So aim of treatment is:

- To control blood pressure by administering antihypertensive agents
- To prevent different complications from raised blood pressure.

Along with management described in mild PE, patient will get any one of the following oral antihypertensive drugs according to response:

Labetalol: 100–400 mg twice daily

Nifedipine: 10–20 mg twice daily

Methyldopa: 1–2 g daily in three to four divided doses.

A. *If patient becomes stable within 24 hours observation* period and baseline parameters are not grossly abnormal pregnancy is to be continued with close monitoring and repeating the tests daily/weekly/fortnightly as indicated:
  - Patient should be instructed to report any headache, visual disturbances, insomnia, oliguria, epigastric pain and less fetal movement.
  - Response to treatment is to be assessed by comparing the baseline parameters with subsequent results and development of new symptoms.
  - If response is good, e.g. blood pressure reduced, all test results do not indicate progression of disease, fetal growth is progressing and there is no development of new symptom pregnancy is to be continued till 34 completed weeks.

- With good control pregnancy can be continued till 37 completed weeks.

B. *If patient is not responding to treatment,* e.g. blood pressure cannot be controlled, all test results are indicative of progressive pathology, static fetal growth and development of new symptoms such as headache, visual disturbances, insomnia, oliguria, vomiting, epigastric pain—pregnancy is to be terminated regardless of gestational age.

RELATED INFORMATION

Severe hypertension is the main risk for pre-eclampsia, which may cause intracranial hemorrhage, left ventricular failure and convulsion. So, objective of antihypertensive therapy is to prevent these consequences. Different oral drugs are used, but during hypertensive emergency intravenous drugs used to cut down the pressure immediately to prevent cerebrovascular accident (CVA), heart failure and convulsion, then oral drugs are used to maintain the reduced pressure. Severe pre-eclampsia presenting with headache, visual disturbances, epigastric pain, excessive proteinuria should be treated with utmost caution. In some cases daily blood testing for liver function test, uric acid and LDH may needed. In case of oligohydramnios and decreased fetal movement daily non-stress testing and ultrasonography should include in fetal monitoring.

Management of Hypertension

Antihypertensive Drugs

Labetalol

Labetalol is the first choice of drug due to its effectiveness and low incidence of side effect. It is both alpha and beta adrenergic blocker at the ratio 1:3 for oral and 1:7 for the intravenous form. Labetalol decreases supraventricular rhythm and slows heart rate, reducing myocardial oxygen consumption. Dizziness, nausea and headache are the side effects of this drug. Almost 75% of the drug is inactivated in the liver.

Dose

1. *Oral:* The dose varies from patient to patient and usually is 100–400 mg every 6–12 hours.

The usual starting dose is 100 mg twice a day (bid) and the dose can be increased weekly to a maximum 2,400 mg daily. Titration increments should not exceed 200 mg bid.
2. *Intravenous:* Labetalol is very effective in the treatment of severe hypertension or hypertensive emergencies and can be given by continuous or intermittent intravenous infusion.
3. *Continuous infusion:* 500 mg (100 mL) labetalol is to be added in 500 mL normal saline (1 mg/mL) and administered at a rate of 20 mg (20 mL)/hour. In 20 minutes observation, if blood pressure does not fall to expected level (<160 mm Hg/80-95 mm Hg), the dose is to be doubled and continued to be doubled every 20 minutes until the desired level of blood pressure, but not exceeding 220 mg/hour. The maximum effect of IV labetalol is usually reached after 5 minutes of injection. The effective dose range is between 50 and 200 mg/hour.
4. *Intermittent dosing:* 20 mg is to be given over a 2-minute period. Dose is to be added 40–80 mg at 20 minutes interval till desired level of blood pressure, but not to exceed 220 mg/hour.

Hydralazine

Hydralazine is another effective and safe drug for hypertensive crisis in obstetrics, where it is used intravenously for rapid reduction of blood pressure. It acts directly on arteriolar smooth muscle to reduce peripheral resistance.

Dose
1. *Intravenous bolus:* Bolus dose is usually given 5 mg IV and increasing by 5 mg every 20 minutes up to 20 mg or until the desired level of blood pressure is achieved.
2. *Intravenous continuous drip:* 20 mg is dissolved in 200 mL normal saline and is given at a rate of 2.5 mg/hour to be doubled every 30 minutes and continued till desired level of blood pressure is achieved. Overshooting hypotension may occur due to arteriolar dilatation and peripheral accumulation of fluid. So 200-500 mL normal saline is to be infused before starting the drip.
3. *Oral:* 10-25 mg twice daily can be given. Its action peaks in 3-4 hours and total duration of action of 6-12 hours. It is effective in oral form in combination with diuretics and beta blocker. After prolonged use, it develops drug resistance.

Side effects
It can cause headache, anxiety, nausea, vomiting, facial flushing and epigastric pain. It causes decreased uteroplacental circulation and fetal distress when the hypotensive effect is rapid or severe. For this reason, electronic fetal monitoring is mandatory when hydralazine is used. After discontinuation of the drug, recovery occurs due to raised blood pressure. Due to this side effect the drug is not recommended as first line when compared with labetalol and nifedipine (Magee et al. 2003).

Nifedipine

Nifedipine is a calcium channel blocker that has been using during pregnancy for tocolysis and treatment of hypertension. It lowers the blood pressure by inhibiting the intracellular influx of calcium into cardiac and vascular smooth muscle and by reducing the peripheral resistance and acts as excellent peripheral vasodilator. It is used in two forms, oral and sublingual.

Dose
1. *Oral:* Initial dose is 10–20 mg bid, may be increased to 10–30 mg every 4–6 hours according to response. It is rapidly absorbed and reaches peak level 30 minutes after ingestion. The half-life of the drug is approximately 2 hours.
2. *Sublingual:* Sublingual drop of nifedipine capsule is used in hypertensive crisis for rapid drop of blood pressure. 3-4 drops stat is given and blood pressure is monitored every 15 minutes to diagnose sudden and severe fall of blood pressure. Dose can be repeated if there is delay in response.

Side effects
It is safe and well tolerated. The most common side effect is headache. Overshoot hypotension may occur with sublingual drop.

Note: The neuromuscular blocking action of magnesium is potentiated by simultaneous calcium channel blockade. So nifedipine should not be used along with magnesium sulfate to avoid respiratory distress or failure.

Methyldopa

Due to its safety methyldopa is recommended by many as first line antihypertensive agent in pregnancy. It is a centrally acting α-adrenergic agonist that appears to inhibit vasoconstrictor impulses from the medullary vasoregulatory center. Response is very slow, so no risk of severe hypotension.

Dose
Dose of 250–500 mg three to four times daily. Maximum 2 g can be used safely. Peak plasma levels occur 2–3 hours after administration and the maximum effect occurs 4–6 hours after an oral dose.

Side effects
Hemolytic anemia, liver function abnormalities, granulocytopenia and thrombocytopenia are rare side effects.

Other antihypertensive medications used in pregnancy include atenolol, metoprolol, prazosin, minoxidil with limited published evidence.

Caution about antihypertensive drugs:
- *Angiotensin-converting enzyme (ACE) inhibitor is contraindicated* during pregnancy due to fetal complications and death.
- *Diuretics is better to be avoided* in PE to reduce hypertension.
- *Beta blocker (propranolol)* reduces blood pressure by reducing cardiac output so *reduces placental circulation* and causes fetal hypoxia and growth retardation.

> *Suppose Maleka at her 33 weeks of pregnancy developed sudden rise of blood pressure 170/120 mm Hg. Dipstick albumin is +++ and complaints of headache and oliguria.*
> *How will you manage her?*

She developed symptoms suddenly. It is called fulminant pre-eclampsia. Blood pressure is very high and it is a state of hypertensive emergency.

Hypertensive emergency should be managed immediately very efficiently to prevent:
- Cerebrovascular accident
- Hypertensive encephalopathy
- Congestive cardiac failure
- Pulmonary edema
- Acute myocardial infarction
- Eclampsia.

Here blood pressure is to be controlled urgently by injection hydralazine or injection labetalol followed by oral maintenance dose (As mentioned earlier).

Injection magnesium sulfate is to be administered urgently to prevent convulsion and development of eclampsia:
- A loading dose of 4 g (100 mL nalepsin) of magnesium sulfate is to be given IV over 20 minutes followed by a continuous infusion of 2 g/hour as the maintenance dose.
Or
- A loading dose 4 g IV and 6 g IM is to be given followed by a maintenance dose of 2.5 g IM every 4 hours till 24 hours:
  - Response to treatment should be watched carefully by monitoring of blood pressure, urine output, proteinuria and hematological parameters.
  - Pregnancy is to be terminated, but can be postponed for 24–48 hours to administer steroids to the mother to accelerate fetal lung maturity.
  - This patient is to be delivered by cesarean (CS) as there are ominous symptoms for developing eclampsia. In addition, in 33 weeks of gestation, cervix is usually unfavorable for induction. In this case, quick delivery is essential to prevent complications. So, CS is logical option.

RELATED INFORMATION

Anticonvulsant Therapy

There are ample of evidences indicating effectiveness of magnesium sulfate in the prevention of convulsion in women with severe pre-eclampsia. The incidence of eclampsia was 3.2% in placebo versus 0.3% in magnesium sulfate (Coetzee et al. 1998), 2.7% in placebo versus 1.1% in magnesium sulfate (Magpie Trial, 2002) 2.6% in placebo vs 0.8% in magnesium sulfate (Belfort et al. 2003).

Though administration of magnesium sulfate reduces the incidence of eclampsia [Magpie Trial, 2002] in current trend it is not recommended to give magnesium sulfate to women with mild pre-eclampsia, as at least 100 women needs to expose to the toxic effect to avoid only one case of eclampsia. Another study shows no difference between the groups of magnesium sulfate and placebo in the development of eclampsia in mild pre-eclampsia cases (Livingston et al. 2003).

Note: Details of $MgSO_4$ is described afterwards.

Termination of Pregnancy

Situations where pregnancy is to be terminated regardless of gestational age in spite of treatment to avoid grave complications of severe pre-eclampsia:
- Persistently raised blood pressure 160/110 or greater despite treatment
- Persistent epigastric or upper right quadrant pain
- Diminished urinary output <400 mL in 24 hours
- Platelet count <50,000/mm^3
- Progressive increase in serum creatinine and uric acid
- Progressive increase in serum alanine transferase (ALT) and aspartate transaminase (AST)
- Lactate dehydrogenase (LDH) >600 U/L
- Minimum or no fetal growth by ultrasound
- Persistent visual symptoms
- Persistent intense headache and insomnia
- Total protein excretion >5 g/L
- Oligohydramnios (AFI <5 cm)
- Repetitive variable or late deceleration with poor variability
- Absent or reversed umbilical artery Doppler.

Precautions of Labor

- Labor should be followed up by using partograph
- During labor, patient's blood pressure is to be recorded repeatedly as it tends to rise during labor and convulsion may occur
- Careful monitoring of fetal heart rate is mandatory during labor
- Labor should not be prolonged in any way. Induction delivery or onset of labor and delivery interval should be minimum (6-8 hours). Prolonged 1st stage of labor should be curtailed by doing CS and second stage of labor should be cut short by application of forceps or ventouse
- During labor, liberal analgesic and sedative is to be given in the form of pethidine.

Fluid Management in Pre-eclamptic Patients

- Careful fluid balance is to be maintained in pre-eclamptic patients.
- Diuretics should be avoided, as patients with pre-eclampsia are volume depleted (exception is pulmonary edema).
- Careful volume resuscitation is to be done to prevent pulmonary edema. Patient should be fluid restricted at least until the period of postpartum diuresis.
- A central venous pressure (CVP) or pulmonary artery pressure monitoring may be indicated in critical cases.
- Total fluid should generally be limited to 80 mL/hour or 1 mL/kg/hour.

Postpartum Management

- Injection ergometrine should be avoided in pre-eclamptic patients after placental delivery, as it may cause heart failure due to sudden increasing volume load by returning blood from retracted uterus. Though it is indicated in postpartum hemorrhage.
- All pre-eclamptic patients should be followed up vigilantly for 48 hours postpartum to prevent postpartum eclampsia. Majority of postpartum eclampsia develops within first 48 hours of delivery.
- Diuretics may be needed in some cases to prevent pulmonary edema and should be initiated shortly after vaginal or cesarean delivery at a dose of 20–40 mg IV every 6–12 hours. Women with severe pre-eclampsia usually have an acute volume expansion due to autotransfusion following the contraction of uterus and mobilization of interstitial fluid into intravascular space after delivery. That may cause heart failure and pulmonary edema.
- Liver function tests, platelet count and urinary albumin must document decreasing values prior to hospital discharge.
- Antihypertensive should be continued till reducing the blood pressure at normal level.
- Patients should be warned about development of complications like convulsion, which may develop up to 4 weeks postpartum.

What are the risks or complications of pre-eclampsia?

Pre-eclampsia is a multiorgan disorder and it causes multiple complications.

Immediate Risks

- Eclampsia
- Cerebrovascular accident (CVA)
- Heart failure
- Pulmonary edema
- Hepatic failure
- Renal failure
- Accidental hemorrhage (abruptio placenta)
- DIC
- HELLP syndrome
- Eye complication (retinal detachment)
- Premature labor.

Remote Risks

- Residual hypertension
- Recurrent pre-eclampsia
- Chronic renal disease.

What are the fetal risks of this disease?

- Prematurity
- Intrauterine growth retardation
- Intrauterine death
- Birth asphyxia
- Acute respiratory distress syndrome (ARDS).

How will you manage a case of severe pre-eclampsia in 28 weeks of pregnancy?

Patient is to be managed in the tertiary hospital with vigilant monitoring and treatment as mentioned before (detailed investigation and treatment is to be described):

- If patient becomes stable within 24 hours observation period and baseline parameters are not grossly abnormal pregnancy is to be continued with close monitoring and treatment repeating the tests daily/weekly/fortnightly as indicated.
- Response of treatment is to be assessed by comparing the baseline parameters with subsequent results.
- If response is good, pregnancy can be continued till 34 completed weeks.
- If patient is not responding to treatment pregnancy is to be terminated.

RELATED INFORMATION

Expected or conservative management in severe PE has no maternal advantages rather it exposes the mother to significant risks. Different researchers showed high stillbirth and neonatal death (33–100%) when they gave conservative treatment to women before 30 weeks of gestation (Martin and Tupper, 1979, Goodlin et al. 1978, Moore and Redman, 1983). The largest published series of expectant management (24–33 weeks) is by Haddad et al. (2004) found median prolongation of pregnancy of 5 days (2–35) with perinatal mortality 5.4%, but incidence of maternal HELLP syndrome was 14.2%. So, conservative management for severe PE developing before 30 weeks is challenging from maternal point of view. Decision should be taken by assessing risk benefit balance between mother and fetus.

How can you prevent the disease?

Pre-eclampsia is not a totally preventable disease and efforts to prevent pre-eclampsia have been disappointing (Sibai, 1998):

- *Low dose aspirin*: 75 mg daily starting from 12 weeks of gestation decreases the incidence of pre-eclampsia (Duley, 2007). Aspirin in low dose inhibits cyclo-oxygenase in platelets thereby preventing the formation of thromboxane A2 without interfering the prostacyclin generation. Aspirin in high doses inhibits both thromboxane and prostacyclin.
- *High dose calcium supplementation*: 2 g daily can prevent the disease to some extent. Although a number of researches did not find a reduction in the incidence of pre-eclampsia with calcium and vitamin C and E supplementation (Villar et al. 2006; Poston et al. 2006; Rumbold et al. 2006).
- *Antenatal check up:* Regular antenatal check up for early detection and treatment can reduce the severity and prevent complication of the disease.

Prediction of Pre-eclampsia/Screening Tests

Several tests can identify the women at risk of developing pre-eclampsia. Some tests detect pathophysiological changes that occur in pre-eclampsia and some detects biochemical alterations peculiar to the disease:

- *Angiotensin sensitivity test:* Though the development of the disease can be predicted by the degree of vascular sensitivity to angiotensin II, high false positive and false negative results limits its use. Moreover, angiotensin II is not available widely.
- *Rollover test:* Elevation of blood pressure 20 mm Hg or more when patient rolls over from lateral decubitus to supine position is indicative of future development of pre-eclampsia. Though it has limited clinical value due to poor sensitivity and specificity.
- *Calcium creatinine ratio:* Low calcium creatinine ratio is useful for identification of patients at risk.
- *Fibronectin:* Elevated plasma fibronectin is a useful prediction of pre-eclampsia.
- *Uterine artery Doppler:* Early diastolic notch in both uterine arteries at uterine artery Doppler velocimetry at 22–24 weeks is a good predictor of development of pre-eclampsia.

What is the recurrence rate of the disease?

The recurrence risk of pre-eclampsia in woman whose previous pregnancy was complicated by pre-eclampsia near term is approximately 10%. The earlier the disease manifests during pregnancy the higher the chance of recurrence. If pre-eclampsia presented before 30th weeks of gestation, the chance of recurrence may be as high as 40% (Sibai et al. 1991).

> **Case scenario:** Mrs Halima a 32-year-old lady of lower socioeconomic class has come to you with history of amenorrhea for 32 weeks, and convulsion (fit) for 5 hours.
> How will you proceed to diagnose the case?

Pregnancy with convulsion is to be considered as eclampsia until and unless proved otherwise.

Detailed history is to be taken to find out the cause of convulsion:

- Before onset of convulsion was there any oliguria, nausea, vomiting, insomnia or epigastric pain, which are symptoms of severe form of pre-eclampsia?
- Number of convulsion
- Whether there is any history of rise of temp? (to exclude febrile convulsion, pontine hemorrhage, encephalitis, meningitis, cerebral malaria)
- Whether there is any predisposing factors for psychological stress (to exclude hysteric convulsion)
- History of epilepsy
- History of antenatal check-up and diagnosis of raised blood pressure
- Family history of hypertension, eclampsia, pre-eclampsia, diabetes mellitus
- History of rapid weight gain
- History of swelling of hands and feet (though edema is not diagnostic for PE/eclampsia, it is associated with these).

To determine gestational age, menstrual history is to be taken:

- Whether menstrual cycle was regular or not?
- What was the length of the cycle?
- When was the last menstrual period?

About obstetric history:

- Is it her first pregnancy?
- If not how was her previous pregnancy? Was there any similar complication?

Physical Examination

General Examination

- Pulse and blood pressure is to be checked
- Heart and lungs are to be auscultated
- Whether there is any pitting edema and generalized edema
- Level of consciousness (Glasgow coma scale).

Obstetrical Examination

Per abdomen (P/A)

- Uterine height to assess gestational age
- Uterine contraction
- Fetal heart sound auscultation
- Assessment of liquor volume.

Per vaginal (P/V)
To assess:

- Position, consistency, effacement and dilatation of the cervix

- Station of fetal head
- Adequacy of pelvis.

Investigation

Dipstick urine test is to be done to assess the presence of albumin in urine.

> On enquiry from attendant, it is revealed that she is a primiparous woman without any antenatal check-up. Her LMP was 32 weeks back. For last 1 month she noticed swelling of legs and hands. She also suffered from headache and insomnia for a few days. No history of previous convulsion. After physical examination it is revealed that her pulse is 78/m, BP is 170/120 mm Hg, heart, lungs clear, pitting edema is present. Patient is conscious. Patient is not in labor and fetal heart rate is 140/m. Dipstick urine test shows +++ albumin.
> What is your diagnosis? Give reason for diagnosis.

It is a case of eclampsia. Pregnancy with hypertension and proteinuria are diagnostic feature for PE. When PE complicates with convulsion, it is called eclampsia.

> What other investigations are needed for management of this patient?

Other Investigations

- Hb%
- Routine urine analysis
- Blood grouping and Rh typing if not known before
- Blood sugar 2 hours postprandial
- Kidney function tests:
  - Blood, urea, creatinine
  - Serum uric acid.
- Liver function tests:
  - SGOT
  - SGPT
  - LDH
  - Serum bilirubin if yellow tint of skin and urine is present.
- Coagulation profile
  - Platelet count
  - PT
  - APTT.
- USG for fetal well-being
- Doppler study of umbilical artery.

RELATED INFORMATION

Eclampsia is a consequence of pre-eclampsia. When pre-eclampsia is complicated with fit or convulsion then it is called eclampsia. Incidence is between 1 in 2,000 and 1 in 4,000 in developed countries, but it is several times higher in developing countries. In Bangladesh, eclampsia is the third major cause of maternal death (16%). In hospital statistics, it is the first cause and more than 50% maternal death is due to eclampsia. Although PPH is the first cause of maternal death nationwise, in hospital due to competent management of PPH with liberal blood transfusion mortality can be prevented. But in case of eclampsia when patient comes with multiple complications then patient's condition goes beyond the scope of management resulting high mortality.

As this is the complication of severe pre-eclampsia the etiology, pathogenesis and risk factors are same as pre-eclampsia. When pre-eclampsia remains neglected and untreated it complicates with convulsion and eclampsia develops. Convulsion occurs due to spasm of cerebral vessels, causing cerebral anoxia, edema and irritation.

Types of Eclampsia

Eclampsia can be classified as:
- *Antepartum eclampsia:* When convulsion occurs before onset of labor (50% cases)
- *Intrapartum eclampsia:* When convulsion occurs for the first time during labor (30% cases)
- *Postpartum eclampsia:* When convulsion occurs for the first time after birth of the baby in puerperal period (20%). Majority occurs within first 48 hours of puerperium. That is why intensive monitoring of severe PE cases is needed during this period. Commonly convulsion occurs within 7 days of puerperium, but rarely may occur any time during puerperium.

Stages of Convulsion

Eclamptic convulsion or fit has four stages:
1. *Premonitory stage:* There is twitching of the muscle of the face, tongue and limbs, and

rolling of eye balls at this stage. This stage persists for 30 seconds **(Fig. 9.1)**.
2. *Tonic stage:* The whole body goes into a tonic spasm (state of opisthotonus). Respiration ceases, tongue protrudes and cyanosis occurs. This stage persists for 30 seconds.
3. *Clonic stage:* At this stage, all the voluntary muscles undergo alternate contraction and relaxation and lasts for 1–4 minutes.
4. *Stage of coma:* After cessation of convulsion patient passes on to the stage of coma, which lasts for a brief period or till another convulsion.

Mechanism of Convulsion

Cerebral edema is the main cause of convulsion in eclampsia. But mechanism of development of edema is different in severe and mild hypertension. In severe hypertension with PE, the normal autoregulatory response to hypertension is exceeded and vasodilatation occurs with hyperperfusion. Due to excessive vasodilatation endothelial capillary damage occurs causing vasogenic edema. On the other hand in mild hypertension, there is abnormal autoregulation with exaggerated vasoconstriction and ischemic changes causing fluid exudation in cortical matter. By these ways, cerebral edema is responsible for convulsion in eclampsia. Intracranial Doppler (Riskin-Mashiah and Belfort, 2005) and MRI (Morris et al. 1997) demonstrated elevated perfusion pressure and lower vascular resistance in the cerebral circulation of pre-eclamptic women.

Differential Diagnosis

There may be convulsion due to other causes during pregnancy which needs to be differentiated from eclamptic convulsion. Other causes of convulsion are:
- Epilepsy
- Hysteria
- Encephalitis
- Meningitis
- Puerperal cerebral thrombosis
- Poisoning
- Cerebral malaria.

> How will you manage Mrs Halima?

Management/Treatment

Management of eclampsia includes:
1. General management
2. Controlling of convulsion
3. Controlling of blood pressure
4. Obstetrical management (delivery by 6–8 hours).

Note: In other cases, where there is complication, treatment of complication will be included.

So for this patient, treatment will be:
1. *General management*:
   - Patient should be kept in a comfortable situation in an isolated room
   - A self-retaining catheter is to be introduced for continuous drainage and measurement of the urinary output. It also helps to collect urine for testing and prevents soiling of bed during convulsion if occurs
   - Pulse, respiratory rate and blood pressure are to be recorded 4 hourly
   - Heart lungs are to be ausculted for added breath sounds and basal crepitation, 4 hourly

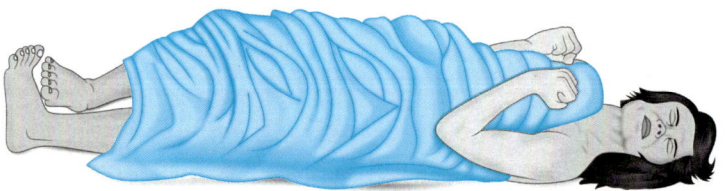

Fig. 9.1 Eclamptic convulsion

- Fluid balance is to be maintained intravenously by 5% D/A 1,000 mL + the amount equivalent to previous days output, but should not more than 2,000 mL in 24 hours
- Antibiotic is to be given to prevent infection
- Oral feeding also is to be given.

2. *Controlling of convulsion (fit)*: MgSO$_4$ is the most potent anticonvulsant used to control convulsion. It can be used in two ways. So, any one of the regimes can be used.

   Criteria for administering MgSO$_4$:
   - Urine output should be at least 30 mL/hour
   - Respiratory rate should be at least 16/minute
   - Patellar reflex (knee jerk) should be present.

   a. **Loading plus maintenance dose:**
      - *Combined intravenous and intramuscular protocol*: The low dose regime injection MgSO$_4$ 4 g IV and 6 g IM, 3 g in each buttock as loading dose is to be administered as quickly as possible, which will be followed by 2.5 g IM every 4 hours till 24 hours of last fit or delivery which occurs later (Eclampsia Working Group, 1996; Shamsuddin, 1997).
        Note: A large series shows same efficacy when MgSO$_4$ administered for 24 hours from the first dose of the drug (Begum et al. 2002). Advantage of this regime is that, the duration of treatment is reduced by few hours.
      - *Only intravenous protocol* (Described in page 120).
   b. **Only loading dose:** Injection MgSO$_4$ 4 g IV and 6 g IM, 3 g in each buttock (Begum et al. 2002). Recurrent convulsion rate is 4%, which is comparable with the rate of 3.5% with standard regimen. Case fatality rate is 4.5 and 5% with only loading dose and standard regimen respectively:
      - For recurrent convulsion injection MgSO$_4$ 2.5 g IM stat is to be given if it occurs beyond 30 minutes of first dose
        Note: Convulsion that occurs within 30 minutes of first dose is not recognized as recurrent convulsion.

- As precaution patient is to be monitored before each administration of MgSO$_4$ to avoid toxic effect of drugs by observing urine output, respiratory rate and patellar reflex (knee jerk) as mentioned earlier.

3. *Controlling of blood pressure*: As blood pressure is very high this is hypertensive emergency, so immediate injection hydralazine or labetalol is to be started to control blood pressure. Then oral form is to be added to maintain blood pressure to a safe level.
   (**Note:** Same protocol, which mentioned in hypertensive emergency in PE).

4. *Obstetrical management*: Eclampsia is a very high-risk pregnancy. Once it is diagnosed there is no scope of continuation of pregnancy. Termination of pregnancy is the definitive treatment for eclampsia:
   - As patient is not in labor, if pelvis is adequate and Bishop's score is favorable it is to be induced by ARM followed by oxytocin drip.
   - Patient should be monitored vigilantly for progress of labor and for detection of any complications.
   - Duration of labor should be curtailed by cesarean section in 1st stage and by forceps or ventouse in 2nd stage.

Labor management, fluid intake during labor and postpartum management are same as management with severe PE patients.

> What other anticonvulsants can be used?

Following anticonvulsants can be used, but in Bangladesh, diazepam is generally used:
- Diazepam
- Phenytoin
- Phenobarbitone
- Lytic cocktails.

RELATED INFORMATION

Magnesium Sulfate

Mechanism of Action of MgSO$_4$

- It causes vasodilatation → Increases cerebral blood flow → Reduces anoxia, cerebral edema and irritation thus prevent convulsion.

- It decreases the acetylcholine release from the nerve endings and reduces the motor end plate sensitivity to acetylcholine. It also blocks calcium channel. As a result prevent convulsion.
- It increases uterine and renal blood flow so improves renal and uteroplacental function.
- It inhibits platelet aggregation so prevents coagulation cascade.

Original Dose of $MgSO_4$

Original Pritchard's regime is 4 g IV and 5 g in each buttock as loading dose followed by 5 g IM every 4 hours till 24 hours of last fit or delivery, which occurs later (Pritchard, 1955). As Bangladeshi women are of low BMI, average 53 kg during pregnancy, a lower dose is equally effective for controlling convulsion. Lighter patients have a lower total body volume, so the drug concentration is accordingly higher in serum during treatment with maintenance regimen (Chesley 1957; Brandt et al. 1958; Chesley, 1979).

Alternate Dosing of $MgSO_4$

Only intravenous $MgSO_4$ can be used for controlling convulsion, but drawback of this regime is that inadvertent high dosing during continuous infusion may occur. Zuspan promotes a 4 g intravenous loading dose over 15 minutes followed by a 2–3 g/hour maintenance infusion (Zuspan, 1978).

According to *Eclampsia Working Group Bangladesh*, the IV dose of $MgSO_4$ is following:
4 g (100 mL) IV rapidly at a rate of 60–70 drops/minute over a period of 20 minutes. Then 2 g (50 mL) IV slowly at a rate of 12 drops/minute within 1st hour. Finally drug is to be maintained by giving 4 g (100 mL) at a rate of 6 drops/minute within next 4 hours.

Diazepam

Mechanism of Action of Diazepam

Diazepam enhances the effect of the neurotransmitter GABA by binding to the benzodiazepine site on the $GABA_A$ receptor leading to central nervous system depression and control convulsion. It acts on the limbic, thalamic and hypothalamic regions of the CNS to potentiate the effects of inhibitory neurotransmitters, raising the seizure threshold in the motor cortex.

Dose of Diazepam

Injection diazepam 10 mg IV and 10 mg IM slowly stat then 40 mg in 500 mL dextrose in aqua IV at a rate of 10–15 drops per minute for 24 hours.

Advantages of $MgSO_4$ over Diazepam

$MgSO_4$ has got some beneficiary effects in comparison to diazepam like:
- $MgSO_4$ is much more effective in terms of controlling convulsion in comparison to diazepam
- Patient becomes deeply sedated with diazepam, but remains alert with $MgSO_4$ so chance of aspiration is less or absent
- Recurrent convulsion rate is less in comparison to diazepam
- No fetal hypotonia occurs like diazepam
- It has got immediate hypotensive effect by causing cerebral vasodilatation
- It inhibits platelet aggregation and coagulation
- It reduces cerebral edema.

> *Why it is necessary to monitor urine output, respiratory rate and tendon reflex (Knee jerk) before administration of $MgSO_4$?*

Magnesium sulfate has serious toxicity causes *cardiac arrest* and *respiratory arrest*. Its window of therapeutic level and toxic level is very narrow (upper limit of therapeutic level is 8.4 mg/dL and lower limit of toxic level is 10 mg/dL). That is why it needs proper selection of the case for using the drug and continuous monitoring throughout the treatment period. During treatment, patient is to be monitored by observing urine output, respiratory rate and patellar reflex (knee jerk) as mentioned earlier. *Drug is contraindicated if any one of the criteria is not fulfilled*. Because $MgSO_4$ is excreted solely through kidney. If renal function is compromised then $MgSO_4$ excretion will be diminished and will cause toxicity. Earliest sign of $MgSO_4$ toxicity is loss of tendon reflexes (knee jerk) at serum level of 10 mg/dL, then respiratory arrest at serum level of 15 mg/dL and cardiac arrest at serum level of 20 mg/dL.

> Suppose upon introduction of catheter you found that scanty urine came only into the catheter, not deposited into the bag. You know that if urine output is <30 mL/hour then MgSO₄ is contraindicated, but you also know that it is very much effective anticonvulsant.
> In this situation how will you manage the patient?

Detailed History is to be Taken

- Whether convulsion was preceded by oliguria?
- Whether the cloth becomes wet during transportation? If wet may be due to passage of urine or rupture of membrane. If membrane is intact then possibility of passage of urine is there:
  - If there is no history of oliguria or history of passage of urine on the way then urine will come soon after a few minutes observation. Then MgSO₄ can be given.
  - If there is history of oliguria or no history of passage of urine then considering the case of oliguria MgSO₄ administration is to be delayed till further assessment. In that case diazepam is to be used for immediate controlling of convulsion.
  - If it is due to *volume depletion* or there is dehydration, infusion of running aqua will give rise to urine production and MgSO₄ can be started thereafter.
  - If it is due to *renal function impairment* due to ischemia resulting from vasospasm urine will not come even after fluid administration. MgSO₄ is *contraindicated in renal function impairment*. Alternate anticonvulsant like diazepam is to be given to control convulsion.

Note: In case of *renal function impairment* urine may come after giving injection furosemide. Coming of urine after giving furosemide is not an indicator of healthy kidney. So even after optimum output with furosemide MgSO₄ is contraindicated as function of the kidney is compromised here and there is chance of accumulation of MgSO₄ in the body.

> During monitoring of MgSO₄ therapy, it is found that Halima's knee jerk could not be elicited or knee jerk is absent.
> What measure would you like to take?

- The earliest sign of MgSO₄ toxicity is absence of knee jerk. As it indicates toxicity next dose of MgSO₄ must be omitted.
- As antidote calcium gluconate 5 mL (1 g) IV is to be given.
- Patient is to be watched to observe whether further convulsion takes place or not; if no further convulsion, no need of any further anticonvulsant
- If there is convulsion switch over to diazepam for anticonvulsant.

> What are the side effects of MgSO₄?

- Feeling of warmth
- Flushing
- Nausea
- Vomiting
- Slurred speech
- Hypotension and arrhythmia.

> Suppose after 2 hours of starting MgSO₄ patient again developed convulsion.
> What do you want to do?

Patient developed recurrent convulsion. For which injection MgSO₄ 2.5 g IM is to be given with usual scheduled injection after 2 hours.

> If she develops convulsion 15 minutes after completion of first dose. What to do?

Nothing is to be done as sometimes it takes a little time to achieve the action of MgSO₄. Usually, it is less intense and subsides quickly. No need of giving further injection if convulsion occurs within 30 minutes of first injection.

> Suppose just at arrival patient has a convulsion for a sustained period. You did not get the chance to take history and perform examination. You do not know the status of kidney function.
> Will you give MgSO₄?

No. To be on safe side it is better to control convulsion by giving injection diazepam 10 mg IV and 10 mg IM. After completion of history and physical examination if there is no contraindication of MgSO$_4$ it is to be started as usual dose. There is no harm of giving diazepam with MgSO$_4$. If MgSO$_4$ is found contraindicated diazepam drip is to be started as per schedule.

> During follow-up of labor suddenly patient became restless and seems to be a stage of convulsion.
> Will you give MgSO$_4$ as recurrent dose?

As patient is in labor per vaginal examination is to be done to assess whether she is in second stage of labor or not. Usually, at second stage of labor patient behaves like this. If it is due to stress of labor nothing is to be given except acceleration of labor.

> Suppose the patient came in a stage of coma. She had repeated convulsion >20 times within last 12 hours. For 2 hours she is unconscious and did not develop any convulsion. On examination you could not elicited the knee jerk. Her respiratory rate and urine output is normal. She did not receive any anticonvulsant.
> Which anticonvulsant would you like to give?

Right at this moment patient does not need any anticonvulsant as she is deeply unconscious. She needs to be kept under close supervision. If she further develops convulsion MgSO$_4$ can be considered. Any neurological problem may be responsible for not eliciting knee jerk. As she did not receive any MgSO$_4$ beforehand so there is no question of toxicity. But she should receive only loading dose as knee jerk monitoring during maintenance schedule may misinterpreted in such a case.

> How will you assess her level of consciousness?

Level of consciousness can be assessed by scoring Glasgow coma scale (**Table 9.1**). It gives reliable, objective way of recording the conscious state of a person. A person is assessed against the criteria of the scale. Score 3 indicating deep unconsciousness (coma) and 15 is fully conscious. Previously score 14 was for conscious people, but the more widely used revised scale used 15 for conscious people. The score is based on the result of three tests like eye response, response on verbal command and motor response.

> Suppose in spite of giving MgSO$_4$ patient developed convulsion, which persisted for >5 minutes. How will you manage her?

This is a case of status eclampticus. It is a condition when brain is in a state of persistent convulsion without any remission for 5 minutes or more. Thiopental sodium is to be given to control convulsion.

> **Case scenario:** Sajeda a 28 years lady gave birth a baby at home per vaginally 12 hours ago. Suddenly she developed convulsion 4 hours after delivery. With this complaint she has come to you. Her blood pressure is 155/110 mm Hg. She has no edema, but her dipstick urine test revealed +++ albumin in urine. She had no antenatal check-up and she did not go to any other facility with this complaints. Number of fit is 12–14 times within these 8 hours. Patient is unconscious, but responded to deep stimulation. There is history of tongue bite. Slight froth is coming and on auscultation basal crepts are present in the lungs. After catheterization 200 mL urine came out, which is accumulation of last 5 hours.
> On the basis of these findings what is your diagnosis? How will you manage this case?

Table 9.1 Glasgow coma scale

	1	2	3	4	5	6
Eye	Does not open	Opens eyes in response to painful stimuli	Opens eyes in response to voice	Opens eyes spontaneously	NA	NA
Verbal	Makes no sound	Incomprehensible sound	Utters inappropriate words	Confused, disoriented	Oriented, converses normally	NA
Motor	Makes no movements	Extension to painful stimuli	Abnormal flexion to painful stimuli	Flexion/withdrawal to painful stimuli	Localizes painful stimuli	Obeys commands

Diagnosis and Management

This is a case of postpartum eclampsia with pulmonary edema.

The line of management is exactly the same as antepartum eclampsia except labor management as she is postpartum.

Additional managements are:
- Per vaginal examination is to be done to exclude lacerations, tear and retention of placental tissue as delivery was conducted at home.
- Patient should be kept in *eclamptic position* in an isolated room:
  - Lateral position with head extended, which will facilitate postural drainage
  - Lower leg straight, upper leg flexed over the abdomen
  - Lower arm free and upper arm flexed over the chest.
- The airway is to be cleaned and a mouth gag is to be placed as patient is unconscious, there is chance of aspiration and tongue fall back
- Posture is to be changed every 2 hours
- Oropharyngeal suction is to be given
- O_2 inhalation
- Care of the eyes and oral hygiene is to be taken
- Diuretics 20–40 mg IV every 6 hours is to be added to reduce pulmonary edema
- As patient is unconscious Ryle's tube feeding is to be given till regain of consciousness.

Note:
- In antepartum cases with pulmonary edema in addition to above mentioned management patient should be managed according to status of labor, whether she is in labor or not. If she is not in labor it should be induced and if she is in labor it should be augmented. Rest will be same as other cases. Precaution should be taken about fluid infusion. Vaginal delivery is preferable. If cesarean section is needed spinal anesthesia is preferable.
- For conscious patient no need of eclamptic position.
- In postpartum eclampsia without any complication and with consciousness controlling of convulsion and blood pressure will be the appropriate management.

RELATED INFORMATION

The indications of diuretics in pre-eclampsia eclampsia are oliguria, anuria and pulmonary edema. Because intravascular fluid volume is already reduced in pre-eclampsia and eclampsia. Diuretics will further reduce the volume, which will reduce both renal and uterine circulation. *So diuretics are not indicated to reduce generalized edema.*

In eclampsia, main causes of development of *pulmonary edema* are:
- Fluid overload
- Left ventricular failure
- Aspiration
- Reduced oncotic pressure causes leakage of fluid from blood vessel.

In Bangladesh, *pulmonary edema* is the most common cause of *maternal death* from eclampsia.

> What are the complications of eclampsia?

Maternal Complications

- Cerebrovascular accident (CVA)
- Pulmonary edema
- Acute left ventricular failure
- Hepatic subcapsular hemorrhage, necrosis and failure
- Renal failure
- Accidental hemorrhage (abruptio placenta)
- DIC
- HELLP syndrome
- Coma
- Eye complication (retinal detachment)
- Premature labor
- Postpartum shock
- Postpartum sepsis
- Postpartum psychosis.

Fetal Complications

- Prematurity
- Intrauterine growth retardation
- Intrauterine death
- Birth asphyxia
- ARDS.

How will you Judge the Prognosis of an Eclamptic Case?

- Prognosis of the patient is good when there is no complication except convulsion
- Prognosis is worse even *death may occur* in the following situation:
  - Duration of convulsive state is more than 8 hours
  - Repeated convulsion
  - Deep coma
  - Infection
  - Cerebrovascular accident (CVA)
  - Heart failure
  - Pulmonary edema
  - Hepatic failure
  - Renal failure
  - Accidental hemorrhage (abruptio placenta)
  - DIC
  - HELLP syndrome.

What are the causes of high perinatal death in pre-eclampsia, eclampsia?

- Prematurity
- Intrauterine growth retardation due to placental insufficiency
- Intrauterine death due to same reason
- Operative interference.

Case scenario: Selina a primiparous 32-year-old woman has come to you with the complaints of 34 weeks pregnancy with convulsion for 8 hours. On taking history she gave history of oliguria, headache and sleeplessness for last three days. She is disoriented. On examination her blood pressure is 160/110 mm Hg, generalized edema is present. After catheterization 150 mL yellowish urine came, which is the accumulation of last 4 hours. On per abdominal examination uterus is 34 weeks size, FHR: 145/m, contraction absent. On per vaginal examination there is no sign of labor, Cx is soft and partially effaced, os closed, presentation Vx deep stick urine test shows +++ albumin.

UTP 4.5 g, uric acid 6 mg/dL, serum bilirubin 3 mg/dL, SGOT 80 IU/L, SGPT 78 IU/L, LDH 850 IU/L, platelet count 90,000/mm^3.

On the basis of these findings, what is your diagnosis?

Eclampsia with HELLP syndrome.

What are the diagnostic points of HELLP syndrome?

- Sign of hemolysis—bilirubin (≥ 1.2 mg/dL) and (LDH > 600 IU/L).
- Elevated liver enzymes (ALT $\geq$ 72 IU/L, LDH >600 IU/L).
- Low platelet count (<100,000/mm^3).

Note: Other signs of hemolysis are:
- Burr cells, schistocytes in the blood smear
- Absent plasma haptoglobin.

How will you manage her?

Patient will be managed following same principle of management of eclampsia. In addition complication (HELLP) will be managed:
- *Anticonvulsant* (As described before)
- *Antihypertensive* (As described before)
- *General management* (As described before)
- *Obstetric management*: Termination of pregnancy is the definitive treatment in case of eclampsia irrespective of gestational age. So, pregnancy is to be terminated. As cervix is soft and favorable, presentation is Vx and fetal condition is good, labor is to be induced by ARM followed by oxytocin drip. But here platelet count is low so caution is to be taken to improve platelet count simultaneously.

Following extra measures are to be taken for complication:
- Administration of fresh frozen plasma to improve platelet count
- Donor should be kept ready for platelet concentration as transfusion of platelet is needed if count falls below 50,000/mm^3
- Administration of corticosteroid betamethasone 12 mg IM 12 hourly for 48 hours or dexamethasone 6 mg intravenously 6 hourly for four doses:
  - It accelerates fetal lung maturity
  - Achieve maternal hemodynamic stabilization through volume expansion
  - It increases platelet count
  - It causes quick normalization of platelet count and LDH, and reduction of blood pressure.

RELATED INFORMATION

Eclampsia with HELLP Syndrome

The HELLP has been recognized as a complication of pre-eclampsia and eclampsia for many years. Incidence is 4–12% among pre-eclampsia, eclampsia. HELLP is classified according to Mississippi triple class system in class 1, 2 and 3, which is used to facilitate management and estimate risk for major maternal morbidity (Magann et al. 1994).

Classification

Patients are classified into:
- *Class 1, severe thrombocytopenia*: 0 to ≤50,000/mm^3, LDH ≥ 600 IU/L, AST and/or ALT ≥70 IU/L (major maternal morbidity 40–60%)
- *Class 2, moderate thrombocytopenia*: >50,000 to ≤100,000/mm^3, LDH ≥ 600 IU/L, and AST and/or ALT ≥ 70 IU/L (major maternal morbidity 20–40%)
- *Class 3, mild thrombocytopenia*: >100,000 to ≤150,000/mm^3, LDH ≥ 600 IU/L, and AST ≥40 IU/L (major maternal morbidity 20%).

Platelet transfusion is necessary when platelet count falls below 25 × 10^9/L. One unit of pooled platelets is expected to increase the platelet count by about 10,000/mm^3. Regional anesthesia is contraindicated when platelet falls below 80 × 10^9/L, owing to the risk of epidural hematoma.

The clinical course of HELLP is one of progressive deterioration of the maternal and fetal conditions with 1% risk of maternal death.

Following are the conditions associated with HELLP syndrome:
- Abruptio placenta
- DIC
- Pulmonary edema
- Acute renal failure
- Adult RDS
- Hepatic rupture
- Death.

Perinatal morbidity and mortality is also significantly high due to prematurity.

Note: Management of acute renal failure, DIC, abruptio placenta, is not different in eclampsia than in other obstetric situation. So details are not described here.

Management of acute left ventricular failure with eclampsia: Patient suddenly develops breathlessness, on auscultation crepitation present. Evidence of hypoxia by pulse oxymetry or arterial blood gas, and chest X-ray findings consistent with pulmonary edema.

Aim of Treatment

Aim of treatment is to:
- Keep airway clear
- Maintain optimum O$_2$ supply
- Maintain fluid volume.

Line of Treatment

- As usual management of eclampsia described earlier
- High flow O$_2$. If saturation cannot be maintained by high flow O$_2$, ventilatory support may needed
- Injection furosemide
- Suction
- Nebulization
- Digitalization
- Fluid restriction
- Delivery should be within short time with minimum exhaustion. Vaginal delivery is preferable. If CS is needed general anesthesia is preferable. No ergometrine after placental delivery except PPH.

> What will you do if patient develops visual disorders?

Blindness may occur in pre-eclampsia eclampsia due to multiple microhemorrhage and microinfarcts in the occipital lobe. By fundoscopy local and generalized vasospasm and retinal edema can be observed. Blindness may persist for several days though quick recovery after delivery is the rule.

> How eclampsia can be prevented?

Regular antenatal check-up and proper management of pre-eclampsia with timely interference can prevent the development of eclampsia.

BIBLIOGRAPHY

ACOG. Committee on Practice Bulletins-Obstetrics. Diagnosis and management of pre-eclampsia and eclampsia. Obstet Gynecol. 2001;98:159-67.

American College of Obstetricians and Gynecologists. Diagnosis and management of pre-eclampsia and eclampsia. Practice bulletin no 33. Washington DC: ACOG; 2002.

American College of Obstetricians and Gynecologists. Hypertension in pregnancy. ACOG Technical Bulletin No. 219. Washington DC; 1996.

Begum MR, Begum A, Quadir E. Loading dose versus standard regime of magnesium sulfate in the management of eclampsia: a randomized trial. J Obstet Gynaecol. 2002;28(3):154-9.

Belfort MA, Anthony J, Saade GR, et al. A comparison of magnesium sulfate and nimodipine for the prevention of eclampsia. N Eng J Med. 2003;248:304-11.

Brandt JL, Glaser W, Jones A. Soft tissue distribution and plasma disappearance of intravenously administered isotopic magnesium with observations on uptake in bone. Metabolism. 1958;7:355-62.

Chesley LC. Parenteral magnesium sulfate and the distribution, plasma levels and excretion of magnesium. AM J Obstet Gynecol. 1979;133:1-7.

Chesely LC, Tepper I. Plasma levels of magnesium attained in magnesium sulfate therapy for pre-eclampsia and eclampsia. Surg Clin North Am. 1957;37:353-67.

Coetzee EJ, Dommisse J, Anthony J. A randomized controlled trial of intravenous magnesium sulfate versus placebo I the management of women with severe pre-eclampsia. Br J Obstet Gynecol. 1998;105:300-3.

Duley L, Henderson-Smart DJ, Meher S, et al. Antiplatelet agents for preventing pre-eclampsia and its complications. Cochrane Database Syst Rev. 2007;(2):CD004659.

Eclampsia working group, Eclampsia in Bangladesh: A review and guideline. B J Obstet Gynaecol. 1996; 12(1):1-25.

Friedman SA, Schiff E, Emeis JJ, et al. Biochemical corroboration of endothelial involvement in severe pre-eclampsia. Am J Obstet Gynecol. 1995;172(1 Pt 1):202-3.

Goodlin RC, Cotton DB, Haesslein HC. Severe edema proteinuria-hypertension gestosis. Am J Obstet Gynecol. 1978;132:595.

Haddad B, Deis S, Goffinet F, et al. Maternal and perinatal outcome during expectant management of 239 severe preeclamptic women between 24 and 33 weeks gestation. Am J Obstet Gynecol. 2004;190:1590-7.

Khedun SM, Moodley J, Naicker T, et al. Drug management of hypertensive disorders of pregnancy. Pharmacol Ther. 1997;74(2):221-58.

Lim KH, Zhou Y, Janatpour M, et al. Human cytotrophoblast differentiation/invasion is abnormal in pre-eclampsia. Am J Pathol. 1997;151(6):1809-18.

Livingston JC, Livingston LW, Ramsey R, et al. Magnesium sulfate in women with mild pre-eclampsia: a randomized controlled trial. Obstet Gynecol. 2003;101:217-20.

Magann EF, Bas D, Chauhan SP, et al. Antepartum corticosteroids: disease stabilization in patients with the syndrome of hemolysis, elevated liver enzymes and low platelets (HELLP). AM J Obstet Gynecol. 1994;171:1148-53.

Magee LA, Cham C, Waterman EJ, et al. Hydralazine in pregnancy. A meta-analysis. Br Med J. 2003;327:955.

Magpie trial Collaborative Group. DO women with pre-eclampsia, and their babies, benefit from magnesium sulfate? The Magpie Trial: a randomized placebo-controlled trial. Lancet. 2002;359:1877-90.

Martin TR, Tupper WR. The management of severe toxemia in patients at less than 36 weeks gestation. Obstet Gynaecol. 1979;54:602-5.

Moore MP, Redman CWG. Case control study of severe pre-eclampsia of early onset. BMJ. 1983;287:580.

Morris MC, Twickler DM, Hatab MR, et al. Cerebral blood flow and cranial magnetic resonance imaging in in eclampsia and severe pre-eclampsia. Obstet Gynaecol. 1997;89:561-8.

Ngoc NT, Merialdi M, Abdel-Aleem H, et al. Causes of stillbirths and early neonatal deaths: data from 7,993 pregnancies in six developing countries. Bull World Health Organ. 2006;84(9):699-705.

NHBPEP: Report of the National High Blood Pressure Education Program Working Group on High Blood Pressure in Pregnancy. Am J Obstet Gynecol. 2000;183(1):S1-S22.

Poston L, Briley AL, Seed PT, et al. Vitamin C and vitamin E in pregnant women at risk for pre-eclampsia (VIP trial): randomized placebo-controlled trial. Lancet. 2006;367(9517):1145-54.

Pritchard JA. The use of the magnesium ion in the management of eclampogenic toxemias. Surg Gynecol Obstet. 1955;100:131-40.

Redman CW, Sargent IL. Latest advances in understanding pre-eclampsia. Science. 2005;308(5728):1592-94. Doi 10. 1126/science. 1111726. PIMD 15947178.

Riskin-Mashiah S, Belfort MA. Pre-eclampsia is associated with global haemodynamic changes. J Soc Gyneco Investig. 2005;12:253-56.

Rumbold AR, Crowther CA, Haslam RR, et al. Vitamins C and E and the risks of pre-eclampsia and perinatal complications. N Engl J Med. 2006;354(17):1796-806.

Samsuddin L. Official publication of the Federation of Scandinavian Societies of Obstetrics and Gynaecology. Acta Obstet Scand. 1997;76 (Supplement 167): 34.

Sibai BM, Mercer B, Sarinoglu C. Severe pre-eclampsia in the second trimester: recurrence risk and long-term prognosis. Am J Obstet Gynecol. 1991;165(5 Pt 1):1408-12.

Sibai BM. Chronic hypertension and pregnancy. Obstet Gynecol. 2002;100:369-77.

Sibai BM. Prevention of pre-eclampsia: a big disappointment. Am J Obstet Gynecol. 1998;179(5):1275-8.

Taylor RN, de Groot CJ, Cho YK, et al. Circulating factors as markers and mediators of endothelial cell dysfunction in preeclampsia. Semin Reprod Endocrinol. 1998;16(1):17-31.

Villar J, Abdel-Aleem H, Merialdi M, et al. World Health Organization randomized trial of calcium supplementation among low calcium intake pregnant women. Am J Obstet Gynecol. 2006;194(3):639-49.

Villar J, Betran AP, Gulmezoglu M. Epidemiological basis for the planning of maternal health services. WHO/RHR, 2001.

Zhou Y, Damsky CH, Chiu K, et al. Preeclampsia is associated with abnormal expression of adhesion molecules by invasive cytotrophoblasts. J Clin Invest. 1993;91(3):950-60.

Zhou Y, Damsky CH, Fisher SJ. Preeclampsia is associated with failure of human cytotrophoblasts to mimic a vascular adhesion phenotype. One cause of defective endovascular invasion in this syndrome. J Clin Invest. 1997;99(9):2152-64.

Zuspan FP. Problem encountered in the treatment of pregnancy induced hypertension. Am J Obstet Gynecol. 1978;131:591-7.

CHAPTER 10

Ectopic Pregnancy

Rashida Begum

INTRODUCTION

Any pregnancy located outside the uterine cavity is defined as an ectopic pregnancy (EP). The vast majority (99%) of EP's occurs in the fallopian tube and account for 1–2% of all pregnancies. Ectopic pregnancies are potentially life-threatening and diagnostic delay may loss the life. The incidence is increasing yearly due to the occurrence of sexually transmitted diseases, prior salpingitis, intrauterine device (IUD) use, pelvic adhesions and others. Although, many reports from different countries indicated a trend in the decline in the incidence (Coste et al. 2000; Irvin and Setchell, 2001). EP remained the leading cause of early pregnancy fatality (Centers for Disease Control and Prevention, 1995). Diagnosis at the earliest stage can prevent the catastrophes from EP. With transvaginal ultrasonography and an experienced ultrasonographer a normal intrauterine pregnancy should be visible by the time a woman is 5 weeks (only sac) and 6 weeks amenorrhoic (embryo with cardiac pulsation) from her last menstrual period (LMP).

> **Case scenario:** A 28-year-old woman married for 3 years has come to you with amenorrhea for 6 weeks and lower abdominal pain for 4 hours.
> How will you proceed for diagnosis?

Detailed History is to be Taken First

Menstrual History

- About her previous menstrual cycles:
  - Length of the cycle
  - Whether cycle was regular or irregular: In reproductive age amenorrhea in a regularly menstruating woman may be due to pregnancy
- When was her LMP?

Signs and Symptoms of Pregnancy

Is there any symptom of pregnancy such as vomiting, morning sickness?

Contraceptive History

History of taking any contraceptives and history of infertility

If she has any history of taking intrauterine contraceptive device (IUCD) or history of infertility then there is possibility of having ectopic pregnancy.

Pattern of Pain

Intensity of pain: Sudden severe agonizing pain with syncopal attack suggests ectopic pregnancy.

Patient is to be examined thoroughly
- *General examination:* Pulse, blood pressure (BP) and pallor is to be looked for to assess sign of hemorrhage.
- *Per abdominal (PA) examination:* Whether abdomen is distended, tense and tender
- *Per vaginal (PV) examination:* Fornices are tender and posterior fornix may be bulged due to intraperitoneal hemorrhage (PV examination should be gentle as it may provoke the rupture of an unruptured tube or bleeding by dislodging the clots from previously ruptured site).

Ectopic Pregnancy

> On enquiry you elicited that her cycle was regular, LMP was 6 weeks back, she is nulliparous and has been trying for pregnancy for three years. Pain started suddenly, which was severe and agonizing. On examination you found her pulse is 98/minute, BP is 100/60 mm Hg. On PA examination no abnormality is detected. On PV examination no lump is felt, Fornix is tender.
>
> On the basis of these findings what might be your diagnosis?

Ectopic pregnancy. Either tubal rupture or tubal abortion.

> How can you confirm your diagnosis?

By doing following investigations:
1. *Serum β-hCG:* For confirmation of pregnancy serum beta human chorionic gonadotropin (β-hCG) is to be done
2. *Ultrasonogram:* To confirm the site of pregnancy transvaginal ultrasonography (TVS) is to be done. TVS will determine whether there is any gestational sac (GS) in the uterus or in tubo-ovarian (TO) region or any free fluid (blood) in abdominal cavity. High resolution transvaginal prob with its close proximity to the target organs offers a unique sharp clear picture of tubes and surroundings (Rottem et al. 1991; Das 1995).

Findings of TVS are the following:
1. Uterus:
   - It is empty **(Fig. 10.1B)**
   - Decidual reaction present, which is indicated by thickened endometrium
   - Pseudo gestational sac may be present (blood in the cavity comes as gestational sac).
2. In TO region and pouch of Douglas (POD):
   - There may be no findings in 20–30% cases
   - Discern GS, Yolk sac and embryo with cardiac pulsation in tube may present **(Fig. 10.1A)**.
   - Complex adnexal mass (in chronic cases) can be found
   - Free fluid (blood) in POD in case of hemorrhage.

Note: If β-hCG test is not available urinary pregnancy test can be done to prove pregnancy. Laparoscopic view of unruptured tubal pregnancy **(Fig. 10.1C)**

> Is there any role of colpopuncture or culdocentesis here to diagnose hemoperitoneum?

There is limited role of colpopuncture in modern management as TVS can diagnose fluid in the peritoneal cavity. TVS along with hormone (β-hCG) tests and clinical findings are good enough for diagnosis. But in the situation where USG is not available still there is some role.

> What other else can confirm the diagnosis?

Laparoscopy/Laparotomy: By direct visualization of dilated tube containing pregnancy sac.

> Is there any role of dilatation and curettage (DC) to diagnose ectopic pregnancy?

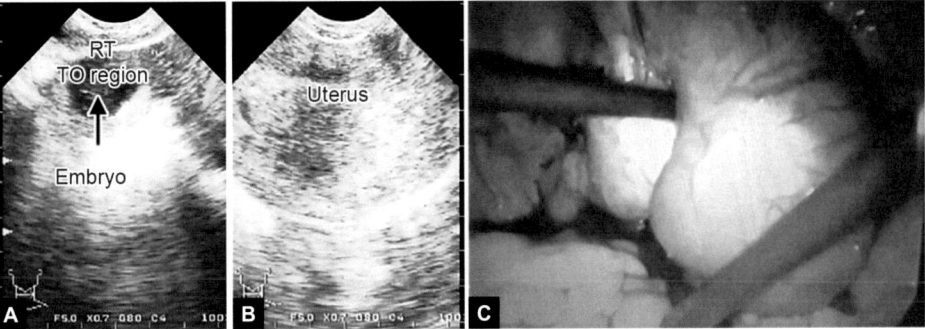

Figs 10.1A to C Tubal ectopic pregnancy: (A) Gestational sac in right tube; (B) Uterus empty; (C) Unruptured tubal pregnancy
(For color version, see Plate 1)

Dilatation and curettage is to be done to rule out intrauterine pregnancy. If the tissue obtained is positive for villi by floating in saline or histologic diagnosis then a nonviable intrauterine pregnancy is diagnosed. In the absence of villi, the diagnosis of ectopic pregnancy is made. But drawback of DC is that it will destroy the desired pregnancy among infertile patient.

RELATED INFORMATION

Possible Sites of Ectopic Pregnancy

- Most common site is fallopian tubes (95–98%)
- Abdominal cavity
- Ovary
- Broad ligament
- Rudimentary horn of uterus
- Cervix.

Risk Factors and Causes of Ectopic Pregnancy

- *Most common risk factor is pelvic inflammatory disease:* Six times increased risk (Westrom et al. 1981) Pelvic inflammatory disease (PID) causes salpingitis resulting peritubal adhesions, partial tubal lumen occlusion, intratubal adhesions, diverticula and disturbed tubal function. It causes epithelial damage and loss of ciliary function and tubal motility. Salpingitis may be due to Chlamydial and gonococcal infection, tuberculosis (forms true diverticula called salpingitis isthmica nodosa), postabortal, post MR, puerperal or secondary to pelvic peritonitis. In 20% cases may give history of previous surgery usually appendicectomy.
- *Prior ectopic pregnancy*: The risk is 7–13 times greater than the overall risk. Since the tubal affection is nearly always bilateral there is a strong tendency for ectopic pregnancy to occur in other side at a later date. Recurrent ectopic may occur in 15–20% cases after linear salpingostomy (Hankins et al. 1995).
- *Use of IUCD's*: IUCD users are more prone to develop ectopic pregnancy (Vessey et al. 1974). IUCD
  - May cause salpingitis
  - Prevent intrauterine pregnancy, hence ratio of ectopic to intrauterine is higher
  - Progesterone containing IUCDs alter tubal motility and polarity and hence lead to abnormal implantation.
- *Smoking (2.5 times risky than nonsmokers)*: Nicotine is thought to alter tubal motility, ciliary activity and blastocyst implantation (Phillips et al., 1992; Saraiya et al., 1998).
- *Assisted reproductive techniques* (3–5% increased risk): This may be due to:
  - Transfer of multiple embryos
  - Direct transfer into fallopian tubes
  - High up transfer beyond midcavity
  - Excessive fluid pushing
  - Retrograde propulsion by uterine contraction
- *Following tubal surgery*: More prone to develop ectopic in scarred tube after recanalization of ligated tube or after tuboplasty in blocked tube. Tubal pregnancy also may occur on the stump of the tube after partial salpingectomy, after tubal ligation and after hysterectomy with conservation of tubes, when operation is performed within 48 hours of coitus.

Other Risk Factors

- Older age.
- Non-white race.
- Endometriosis causes patchy differentiation of endosalpings to endometrium provides site for implantation. Adhesion and faulty transport within the tube is also responsible.
- Developmental errors of the tube such as hypoplasia, undue tortuosity and length, diverticula, accessory lumen-all trap the traveling embryo and impede its progress leading to a faulty implantation.
- Over development of the ovum and external migration.

Most Common and Dangerous Site of the Tube where Ectopic Implantation Occurs (Fig. 10.2)

- Ampulla is the most common site where 55% implantation occurs, but least dangerous as this part is dilated so takes time to rupture.
- Isthmus is less common site (25%), but is more dangerous because it is the narrowest part of the tube and get ruptured within very short duration even before diagnosis of pregnancy.

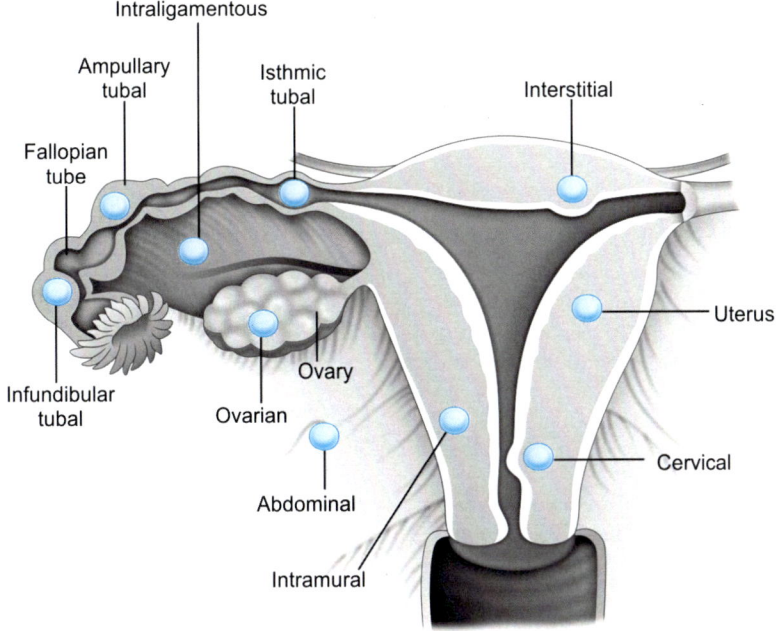

Fig. 10.2 Different sites of ectopic pregnancy

Other Sites of the Tube for Ectopic Implantation

Other sites are not very common:
- Fimbriated opening (17%)
- Interstitial part (3%)
- Diverticula.

> Her β-hCG is 1,900 IU/L. TVS shows thick hypoecoic endometrium, but no gestational sac in the cavity. Nothing abnormality could be detected in TO region. But there is free fluid in POD. Still lower abdominal pain is there.
> How will you manage the patient?

Positive β-hCG, empty uterus, lower abdominal pain, free fluid in POD all are suggestive of bleeding from ectopic pregnancy either due to tubal rupture or tubal abortion. So immediate intravenous (IV) channel with wide bored needle is to be established and intravenous (IV) fluid is to be started, blood is to be sent for grouping and cross matching and after proper counseling patient is to be prepared for laparoscopy/laparotomy.

> You arranged operation and after laparoscopy you found that there is free and clotted blood in the abdominal cavity and left tube is swollen with active bleeding from fimbriated end.
> What do you like to do?

Management depends on patient's future fertility desire and condition of the tubes. Before taking decision other tube should be examined.

As patient has no children and affected tube is not ruptured irrespective of condition of other tube linear salpingotomy is the choice, which is done by giving an incision over the distended segment of the tube using needle tip cautery (can also be done by laser, scalpel or scissors), and the product of conception is to be removed. The tube will be irrigated to remove all trophoblastic tissue and to ensure hemostasis.

> Why not segmental resection or milking instead of salpingotomy?

As the result of segmental resection and linear salpingotomy is same, but latter is an easier and shorter procedure, linear salpingotomy is preferable. Milking was advocated in the past, if the pregnancy is fimbrial and hemorrhage is easy to control. But the risk of recurrent ectopic pregnancy is twice as high as linear salpingotomy, so it is not a preferred choice now-a-days.

> Will you do the same for a patient having one children?

No. If patient has a child and condition of other tube is good then salpingectomy is the choice of surgery. But if other tube is not healthy looking, again linear salpingotomy is ideal option.

> Why did you choose laparoscopy rather than laparotomy?

So far patient's condition is stable laparoscopy is superior to laparotomy as blood loss is less, hospital stay and convalescence are shorter, postoperative analgesic requirement is less, postoperative adhesion is less and cosmetic results are better. On the other hand subsequent pregnancy and tubal pregnancy rates are similar.

> **Case scenario:** Mrs Moyna has amenorrhea for 6 weeks. Her cycle was regular. So she did pregnancy test by strip yesterday due to missed period and it came positive. That is why she has come to you for check up. You did TVS and found no gestational sac in the uterus, but there is decidual change. TO region is normal. You did β-hCG and serum progesterone, which are 2,000 IU/L and 10 ng/mL respectively.
> What do you want to do next?

Most likely it is ectopic pregnancy: Although, intrauterine sac should appear when β-hCG level is more than 1,500 IU/L (Barnhart, 1999), sometimes intrauterine sac may appear at later period. Besides a series of investigations demonstrated that neither a single β-hCG cut-off of 2,000 IU/L nor a doubling of β-hCG <50% with two samples taken 48 hours apart is a guarantee of ectopic pregnancy (Condous 2007). So to avoid confusion β-hCG should be repeated after 48 hours. In intrauterine pregnancy it should be doubled or at least 66% increment after 48 hours. If doubling does not occur it will indicate ectopic pregnancy. Serum progesteron level also is indicative. In intrauterine pregnancy it should be at least 25 ng/mL. So lower level indicates ectopic pregnancy (Ankum et al. 1995). At that time *patient should be warned* that anytime, if any pain occurs she should be hospitalized.

Note: Controversies in measurement of β-hCG and progesterone:
1. *β-hCG:* In a healthy intrauterine pregnancy usually doubled or at least 66% increased within 48–72 hours.
   An increase in β-hCG of less than 66% would be associated with an abnormal intrauterine pregnancy or an extrauterine pregnancy (Kadar et al. 1994). But there are exceptions:
   - About 15% of healthy intrauterine pregnancies do not increase by 66%
   - About 13% of all ectopic pregnancies have normally rising β-hCG levels of at least 66% in 2 days
   - In multiple pregnancy levels of β-hCG is much above the discriminatory zone of 1,500 IU/L, before any ultrasonographic evidence of the gestation is apparent. Gestational sac may not appear in the uterine cavity even with β-hCG 2,300 IU/L and suspicion arises about ectopic pregnancy. In multiple pregnancies doubling may not occur, if growth of one sac stops.
2. *Serum progesterone:* Progesterone value less than 15 is probably an abnormal pregnancy of some kind and a single value over 25 is probably a normal pregnancy.

Following are the exceptions:
- A progesterone level of less than 15 ng/mL is seen in 11% of normal intrauterine pregnancies.
- Less than 2% of ectopic and less than or equal to 4% of abnormal intrauterine pregnancies will have a progesterone level greater than or equal to 25 ng/mL.
- Also, this test is unreliable in differentiating between normal and abnormal pregnancies in patients who conceive after assisted reproductive technology (ART), because of excessive progesterone production from multiple corpora luteal, as well as the practice of exogenous progesterone supplementation.

Serum progesterone levels have the following characteristics:
- They are not gestational age-dependent
- They remain relatively constant during the first trimester of normal and abnormal pregnancies
- They do not return to the reference range, if initially abnormal
- They do not correlate with β-hCG levels.

> You repeated the test and β-hCG is not doubled and serum progesterone level is 15 ng/mL. So you diagnosed the case as ectopic pregnancy. Though sonographically nothing could be detected.
>
> How will you manage the patient?

Ultrasonogram sometimes fails to diagnose the extrauterine sac at very early stage. As biochemical test is indicative here the case will be dealt as ectopic pregnancy. For this case medical treatment will be appropriate.

Methotrexate (MTX) is the commonly used drug. At this level of β-hCG a single IV/IM injection methotrexate 50 mg/m² or 1 mg/kg body weight is enough for resolution of pregnancy. In that case no folinic acid rescue is necessary. Monitoring by β-hCG is done every 3 days until negative. A fall of 15% between day 4 and 7 should occur, otherwise a second dose is to be administered (Rozenberg, 2003).

RELATED INFORMATION

Depending upon the patient's general condition, size of ectopic sac and level of β-hCG, following are the treatment options of ectopic gestation:
A. Expectant
B. Medical
C. Surgical treatment can be done.

A. Expectant Treatment

It can be given with regular monitoring under certain circumstances. About 20–30% EP resolves spontaneously (Ylostalo et al. 1993). Close monitoring with clinical findings and serum β-hCG is essential as EPs have been known to rupture even when the serum β-hCG levels are low (Tulandi et al. 1991). Slow resolution and prolonged follow-up may need treatment.

Criteria for Selection for Expectant Treatment

- If there is slight or no symptom or symptom is subsiding
- β-hCG level is less than 1,000 mIU/mL (Shalev 1995)
- Falling level of serum β-hCG at 2 days interval
- The size of the sac is less than 2 cm on TVS and
- There is no hemoperitoneum or less than 50 mL collection in POD.

B. Medical Treatment

Medical treatment can be given:
- In early and unruptured pregnancy.
- Where surgery is contraindicated or likely to be difficult.
  - Medically unfit
  - Cervical ectopic
  - Cornual ectopic
  - Pelvic adhesions.
- Failed surgical treatment:
  - Persistent ectopic after conservative tubal surgery.

Criteria for Selection of Medical Treatment

Following criteria must be fulfilled for medical treatment (Shalev 1998):
- Patient should be clinically stable
- Patient is able and willing to attend for follow-up scans and blood tests
- Under 8 weeks gestation
- No free fluid on ultrasound scan
- Sac size is less than 3.5 cm
- No fetal cardiac pulsation in ectopic sac
- β-hCG level is <4,000 mIU/mL

Methotrexate can be given in single and multiple doses. Other drugs such as KCL, prostaglandins, RU 486, hyperosmolar glucose, vasopressin and actinomycin have also been tried for medical treatment. Before application of methotrexate investigations like complete blood count (CBC), liver and kidney function tests are needed. Patient is advised not to take folic acid-containing vitamins and alcoholic beverage, and abstinence from coitus during treatment **(Table 10.1)**.

Table 10.1 Protocols and monitoring of methotrexate therapy

Protocol	Monitoring
Single dose Methotrexate 50 mg/m² IM	• Measurement of β-hCG on day 4 and 7 • If fall of 15% occurs repeat β-hCG weekly until undetectable • If β-hCG fall is <15% repeat methotrexate and begin new day 1
Multiple doses Methotrexate 1 mg/kg IM, Days 1, 3, 5, 7 Leukovorin 0.1 mg/kg IM, Days 2, 4, 6, 8	Continue alternate day injection until β-hCG level decreases 15% in 48 hours or four doses methotrexate given, then weekly β-hCG until undetectable

Advantages of Methotrexate Treatment

- Can be treated on outpatient basis. If hospitalization needed it is minimum
- Avoid surgery in 85% cases
- Less costly
- Lower risk of tubal injury
- Not skill dependent
- Higher future fertility than with surgery
- Can be used in persistent placental tissue, which may remain following failed conservative surgical treatment
- Quick recovery
- >90% cure rate in properly selected cases when β-hCG at a lower level (91% when β-hCG is <5,000 IU/L, 98% when β-hCG is <1000 IU/L) (Lipscomb 1999).

Disadvantages of Methotrexate Treatment

- *Risk of toxicity*: Nausea, stomatitis, bone marrow suppression, pneumonitis, elevated liver enzyme
- So cannot be used in abnormally low blood count or abnormal liver function and renal function tests
- Requires repeated visit for follow-up than does surgery to ensure resolution of pregnancy
- In 15% cases the ectopic persists, may rupture and requires surgical treatment
- Some patients develop side effects such as dermatitis, pleuritis and conjunctivitis.
- It cannot be used in heterotopic pregnancies (when pregnancies occur both in intrauterine and extrauterine site).

Note: In heterotopic pregnancy surgical treatment is to be done without disturbing intrauterine pregnancy, if it is viable.

Contraindications of MTX are:
- Hemodynamically unstable
- Suspected ruptured EP
- Sensitivity to MTX
- Intrauterine pregnancy
- Breastfeeding
- Active pulmonary disease
- Renal disease
- Chronic liver disease
- Pre-existing blood dyscrasia
- Immunodeficiency
- Peptic ulcer disease
- Unable to comply with visits and follow-up

Time Taken to Resolute Ectopic Pregnancy

It can take upto 4 weeks for an ectopic pregnancy to resolute completely (Vitthala 2007).

C. Surgical Treatment

Laparoscopy or laparotomy followed by any one of the following:
- Salpingectomy
- Salpingotomy
- Segmental resection or milking.

Note: Irrespective of treatment of EP anti-D immunoglobulin 50 mg IM stat is to be given in

Rh-negative woman, if she is not immunized previously.

> **Case scenario:** Mrs Aleya is diagnosed as a case of cornual ectopic pregnancy. Gestational age is 9 weeks and fetus is alive.
> What measure do you like to do for her?

Salpingocentesis, e.g. intracardiac injection KCL or methotrexate in sac can be given for feto reduction. In case of cornual and interstitial pregnancy where embryo is present with cardiac pulsation IV injection will not be effective and surgery carry the risk of hemorrhage. In that case TVS guided administration of KCL in embryonic heart or methotrexate in sac is directly administered. So sac and fetus is reduced by this manner. Patient should be followed up by TVS and β-hCG.

> **Case scenario:** Mrs Nadira came with amenorrhea with signs and symptoms of pregnancy, with sudden severe lancinating pain and shock. Her abdomen is distended, tense and tender, she is pale and her PV examination elicited that Fornices are tender, cervical motion tenderness is present and uterus cannot be felt due to fluid in abdomen.
> What will be your treatment of choice?

She has obvious acute clinical picture. She is a case of ruptured ectopic with hemodynamic instability, which is diagnosed by clinical findings only. So immediate resuscitation and decision of laparotomy is to be taken. Laparoscopy is not suitable in hemodynamically unstable case. Immediately following should be done:
- Opening up of IV channel and blood should be sent for grouping and cross matching
- Transfusion of IV fluid and plasma expander by the time of getting blood
- Transfusion of blood
- Catheterization
- Laparotomy under GA.

After laparotomy bleeding point should be caught first then after removing the clots and free blood salpingectomy is to be done; provided other tube is healthy.

Note: Care should be taken to clamp infundibulopelvic ligament in such a way that ovarian vessel is not included. It may reduce ovarian reserve by interfering ovarian blood supply.

> **Case scenario:** Mrs Halima has come to you for booking visit. You did USG and diagnosed a pregnancy sac in the TO region having seven weeks sized embryo with cardiac pulsation and uterine cavity is empty.
> What do you want to do?

It is an unruptured ectopic pregnancy, which does not meet the criteria of medical treatment as embryo having cardiac pulsation is found. So surgery should be the mode of treatment. As patient has no emergency situation laparoscopy should be the choice of surgery.

RELATED INFORMATION

Usual Outcome of Tubal Pregnancy

- *Tubal abortion*
  - Complete
  - Incomplete
- *Tubal rupture*: Tube is incapable of distension; wall is eroded easily by chorionic villi and gets ruptured.
  - When rupture occurs in roof or sides of the tubes then it is called intraperitoneal rupture where bleeding occurs in peritoneal cavity. This is the most common.
  - When rupture occurs in the floor of the tube then it is called extraperitoneal rupture where bleeding occurs between the layers of broad ligament producing broad ligament hematoma. This is very rare.
- *Missed abortion (tubal mole)*: Embryo dies due to faulty environment and faulty implantation and is converted into a carnious mole. Finally may produce symptomless hematosalpinx, peritubal hematocele and even pelvic hematocele.
- *Chronic ectopic adnexal mass*: Some products of conception are partially extruded through the fimbria or through a partial rupture. After a slight or mild to moderate bleeding, it may get arrested and form adnexal mass involving the tube, ovaries and clots causing chronic pelvic pain and irregular PV bleeding.

> **Case scenario:** Mrs Rokeya has come with the complaints of irregular PV bleeding for 1 month. Bleeding is altered colored. On enquiry you elicited that she is a regularly menstruating woman, which occurred 30 days interval. But last cycle took place 15 days after due date of menstruation. Before starting the bleeding there was severe agonizing pain persisted for 1 day, for which she took suppository as pain killer. Afterwards pain subsided and menstruation started, but bleeding was less than that of previous cycles, and is continuing till today. A dull ache present. On general examination patient is mildly anemic, abdomen is soft nontender, on PV examination fornices slightly tender and an ill-defined lump is felt through left fornix. Uterus bulky, mobility restricted, cervical motion tenderness present. TVS revealed a mass of about 3 cm × 2.9 cm in left TO region and enlarged left ovary is entrapped within it.
>
> Her β-hCG is 12 IU/L.
>
> *What is your diagnosis? Explain the points in favor of your diagnosis.*

This is a case of chronic ectopic pregnancy. Points in favor:
- Short period of amenorrhea
- Sudden severe pain
- Irregular PV bleeding
- Dull ache in lower abdomen
- Cervical motion tenderness
- Restricted mobility of the uterus
- Ill-defined lump in bimanual exam
- Lump in TO region by USG
- β-hCG is more than non-pregnant level.

RELATED INFORMATION

Diagnostic dilemma of chronic ectopic pregnancy

Amenorrhea, severe abdominal pain and vaginal bleeding are the classical triad for diagnosis of ectopic pregnancy. But always the typical features may not be present. For example:
- 85–90% patients have abdominal pain
- 80–85% have amenorrhea
- 80–85% have vaginal bleeding.

So all women in reproductive age having any one of the three symptoms should raise the suspicion of ectopic pregnancy even though the patient is on an effective contraception or has had a tubal occlusion operation or she is single. Because the picture of ectopic pregnancy is extremely variable and remains the great mimic of gynecology. No other pelvic condition gives rise to more diagnostic errors.

- Patients may or may not have symptoms pointing to pregnancy
- With or without a period of amenorrhea she typically complains of pelvic pain and irregular vaginal bleeding
- Most patients present with amenorrhea and the LMP is often described as lighter than normal. This is not a true period and probably represents withdrawal bleeding secondary to inadequate ovarian steroids.

Conditions Raise Confusions Regarding Diagnosis (D/D)

Diagnosis of EP is sometimes misleading due to some other obstetrical, gynecological and non-gynecological conditions:

Obstetrical

- Abortion of an early intrauterine pregnancy
- Abortion followed by salpingitis
- Early pregnancy with pelvic tumors
- Threatened abortion.

Gynecological

- Dysfunctional uterine bleeding
- Degenerated fibroid
- Endometriosis
- Ruptured corpus luteum (typical acute symptom except amenorrhea)
- Ovulation pain
- Torsion of adnexal mass
- Acute or subacute salpingitis (PID).

Nongynecological (Not Very Common)

- Appendicitis
- Gastroenteritis
- Mesenteric thrombosis
- Perforated peptic ulcer
- Renal colic
- Intraperitoneal hemorrhage from any source (rupture splenic aneurysm/tumors).

Differentiating the Situations from Ectopic Pregnancy?

Signs and symptoms of pregnancy and positive pregnancy test will exclude the other situations. It is unusual for an extrauterine pregnancy to advance beyond 6–8 weeks without pain, bleeding or both. So any one of the feature along with positive β-hCG test, which does not show doubling and ultrasonographic findings will give confirm diagnosis of ectopic pregnancy.

> You diagnosed the case as a chronic EP as you found a lump in TO region following a history of short period of amenorrhea with a positive pregnancy test, severe pain and slight PV bleeding. Now she has slight bleeding, which is altered in color and there is dull pain at this moment.
> How will you manage this case?

In-spite of subsidence of pain laparoscopy/laparotomy is the treatment of choice. After adhesiolysis salpingectomy is to be done.

Note: Ovary may look unhealthy due to entrapment within the clot, must be preserved.

> If you do not do surgery then what will happen about PV bleeding?

As it is due to shedding of decidua it will stop after complete resolution of corpus luteal function. If it is annoying for the patient progesterone can be given to stop the bleeding.

> **Case scenario:** Mrs Naila has a history of EP pregnancy 2 years back for which right-sided salpingectomy was done. Again she has come with feature of ruptured ectopic pregnancy and after laparotomy you confirmed it. Patient is nulliparous.
> What do you want to do this time?

As tube is ruptured there is no option except salpingectomy. For child bearing she will have to go for ART.

> When will you say that pregnancy is cornual? What are the risk factors? How will you diagnose and manage such a case?

The term cornual pregnancy is used interchangeably as a synonym for interstitial pregnancy. It refers to a pregnancy in the interstitial segment of a unicornuate or bicornuate uterus. Though, previously pregnancy in the rudimentary horn of bicornuate uterus was called cornual pregnancy.

Risk Factors

Risk factors for development of interstitial pregnancy include:
- Previous ectopic pregnancy
- Previous ipsilateral salpingectomy
- Uterine anomaly
- *In vitro* fertilization (IVF)
- Ovulation induction
- STD.

Diagnosis

Ultrasonography can diagnose easily at any gestational period. Ultrasound frequently shows a thin rim of myometrial tissue surrounding the ectopic pregnancy sac. Laparoscopic evaluation can confirm the diagnosis.

As pregnancy grows in the area of the fallopian tube that enters the uterus, surrounding myometrial tissue allows for further development of the pregnancy into the second trimester (12–20 weeks). So sometimes diagnosis cannot be done before any catastrophes.

Treatment

The traditional treatment of cornual pregnancy has been cornual resection or hysterectomy in severely damaged uterus by laparotomy.

In modern view ruptured interstitial pregnancy with hypovolemic shock necessitating emergent laparotomy. In the stable patient laparoscopy can be done for resection.

Medical treatment can be done by *single dose or multidose systemic methotrexate*. As interstitial pregnancies are less susceptible to methotrexate because of their increased blood supply and size of gestation is usually bigger *both systemic and local methotrexate give good result* (Fisch et al. 1998). *Intracardiac KCL and systemic methotrexate* also give good result. In both the situations close monitoring (and even hospital admission) should be considered because rupture is possible even after treatment has begun. Future fertility is possible for interstitial pregnancy treated conservatively, though muscles become weakened (Tolland and Al-Jaroudi 2004).

> **Case scenario:** Mrs Rahela has come to you with history of amenorrhea for 24 weeks, and loss of fetal movement for 10–12 hours. She also complaints of slight lower abdominal pain. She mentioned that when she perceived fetal movement it was painful. On further enquiry she told that in early weeks of pregnancy she had an attack of lower abdominal pain and slight vaginal bleeding. On examination you did not feel the uterine contour clearly. On bimanual examination Cx is not typically soft and is displaced upwards and forwards with fetal parts lying below and behind it. A separate lump other than uterus is felt in the abdomen.
>
> What do you think about the case?

Most probably it is the case of an abdominal pregnancy.

> Why did you think so?

Because
- There is a history of lower abdominal pain and vaginal bleeding in early weeks, which may be due to complete tubal abortion.
- As pregnancy is not in the uterus so there is no Braxton–Hicks contraction. That is why uterine contour could not be felt.
- Separate pelvic lump other than uterine lump and painful fetal movement is suspicious.

> How will you confirm it?

Ultrasonography, X-ray and magnetic resonance imaging (MRI) findings can make diagnosis:
- The classic ultrasound finding is the absence of myometrial tissue between the bladder and pregnancy (Varma et al. 2003).
- Lateral X-ray on standing position shows superimposed fetal skeleton shadow with the maternal spinal shadow. X-ray also reveals unusual fetal attitude and position.
- The MRI holds a promising diagnostic tool.
- Elevated serum alpha-fetoprotein has also been associated with abdominal pregnancy (Tromans et al. 1984).

> Ultrasonography failed to diagnose the pregnancy as extrauterine and diagnose the case as missed abortion. So you have given prostaglandin or oxytocin for induction of missed abortion.
>
> What problem you might face after induction?

There will be failure of initiation of uterine contraction and labor after repeated induction. This is the suggestive feature of abdominal pregnancy.

> How does abdominal pregnancy occur?

Abdominal pregnancy is almost always secondary to tubal, ovarian or uterine pregnancy. The pregnancy escapes out in a mass with intact chorionic attachment and intact amniotic sac through abdominal ostium or a rent of the tube or uterine scar and gets attached into the abdominal structure such as omentum, intestine, pelvic peritoneum and broad ligament.

> What are the fates of abdominal pregnancy?

- Sometime fetus can grow up to maturity with serious maternal risk involvement. Because the structures react by developing large blood vessels to serve the placenta. Anatomy of abdominal organs where it attached is grossly disturbed. The fetus develops in the peritoneal cavity, its amniotic sac becoming supported by an outer coat of organized lymph and blood exudates. The placental attachment is so insecure and the local decidual reaction so weak that retroperitoneal and intra-abdominal hemorrhage is likely at any time.
- Due to scanty liquor and placental insufficiency fetal death and malformation is more common.
- Some pregnancies proceed to term and ensues spurious labor pain. Uterus contracts painfully and there are some dilatation of the cervix with a discharge of blood and decidua. Usually fetus dies and remains in the abdominal cavity where it undergoes maceration or calcified to form lithopedion.

> How will you manage once you will diagnose the case as abdominal pregnancy?

Once the diagnosis is made urgent laparotomy irrespective of gestational age is the treatment of choice to avoid the risk of catastrophic hemorrhage:
- The ideal surgery is to remove the entire sac, fetus, placenta and the membranes, if the placenta is *attached to removable organ such as uterus or broad ligament.*

- If placenta is *attached to the vital organs only fetus is taken out* leaving behind the placenta and the sac after tying and cutting the cord flushed with its placental attachment. Complete absorption of the placenta occurs through aseptic autolysis.

> How can you manage and diagnose a case of cervical pregnancy?

When implantation takes place in the cervical canal it is called cervical pregnancy. The condition can be mistaken as an abortion in progress of a normally sited pregnancy. Ultrasound diagnosis is integral to the early detection of cervical pregnancy. This include:
- Empty uterine cavity.
- Hour glass uterine shape.
- Ballooned cervical canal containing the gestational sac with or without embryo.

The use of Doppler flow sonography is only helpful in distinguishing abortion in progress from those with vascular implantation in the cervix.

Management

In the past cervical ectopic pregnancy was associated with significant hemorrhage and was treated presumptively with hysterectomy. Improved ultrasound resolution and early detection of these pregnancies has led to the development of more conservative treatments that attempt to limit morbidity and preserve fertility.

Conservative modalities with varying degree success were described by many researchers (Ceplin et al. 2004; Jurkovic et al. 1996; Stovall et al. 1991; Stovall and Ling 1993; Bagga et al. 2001; Frates et al. 1994) are:
- Systemic methotrexate single or multidoses depending on β-hCG level
- Systemic methotrexate in combination with cervical evacuation and the use of hemostatic techniques (balloon tamponade, packing and cerclage)
- Cervical evacuation and the use of hemostatic techniques (balloon tamponade, packing and cerclage)
- Cervical curettage followed by injection of prostaglandin F2α (believed to increase uterine contraction, promote vasoconstriction and therefore reduce hemorrhage.
- Intra-amniotic injection of methotrexate
- Intracardiac injection of KCL when cardiac activity present.
- Uterine artery ligation and embolization as adjunctive techniques to control hemorrhage from curettage procedures.

There are several reports of successful live births after conservative management of cervical pregnancy. Incidence of cervical incompetence is more requiring cerclage.

> How will you diagnose and manage a case of ovarian pregnancy?

Ovarian pregnancy is a rare event. Diagnosis can be made by USG and laparoscopy. Positive β-hCG and empty uterus raise suspicion for ectopic. In early weeks lower abdominal pain and light vaginal bleeding may present. In advanced stage, hemorrhage may occur and gives the typical features of acute ectopic pregnancy.

Ultrasonography

A wide echogenic ring on the ovary with yolk sac or fetal parts can be seen. Ovarian pregnancies are confused with corpus luteal cyst in early weeks of pregnancy. Three dimensional ultrasound imaging can distinguish ovarian pregnancy from corpus luteal cyst.

Laparoscopy

Laparoscopy requires to make the confirm diagnosis by direct visualization of gestational sac on the ovary.

Management

- **Resuscitation:** If there is acute symptom it should be managed by other acute case of ectopic pregnancy.
- **Definitive measure:**
  - Wedge resection of the ovary, if gestational sac is small
  - Oophorectomy in advanced gestation.

> **Case scenario:** Miss Nasima, a 17 years old girl has come to you with her mother with history of severe pain in the lower abdomen 6 hours back followed by a fainting attack. After history taking it was found that she is unmarried with regular 30 days menstrual cycle. Last menstrual period was 25 days back. On examination, it was found that she is pale, sweating present in the face and she is in a state of shock. Her abdomen is distended, tense and tender. On per vaginal examination her hymen was found intact.
>
> What is the diagnosis? How will you confirm it? How will you manage her?

Most probable diagnosis is corpus luteum cyst rupture, which is called ovarian apoplexy. β-hCG can diagnose it by excluding ectopic pregnancy. Laparoscopy or laparotomy is also diagnostic.

As this is an emergency situation there is no time to wait for β-hCG report. Patient should be managed exactly as the management of acute ectopic pregnancy. After laparotomy or laparoscopy, ruptured area should be ligated or cauterized as appropriate.

Note: You need to mention all steps of management. Corpus luteum cyst rupture has same feature as ectopic pregnancy except short period of amenorrhea.

RELATED INFORMATION

Sudden rupture of the ovary at the site of cyst accompanied by hemorrhage in the ovary or into peritoneal cavity is known as ovarian apoplexy. Pain, which occurs primarily in the mid-cycle or just before menstruation or after a minor delay in menstruation. It may occur after intercourse or training in the gym, when pressure in the abdomen has increased or when ovarian tissue has experienced some stress. It usually occurs due to dystrophic and sclerotic changes in ovarian tissue due to acute and chronic inflammatory processes or due to production of multiple big follicles due to ovarian stimulation. As a result, hemorrhage can occur in the corpus luteum due to the fragility of blood vessels, causing a hematoma. Other possible causes of ovarian rupture include abdominal trauma, excessive physical stress, vigorous sexual intercourse, horseback riding, etc.

BIBLIOGRAPHY

Ankum WM, Van der Veen F, Hamerlynck JV, Lammes FB. Suspected ectopic pregnancy. What to do when human chorionic gonadotropin levels are below the discriminatory zone. J Reprod Med. 1995;40:525-8.

Bagga R, Jain V, Kalra J, Gopalan S. Cervical pregnancy and therapeutic options. Acta Obstet Gynaecol Scan. 2001;80(7):663-4.

Barnhart KT, Simhan H, Kamelle SA. Diagnostic accuracy of ultrasound above and below the beta-hCG discriminatory zone. Obstet Gynecol. 1999;94(4):583-7.

Center for Disease Control and Prevention (CDC) Ectopic pregnancy—United States, 1990, 1992. MMWR Morb Mortal Wkly Rep. 1995;44(3):46-8.

Cepnil, Ocal P, Erkan S, Erzik B. Conservative treatment of cervical ectopic pregnancy with transvaginal ultrasound-guided aspiration and single-dose methotrexate. Fertil Steril. 2004;81(4):1130-2.

Condous G, Van Calster B, Kirk E, et al. Prediction of ectopic pregnancy in women with a pregnancy of unknown location. Ultrasound Obstet Gynecol. 2007;29(6):680-68.

Coste J, Bouver J, Germain E, et al. Recent declining trend in ectopic pregnancy in France: evidence of two clinicoepidemiologic entities Fertil Steril. 2000;74(5):881-6.

Das KK, Mitra BK. Can the status of tubal pregnancy is predicted with transvaginal sonography? A prospective comparison of sonography, beta hCG level and operative findings. J Obstet Gynaecol Ind. 1995;45:689-96.

Fisch JD, Ortiz B, Tazuke S, et al. Medical management of interstitial ectopic pregnancy: a case report and literature review. Hum Reprod. 1998;13(7):1981-6.

Frates MC, Benson CB, Doubilet PM, et al. Cervical ectopic pregnancy: results of conservative treatment. Radiology. 1994;191(3):773-5.

Hankins GD, Clark SL, Cunningham FG, Gilstrap LC. Ectopic pregnancy. In: Operative obstetrics. Norwalk, Conn, Appleton and Lange. 1995;437:56.

Irvine LM, Setchell ME. Declining incidence of ectopic pregnancy in a UK city health district between 1990 and 1999. Hum Reprod. 2001;16(10):2230-4.

Jurkovic D, Hacket E, Campbell S. Diagnosis and treatment of early cervical pregnancy: a review and report of two cases treated conservatively. Ultrasound Obstet Gynaecol. 1996;8(6):373-80.

Kadar N, Bohrer M, Kemmann E, Shelden R. The discriminatory human chorionic gonadotropin zone for endovaginal sonography: a prospective, randomized study. Fertil Steril. 1994;61(6):1016-20.

Lipscomb G. Presented at ACOG Annual Meeting; 1999.

Lipscomb GH, McCord ML, Stovall TG, Huff G, Portera SG, Ling FW. Predictors of success of methotrexate treatment in women with tubal ectopic pregnancies. N Engl J Med. 1999;341:1974-8.

Phillips RS, Tuomala RE, Feldblum PJ, et al. The effect of cigarette smoking, Chlamydia trachomatis infection, and vaginal douching on ectopic pregnancy. Obstet Gynecol. 1992;79(1):85-90.

Rottem S, Thayer I, Timor Tritsh EI. Classification of tubal gestations by transvaginal sonography. Ultrasound Obstet Gynecol. 1991;1(3):197-201.

Rozenberg P, Chevret S, Camus E, et al. Medical treatment of ectopic pregnancies: a randomized clinical trial comparing methotrexate-mifepristone and methotrexate-placebo. Hum Reprod. 2003;18(9): 1802-8.

Saraiya M, Berg CJ, Kendrick JS, et al. Cigarette smoking as a risk factor for ectopic pregnancy. Am J Obstet Gynecol. 1998;178(3):493-8.

Shalev E, Peleg D, Tsabari A, et al. Spontaneous resolution of ectopic tubal pregnancy: natural history. Fertil Steril. 1995;63(1):15-9.

Shalev E, Yarom I, Bustan M, et al. Transvaginal sonography as the ultimate diagnostic tool for the management of ectopic pregnancy: experience with 840 cases. Fertil Steril. 1998;69(1):62-5.

Stovall TG, Ling FW. Single-dose methotrexate: an expanded clinical trial. Am J Obstet Gynecol. 1993; 168:1759-62.

Stoval TG, Ling F, Gray l. Methotrexate treatment of unruptured ectopic pregnancy: a report of 100 cases. Obstet Gynecol. 1991;77(5):749-53.

Stoval TG, Ling F. Single doses methotrexate: an expanded clinical trial. Am J Obstet Gynecol. 1993;168: 1762-5.

Tolland T, Al-Jaroudi D. Interstitial pregnancy: results generated from The Society of Reproductive Surgeons Registry, Obstet Gynecol. 2004;103:47-50.

Tromans PM, Coulson R, Lobb M. Abdominal pregnancy associated with extremely elevated serum alpha-fetoprotein: case report. Br J Obstet Gynecol. 1984;91:296-8.

Tulandi T, Hemmings R, Khalifa F. Rupture of ectopic pregnancy in woman with low and declining serum β-hCG concentrations. Fertili Steril. 1991;56:786-7.

Varma R, Mascarenhas R, Jame D. Successful outcome of advanced abdominal pregnancy with exclusive omental insertion. Ultrasound Obstet Gynecol. 2003;21:192-4.

Vessey MP, Johnson B, Doll R, Peto R. Outcome of pregnancy in women using an intrauterine device. Lancet. 1974:i495.

Vitthala S, Cheema MK, Misra PK. Medical Management of Ectopic Pregnancy using Methotrexate. The Internet Journal of Gynecology and Obstetrics. 2007;6:(2). DOI: 10.5580/1637.

Westrom L, Bergstssan LPH, Mardh PA. Incidence, trends and risks of ectopic pregnancy in a population of women. Br Med J. 1981;282:15.

Ylostalo P, Cacciatore B, Korhonen J. Expectant management of ectopic pregnancy. Eur J Obstet Gynaecol Reprod Biol. 1993;49:83-84.

CHAPTER 11

Gestational Trophoblastic Diseases

Farhat Hossain, Rashida Begum

INTRODUCTION

Gestational trophoblastic disease (GTD) can be benign or malignant. Histologically, it is classified into hydatidiform mole, invasive mole (chorioadenoma destruens), choriocarcinoma, and placental site trophoblastic tumor (PSTT). Those invade locally or metastasize are collectively known as gestational trophoblastic neoplasia (GTN) or gestational trophoblastic tumor (GTT). Hydatidiform mole is the most common form of GTN. While invasive mole and choriocarcinoma are malignant, a hydatidiform mole can behave in a malignant or benign fashion. These tumors are unique in that they develop from an aberrant fertilization event and hence arise from fetal tissue within the maternal host. These tumors are highly curable with chemotherapy even with widespread metastasis. They elaborate a unique and characteristic tumor marker, human chorionic gonadotropin (hCG).

The disease is quiet common in South-East Asia including Bangladesh where the diagnosis is missed quiet often particularly in the rural area or the patient reports late with complications. Thus mortality from the disease is seen in spite of its high cure rate.

> **Case scenario:** Nasima a young primipara of 22 years presents with 10 weeks of amenorrhea, excessive vomiting and per vaginal bleeding.
>
> How will you proceed to diagnose the case?

History Taking

First of all detailed history is to be taken:
- Whether per vaginal (PV) bleeding is associated with pain or not
- Amount of bleeding
- Whether vomiting is protracted or not
- Whether she can take usual food or not
- Exact date of last menstrual period.

Examination

Then the patient is to be examined thoroughly:
- General examination
- Per abdominal examination
- Inspection of vulva to assess the amount of bleeding
- Per vaginal examination.

> On enquiry it is elicited that bleeding is small in amount and does not soak the cloth. There is slight lower abdominal pain. Vomiting takes place frequently. But it is not protracted. On examination her pulse, blood pressure (BP) and other systemic functions are normal. Per abdominally uterus is 18 weeks size. No fetal heart sound is audible. Gentle PV examination is done and cervical os found closed.
>
> On the basis of these findings what is your assumed diagnosis?

Most probable diagnosis is hydatidiform mole. Other possibilities are:
- Threatened abortion with multiple pregnancy and hyperemesis
- Threatened abortion with mistaken date and hyperemesis
- Threatened abortion with polyhydramnios and hyperemesis
- Threatened abortion with pregnancy with fibroid and hyperemesis.

> What investigations will be helpful for diagnosis of molar pregnancy?

Gestational Trophoblastic Diseases

1. Ultrasonography is the first test as it is readily available, reliable (90% sensitivity), simple, safe, cheaper and will give adequate information about fetus, placenta and liquor amni.
2. Quantitative measurement of serum β-hCG. Rapidly increasing value of serum β-hCG >100,000 mIU/mL are usual with molar pregnancy. β-hCG is raised two multiples of the mean.
3. Histological examination of the product of conception gives a confirmatory diagnosis.

If it is hydatidiform mole what features do you expect in ultrasonography?

The characteristic feature of molar pregnancy is 'snowstorm' appearance **(Fig. 11.1)** due to diffuse hydropic swelling of chorionic villi without any existing fetus or gestational sac.

What are the other conditions, which can be confused with this snowstorm appearance?

- Missed abortion
- Degenerated fibroid.

How will you differentiate these situations from hydatidiform mole?

By estimating serum β-hCG, which will be higher in molar pregnancy and absent in degenerated fibroid.

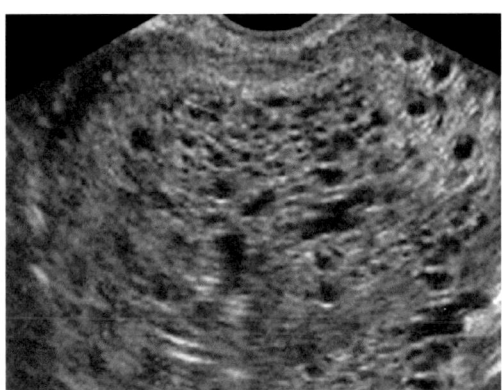

Fig. 11.1 Sonographic image of molar pregnancy snowstorm appearance

Mrs Nasima's ultrasonography shows snowstorm appearance of the contents of the uterus and bilateral lutein cysts. Her β-hCG level is 150,000 mIU/mL.
What other investigations are essential for management?

- X-ray chest is essential to see the sign of dissemination of molar tissue. If there is dissemination cannon ball shadow is present in X-ray.
- Full blood count, ABO grouping and rhesus (Rh) typing if not known beforehand. Liver and kidney function tests.

RELATED INFORMATION

Gestational trophoblastic disease includes:
- Molar pregnancy
- Invasive mole
- Placental site trophoblastic tumor
- Chorio carcinoma.

Incidence of GTD

Incidence of GTD varies and in South East Asia, the incidence is 1 in 200 hospital deliveries. Occurrence of molar pregnancy is more in rice eaters. The reported frequencies range from 1 in 100 pregnancies in Indonesia to 1 in 200 pregnancies in Mexico to 1 in 1,200 pregnancies in USA and 1 in 5,000 pregnancies in Paraguay (Atrash 1986, Grimes 1984). In Bangladesh we do not have any GTT registry. But observational study in hospital suggests that incidence will be higher.

Features of Molar Pregnancy

Features of molar pregnancy are:
- Short period of amenorrhea.
- Vaginal bleeding is the most common presentation and found in about 90% cases. May confuse with incomplete or threatened abortion. Due to mixture of ruptured vesicular gelatinous fluid blood appears as 'white currant in red currant juice'.
- Hyperemesis due to excessive production of β-hCG by hyperproliferative trophoblastic cells. About 10% may have severe enough to require hospitalization.
- Undue enlargement of uterus in 50% cases, which does not correspond with period of

amenorrhea due to excessive proliferation of trophoblastic tissue.
- Lower abdominal pain due to
  - Uterine distension
  - Concealed bleeding due to separation of trophoblastic tissue.
  - Rarely perforation of the uterus due to invasive mole
  - Infection
  - Uterine contraction to expel the contents
  - Bilateral enlargement of ovaries.
- Expulsion of grape-like vesicles **(Fig. 11.2)** per vaginum (conclusive for diagnosis).
- Features of pre-eclampsia is seen in one third of cases and develop earlier than usual.
- Consistency is doughy due to absence of amniotic fluid sac and uterus does not contract.
- History of quickening and fetal movement absent.
- Fetal parts are not felt.
- Fetal heart sound is absent.
- Pallor is present and may be out of proportion of the visible blood loss.
- Bilateral ovarian enlargement producing theca/lutein cyst is found in 25–50% cases due to effect of high β-hCG.
- Ascitis due to extravasation of fluid due to increased capillary permiability by vascular endothelial growth factors released from hyperstimulated ovaries.
- Pleural effusion rarely due to same reason.

- Features of thyrotoxicosis (7–10%) as alpha subunit of hCG is identical to thyroid-stimulating hormone (TSH) and therefore has an inherent capacity to stimulate the thyroid.
- Ascites, pleural effusion and thyrotoxicosis are uncommon presentations
- On rare occasion respiratory distress develops in 2% cases, which present with chest pain, dyspnea, tachypnea and tachycardia. This is due to trophoblastic embolization or thyroid storm or toxemia and massive fluid replacement.

Types and Causes of Molar Pregnancy

Two types of molar pregnancy exist. Complete or classic mole, where no fetus exists and partial mole, where along with mole fetus exists.

Complete mole occurs due to fusion of nucleus of spermatozoa with an empty ovum. The ovum nucleus may be either absent or inactivated. In 90% cases of complete mole there is 46XX karyotype, which results from fertilization of this empty ovum by a haploid sperm (23X), which then duplicates its own chromosomes. In 10% cases of complete mole, the karyotype is 46XY, which arises from fertilization of an empty ovum by two sperms (Yamashita et al. 1979).

Partial mole results from the fertilization of an apparently normal ovum by two sperms (Szulman et al. 1978). The fetus is associated with chromosomal abnormalities, which are triploid in the majority of the cases. The extra haploid sets of chromosomes generally being derived from father.

Though the fetus exists, if survives it exhibits the stigma of triploidy like intrauterine growth restriction (IUGR) and congenital anomaly, e.g. syndactyly, hydrocephalus.

New Concept of Development of Hydatidiform Mole

Hydatidiform mole is supposed to be developed from embryonic trophoblast. But sometimes it may develop from embryonic inner cell mass. At bilaminar stage of embryogenesis inner cell mass has the potential to differentiate to trophoblast, ectoderm or endoderm. If normal embryogenesis is interrupted inner cell mass loss its capacity to differentiate ectoderm and endoderm instead

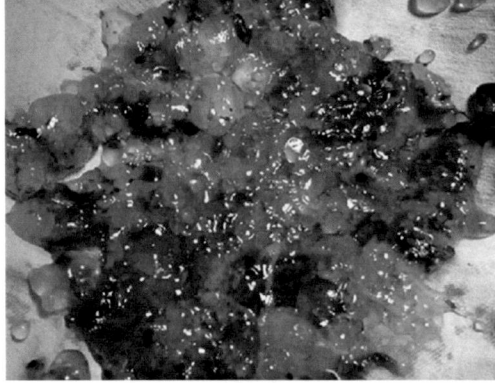

Fig. 11.2 Grape-like vesicles
(For color version, see Plate 2)

a divergent differentiation to trophoblast takes place. Subsequently cytotrophoblast and syncytiotrophoblast develop and differentiate extraembryonic mesoderm and molar vesicle with loose mesoderm, in their villous core.

Pathological Changes in Chorionic Tissue

It is the neoplasm of trophoblast, which involves both cytotrophoblast and syncytiotrophoblast. Complete mole shows proliferation and pleomorphism of epithelial cells whose nuclei are hyperchromatic and actively mitotic.

Pathological changes are:
- Edema of villous stroma
- Loss of central core and blood vessel
- Proliferation of cytotrophoblast and syncytiotrophoblast.

The villus is then swells to form rounded cysts filled with watery fluid. The chorion thus becomes converted into a mass of grape-like structures attached by a fine stalk.

Basic causes of this mechanism is not known, but there are certain theories:
- Primarily death of the fetus resulting in failure of the villus circulation and consequent edema and liquefaction of the stroma.

Or
- Primary error in the development of the vessels in the core causes the villus to become overloaded with fluid and foodstuffs. These foodstuffs stimulate the covering epithelium of the villus or primary over activity of the epithelium of the villus in response to anoxia causes cellular hyperplasia and active secretion of fluid into the core of the villus resulting in cyst formation.

Microscopically
- Marked proliferation of the syncytial and cytotrophoblastic epithelium
- Marked thinning of the stromal tissue due to hydropic degeneration
- Absence of blood vessels in central core
- Pleomorphism of the epithelium, hyperchromatism of the nucleus and active mitosis present
- The villus pattern is distinctly maintained.

Differences between Complete and Partial Mole (Table 11.1)

Complete and partial mole can be differentiated by ultrasonography. USG is a reliable, sensitive and safe test for diagnosis of hydatidiform mole. The characteristic 'snowstorm' appearance is seen in the uterine cavity in complete mole due to diffuse hydropic swelling of chorionic villi. On the other hand, in partial mole:
- There will be focal cystic changes in the placenta
- The transverse diameter of the gestational sac will be increased, as a result of which the ratio of transverse to anteroposterior diameter of gestational sac will be >1.5. These two sonographic findings are significantly associated with the diagnosis of partial mole.
- On rare occasions, the sonogram will show the presence of a fetus with multiple congenital anomalies associated with a focally hydropic placenta (Fine et al. 1989; Benson et al. 2000). Sometimes complete mole may coexist with fetus. With the increased availability of ovulation inducing drugs, twin pregnancy consisting of a complete mole and a coexisting fetus has been reported.

Importance of Differentiation of Complete and Partial Mole

Complete moles are well recognized to have a potential for developing choriocarcinoma and distant spread. If one knows about the type of mole, patients with complete mole will be advised for a longer and close follow-up.

> How will you manage Mrs Nasima's problem?

Suction evacuation is the preferred method of evacuation regardless of uterine size. Before starting the procedure consent of laparotomy is to be taken and laparotomy setup should be kept ready, as hysterotomy, hysterectomy or bilateral hypogastric artery ligation may be necessary if perforation or hemorrhage occurs:
- An IV channel is to be opened and intravenous infusion with Ringers lactate solution is to be started
- Parenteral antibiotic is to be started

Table 11.1 Complete versus partial mole

Sl. No.		Complete mole	Partial mole
1.	Fetal or embryonic tissue	Absent	Present
2.	Chorionic villi swelling	Diffuse	Focal
3.	Trophoblastic hyperplasia	Diffuse	Focal
4.	Implantation site trophoblast	Diffuse, marked atypia	Focal, mild atypia
5.	Scalloping of chorionic villi	Absent	Present
6.	Trophoblastic stromal inclusions	Absent	Present
7.	Karyotype	46 XX (mainly) 46 XY	Triploid/Occasionally tetraploid
8.	Pre-evacuation human chorionic gonadotropin (hCG) levels	Markedly elevated	Less elevation
9.	Free β-and α-subunits of hCG	Higher percentage of β-hCG	Higher percentage of α-hCG
10.	Sign/Symptoms	Uterus enlarged and vaginal bleeding takes place earlier	• Uterus is often not enlarged • Vaginal bleeding tends to occur in the second trimester • Occasionally present with a missed or incomplete abortion
11.	Chemotherapy	Malignant change is higher about 16–20% so need chemo-therapy	• Less chance of malignancy • Only 0.5% require chemotherapy for postmolar gestational trophoblastic disease (GTD) (Seckl et al. 2000)

- Blood is to be kept ready at hand to combat situations as blood loss may be excessive
- The procedure should be done under spinal or general anesthesia
- A negative pressure up to 200–250 mm Hg is to be applied
- Oxytocin drip should be started after a moderate amount of tissue has been removed and may be continued for 24 hours postevacuation depending upon the amount of bleeding and uterine contractility
- When evacuation is complete, a sharp curettage is to be performed with caution, keeping the chance of perforation in mind, to remove any residual chorionic tissue
- Curettage specimen must be sent for histopathological examination to identify complete and partial mole and to exclude choriocarcinoma.

Note: A pre-evacuation β-hCG and X-ray chest should be done routinely as baseline assessment:
- To categorize the patient into low risk and high risk
- For assessment of the patient for monitoring during treatment.

Why suction evacuation is the first choice for evacuation of molar pregnancy?

Suction evacuation is the preferred choice of treatment in molar pregnancy as:
- It is safe and rapid and effective almost in all cases
- Usually cervical dilatation is not needed
- It effectively removes the chorionic tissue form the uterus under negative pressure; so the process becomes complete
- No chance of dissemination as it done under negative pressure
- The time needed to perform the procedure is short and minimum amount of blood is lost
- There is less chance of injury or perforation of uterus as the process is done under negative pressure.

Is there any role of oxytocin or prostaglandin in the management of hydatidiform mole?

Prostaglandin and oxytocin are not recommended for cervical dilatation or expulsion of molar tissue to avoid the risk of dissemination and pulmonary embolization of trophoblastic tissue due to forceful contraction of myometrium. It is noted that prolonged use of agents that stimulate the uterus has rarely been associated with embolization of trophoblastic tissue (Tidy et al. 2000).

But oxytocin and prostaglandin can be used during procedure of suction curettage if there is life-threatening bleeding. Otherwise these are not recommended before completion of the evacuation.

> Can medical evacuation with mifepristone be tried in molar pregnancy?

It also should be avoided to prevent the potential risk of embolization of trophoblastic tissue in the venous system (Stone et al. 1979; Tidy et al. 2000).

> Suppose Mrs Nasima came to you with moderate PV bleeding with passage of grape-like structures. She is pale with feature of shock.
> What investigation will you do for her diagnosis and how will you manage her?

Passage of grape-like vesicle is conclusive for diagnosis. So nothing is needed to establish diagnosis. But for future management baseline β-hCG and X-ray chest is to be done:

- Immediately IV channel is to be opened and blood is to be sent for complete blood count (CBC), grouping Rh typing and crossmatching for blood transfusion
- By the time of arrangement of blood, Ringer's lactate solution and plasma expander is to be started to keep the patient hemodynamically stable
- Parenteral antibiotic is to be started
- A self-retaining Foley's catheter is to be introduced to assess urine output
- Simultaneously suction evacuation is to be done under general anesthesia (GA) to complete the expulsion and control bleeding
- Injection oxytocin drip can be added to combat excessive bleeding and help the expulsion
- A gentle curettage can be done with caution to remove residual molar tissue
- Specimen is to be sent for histopathology, which will diagnose the type of mole
- Injection oxytocin drip is to be continued or ergometrine is to be given depending upon bleeding and uterine contractility.

> Is there any other procedure for evacuation of molar contents from the uterus?

1. If cannula for suction evacuation cannot be introduced due to closed and tubular cervix laminaria tent can be used to ripe the cervix before the procedure. Alternatively vaginal misoprostol 400 µg 2–3 hours before surgery can be given to ripe the cervix.
2. If molar tissue is in the process of expulsion removal of mole by ovum forceps under general anesthesia (GA) can also be done.
3. MVA tool can be used if the size of uterus is less than 12 weeks.

> Suppose after 7–10 days of evacuation patient has no complain. Is there any role of check dilatation and curettage (D&C) after evacuation?

No. There is no clinical indication for the routine use of second uterine evacuation in the management of molar pregnancies. If symptoms are persistent, evaluation of the patient with hCG estimation and ultrasound examination is advised. There is no role of check D&C as patient has no complaint of bleeding, since evacuation is done by suction curettage and residual chorionic tissue is finally removed by gentle curettage. But individualization of patient is required. Approximately 80% of women undergoing a further evacuation subsequently requiring chemotherapy (Savage and Seckl, 2005). Moreover, each procedure carries a risk of infection, triggering hemorrhage and rarely uterine perforation either due to instrumental or due to possibility of invasive or perforating mole.

> She has complete mole and her blood group is Rh negative. Does she need Rh anti-D immunization?

No she does not need anti-D prophylaxis. Because of poor vascularization of the chorionic villi and absence of the anti-D antigen in complete moles, anti-D prophylaxis is not required. It is, however, required for partial moles. So administration of anti-D can be delayed till histopathologic confirmation.

> If there is twin pregnancy with one molar (complete) and other with normal baby, what should be your decision?

With the increased availability of ovulation induction drugs, twin pregnancy consisting of a complete mole and a coexisting fetus has been reported (Vejerslev, 1991) In the situation of a twin pregnancy where there is one viable fetus and the other pregnancy is molar, the woman should be counseled about the increased risk of perinatal morbidity and outcome for GTN. Prenatal invasive testing for fetal karyotype should be considered in cases where it is unclear if the pregnancy is a complete mole with a coexisting normal twin or a partial mole. The outcome for a normal pregnancy with a coexisting complete mole is poor, with an increased risk of early fetal loss (40%) premature delivery (36%) and greater risk of developing persistent trophoblastic disease (50–60%) and progression to metastatic disease. So considering poor outcome of complete mole, pregnancy can be terminated after proper counseling of the patient with usual follow-up.

> She has no complain after evacuation and curettage. So do you think that this management is enough for this patient?

No. Routine follow-up is mandatory for all cases. She needs to be followed up for at least 1 year to diagnose persistent trophoblastic disease or choriocarcinoma, which may occur in 4–15% of cases (Berkowitz et al. 1993).

> How will you follow-up Mrs Nasima?

Patient should be followed up for at least 1 year. During this period she should take an effective contraceptives to avoid pregnancy. The follow-up should include:
- Details history
- Physical examination
- Estimation of β-hCG
- X-ray chest.

Schedule of Follow-up

Follow-up depends upon β-hCG level
- Weekly until β-hCG are normal for three consecutive weeks.
- Monthly for six consecutive months
- About 3 monthly for rest of the time.

Protocol

A. History:
   - In the history well-being of the patient, complaints of irregular PV bleeding, chest complains such as persistent cough, breathlessness or hemoptysis, brain complains such as headache, convulsion, complaints of liver involvement such as epigastric pain and jaundice are important.
B. Physical Examination:
   - Physical examination will depend upon patients' complaints. Pelvic examination includes careful search for uterine size and bilateral theca-luteal cyst. Lutein cysts should regress within 2 months.
C. Investigation
   - Serum β-hCG estimation
   - *X-ray chest*:
     – Only if pre-evacuation X-ray shows metastasis it should be repeated at 4 weeks interval until remission is confirmed. It is then repeated at 3 months interval during the rest of the follow-up period.
     – If pre-evacuation X-ray is normal it is repeated only when hCG titer plateaus or rises.

> Why the patients should not conceive during follow-up?

Pregnancy means rise in β-hCG level. This will arise confusion whether the rise is due to pregnancy or for the recurrence of disease itself. So to avoid any confusion about the development of malignant disease, the patient must avoid pregnancy during the period of follow-up described above. Effective contraception should be used. If a pregnancy occurs, the elevation in β-hCG levels cannot be differentiated from the disease process.

> What contraception is ideal?

- Barrier method or oral contraceptives can be safely used during the follow-up period.
- IUCD should not be used till normalization of the uterus and the β-hCG has returned to normal because of potential risk of uterine perforation, infection and bleeding. Moreover,

IUCD is associated with irregular PV bleeding, which is a feature of choriocarcinoma.
- If family is complete permanent sterilization can be done.

When she should get pregnant?

Women should be advised not to conceive until their follow-up is complete or pregnancy should be delayed at least for 1 year after molar pregnancy. The risk of a further molar pregnancy is low (1.25%). More than 98% of women who become pregnant following a molar pregnancy will not have a further molar pregnancy and there is no increased risk of obstetric complication.

What are the complications of molar pregnancy?

Immediate Complications

- *Hemorrhage:* Due to detachment of vesicles, perforating mole (intraperitoneal), uterine atonicity, uterine perforation during evacuation.
- *Uterine perforation:* Due to perforation mole or during surgical procedure of evacuation.
- *Shock:* Due to excessive hemorrhage.
- *Sepsis*
- *Pre-eclampsia*
- *Thyroid storm:* In presence of hyperthyroid state if evacuation is done under general anesthesia (GA), the acute features such as hyperthermia, delirium, convulsion, coma and cardiovascular collapse may develop.
- *Acute pulmonary insufficiency:* Due to pulmonary embolization of trophoblastic cells. Usually develops within 4–6 hours of evacuation.
- *Coagulation failure:* Due to pulmonary embolization of trophoblastic cells.

Late Complication

- *Choriocarcinoma:* Develops in 16–20% from complete mole and 0.5% from partial mole.

What are the risk factors for malignant change?

- *Patients age:* More than 40 or less than 20 years irrespective of parity
- *Parity:* Multiparous more than para 3
- *Asian women* are more risky than other ethnic groups
- *Complete moles* are more risky than partial moles
- *Recurrent mole or previous history of molar pregnancy*: Patients with repetitive molar disease have three fold increased risk of developing postmolar tumors.
- *Serum β-hCG:* >100,000 mIU/mL
- *Uterine size:* If size is bigger than 20 weeks
- *Larger theca-lutein cysts:* Larger than 6 cm.
  These patients have higher chance of developing uterine invasion and metastasis and are categorized as high-risk patients.

Is there any chance of developing hydatidiform mole in next pregnancy?

Yes. After a hydatidiform mole, the risk of developing a second mole is 1.2–1.4%. The risk increases to 20% after 2 moles (Garner et al. 2002).

Suppose during follow-up you found that Mrs Nasima's β-hCG level remained the same after 2 months of evacuation.
What do you want to do now?

Patient should be followed-up till 15 weeks postevacuation provided there is no other symptom or pathology except increased β-hCG. In spite of high β-hCG still patient should be followed up because of the following reasons:
- About 70% patients achieve normal β-hCG level within 8 weeks postevacuation
- About 15% patients demonstrate a slow decline in titers, but ultimately achieve normal titers without treatment within 15 weeks
- Remaining 15% patients who have elevated titers at 8 weeks postevacuation demonstrate a rising or plateau titer. Nearly half of these have histologic evidence of invasive mole and other half will have choriocarcinoma
- Thus treatment should be instituted when β-hCG remains elevated at 15 weeks postevacuation.

If remained elevated after 15 weeks, what is the treatment?

Single agent chemotherapy either methotrexate or actinomycin D can be given for three courses at weekly interval.

Note: Dose schedule is discussed under persistent GTT.

> What are the indications of chemotherapy after evacuation of molar pregnancy?

Indications of chemotherapy after evacuation of molar pregnancy are:
- Rising β-hCG level for two successive weeks
- Constant level for three successive weeks
- If β-hCG level fails to become normal by 15 weeks
- Rising β-hCG level after reaching normal level
- Any detectable level of hCG not showing a tendency to disappear 4–6 months postpartum
- Evidence of metastasis with any level of hCG.

> Suppose a patient who is mother of two children and no longer desires to preserve fertility.
> Can hysterectomy be an option of treatment of molar pregnancy, as there is chance of developing choriocarcinoma from it?

No. Hysterectomy is not considered as an option of treatment. Although hysterectomy eliminates the risk of local invasion, it does not prevent metastasis. Thus hysterectomy does not obviate the need of follow-up. In addition since most of the patients belong to the younger age groups, even though she does not desire pregnancy, preservation of uterus means maintenance of menstruation, which will give a sense of well-being to the patients. Moreover, for young patients nobody assures about the need of future fertility. On these grounds, hysterectomy is discouraged in molar pregnancy.

> But sometimes it is needed to do the hysterectomy.
> What are the situations when hysterectomy is needed?

Following are the situations when hysterectomy is indicated:
- Profuse bleeding, which is not controlled by evacuation
- Uterus is perforated during evacuation
- Intraperitoneal hemorrhage due to perforating mole.
- Placental site trophoblastic tumor.

> Following molar evacuation, what is the percentage of invasion and metastasis?

Following molar evacuation, uterine invasion and metastasis occur in 15% and 4% of patients, respectively (Berkowitz et al. 1993).

> **Case scenario:** A lady of 28 years has been evacuated for hydatidiform mole. Her histopathologic review shows complete mole. Her pre-evacuation β-hCG level was 2,38,000 mIU/mL, size of uterus was 18 weeks against 12 weeks amenorrhea, there were bilateral football size theca-lutein cysts in the abdomen.
> How will you manage her?

This patient belongs to high-risk category. Prophylactic chemotherapy can be used. Chemoprophylaxis significantly reduces the incidence of postmolar tumor from 47% to 14% and it is beneficial when hormonal follow-up is unavailable or unreliable (Berkowitz et al. 1993).

Note: There is a role of prophylactic chemotherapy in molar pregnancy in rare occasion particularly when the patient is high-risk category and serum β-hCG is not falling satisfactorily. The chemotherapy is single agent–methotrexate or actinomycin for 2–3 weeks.

> Patient's ovaries are so big that looks like ovarian cyst.
> Is surgery indicated for this patient?

No. Surgery is not indicated for lutein cysts. It is the effect of β-hCG from surviving trophoblastic disease. Once trophoblastic tissue dies in response to chemotherapy β-hCG levels will reduce and ovaries will return to normal size in due course of time.

> Other than ovarian hyperstimulation syndrome, what complication may happen if ovarian size becomes bigger?

Ovarian torsion, rupture and hemorrhage may occur.

> What should be done if such situation occurs?

- If there is torsion, untwisting is the preferred option of treatment where significant viable ovarian tissue is present

- In case of rupture and hemorrhage blood transfusion, laparotomy followed by peritoneal toileting and hemostasis either by cautery or ligature is to be done.

> *What is invasive mole? How it can be confirmed?*

Invasive hydatidiform mole, also known as *chorioadenoma destruens* is a type of neoplasia that grows into the muscular wall of the uterus. In 20% cases the hydatidiform mole invades the myometrium or adjacent structure. Although it is considered benign neoplasm, invasive mole is locally invasive and may produce distant metastasis. It may spread to other parts of the body, such as the vagina, vulva, and lung. It has the potential to completely penetrate the myometrium and causes subsequent uterine rupture and hemoperitoneum. It can regress spontaneously. Microscopically it is similar to hydatidiform mole.

Doppler color flow mapping can reveal an abnormal color blood flow within the echo-free space in the uterine myometrium, and pulsed Doppler ultrasound can show a prominent arteriovenous shunt flow. Though definite diagnosis can be made on the basis of myometrial invasion on histology.

Note: Line of management is same as hydatidiform mole in addition chemotherapy is to be given.

> *What is placental site trophoblastic tumor (PSTT)? What is its treatment and prognosis?*

The PSTT is a rare slow growing form of gestational trophoblastic disease that has been proposed to arise from intermediate trophoblast at the implantation site (Shih and Kurman, 2001). It may arise from hydatidiform mole, non-molar abortion or rarely from a normal term pregnancy (Palmieri, 2005). It form local mass and confined to the uterus and metastasizes late in its course. Syncytiotrophoblast is usually absent from the tumor, so β-hCG secretion is minimum in relation to volume of the tumor. hCG elevation at diagnosis has been found to be less than 500 IU/L in over 50% of cases (Papadopoulos et al. 2002). However, placental human lactogen is secreted and its level can be monitored to follow-up.

Peculiarities of PSTT

- It differs from other GTN in that it produces relatively little hCG and human placental lactogen (hPL) in relation to the size of tumor. Thus tumor burden may be present before human placental lactogen hCG levels are detectable.
- The tumor tend to remain confined to the uterus, metastasizing late in their course. Metastases may occur in the vagina, extrauterine pelvic tissues, retroperitoneum, lymph nodes, lungs and brain (Papadopoulos et al. 2002).
- PSTT are relatively insensitive/resistant to chemotherapy. Thus once diagnosed hysterectomy is the treatment of choice.

Note: Chemotherapy is given in disseminated disease with late diagnosis. The preferred combination therapy is etoposide, cisplatinum-etoposide, methotrexate and actinomycin D (EP-EMA) which is given for 2–3 additional courses after β-hCG level has returned to normal. This is then followed by hysterectomy.

Prognosis

The most important prognostic factors for patients with PSTT are stage, myometrial invasion and date from antecedent pregnancy (better for those with an interval <4 years). Hyperprolactinemia can occur, resulting in amenorrhea or galactorrhea (Young and Scully, 1984).

High cure rate is achieved with early diagnosis and surgical reaction. Since, the diagnosis is late, the overall prognosis is not satisfactory. The greatest adverse outcome is associated when the interval from antecedent pregnancy to diagnosis is >4 years.

> *What is epithelioid trophoblastic tumors?*

Epithelioid trophoblastic tumor (ETT) is a recently described neoplastic proliferation of intermediate trophoblast that is thought by some investigators to be distinct from PSTT and choriocarcinoma (Hui et al. 2005; Shih and Kurman, 1998).

It has been proposed that ETT arises from the intermediate trophoblasts of the chorionic leave.

The cells are positive for cytokeratin, epithelial membrane antigen and inhibin-a, whereas the trophoblastic markers hPL, hCG and melanoma cell adhesion molecule are only focally expressed (Hui et al. 2005).

The presenting signs are vaginal bleeding with a low level of hCG (<2,500 IU/L). A total of 50% of cases present with a lower uterine or cervical lesion, which is important to differentiate from squamous cell carcinoma of the cervix. Like PSTT it is less responsive to conventional chemotherapy and the current accepted management is hysterectomy, and close follow-up.

> **Case scenario:** Mrs Hasina 24 years old lady gives history of hydatidiform mole evacuation 4 months back. She is having irregular PV bleeding on and off since then with cough and occasional hemoptysis for the last 15 days. What is your diagnosis?

Persistent gestational trophoblastic tumor or choriocarcinoma.

> How will you define persistent GTT?

In United States persistent GTT is defined as a re-elevation or persistent plateau in hCG for at least 3 consecutive weeks following molar evacuation.

In western Europe, the criteria for persistent GTT is more stringent. It includes:
- hCG >20,000 IU/L, >4 weeks after evacuation
- Progressively rising hCG levels, with a minimum of three rising valves over 2–3 weeks
- Persistent high hCG level 4–6 weeks after evacuation
- Metastasis to the liver, kidney, brain or GIT
- Metastasis to the lung >2 cm in diameter or three or more in number.

Persistent GTT Follows

- Molar pregnancy
- Non-molar pregnancy
  - Abortion
  - Ectopic pregnancy
  - Full-term pregnancy.

> Mrs Hasina is suffering from persistent GTT that has originated from hydatidiform mole.
> What measures will you take for her?

Evaluation by history and physical examination is to be done first.

Detailed History

- History of antecedent pregnancy: Here history is given about molar pregnancy. Most common is molar pregnancy (80%) (choriocarcinoma following a full-term pregnancy is more often associated with aggressive disease).
- History about first X-ray chest and pre-evacuation hCG level.
- History of intermittent, but heavy vaginal bleeding lasting longer than normal.
- History of abdominal swelling due to bilateral theca-lutein cysts.
- Symptoms due to *metastatic* involvement of the following organs:
  - *Lung:* Chest pain, dyspnea, hemoptysis
  - *Brain:* Vomiting, headache, convulsion, hemiparesis, visual disturbances, intracranial hemorrhage, symptoms of raised intracranial pressure.
  - *Liver:* Epigastric pain, referred pain to the right shoulder tip, jaundice, intra-abdominal bleeding following hepatic rupture.

Thorough Physical Examination

- *General examination:* Patient looks ill with pallor of varying degrees, jaundice due to hepatic involvement, lethargy and coma due to brain involvement.
- *PA examination:*
  - Abdominal tenderness may present if liver or gastrointestinal metastases have occurred.
  - Bilateral luteal cysts can be palpable.
  - Abdominal distension and tenderness may present if a hemoperitoneum has occurred due to bleeding from an abdominal metastasis. Bleeding from a metastasis could also result in signs and symptoms of hemorrhagic shock.
- *PV examination*
  - Metastasis to the lower genital tract present as *purple to blue-black* papules or nodules in *fornices and suburethral* region. These are extremely vascular.

- Uterus may be bulky
- Respiratory and cardiovascular (CVS) examination depending upon the site of metastasis.

Note: *Common site of metastasis:* Lungs—80%, vagina—30%, pelvis—20%, brain—10%, liver—10%, rarely in skin, heart, kidney and cauda equina.

Important points to note here are:
- Virtually all patients with brain metastasis have concurrent pulmonary and/or vaginal metastasis
- Patients with liver metastasis generally present with pulmonary, vaginal or cerebral involvement.

> After taking history you explored that she has no other complaints except cough, hemoptysis and slight weakness. On physical examination you found her anemic, otherwise normal.
> How will you evaluate this case before starting treatment?

Investigations

Following investigations are to be done:
- CBC and platelet count
- β-hCG
- Ultrasonography of whole abdomen
- X-ray of chest/computed tomography (CT) scan of chest
- Hepatic and renal function test
- CT scan of abdomen and CT/magnetic resonance imaging (MRI) of brain.

> Why pelvic USG is an essential aid in evaluation of the patients?

Color Doppler USG can noninvasively detect extensive uterine tumor. Thus it helps to select patients who will benefit from hysterectomy. When the uterus contains large amounts of tumor, hysterectomy may substantially reduce the tumor burden and limit the requirement for chemotherapy, as well as eliminate the potential for hemorrhage or infection. Also perforating mole on diagnosis by USG can be subjected to hysterectomy.

> What are the different radiographic patterns in the lungs, in persistent GTTs/choriocarcinoma?

The GTT produces four principal radiographic patterns in the lungs:
- Alveolar or snow-storm appearance
- Discrete rounded densities—Cannonball appearance
- Pleural effusion
- Embolic pattern caused by pulmonary arterial occlusion.

> As Mrs Hasina diagnosed as persistent GTT, would you like to do D&C for histopathological confirmation?

No. Following molar pregnancy, persistent GTTs may have histopathological evidence of either molar tissue or choriocarcinoma, but diagnosis of GTT or choriocarcinoma can be confirmed by high level of serum hCG only.

Diagnostic curettage for histopathological confirmation is not essential as:
- It usually gives negative findings because the growth does not always present in the uterine cavity.
- In one third of metastatic choriocarcinoma there is no evidence of disease in the uterus.

Development of metastasis is a sufficient justification for chemotherapy.

> Suppose you have seen a suburethral nodule. How will you confirm vaginal metastasis?

Vaginal metastasis in persistent GTT/choriocarcinoma are usually highly vascular and might bleed profusely if biopsied. So attempts at histopathologic confirmation of the diagnosis should be absolutely avoided. Suburethral nodule with a high serum β-hCG is enough to confirm vaginal metastasis and should proceed for treatment.

RELATED INFORMATION

More investigations in some cases:
- *CT scan of abdomen and CT or MRI of head*: Patients with no relevant symptomatology, normal pelvic examination and normal chest radiograph are very unlikely to have liver or brain metastasis. CT scan of abdomen is done to exclude liver involvement in patients with abnormal liver function test and CT or MRI scan of the head is indicated in suspected cases.

- *Lumbar puncture*: Patients with pulmonary disease are at risk of developing brain metastases. Cerebrospinal fluid (CSF) hCG estimations are useful in detecting tumor involvement of the neuroaxis, which can lead to the secretion of hCG into the CSF, reducing the serum to CSF hCG ratio to less than 60:1 (Bagshawe and Harland, 1976; Athanassiou et al. 1983). Despite advances in CT and MRI scanning, occasionally metastatic disease can be detected by this simple technique when the scans are normal. However, in the era of MRI and 18-fluorodeoxyglucose- positron emission tomography (18-FDG PET), the need of CSF determination is limited.
- *18-FDG PET*: Patients presenting with relapsed disease or with unexplained elevated hCG can occasionally benefit from 18-FDG PET scanning. This can help to identify the site of active disease. However, false positive and false negative results are possible (Dhillon et al. 2006). Still this is a useful technique and can still provide helpful data even when the hCG is <10I U/L (Dhillon et al. 2006).
- *Genetic testing*: Women who develop choriocarcinoma or PSTT some years after a pregnancy are often assumed to have gestational tumors. However, sometimes these tumors have arisen from a nongestational source and subsequently differentiate to resemble GTN. Prognostically these are very aggressive tumor. Genetic analysis to determine the presence or absence of paternal genes will distinguish between gestational and nongestational choriocarcinoma and/or PSTT. The results are clearly helpful in providing prognostic and therapeutic information in such cases (Fisher et al. 2007).

> How patients are categorized in to low risk and high risk?

Patients are categorized for chemotherapy as low (good prognostic) and high risk (poor prognostic) depending on their prognostic scores using the WHO/FIGO scoring system **(Table 11.2)**.

A total score of 0-6 is considered low-risk and single agent chemotherapy is selected while a total score ≥7 is considered as high-risk and requires combination chemotherapy to achieve remission.

Now International Federation of Obstetrics and Gynecology revised the scoring system combining the use of both anatomic and non-anatomic factors.

According to FIGO, patient is assigned a stage **(Table 11.3)** based on anatomic location of the disease and given a risk score based on WHO prognostic scoring system. This is done to:
- Improve the assessment and assist in selecting appropriate chemotherapy, thus avoiding drug resistance.

Table 11.2 Modified WHO prognostic scoring system as adapted by FIGO (FIGO Report: 2009)

Prognostic factor	Score			
	0	1	2	4
Maternal age	<40	≥40		
Antecedent pregnancy (AP)	Mole	Abortion	Term	
Interval between AP and chemotherapy (M)	<4	4–6	7–12	>12
hCG IU/L	$<10^3$	10^3–10^4	10^4–10^5	$>10^5$
Number of metastasis	0	1–4	5–8	>8
Site of metastasis	Lung	Spleen, kidney	Gastro-intestinal (GI) tract	Brain, liver
Largest tumor mass		<3	3–4 cm	≥5 cm
Prior chemotherapy			Single drug	≥2 drugs

Table 11.3 FIGO anatomic staging (FIGO report, 2009)

Stages	Diseases
Stage I	Disease confined to the uterus
Stage II	GTN extends outside the uterus, but limited to the genital structures (adnexa, vagina broad ligament)
Stage III	GTN extends to the lungs, with or without known genital tract involvement
Stage IV	All other metastatic sites

- It also allows comparable reporting of data, which is important for comparison of treatment results.

Relation of WHO prognostic scoring and staging
WHO prognostic scoring can be predicted by staging. It is evident that stage I GTT have low-risk score, while stage IV patients have high-risk scores. The scoring is mostly applicable for patients with stage II or III disease to categorize low risk or high risk.

A patient of GTT with stage IV has poor prognosis. Stage IV disease in most cases follow a non-molar pregnancy with delays in diagnosis and large tumor burdens. The histopathologic pattern is mostly choriocarcinoma. They are likely to be resistant to chemotherapy and thus have a poor prognosis.

Format of writing the diagnosis in GTT
The stage and WHO prognostic risk score is allotted for each patient. For example GTT stage II : 6.

> Mrs Hasina's CBC is within normal range, β-hCG is 35,000 IU/L, lung field shows cannonball appearance. Baseline chest X-ray was normal and β-hCG was 80,000 IU/L. Other test reports including CT scan of abdomen and brain are normal.
> How will you manage Mrs Hasina?

According to WHO prognostic scoring system Mrs Hasina has *low risk or good prognostic* disease. So single agent chemotherapy will be effective for her.

Single agent chemotherapy with either *methotrexate or actinomycin-D* induces excellent remission rate in non-metastatic and low-risk metastatic GTTs. It induces excellent remission rate with minimum toxicity, but also effectively limits chemotherapy exposure.

Side effects: Alopecia, sepsis, thrombocytopenia, granulocytopenia and hepatotoxicity is minimum.

First-line therapy: Methotrexate and folinic acid.

Dose and regime: 8 days regimen
- Injection methotrexate 1 mg/kg intramuscularly (IM) on day 1, 3, 5 and 7 every 48 hours.
- Injection folinic acid 0.1 mg/kg IM on day 2, 4, 6 and 8, 24 hours after injection methotrexate.

Note: Folinic acid nullifies the toxic effect of methotrexate to healthy tissue. But to act on malignant cell a 24 hours window is given for methotrexate.

Duration of Rx: Therapy should be given until the patient achieve normal hCG. Each course is to be repeated at 1 week interval because treatment gap of 2 weeks or more allows tumor regrowth. After normal hCG levels are attained, at least one additional course of chemotherapy are undertaken as consolidation therapy to reduce the risk of relapse.

Second line therapy: Actinomycin D

Dose: 0.5 mg by intravenous (IV) daily for 5 days.

Duration: Same as methotrexate.

2nd line (or changing of the drug) is given when:
- There is no response or resistant to the treatment, manifested by:
  - Rising or plateauing hCG titers
  - By the development of new metastasis
  - If negative titers are not achieved by the fifth course of methotrexate.
- There is development of toxicity.

Note:
- *Failed response:* It is defined as appearance of metastasis or plateau of serum β-hCG. (*Plateau:* Any fall in serum β-hCG of <10% of previous week in 3 consecutive weeks)
- *Drug resistance:* It is diagnosed when there is plateau or rise of serum β-hCG. (*Rise:* Any rise in serum β-hCG of >10% of previous week in 3 consecutive weeks)
  If second line does not work combination (MAC) therapy is indicated.

> How will you monitor Mrs Hasina in between treatment?

Patient must be monitored carefully between two courses of chemotherapy.
Monitoring is essential to:
- Evaluate the response to treatment and
- Evaluate toxicity.

Evaluation of Response

This is done by doing serum β-hCG on the weekly basis that is in the window of the course. If the fall of serum β-hCG is >10% of the previous week it is satisfactory and further chemotherapy is continued as per schedule.

Then test is to be continued:
- Weekly until 3 consecutive normal titers
- Monthly for 12 months
- Two monthly for 1 year
- Every 6 months for life long.

Note: If titer rises 10-fold or more, titer plateaus at an elevated level or new metastasis appears, alternate regime is indicated.

Evaluation of Toxicity

- Systemic side effects of methotrexate (MTX) like stomatitis, skin rash, alopecia, conjunctivitis and gastrointestinal disturbances are regularly excluded.
- Regular checks are made on white cell count, platelet count, liver function and renal function tests on second week of chemotherapy.

Toxicity is diagnosed if:
- Systemic side effects are prominently evident
- White cell count <3000 mL for >21 days after the last cycle
- Platelet count <1,00,000 mL for >21 days after the last cycle
- Liver function test (LFT) are elevated more than twice normal
- Blood urea is raised

Baseline *CBC*, LFT and *kidney function* tests are to be repeated before each course of treatment.

Treatment course should not be repeated if:
- WBC falls below 3,000 cumm and neutrophils below 1,500 cumm
- Platelet falls below 100,000 cumm
- Significant elevation of blood urea nitrogen (BUN) and serum glutamic pyruvic transaminase (SGPT).

> Suppose Mrs Hasina did not respond to single agent chemotherapy. Moreover, she developed neurological symptoms.
> What treatment would you like to give?

According to risk category she is now poor prognostic or high-risk score group. Failure of single agent chemotherapy or metastasis to brain or lungs falls under score 7 or more. She has two risk factors now and she needs combination chemotherapy. As combination therapy methotrexate, actinomycin D and chlorambucil (MAC) or modified Bagshaw (*CHAMOCA*, cyclophosphamide, hydroxyurea, methotrexate, vincristine, and actinomycin) can be used. But *currently EMACO* [etoposide, methotrexate, actinomycin D, cyclophosphamide and oncovin (vincristine) provides the best response and with low side effects.

EMACO Therapy

EMACO is currently the preferred treatment for patients with high-risk score. EMACO induces complete remission in 70–90% patients.

Regime of EMACO Therapy

The regime consists of two courses:
- Course I (EMA) is given on day 1 and day 2, which require overnight hospital stay
- Course 2 (CO) is given on day 8 as outpatient procedure. The courses are again repeated in the second cycle on day 15.

Duration

Combination chemotherapy is given until normal hCG is achieved. After normal hCG levels are attained, at least two additional courses of chemotherapy are undertaken as consolidation therapy to reduce the risk of relapse.

> Can other combination therapy be used?

Modified triple therapy (MAC III) with MT X FA, Act-D, cyclophosphamide was used. But it was proved to be inadequate as an initial treatment in patients with metastasis and high-risk score. The remission rates are low.

> In case of resistance and toxicity to EMACO what other chemotherapy can be used?

If patients experience resistance to EMACO, they can be successfully treated with modification of this regimen called *salvage therapy* by substituting etoposide and cisplatin on day 8 for cyclophosphamide and vincristine (EMA-EP) or *surgical intervention* may be necessary to remove sites of resistant tumor. This chemotherapy needs extremely careful monitoring of renal function since cisplatin is nephrotoxic and methotrexate is excreted in the urine. Second-line therapy with cisplatin, vinblastine, and bleomycin (PVB) is also effective in patients with drug resistant GTT. Paclitaxel is another agent, which has activity in GTN.

Note: With failure of EMA-EP, BEP (cisplatin, etoposide, bleomycin) and VIP (etoposide, ifosfamide, cisplatin) can be used.

What are the toxicities with the use of chemotherapy? Particularly of etoposide?

Patients treated with single agent MTX do not appear to have increased risk of secondary tumors. But there is 1.5 fold increased risk of developing secondary tumors including myeloid leukemia, colon cancer, melanoma and breast cancer in patients treated with EMACO. That is why etoposide is included to combination chemotherapy as secondary tumors develop 10–25 years after therapy in patients who received a total dose of at least 2 g/m^2.

Can one predict, the number of cycles needed to induce remission?

The number of cycles needed to induce remission is proportionate to the burden of serum β-hCG at the start of treatment. More is the pretreatment hCG, more is the cycle needed. An average of 4–6 cycles are needed to achieve remission. In low-risk group one additional course and high-risk group two additional courses are given after serum β-hCG has become negative to reduce the risk of relapse.

What does remission means?

Remission or complete response is defined as 3 consecutive weekly normal serum β-hCG values measured over 2 consecutive weeks.

When is the disease declared as cured?

Cure is said to have occurred after a period of 5 years in remission.

What is the effect of chemotherapy in reproduction?

Patients with GTT who are treated successfully with chemotherapy can expect normal reproduction in future. There is no evidence of infertility or subfertility in these patients. Regular menstruation resumes 2–6 months after the end of chemotherapy.

After recovery when patient should get pregnant?

Patient should avoid pregnancy at least for 1½ years because the mutogenic and teratogenic effects of chemotherapy persist in the ova of the ovaries for at least 1 year following chemotherapy. So if pregnancy can be avoided for 1½ years, all mature ova, which were exposed to chemotherapy will be eliminated from the body by the time the patient tries for conception. Usually the resting oocytes are not affected by the drugs. Patient should receive contraceptives during this follow-up period. Both barrier method and oral contraceptives are safe during this period. In stage III or IV disease there is increased risk of late recurrences, then contraception should be continued for 2 years.

Is there any effect of chemotherapy in future pregnancy?

In a study of 230 women who conceived within 12 months of completing chemotherapy, there was an increased risk of miscarriage and higher rate of termination in women who received multiagent chemotherapy. The rate of congenital abnormality was low (1.8%), irrespective of the type of chemotherapy used (Blagden, 2002). The rate of stillbirth was elevated compared with the normal population (18.6/1,000 births) (Woolas, 1998). But if pregnancy can be delayed the abortion rate, stillbirth, premature deliveries, cesarean section rate and congenital malformations are consistent with the general population. The explanation is that conception resulting from resting oocytes are not affected by chemotherapy drugs.

What special precaution should be undertaken antenatally and postnatally if patient conceives following successful treatment of GTT?

- An USG should be done in the first trimester to confirm normal gestational development.
- A sample of placenta should be sent after delivery for histopathology to confirm normal placental tissue.

- Serum hCG should be measured at 6 weeks postpartum to exclude occult trophoblastic disease.

> What is the long-term outcome of women treated for GTN?

Early Menopause

Women who receive chemotherapy for GTN are likely to have an earlier menopause. The age at menopause for women who receive *single-agent chemotherapy is advanced by 1 year and by 3 years if they receive multiagent chemotherapy* (Seckl and Rustin, 2003). Hormone replacement therapy may be used safely once hCG levels have returned to normal.

Cancer

Women with high-risk GTN who require multi-agent chemotherapy, which includes etoposide should be advised that they may be at increased risk of developing secondary cancers. Study among 1,377 women showed a relative risk 16.6 for developing acute myeloid leukemia, 4.6 for colon cancer, 3.4 for melanoma and 5.79 for breast cancer in women surviving for more than 25 years (Rustin et al. 1996). If combination chemotherapy is limited to less than 6 months there appears to be no increased risk of secondary cancers (McNeish et al. 2002).

> **Case scenario:** A 30-year-old lady with one child had molar pregnancy and underwent D&C 5 months back. She is having irregular PV bleeding since then. On bimanual examination her uterus is just bulky otherwise normal. USG shows normal ovaries and bulky uterus with bright ecogenic structure within it. Her serum β-hCG is 122,000 IU/mL and chest X-ray reveals multiple discrete nodules in the lung field.
>
> How will you evaluate her? What is her diagnosis?

Evaluation includes more details history, physical examination including per speculum and bimanual examination to exclude metastasis in the vagina and presence of bilateral theca-lutein cysts. Her serum β-hCG and chest X-ray report are known, but USG of lower abdomen is needed to exclude tumor burden. Blood for CBC, renal and hepatic function tests should be done to exclude any abnormality.

Now the patient is subjected to FIGO staging and WHO prognostic scoring. The diagnosis of the disease is *GTN stage III:5*.

> USG shows bright ecogenic structures in the uterine cavity suggestive of retained product of conception.
>
> Is repeat D&C indicated?

Repeat D&C is not indicated in this situation, because chorionic tissue will persist in the uterine cavity no matter repeat D&C is done or not. The uterine cavity becomes clear once the disease is cured and serum β-hCG comes down to normal.

> What will be the treatment option for this patient?

Since the WHO prognostic score is 5, the patient falls in the low-risk group. So, the treatment of choice for this patient will be single agent chemotherapy. Injection MTX alternating with folinic acid on 8 day course is given and repeated every 2 weeks till the serum β-hCG comes to normal (i.e. 0–5 MIU/mL). In addition one more course will be given since the disease belongs to low-risk groups.

> How will you follow-up this patient?

Since this patient is in stage III she will be closely followed up for 1 year. Then the follow-up is for 5 years. Apart from history and physical examination, she needs to do serum β-hCG:
- Every week until they are normal for 3 weeks
- Every month for 12 consecutive month
- Every 3 month for the next 5 years.

Since the patient had chest metastasis, chest X-ray need to be:
- Repeated every month till the lung shadow disappears
- Every 6 months for the next 2 years.

> If the patient is in stage IV, how long she will be followed up?

Close follow-up will be for 2 years. Then the follow-up be for 5 years. Apart from history and physical examination, serum β-hCG is done:
- Every week till it is normal for 3 weeks
- Every month for 24 months
- Every 6 months for the rest of 5 years.

> **Case scenario:** About 40-year-old lady had incomplete abortion and underwent D&C 6 months back. She had irregular PV bleeding on and off after D&C. She went to a local doctor in the Upazila after 3 months. USG of lower abdomen was done, which showed retained product of conception. The local doctor did repeat D&C. But PV bleeding continued. After one more month she started having cough and hemoptysis along with PV bleeding. She then went to the District Hospital where the concerned doctor advised her for a chest X-ray, which revealed cannonball appearance in the lung field and serum β-hCG was 465,000 IU/mL. The doctor started single agent chemotherapy with injection methotrexate and folinic acid (MTXFA) cyclically on a 8 days course. She received five cycle of MTXFA but her lung shadow persisted and serum β-hCG remained as high as 318,000 IU/mL. Now she came to Dhaka for better management.
>
> On the basis of this scenario what is your opinion? Did she get right treatment? If not, what were the pitfalls and what should be her next treatment?

No, she did not get right treatment.

Pitfalls

- A repeat D&C at 3rd month was unnecessary. Rather the patients should have been subjected to serum β-hCG, which would have been raised. This would have suggested the doctor about the diagnosis of persistent GTT and she could have started chemotherapy.
- The selection of chemotherapy by the district doctor was not appropriate. The patient should have undergone staging and WHO prognostic scoring to select the appropriate chemotherapy. In this situation, the WHO risk score was 7 and she should have received combination chemotherapy EMACO to achieve remission.

Proposed Present Treatment

At present scenario, this is a case of failed response due to previous failed chemotherapy. Now the scoring will go up high. Previous 7 + 6 (failed CT) = 13. The patient now needs to be thoroughly assessed in regards to the size of uterus. If the uterine size is bulky the chemotherapy can be changed to EMACO, which is repeated every 2 weeks, until the hCG becomes normal, then two additional cycles of EMACO should be given.

But if the uterus is enlarged with packed chorionic tissue, the patient should be subjected first to hysterectomy to reduce the tumor burden followed by EMACO therapy.

> *If the patient still does not response to EMACO showing either plateau or rising β-hCG titer (drug resistance). What alternative chemotherapy can be tried?*

In such situations of drug resistance salvage therapy with (EP-EMA) can be tried where cyclophosphamide and vincristine (CO) is replaced by etoposide and cisplatin (EP).

> *Why EMACO is the preferred combination therapy instead of MAC therapy for GTT?*

EMACO regimen is well tolerated and treatment seldom has to be suspended because of toxicity. Moreover, the response rate is as high as 80%. On the other hand MAC III (triple therapy) has a remission rate of 50% and patient experiences high side effects. As a result EMACO is now the preferred primary treatment in high-risk GTT.

> *What is the role of surgery in persistent GTT?*

After the advancement of chemotherapy, surgery has limited role in persistent GTT:
- *Total abdominal hysterectomy*: Its role is confined in patients:
  - Who are resistant to chemotherapy
  - Who have uncontrolled uterine bleeding
  - Extensive uterine tumor, to reduce tumor burden and thereby limit the need of multiple courses of chemotherapy
  - Placental site trophoblastic tumors.
- Hepatic resection is indicated in stage IV disease to control intraperitoneal bleeding from hepatic source or to excise resistant tumor.
- Craniotomy may be necessary to provide acute decompression or to control bleeding or to excise resistant tumor.

> *If a patient of persistent GTT manifests signs and symptoms relevant to cerebral metastasis. How will you treat her?*

If cerebral metastasis is diagnosed by CT scan, whole brain *irradiation* (3000 CGy) in 10 fraction is instituted promptly. Brain irradiation is both hemostatic and tumoricidal. Concurrent use of combination chemotherapy and brain irradiation lessens the risk of spontaneous cerebral hemorrhage. In very few instances where cerebral hemorrhage has already started, craniotomy can be done to provide acute decompression or to control bleeding or resect chemotherapy resistant tumor.

> What is the prognosis of patients suffering from cerebral metastasis?

In contrast to most other malignancies cerebral metastasis are associated with a very poor prognosis. Persistent GTT with cerebral metastasis can be cured of the disease with the available treatment. Once they achieve remission generally they have no residual neurologic deficits.

> What is the risk of relapse in patients treated for persistent GTT or choriocarcinoma?

Once the patient achieves biochemical remission the outlook is very bright in terms of future risk of relapse, possibility of future pregnancy and long-term health risks from chemotherapy exposure.

The risk of relapse is <5% for patients treated with single agent chemotherapy and only 3% for patients treated with combination therapy. Generally these recurrences occur within first 12 months after treatment and retain the possibility of cure.

> **Case scenario:** A young nulliparous lady of 23 years, presents with the history of D&C twice for molar pregnancy. Her serum β-hCG is 154,000 IU/mL and USG shows bilateral ovarian cyst of 10 × 12 cm (right ovary) and 8 × 9 cm (left ovary) size.
>
> What will you do for ovarian cyst?

According to WHO prognostic risk category, the patient belongs to a high-risk group. She should be treated with combination (EMACO) chemotherapy till negative β-hCG. A few cycles of EMACO will bring her serum β-hCG to normal. Additional two more cycles will reduce the risk of relapse. Bilateral ovarian cyst will regress to normal within 3-4 cycles of chemotherapy. After 1½ years of follow-up, this patient will be fit to conceive if she desires.

Note: In no way ovarian surgery is indicated in this case as it occurs due to excessive β-hCG and it will regress with regression of β-hCG.

RELATED INFORMATION

Possible Side Effects of the Drugs

Cancer cells tend to grow fast and chemotherapeutic drugs kill fast-growing cells. As drugs are systemic, they can affect normal any healthy cells that are fast-growing too. Damage to healthy cells causes side effects.

Most commonly affected cells are blood-forming cells in the bone marrow, hair follicles, cells in the mouth, digestive tract and reproductive system. Some drugs can damage cells in the heart, kidneys, bladder, lungs and nervous system.

Every person does not get every side effect, and some people get few if any. The severity of side effects varies greatly from person to person.

Chemotherapy Drugs

All chemotherapy drugs have different side effects. The side effects depends on:
- The type of drugs
- The dose of the drugs
- Individual reaction.

Some people have more side effects than others. And different drugs have different side effects such as the followings:
- Changes in sense of taste
- Nausea
- Vomiting
- Mouth sores and ulcers
- Diarrhea
- Pain in chest and abdomen
- Increased risk of infection
- Fatigue (tiredness)
- Feeling and being sick.

How Long do Side Effects Last?

Most side effects slowly go away after treatment ends because the healthy cells recover over time. The time it takes to get over some side effects varies from person to person. It depends on many factors, including overall health and the drugs were given.

Many side effects go away fairly quickly, but some may take months or even years to completely go away. Sometimes the side effects can last a lifetime, such as when drug causes long-term damage to the heart, lungs, kidneys or reproductive organs.

BIBLIOGRAPHY

Athanassiou A, Begent RH, Newlands ES, et al. Central nervous system metastases of choriocarcinoma: 23 years' experience at Charing Cross Hospital. Cancer. 1983;52(9):1728-35.

Atrash HK, Hogue CJ, Grimes DA. Epidemiology of hydatidiform mole during early gestation. Am J Obstet Gynecol. 1986;154(4):906-9.

Bagshawe KD, Harland S. Immunodiagnosis and monitoring of gonadotrophin-producing metastases in the central nervous system. Cancer. 1976;38(1):112-8.

Benson CB, Genest DR, Bernstein MR, et al. Sonographic appearance of first trimester complete hydatidiform moles. Ultrasound Obstet Gynecol. 2000;16(2):188-91.

Berkowitz RS, Goldstein DP. The management of molar pregnancy and gestational trophoblastic tumours. In: Knappe RC, Berkowitz RS (Eds). Gynaecologic, 3rd edition Oncology. New York; McGrow-Hill; 1993. pp. 328-38.

Blagden SP, Foskett MA, Fisher RA, et al. The effect of early pregnancy following chemotherapy on disease relapse and fetal outcome in women treated for gestational trophoblastic tumours. Br J Cancer. 2002;86(1):26-30.

Dhillon T, Palmieri C, Sebire NJ, et al. Value of whole body 18FDG-PET to identify the active site of gestational trophoblastic neoplasia. J Reprod Med. 2006;51(11):879-87.

FIGO Committee on Gynecologic Oncology. Current FIGO staging for cancer of the vagina, fallopian tube, ovary, and gestational trophoblastic neoplasia. Int J Gynaecol Obstet. 2009;105(1):3-4.

Fine C, Bundy AL, Berkowitz RS, et al. Sonographic diagnosis of partial hydatidiform mole; Obstet Gynecol. 1989;73(3 pt 1):414-8.

Fisher RA, Savage PM, MacDermott C, et al. The impact of molecular genetic diagnosis on the management of women with hCG-producing malignancies. Gynecol Oncol. 2007;107(3):413-9.

Garner EI, Lipson E, Bernstein MR, et al. Subsequent pregnancy experience in patients with molar pregnancy and gestational trophoblastic tumor. J Reprod Med. 2002;47(5):380-6.

Grimes DA. Epidemiology of gestational trophoblastic disease. Am J Obstet Gynecol. 1984;150(3):309-18.

Hui P, Martel M, Parkash V. Gestational trophoblastic diseases: recent advances in histopathologic diagnosis and related genetic aspects. Adv Anat Pathol. 2005;12(3):116-25.

McNeish IA, Strickland S, Holden L, et al. Low-risk persistent gestational trophoblastic disease: outcome following initial treatment with low dose methotrexate and folinic acid 1992 to 2000. J Clin Oncol. 2002;20(7):1838-44.

Palmieri C, Fisher RA, Sebire NJ, et al. Placental site trophoblastic tumour arising from a partial hydatidiform mole. Lancet. 2005;366(9486):688.

Papadopoulos AJ, Foskett M, Seckl MJ, et al. Twenty-five years' clinical experience of placental site trophoblastic tumors. J Reprod Med. 2002;47(6):460-4.

Rustin GJ, Newlands ES, Lutz JM, et al. Combination but not single-agent methotrexate chemotherapy for gestational trophoblastic tumors (GTT) increases the incidence of seconds tumors. J Clin Oncol. 1996;14(10):2769-73.

Savage P, Seckl MJ. The role of repeat uterine evacuation in trophoblast disease. Gynecol Oncol. 2005;99(1): 251-2.

Seckl MJ, Fisher RA, Salerno GA, et al. Choriocarcinoma and partial hydatidiform moles. Lancet. 2000; 356(9223):36-9.

Seckl MJ, Rustin GJS. Late toxicity after therapy for gestational trophoblastic tumours. In: Hancock BW, Newlands ES, Berkowitz RS, Cole LA (Eds). Gestational Trophoblastic Disease, 3rd edition. London: International Society for the Study of Trophoblastic Disease; 2003. pp. 470-84. [www.isstd.org/isstd/book.html].

Shih IM, Kurman RJ. Ki-67 labeling index in the differential diagnosis of exaggerated placental site, placental site trophoblastic tumor, and choriocarcinoma: a double immunohistochemical staining technique using Ki-67 and Mel-CAM antibodies. Hum Pathol. 1998;29(1):27-33.

Shih IM, Kurman RJ. The pathology of intermediate trophoblastic tumors and tumor-like lesions. Int J Gynecol Pathol. 2001;20(1):31-47.

Stone M, Bagshawe KD. An analysis of the influence maternal age, gestational age, contraceptive method, and the mode of primary treatment of patients with hydatidiform moles on the incidence of subsequent chemotherapy. Br J Obstet Gynaecol. 1979;86(10): 782-92.

Szulman AE, Surti U. The syndromes of hydatidiform mole. 1. Cytogenetic and morphologic correlations. Am J Obstet Gynecol. 1978;131(6):665-71.

Tidy JA, Gillespie AM, Bright N, et al. Gestational trophoblastic disease: a study of mode evacuation and subsequent need for treatment with chemotherapy. Gynecol Oncol. 2000;78(3 pt. 1):309-12.

Vejerslev LO. Clinical management and diagnostic possibilities in hydatidiform mole with coexistent fetus. Obstet Gynecol Surv. 1991;46(9):577-88.

Woolas RP, Bower M, Newlands ES, et al. Influence of chemotherapy for gestational trophoblastic disease on subsequent pregnancy outcome. Br J Obstet Gynaecol. 1998;105(9):1032-5.

Yamashita K, Wake N, Araki T, et al. Human lymphocyte antigen expression in hydatidiform mole, androgenesis following fertilization by a haploid sperm. Am J Obstet Gynecol. 1979;135(5):597-600.

Young RH, Scully RE. Placental-site trophoblastic tumor: current status. Clin Obstet Gynecol. 1984;27(1): 248-58.

CHAPTER 12

Ovarian Masses

Rashida Begum, Rehana Parveen

INTRODUCTION

Ovarian mass is a tissue mass in the ovaries. Ovarian mass is responsible for surgery in about 10% women of reproductive age. Almost all ovarian masses in premenopausal women are ovarian cysts and mostly are benign. These cysts fall under five groups:
1. Follicular or retention cysts.
2. Inflammatory cysts.
3. Chocolate cysts.
4. Ectopic pregnancy
5. Neoplastic cysts.

> **Case scenario:** Mrs Ayesha is a multiparous woman of 32 years has come to you with the complaints of heaviness and slight bulging of the lower abdomen. She is confirmed that she is not pregnant as her cycle is regular and strip test is also negative.
> How will you proceed for diagnosis?

Detailed History is to be Taken

- Whether menstruation is associated with dysmenorrhea—may be endometriosis
- History of any dyspareunia—may be endometriosis
- Pain during defecation—may be endometriosis
- Frequency of micturition due to pressure symptom
- Any abdominal fullness and bloating
- History of indigestion, heartburn or early satiety—these are symptoms of malignancy
- Any pain in the abdomen apart from menstrual pain. Nature of the pain is to be elicited. Sudden severe pain with nausea, vomiting without history of amenorrhea may be due twisted ovarian cyst or corpus luteum rupture
- History of risk factors and protective factors for ovarian neoplasia (mentioned in Chapter 13)
- Family history of ovarian and breast cancer.

Thorough Examination

Next she should be examined thoroughly
- General examination
- Perabdominal examination.

If any lump felt following points need to be assessed to differentiate origin of lump and nature of lump, that is whether it is benign or malignant:
- *Size:* Size of the lump is to be assessed
- *Consistency:* Cystic or solid
- *Mobility:* Free or restricted. Side to side and above downwards movement. Benign ovarian cyst usually moves freely in all direction
- *Surface:* Smooth or rough and nodular
- *Margin:* Regular or irregular
- *Tenderness:* Present or not
- *Ascites present or not:* This can be best elicited by fluid thrill and shifting dullness test.

Bimanual Examination

- *Size of the uterus*
- *Origin of lump:* Is there any cleft between lump and suprapubic region to assess origin of lump, whether uterine or ovarian; no cleft is felt, if lump is uterine origin
- *Mobility of the cervix:* In case of fibroid uterus cervix moves along with movement of the lump
- *Cervical motion tenderness:* It is positive in case of endometriosis
- *Any lump felt through fornixes:* If present its size, consistency, tenderness and fixity is to be assessed

- *Nodularity in posterior fornix:* This is felt in endometriosis, tuberculosis and in malignant ovarian tumor.

> On enquiry it is revealed that she has no complaints except slight bulging and heaviness of the abdomen. On per abdominal examination, a lump of about 20 weeks size is felt in the midline, which is cystic in consistency, freely mobile in all direction, surface is smooth, margin is regular, tenderness absent, a cleft found between lower pole of the lump and suprapubic region. No ascites present. Per vaginal examination revealed a lump of same feature, which is separate from the uterus but side cannot be determined. No deposit is felt through posterior fornix.
> What is your provisional diagnosis?

Benign ovarian tumor (cyst). All characteristic features go in favor of benign ovarian cyst.

> How will you confirm that this is an ovarian mass?

By Doing Ultrasonogram

Ultrasonogram can confirm the origin of the cyst and is the single most effective way of evaluation of ovarian mass. Transvaginal ultrasonography (TVS) is preferable due to its increased sensitivity over transabdominal ultrasound. But, any lump of more than 10 cm cannot be visualized by TVS. Transabdominal ultrasonogram is needed for these cases. Except complex mass such as malignant ovarian tumor and twisted ovarian tumor, color Doppler ultrasonography has no role. In those cases details of morphologic characteristics can be determined, but to confirm the nature of ovarian tumor histopathological examination is mandatory.

This is the primary imaging tool for a patient considered to have an ovarian cyst. Findings can help to define a cyst's morphologic characteristics.

Ultrasonographic Findings of Ovarian Tumor

Benign ovarian cysts have
- A uniformly thin and rounded wall
- A unilocular appearance (no septation)
- Hypoechoic or anechoic shadow, which indicates cystic nature

They usually measure 2.5–15 cm in diameter and posterior acoustic enhancement (a hyperechoic area) may be visible deep to the fluid-filled cyst. These cysts are unlikely to be cancerous. Most commonly, they are functional follicular or luteal cysts, or less commonly serous cystadenomas or inclusion cysts. If the ultrasonographic features are not typical of an ovarian cyst, follow-up ultrasonography can be performed to exclude ovarian neoplasm.
- Malignant cysts are:
  - Multilocular/septed
  - Thick walled, papulations sticking into the lumen or on the surface, or abnormalities within the cyst contents.
  - Hyperechoic or hyperechoic and hypoechoic mixed shadow.

Hemorrhagic cysts, endometriomas, and dermoids tend to have different characteristic features on ultrasonograms that may help to differentiate them from malignant complex cysts.

Note: There is no role of routine use of color Doppler ultrasonography, computed tomography (CT) or magnetic resonance imaging (MRI) in simple ovarian cyst, where transabdominal or TVS is enough. However, these modalities will have a place in the evaluation of malignant ovarian tumor.

> What other tests can be done to assess whether it is benign or not?

Tumor Markers

When clinical and USG evidence suggest simple ovarian cyst, there is no need to do tumor markers. But, in suspected malignant cases in particular above 20–25 years and complex ovarian masses tumor markers are indicated. Young patients below the age of 25 years, the probability of germ cell tumor is more. So α-FP, hCG and LDH tumor markers are indicated. Tumor markers, which are relevant for malignant epithelial ovarian tumors are serum CA 125 and serum CA 19.9I. CA-125 rises in serous cystadenocarcinoma, while serum CA-19.9 in mucinous cystadenocarcinoma. In reproductive age CA-125 increases due to many non-neoplastic causes such as fibroids, endometriosis, adenomyosis and pelvic infection. So it's sensitivity is low. But, if it is high and on serial monitoring increases rapidly then it is more likely to be associated with malignancy.

What are the conditions with which a benign ovarian cyst can be confused? Differential diagnosis (D/D)

- Pregnancy
- Full bladder
- Hydrosalpinx
- Paraovarian cyst
- Pedunculated leiomyoma
- Pelvic kidney
- Pelvic lymphocele
- Peritoneal cyst
- Psoas abscess
- Tubo-ovarian abscess
- Tubal disease
- Diverticular disease
- Hydronephrosis
- Chocolate cyst.

Ultrasonographic findings show the right ovarian mass of about 20 × 18 cm size with features suggestive of benign ovarian cyst.
What will be the option of treatment?

Only surgery is the mode of treatment. For ovarian neoplasia surgery is to be done immediately after making diagnosis, as actual nature of tumor is not known until and unless histopathology is done.

Surgery can be done by either laparoscopy or laparotomy. Whatever may be the process, the modality of surgery is same for this patient:
- After surgical evaluation of tumor (intactness of surface, adhesion and vascular engorgement), other ovary, peritoneal fluid, paracolic gutters and omentum—if everything is found satisfactory *unilateral salpingo-oophorectomy is to be done* as she is multiparous woman
- Frozen section biopsy can be done, if facilities are available to exclude malignancy
- Removed specimen is to be sent for histopathology.

If the patient is nulliparous or has one child, any other conservative surgery can be done here?

Yes alternatively cystectomy can be done. Though reproduction is possible with one ovary, to keep better fertility potential affected ovary can also be preserved in this case by doing cystectomy. If facilities available cyst wall is to be sent for frozen section before the abdomen is closed. Otherwise routine histopathological test is to be done afterwards.

Suppose similar cyst occurs in 20 years unmarried girl. What will be the option of treatment?

For unmarried girls or nulliparous women cystectomy followed by frozen section biopsy, if facility available or subsequent histopathology of the specimen is the ideal option.

What will be the surgery of same type of cyst in a woman of ≥ 45 years of age?

As malignant potential is more in advanced age, in spite of benign cyst bilateral salpingo-oophorectomy (BSO) and hysterectomy is the ideal option for this group of women. There is no justification of conserving the other ovary, which can be the seat of future pathology.

Note: Summary of surgical options for benign ovarian cyst according to age and parity of the patients:
- *In young girl:* Cystectomy is the choice of surgery in young girl for preserving fertility potential.
- *Mother of one child and age less than 40:* Cystectomy for preserving fertility potential.
- *Family completed and age more than 35 years:* Unilateral salpingo-oophorectomy.
- *Family completed and age less than 35:* Unilateral salpingo-oophorectomy/cystectomy, if patient desires to preserve ovary.
- *Postmenopausal women and women of ≥ 45 years:* Bilateral salpingo-oophorectomy with abdominal hysterectomy irrespective of family size.

RELATED INFORMATION

Etiology of Ovarian Cysts

- *Neoplastic cysts:* Only a subset of primary ovarian malignancy are de novo. Rest develop as a consequence of benign epithelial tumor. So, etiology and risk factors of primary ovarian neoplasia remains the same for both

benign and malignant tumors. Dermoid cysts arise from oocytes (etiology and risk factors discussed in chapter 13).
- *Retention cysts:* Functional ovarian cysts arise from ovulatory failure, growth and rupture of the Graafian follicle.
- *Luteal cysts:* From corpus luteum of menstruation and pregnancy.
- *Chocolate cysts:* Endometriomas arise from cyclic bleeding of ectopic endometrium.
- *Inflammatory cysts:* From chronic pelvic inflammatory diseases.

General Classification of Ovarian Tumor

According to the World Health Organization (WHO) histological classification for ovarian tumors are:
- Surface epithelial tumor (65%)
- Germ cell tumor (15%)
- Sex cord-stromal (10%)
- Metastatic (5%)
- Miscellaneous.

Surface epithelial tumors are further classified by cell type serous, mucinous, endometrioid, etc. and atypia–benign (atypical proliferation) borderline (low malignant potential) or malignant. Malignant may be invasive or noninvasive. Majority (90%) malignant ovarian tumors are surface epithelial in origin.

A. Surface Epithelial Stromal Tumors

Serous tumors
- Benign (cystadenoma)
- Borderline tumors (serous borderline tumor)
- Malignant (serous adenocarcinoma).

Mucinous tumors, endocervical-like and intestinal type
- Benign (cystadenoma)
- Borderline tumors (mucinous borderline tumor)
- Malignant (mucinous adenocarcinoma).

Endometrioid tumors
- Benign (cystadenoma)
- Borderline tumors (endometrioid borderline tumor)
- Malignant (endometrioid adenocarcinoma).

Clear cell tumors
- Benign
- Borderline tumors
- Malignant (clear cell adenocarcinoma).

Transitional cell tumors
- Brenner tumor
- Brenner tumor of borderline malignancy
- Malignant Brenner tumor
- Transitional cell carcinoma (non-Brenner type).

Epithelial stromal
- Adenosarcoma
- Carcinosarcoma (formerly mixed Müllerian tumors).

B. Sex Cord-stromal Tumors

Granulosa tumors
- Fibromas
- Fibrothecomas
- Thecomas.

Sertoli cell tumors
- Leydig cell tumors
- Sex cord tumor with annular tubules
- Gynandroblastoma
- Steroid (lipid) cell tumors.

C. Germ Cell Tumors

- Dysgerminoma
- Yolk sac tumor (endodermal sinus tumor)
- Embryonic carcinoma
- Polyembryoma
- Choriocarcinoma
- Teratomas:
  - Immature
  - Mature
  - Solid
  - Cystic (Dermoid cyst).
- Monodermal and highly specialized:
  - Struma
  - Carcinoid
  - Strumal carcinoma
  - Mucinous carcinoid
  - Neuroectodermal tumors.

D. Malignant, not Otherwise Specified

Metastatic cancer from nonovarian primary
- Colonic, appendiceal
- Gastric
- Breast.

Pathogenesis of Ovarian Tumor

The majority of primary ovarian tumors derive from epithelial cells on the surface of the ovary, which is derived from the coelomic epithelium. These cells are a product of primitive mesoderm, which can undergo neoplastic transformation when they are genetically predisposed to oncogenesis. Thus, five main histologic subtypes, which are similar to carcinoma arising from epithelial lining of fallopian tube, endometrium and cervix as follows:
1. Serous—from fallopian tube
2. Endometrioid—from endometrium
3. Mucinous—from cervix
4. Clear cell—from mesonephrons
5. Brenner—from mesonephrons.

Two General Hypotheses have been Proposed to Explain the Pathogenesis of EOT

1. Regular ovulation with repeated trauma and repair to the ovarian epithelium, which afford an opportunity for genetic mutation and cellular neoplasm. The protective effect of oral contraceptive use and multiparity supports this theory.
2. Excess gonadotropins lead to high-estrogen concentrations, which gives rise to epithelial proliferation and probably neoplastic, and malignant transformation.

The molecular events leading to the development of EOT are unknown mutations and/or over expression of the oncogenes HER2, tumor suppressor gene *P53* have been observed in sporadic ovarian cancer.

Germline mutations in BRCA1 and BRCA2 have been implicated in genetically predisposed breast ovarian cancer syndrome.

Serous Tumors

Next to dermoid cysts, these are the second most common cysts accounts for 20% of all benign ovarian neoplasia:

- Usually unilateral, but may be bilateral.
- Size is variable, may be up to 20–30 cm.
- May be cystic (serous cystadenoma), papillary (papillary serous cystadenoma) or adenofibromatous (serous adenofibroma).
- Cyst wall of serous cystadenoma is usually thin, translucent, unilocular. Some daughter cysts may be present in the wall. Walls lined by a single layer of flattened or cuboidal cells, but in places columnar cells may be present resembling tubal epithelium. Psammoma bodies may be seen in the stroma of these tumor.
- Papillary serous cystadenoma has papilla on the inner wall or outer wall (exophytic) gives the impression of malignancy and are 5–10% malignant potential.
- Serous adenofibroma are lobulated, hard knobby solid mass.
- About 25% percent are malignant and accounts for 75% of epithelial cancer.

Mucinous Cystadenoma

These are also common and accounts for 20% of all ovarian tumor:
- Usually unilateral, but 10% may bilateral.
- Size may be larger.
- Cyst wall is thick and outer wall is white, gray or silvery blue in color.
- Cyst is multilocular or septed. Locules may be larger due to rupture of septum.
- Inner wall is smooth, but few intracystic papillae may present.
- Cyst wall lined by tall columnar cells resembling the epithelium of cervix or intestine.
- Cells secrete mucus-containing glycoprotein with high content of neutral polysaccharides.
- Cystic fluid is thick, glairy and colorless. May be yellow, green or brown depending upon the presence of blood pigments of previous intracystic hemorrhage, if any.
- If this fluid spills in the abdominal cavity, the cells invade the omentum and peritoneum from where semisolid mucin secrets into the abdominal cavity causing distension, pain, aching and vomiting. The condition is called **pseudomyxoma peritonei**. Even the tumor is benign, there is a strong tendency to refilling after removal of tumor and contents. The same

features may develop from complication of mucocele or adenocarcinoma of the appendix and colon. So may be found in men also.
- Malignant transformation is less than serous cysts about 5-10% and accounting for 20% of epithelial cancers.

Mature Cystic Teratoma (Dermoid Cyst)

It is germ cell tumor, which comprises 10-15% of all ovarian tumors. It usually occurs at earlier age:
- It is usually unilateral, but in 12% cases it is bilateral.
- Size is medium and rarely grows than a melon.
- It is unilocular and has very few locules.
- It has thick and smooth capsule, and due to presence of sebaceous material it gives grayish, yellow color.
- The cyst is lined by stratified squamous epithelium and contains the derivatives of ectoderm, mostly cutaneous elements such as sebaceous glands, hair follicles and sometimes teeth (incisor, bicuspid and molar). Tissues of central nervous system, i.e. choroid plexus are often seen.
- The cyst is filled with thick, yellowish, greasy-sebaceous fluid, which is secreted by the glandular tissue of the cyst wall.
- There is a node and tissues are distributed around the nodal point. Hair follicles grow from the nodal point.
- Chemical changes that take place between sebaceous material and fragmentation of hair follicles, sometimes form balls and pellets of fat and hair.
- Though, it is mostly ectodermal, tissue of thyroid can be found in active stage and can cause hyperthyroidism. The condition is known as *Struma ovary* (Lavine, et al, 2010).
- It can undergo malignant changes in few cases.

Clinical Presentation

- Most of the benign ovarian cyst remains symptomless. Usually can be diagnosed incidentally by ultrasonogram due to other purpose.
- Lump in the abdomen may be complaining feature, which is slowly growing.
- Other complaints associated with complications.

Characteristics of Benign Ovarian Tumor

Physical examination

P/A: Tumors are smooth surfaced with regular outline, usually cystic in consistency except ovarian fibroma; unilateral and freely mobile from side to side and above down wards. Usually not associated with pain and tenderness. Size of the tumor may be larger. Ascites is not common. Lower pole of the tumor can be felt and a cleft felt between tumor and uterus.

Bimanual: Lump can be felt through fornixes clearly as there is no ascites, can be separated from uterus except twisted benign ovarian tumor, which becomes adherent with the uterus. No nodularity felt in pouch of Douglas.

Ultrasonogram: Clear cyst <10 cm with septation, <3 mm in thickness present. Unilateral distribution. Hypoechogenicity, calcification and teeth can be found in dermoid cysts.

Surgical evaluation: Simple cysts, unilateral in distribution, no adhesion (except twisted benign ovarian tumor) and smooth surface with intact capsule.

Complications of Ovarian Cysts

- *Torsion of the pedicle:* Freely mobile medium sized cysts undergo axial rotation and torsion.
- *Intracystic hemorrhage:* Rupture of small vessel of cyst can cause intracystic or intraperitoneal bleeding.
- *Rupture of a cyst:* Sometimes due to intracystic increased pressure and weak wall of the cyst, it may rupture and can cause acute symptom. Sebaceous content of dermoid cyst and mucinous content of mucinous cyst produces more symptoms. Rupture of mucinous cystadenoma causes pseudomyxoma peritonei.
- *Degeneration:* It is usually rare, if it is truly cystic, but may occur in solid tumor causing necrosis and hemorrhage.
- *Infection:* Infection may occur after torsion and after cyst aspiration.
- *Intestinal obstruction:* Rarely occur in benign cyst. When huge benign cyst compressed or becomes adherent, and press the lumen of the gut may cause intestinal obstruction.

- *Malignancy:* All benign ovarian tumor can become malignant, if left untreated. But, usually 5–10% undergo malignant transformation by the time of diagnosis and treatment.

> Suppose Halima has a solid freely mobile tumor in the ovary associated with right-sided hydrothorax and ascites.
> What treatment will you offer her?

Solid freely mobile tumor associated with hydrothorax and ascites, the most likely diagnosis is fibroma and is called Meigs' syndrome. After laparotomy, if there is no sign of malignancy unilateral salpingo-oophorectomy is to be done. Ascites developed due to peritoneal irritation by mobile tumor and hydrothorax due to leakage of fluid through defect in the diaphragm. Both hydrothorax and ascites will subside spontaneously after removal of the tumor. Hydrothorax can be bilateral, but mostly right-sided due to more diaphragmatic defect in the right side.

RELATED INFORMATION

Connective Tissue Tumor

Fibroma

Fibroma of the ovary represents 3–5% of the ovarian tumor. It is small in size, rarely exceed the size of the fetal head, solid and hard in consistency; cut surface is white and whorled-like myoma uterus. It may occupy the whole ovary or may protrude in any pole of the ovary. Usually, unilateral ovoid or spherical shaped may be lobulated. It has got no muscular tissue like fibroid uterus, but it behaves like it. It may degenerate undergo fatty change and calcification. Other mobile tumor (ovarian or uterine) may cause ascites and hydrothorax, which is called pseudo-Meigs' syndrome.

Adenofibroma, leiomyoma, lipoma, chondroma, osteoma, hemangioma and lymphangioma are other benign connective tissue tumors.

Role of laparoscopy in managing ovarian tumor

Benign ovarian cyst can be managed by laparoscopy, which needs shorter recovery time and reduces postoperative morbidity. It is cost effective due to short hospital stay and return to work earlier. Masses should be removed through umbilical port by using a tissue retrieval bag rather extending the side ports. Benefits of removing through umbilical ports are; it reduces retrieval time and postoperative pain, there is no chance of epigastric vessel injury and scar marking, which occur in lateral port extension. But, there should be certain limitations:

- Laparoscopy should be performed by a surgeon with experience and appropriate equipment.
- Very large ovarian cyst may require extension of the port or minilaparotomy for drainage, and removal of cyst or ovary, which minimizes the advantages of laparoscopic approach. So, laparotomy would be better option.
- Large masses with solid components such as large dermoid cyst should be managed by laparotomy to avoid chemical peritonitis, which might occur in few cases (0.2%) (Kocak et al. 2004; Nezhat et al. 1993; Shawki et al. 2007)
- In postmenopausal women risk of malignancy index (RMI) is to be done:
  - If there is no risk or very low risk of malignancy after assessing by RMI hysterectomy and BSO can be done by laparoscopy. In that case, cyst must be removed intact by using a cyst removal bag.
  - If there is high risk for malignancy, BSO and hysterectomy with comprehensive surgical staging is to be done. So laparotomy would be preferred mode of surgery. Besides inadvertent cyst rupture into peritoneal cavity may have an unfavorable impact on disease free survival, if it is malignant.

Risk of Malignancy Index

Preoperative assessment of risk of malignancy in clinically diagnosed benign ovarian tumor with suspicion can be calculated and it is particularly important for postmenopausal women whose chance of malignancy is more.

Estimation of RMI is a calculation of intensity of risk of malignancy in premalignant cases. Though 4 types of RMI exists, RMI-I is the most effective for women with suspected ovarian malignancy (Geomini et al. 2009).

Calculation of RMI-I

It is done by combining three pre-surgical features.
Serum CA-125, ultrasonogram score (U) and menopausal status (M)
RMI = U × M × CA-125

- *Ultrasound score:* It is done by assessing the following characteristics of the tumor—multilocular, solid areas, metastases, ascites and bilateral lesion. One point for each characteristic. U = 0 for an ultrasound score 0. U = 1 for an ultrasound score 1 and U = 3 for an ultrasound score 2–5.
- *Menopausal status:* Score is 1 for premenopausal women and 3 for postmenopausal (absence of menstruation for > 1 year or age 50 years or more, who have hysterectomy) women.
- *Serum CA-125:* Score will be more, when level will be higher. Measure in IU/mL and can vary between 0 and 1,000 of units.

The RMI score 200 or more has 78% sensitivity and 87% specificity for detection of malignancy (Bourne et al. 1993; Morgante et al. 1999; Aslam et al. 2000; Ma et al. 2003).

Alternate Way of Estimating Risk of Malignancy

International ovarian tumor analysis (IOTA) group estimated risk index only by ultrasound morphologic findings without showing CA-125. Following characteristics are considered as benign (B-rules) and malignant (M-rules) with sensitivity 95% and specificity 91% (Timmerman et al. 2008; Timmerman et al. 2010).

B-rules (Benign)

- Unilocular cysts
- Presence of solid components where the largest solid component <7 mm
- Presence of acoustic shadowing
- Smooth multilocular tumor with largest diameter <100 mm
- No blood flow.

M-rules (Malignant)

- Irregular solid tumor
- Ascites
- At least four papillary structures
- Irregular multilocular solid tumor with largest diameter ≥100 mm
- Very strong blood flow.

> **Case scenario:** Miss Laila 26 years old has come with severe excruciating right lower abdominal pain, nausea and vomiting.
>
> *How will you proceed for diagnosis?*

Detailed History is to be Taken

Pregnancy should be excluded no matter married or unmarried:

- Menstrual history:
    - *LMP:* Menstruation regular or not and pregnancy should be kept in mind to exclude ectopic
    - *History of dysmenorrhea:* May be endometriosis and adenomyosis.
- History of any heavy work such as exercise or other works.
- Presence of any lump beforehand
- Pain around the umbilicus: Presence is suspicious of appendicitis.

Physical Examination is to be Done

- *General examination:* Pulse, blood pressure, temperature, anemia, pallor and sweating
- Perabdominal examination:
    - Tenderness and rigidity of the abdomen
    - Tenderness in McBurney's point
    - Presence of any lump, ovarian or uterine
    - If any lump is felt, it is to be assessed by its size, mobility, tenderness, consistency, smoothness of surface and regularity of the margin
    - Whether there is any distension of abdomen and flanks, may be due to fluid, blood or big lump. Presence of fluid can be assessed by fluid thrill and shifting dullness test.

As girl is unmarried bimanual examination is replaced by per rectal (P/R) examination.

Note:
If there is any lump, its characteristics including adhesion and freeness of rectal mucosa is to be assessed by PR examination in unmarried girls.

> From history taking and examination, you found that her menstrual cycle is regular with normal flow and LMP was just 7 days back. She has no history of dysmenorrhea. On examination, her pulse is rapid, temperature 99°F BP is normal, but slight sweating is present. Pain is just in right iliac fossa, but not around the umbilicus. McBurneys' point tenderness is absent. Abdomen is tense and tender, but no free fluid is present. Both by P/A and P/R an ill-defined lump is felt, whose characteristics could not be delineated properly, but it is not mobile.
>
> What might be your clinical diagnosis and what investigations do you like to do for confirmation?

Most probable diagnosis is twisted ovarian tumor suggested by age and sudden onset of severe pain. Twisted ovarian tumor is a gynecological emergency, which needs immediate treatment.

Investigations

- *Blood for CBC:* WBC may rise due to invading infection.
- *Blood for CA-125:* Not so significant in this age, but may be raised due to endometriosis.
- *Ultrasonography:* Can diagnose origin of lump. So, ultrasonography should be the first test to be performed. The affected ovary is enlarged, with multiple immature or small follicles along its periphery. If color Doppler ultrasonography is available, it is the method of choice for evaluation of adnexal torsion, because it can show morphologic and physiologic changes in the ovary and can help in determining whether blood flow is impaired or not (Lee et al. 1998; Fleischer et al. 1995; Peña et al. 2000; Zanforlin Filho et al. 2008). The presence of an enlarged ovary with small peripheral cysts with lack of intraovarian arterial or venous flow is highly indicative of torsion. However, the presence of adnexal flow should not be considered as ruling out the diagnosis. Gray-scale and spectral findings are correlated with the age of the torsion (i.e. acute torsion or chronic torsion) and the degree of the twist or torsion. Combined use of transvaginal ultrasonography and color flow mapping, and 3D imaging may improve sensitivity in complex masses.
- *CT scan MRI:* If ultrasonographic findings are nondiagnostic, *rarely* CT or MRI is needed to make a definitive diagnosis.

RELATED INFORMATION

What is Ovarian Torsion?

An ovarian torsion is the rotation or twisting of an enlarged ovary and occluding ovarian blood supply causing ovarian ischemia, degeneration and finally necrosis. Due to cutting off its blood supply leads to degeneration and necrosis, which causes severe abdominal pain. It is a gynecological emergency with a diagnostic dilemma. Due to similar features of some other gynecological and nongynecological conditions diagnosis is sometimes misleading and delayed. Incidence is high between 20 and 30 years of age though it may occur beyond this age.

Characteristic Features

- Sudden onset of excruciating unilateral lower abdominal pain, which often radiates towards the groin.
- This may be accompanied by nausea and vomiting.
- History of exercise or aggressive physical movement may be present. On examination, severe abdominal tenderness is found. Exact features of lump may be obscured due to tenderness.
- Temperature may be raised due to inflammatory changes.

Predisposing Factors for Ovarian Torsion

- Enlarged ovarian cyst
- Larger ovaries than normal
- Excessively long fallopian tube
- Presence of an ovarian tumor
- Pregnancy, particularly during the first 3 months
- Prior tubal ligation
- Taking medications to induce ovulation (stimulation of ovary)
- History of pelvic surgery.

Differential Diagnoses of Twisted Ovarian Tumor

- Ectopic pregnancy
- Endometriosis
- Pelvic inflammatory disease
- Torsion of paraovarian cyst
- Tension of large ovarian cyst
- Tubo-ovarian abscess
- Appendicitis
- Diverticulitis
- Large-bowel obstruction
- Mesenteric ischemia in emergency medicine
- Small-bowel obstruction in emergency medicine
- Nephrolithiasis
- Urinary tract infection.

Investigations shows WBC count 11,000, CA-125 < 35 IU/L, color Doppler ultrasonography shows an ovarian lump 10 × 8 cm in size absent intra-ovarian blood flow.
How will you manage the case?

This is the twisted ovarian tumor with necrosis. Necrosis is the cause of exudation and infection causing raised temperature, pain and adhesion:
- Surgery is the only option of treatment
- Simultaneously pain killer and broad spectrum antibiotic are to be started
- Laparoscopy will be the ideal approach, but laparotomy can be done
- Type of surgery will depend upon the degree of torsion:
  - If ovary is totally necrosed, salpingo-oophorectomy is to be performed
  - If ovary is not necrosed, only untwisting and cystectomy will cure it
- Specimen should be sent for histopathology.

Histopathology report shows benign epithelial tumor. Does she need further treatment?

No, she does not need further treatment and follow-up.

What is the fate of ovarian torsion?

Fate of ovarian torsion depends upon:
- Number of torsion
- Extent of vascular occlusion
- Promptness of management.

- The fate of ovarian torsion is excellent with early diagnosis and treatment, when there is one or two torsion with incomplete occlusion, early diagnosis allows conservative laparoscopic cystectomy and reduction in complications.
- Delayed diagnosis often results in infarction and necrosis of the ovary, when ovary must needs to be removed.
- Loss of a single ovary is unlikely to result in significantly reduced fertility.
- Death due to ovarian torsion is highly unlikely.

What are the complications of ovarian torsion?

Complications of ovarian torsion include the following:
- Infection
- Peritonitis
- Sepsis
- Adhesions
- Chronic pain
- Reduced ovarian reserve.

Case scenario: Mrs Laboni, a multiparous 35-year-old woman, has a cyst of about 42 mm in her right ovary. Cyst was diagnosed incidentally.
How will you manage the case?

Nothing to be done for this patient, as this is most likely physiological cyst. In luteal phase, 4% patients develop cyst more than 30 mm [Teichmann, 1995]. Cystic structure less than 50 mm are most likely physiological and they usually regress within 3 menstrual cycles. So asymptomatic simple cysts of 30–<50 mm does not need strict follow-up.

Suppose after 6 months Laboni did a follow-up ultrasonography and found that there is increment of the size of the cyst (75 mm).
What do you want to do now?

Persistent cysts or increasing cysts are unlikely to be functional. So, surgical management will be appropriate with preoperative assessment using RMI. As nature of the cyst is not known and mature cystic teratoma grows over time it is better to remove the cyst and must be tested by histopathology.

Note: Usually asymptomatic cysts of 30–<50 mm in diameter do not require follow-up, cysts of 50–70 mm require follow-up, and cysts more than 70 mm in diameter should be considered for further evaluation by MRI or surgery can be done with preoperative assessment using RMI.

> Is there any role of oral contraceptive to reduce the cyst?

No, oral contraceptive has no role in reducing the size of the cyst. But, it can be used to keep the ovary quiescent and to prevent development of new cyst. Because stimulation may increases the size of existing cyst.

> Is there any role of aspiration of cyst?

Aspiration of ovarian cyst either ultrasono guided vaginally or laparoscopically has limited role in the treatment of benign ovarian cyst. As cyst wall remained in situ refilling is the logical sequence. So, recurrence is obvious in neoplastic situation. In highly selected cases, where patient is not willing to do surgery, aspiration can be done for cytological test. In that case, if it is neoplastic spillage of fluid is harmful for the patient. If one is sure that it is a functional cyst and is regressing very slowly, but patient needs ovarian stimulation only in that situation cyst aspiration can be done.

Note: Aspiration of asymptomatic cyst is absolutely contraindicated in postmenopausal women. Sensitivity of cytological examination of cystic fluid to distinguish benign and malignant is low. Moreover, there is spillage of fluid and risk of rupture of the cyst, and if the cyst is malignant it would have unfavorable impact on disease free survival.

> **Case scenario:** Mrs Rahila, a nulliparous woman has come to you for fertility treatment. During 6th day of her cycle you found her both ovaries are cystic giving an impression of septated ovarian cyst. Maximum size of the cyst is 39 mm. She had history of taking clomiphene citrate in her last cycle.
>
> How will you manage her?

Nothing is to be done for regression of cysts except omission of further stimulation till subsidence of those. Due to stimulation, multiple follicles developed, which did not regress and formed luteal cysts. As a result of multiple cysts ovaries became larger and gave an impression of complex septated cyst. These are functional or physiological cysts. It will regress within 2–3 months. If there is urgency of treatment GnRHa can be used to accelerate regression by totally suppressing pituitary activities. *In no way surgery is indicated in this type of case.*

> **Case scenario:** Mrs Anjuman, a 28 years lady had evacuation of molar pregnancy 1 week back. Now she reports with dull ache and heaviness in lower abdomen. On examination by both per abdominal (P/A) and per vaginal (P/V) you found bilateral ovarian enlargement. Ultrasonography shows bilateral ovarian complex cyst of about 14 × 16 cm each. Patient is very worried about cysts.
>
> How will you manage her?

Pain-killer can be given. But, it should be kept in mind that severe pain may occur due to torsion, which might occur due to enlargement of the ovaries.

According to history and findings, these cysts are luteal cyst due to over stimulation by excessive hCG, which is released from molar tissue. As molar tissue has been evacuated, hCG will fall gradually and ovaries will return to their normal size in due course of time.

But, patient needs to keep under regular follow-up for molar pregnancy, which is discussed under the chapter trophoblastic tumor.

> **Case scenario:** Mrs Laizu a, 34-year-old lady—mother of two children complaints of slight pain in lower abdomen. You examined her and found a cystic lump of about 7–8 cm in left adnexal region. Ultrasonography showed a simple cyst of about 10 cm in size arising from left adnexal region, but may not from ovary, as it seems separated from the ovary.
>
> How will you manage her?

Most likely diagnosis is paraovarian cyst. As it is quite big and symptomatic, laparoscopy is to be done to diagnose as well as to do cystectomy.

RELATED INFORMATION

A paraovarian cyst, also sometimes known as a para tubal cyst or a hydatid cyst of Morgagni, is a type of adnexal cyst that does not arise from the ovary. They account for 10–20% of adnexal masses

(Kier, 1991; Athey and Cooper, 1985). They typically occur in women in their 3rd to 4th decades. They usually occur around the broad ligament and arise from paramesonephric, mesothelial, or mesonephric remnants.

They are usually simple cysts, very small ranges from 2 to 20 cm. Although known for their small size, paraovarian cysts will sometimes grow larger, especially during pregnancies. Unlike small cysts, the larger cysts are symptomatic. Depending on their size and location, large paraovarian cysts may produce symptom. The smaller cysts are commonly found in middle-aged women (in between 30 and 40 years) and are often indistinguishable from simple ovarian cysts.

Due to close proximity to ovary small paraovarian cyst makes confusion with follicle of ovary, which interfere with follicular monitoring during induction of ovulation.

Symptoms

Small cysts are symptomless.

Larger paraovarian cysts will show some symptoms:
- Frequent complain of pelvic pain usually on one side (unilateral)
- Irregular periods
- Abnormal uterine bleeding.
- Pain during sexual intercourse (dyspareunia).

Diagnosis

- *Ultrasonogram*: They are typically thin-walled and smoothly marginated. They most often appear as unilocular 'simple' cysts (in 66%) and rarely as multilocular (4%).
- *Laparoscopy*: Clearly identify the site and number of cysts.

Differential Diagnosis

- Ovarian follicular cyst
- Ovarian neoplastic simple cyst
- Paraovarian cystadenoma
- Pelvic peritoneal inclusion cyst.

Treatment

- Smaller lesions can be followed expectantly and no need of treatment.
- Following cases need treatment, option of treatment is surgery (cystectomy) by laparoscopy.

If the cyst is:
- Larger lesions: Greater than 4 inches (10 cm)
- Complex
- Symptomatic
- Increasing in size
- Persisting after several months
- Sonographically suspicious findings like septation, papillations, fluid and solid components, dense and irregularly shaped
- Infected, ruptured or there is bleeding.

According to a consensus statement by the society of radiologists in ultrasound [Levine, 2010] follow-up is recommended for cysts that are:
- 5–7 cm in a woman of reproductive age
- 1–7 cm in a postmenopausal woman
- Irrespective of age, cysts larger than 7 cm warrant further evaluation (with MRI) or surgical review.

Hydatid Cysts of Morgagni

Hydatid cysts of Morgagni, also hydatids of Morgagni or Morgagni's cysts, are common and appear as pedunculated, often tiny, frequently multiple cysts connected to the fimbriae of the fallopian tubes. While usually asymptomatic, it has been noted that these cysts tend to be more common in women with unexplained infertility (52.1% vs 25.6% in unexplained and controls respectively, $p < 0.001$) and suggested that they may play a role in infertility (Rasheed and abdelmonem, 2011). It has been proposed that these cysts interfere with tubal pick-up and function (Abd-el-maeboud, 1997, Cebesoy et al. 2010).

> **Case scenario:** Mrs Akhi, a postmenopausal woman of 48 years, incidentally diagnosed as having a unilocular cyst in left ovary, whose size is 35 × 37 mm. She never felt it or she has no complaints about this.
> How will you mange her?

Though chance of malignancy is more in postmenopausal women, risk of malignancy of cyst less than 5 cm, unilateral, unilocular and ceho-free with no solid parts or papillary formation is less than 1% (Roman et al. 1997). More than 50% cases these cysts resolves spontaneously within 3 months (Levine et al. 1992). So conservative treatment for cyst 2–5 cm can be done with regular follow-up at 4 months interval. Though patient's choice and gynaecologist's view matters.

> **Case scenario:** Mrs Sufia, a 22-year-old primigravid patient carrying 12 week pregnancy came to you. She is anxious about her dating. Ultrasonography report shows 12 weeks viable intrauterine pregnancy and a 6 cm sized right adnexal cyst. She has complains suggestive of early pregnancy and her uterus is gravid, 12 weeks size. There is right ovarian cystic enlargement of about 5–6 cm, which is well-defined, nontender and separated from the uterus. All tumor markers are normal. For fear of malignancy patient wants her tumor to be removed.
>
> What is your decision regarding the desire of Mrs Sufia?

She will be counseled for follow-up rather than straight surgery, because approximately 90% of adnexal masses diagnosed in the 1st trimester of pregnancy are corpus luteal cysts of pregnancy and resolve spontaneously (Sharard, 2003). So, surgical intervention is not recommended in this situation. Therefore, follow-up scan can be considered after 1 month to see whether the cyst disappears or not. So, the patient is to be counseled accordingly to alleviate her fear.

> She is agreed to follow-up rather than surgery, but she wants to do MRI or CT scan to detect the nature of tumor.
>
> What is your suggestion?

In simple cyst ultrasonogram is enough for diagnosis. CT scan or MRI will not give more information about the nature of the tumor. Rather it is better to avoid CT scan and MRI during pregnancy.

Note:
Both CT scan and MRI can be done during pregnancy, but better to avoid. MRI is safer than CT scan.

> Suppose the size of the cyst did not subside till 20 weeks of pregnancy rather it increased.
>
> What will be your decision?

Cyst should be removed and tested histopathologically.

> What are the possible types of this adnexal cyst?

- Simple follicular cyst
- Corpus luteum cyst
- Serous cystadenoma
- Mucinous cystadenoma
- Mature teratoma
- Theca lutein cysts
- Endometrioma
- Germ cell tumor
- Hydrosalpinx with septation
- Rarely epithelial ovarian carcinoma.

RELATED INFORMATION

The majority of lesions that perish are benign and includes teratoma and other benign ovarian neoplasms. Malignant and borderline ovarian tumors are rare during pregnancy. There is recommendation for surgical intervention for adnexal masses that have any of the following characteristics:

- Size of the tumor is 8 cm and persist up to the second trimester
- Are larger than 10 cm in diameter
- Have solid or mixed solid and cystic ultrasound characteristics, highly suspicious for malignancy on imaging.

The rationale for surgery is to diagnose malignancy at an early stage and to prevent complications of labor.

The optimal time for surgery during pregnancy is in the *early second trimester due to following reasons.*

- Organogenesis is completed by this time, thus minimizing the risk of anesthesia and other drug-induced teratogenesis.
- The hormonal function of the corpus luteum has been replaced by the placenta, so the risk of pregnancy loss is low.
- Almost all functional cysts will be resolved by this time.
- At the end of 2nd trimester and in third trimester, tumor is not readily accessible and may precipitate premature labor.

According to gestational age following are to be done

- In first trimester—follow-up.
- In 2nd trimester—surgery.

- In 3rd trimester the surgery can be deferred until term:
    - As labor may turned to cesarean section due to many reasons and tumor can be removed at the time of cesarean section.
    - If tumor itself becomes a cause of obstruction of labor cesarean section is to be done. Baby is to be deliver first and then tumor should be removed.
    - If delivery takes place vaginally, then tumor should be removed during the 1st week of the puerperium.
- An adnexal mass identified incidentally at the time of cesarean section should be removed.

Note: In all cases frozen section biopsy is ideal.

> What is the risk after delivery, if tumor remains in situ?

Torsion of the tumor is a common risk of in situ tumor during postpartum period.

BIBLIOGRAPHY

Abd-el-Maeboud KH. Hydatid cyst of Morgagni: any impact on fertility? J Obstet Gynaecol Res. 1997;23(5):427-31.

Aslam N, Tailor A, Lawton F, et al. Prospective evaluation of three different models for the pre-operative diagnosis of ovarian cancer. BJOG. 2000;107(11):1347-53.

Athey PA, Cooper NB. Sonographic features of para-ovarian cysts. Am J Roentgenol. 1985;144(1):83-6.

Bourne TH, Campbell S, Reynolds KM, et al. Screening for early familial ovarian cancer with transvaginal ultrasonography and colour blood flow imaging, BMJ. 1993;306(6884):1025-9.

Cebesoy FB, Kutlar I, Dikensoy E, et al. Morgagni hydatids: a new factor in infertility? Arch Gynecol Obstet. 2010;281(6):1015-7.

Fleischer AC, Stein SM, Cullinan JA, et al. Color Doppler sonography of adnexal torsion. J Ultrasound Med. 1995;14(7):523-8.

Geomini P, Kruitwagen R, Bremer GL, et al. The accuracy of risk scores in predicting ovarian malignancy: a systematic review. Obstet Gynecol. 2009;113:384-94.

Kier R. Nonovarian gynecologic cysts: MR imaging findings. Am J Roentgenol. 1992;158(6):1265-9.

Kocak M, Dilbaz B, Ozturk N, et al. Laparoscopic management of ovarian dermoid cysts: a review of 47 cases. Ann Saudi Med. 2004;24(5):357-60.

Lee EJ, Kwon HC, Joo HJ, et al. Diagnosis of ovarian torsion with color Doppler solography: depiction of twisted vascular pedicle. J Ultrasound Med. 1998;17(2):83-9.

Levine D, Brown DL, Andreotti RF, et al. Management of asymptomatic ovarian and other adnexal cysts imaged at US: Society of Radiologists in Ultrasound Consensus Conference Statement. Radiology. 2010;256(3):943-54.

Ma S, Shen K, Lang J. A risk of malignancy index in preoperative diagnosis of ovarian cancer. Chin Med J (Engl). 2003;116(3):396-9.

Morgante G, La marca A, Ditto A, et al. Comparison of two malignancy risk indices based on serum CA125, ultrasound score and menopausal status in the diagnosis of ovarian masses. Br J Obset Gynaecol. 1999;106(6):524-7.

Nezhat CR, Kalyoncu S, Nezhat CH, et al. Laparoscopic management of ovarian dermoid cysts: ten years experience. JSLS. 1999;3:179-84.

Peña JE, Ufberg D, Cooney N, et al. Usefulness of Doppler sonography in the diagnosis of ovarian torsion. Fertil Steril. 2000;73(5):1047-50.

Rasheed SM, Abdelmonem AM. Hydatid of Morgagni: a possible underestimated cause of unexplained infertility. Eur J Obstet Gynecol Reprod Biol. 2011;158(1):62-6.

Sharard GB, Hodson CA, Williams HJ, et al. Adnexal masses and pregnancy: a 12-year experience. Am J Obstet Gynecol. 2003;189(2):358-62.

Shawki O, Ramadan A, Askalany A, et al. Laparoscopic management of ovarian dermoid cysts: potential fear of dermoid spill, myths and facts. Gynaecol Surgery. 2007;4:255-60.

Teichmann AT, Brill K, Albring M, et al. The influence of the dose of ethinylestradiol in oral contraceptives on follicle growth. Gyncol Endocrinol. 1995;9(4):299-305.

Timmerman D, Ameye L, Fischerova D, et al. Simple ultrasound rules to distinguish between benign and malignant adrenal masses before surgery: prospective validation by IOTA group. BMJ. 2010;341:c6839.

Timmerman D, Testa AC, Bourne T, et al. Simple Ultrasound-based rules for the diagnosis of ovarian cancer. Ultrasound Obstet Gynecol. 2008;31(6):681-90.

Zanforlin Filho SM, Araujo Júnior E, Serafini P, et al. Diagnosis of ovarian torsion by three-dimensional power Doppler in first trimester of pregnancy. J Obstet Gynaecol Res. 2008;34(2):266-170.

CHAPTER 13

Ovarian Malignancy

Rehana Parveen, Rashida Begum, Farhat Hossain

INTRODUCTION

Ovarian cancer is the second most common gynecologic malignancy and the most common cause of death among women with gynecologic cancer. The disease has a poor prognosis, which is due to the fact that 75-80% of patients with epithelial ovarian cancer (EOC) are diagnosed at an advanced stage when their disease has spread throughout the peritoneal cavity. Diagnosis of EOC at early stages of the disease are potentially curable. Unfortunately, attempts to develop screening procedure for EOC using pelvic examination, pelvic imaging or tumor markers have not yet been successful. The goal of early detection is to reduce ovarian cancer mortality by diagnosing the disease, while it is confined to the ovary with a 5-year survival rate 80-90%. Almost, 80% of women have lymph node or distant metastases at the time of diagnosis with a 5-year survival rates falling to 19-32%.

> **Case scenario:** Mrs Aklima an old, multiparous, menopausal lady presented to you with the complaints of lump in abdomen for 8 months, abdominal swelling and pain for 2 months.
> How will you proceed for diagnosis?

Detailed History

First of all, a detailed history is to be taken:
- *Age:* Any pelvic lump at this age is suspicious of malignancy. Age is the most important risk factor for developing ovarian cancer. Almost 50% of all ovarian cancers occur over the age of 65. Tumor of uterus is rare at this age.
- *Parity (number of child birth):* Parity is an important risk factor for ovarian cancer. Women who were pregnant have a 30-60% less risk of ovarian cancer than nulliparous women. So low parity is a risk factor than multiparous women. Low parity also favors the development of uterine fibroids, but it is rare at this age.
- *Age of menarche and menopause:* Early menarche (before age 12) and late menopause (after age 50) also increases the risk of ovarian cancer. It is presumed that due to long continued ovarian stimulation by pituitary gonadotropins may provoke the development of ovarian tumor. Fibroids become smaller in menopausal age.
- *Per vaginal bleeding:* Ovarian cancer never interferes menstrual function in reproductive age except in hormone-producing tumor of ovary or misfit tumor.
- About lump:
  - When was it first noticed? Duration of the disease.
  - Rapidity of growth:
    - Benign ovarian tumors usually grow slowly.
    - Sometimes initially a tumor grows slowly for certain duration and then grows rapidly. If benign tumor turns into malignancy, it then grows rapidly.
    - Malignant ovarian tumors may grow rapidly from the beginning.
    - Uterine tumors rather regress after menopause.
- *Abdominal pain:* It is characteristic feature of malignant ovarian tumor. Benign ovarian

tumors are usually not painful. Pain develops when some complications develop in the tumor. There may be torsion of the pedicle of ovarian tumor and the patient presents with the features of acute abdomen.
- *Swelling of abdomen:* Whether abdomen is distended and distension is gradual, suddenly and whether it is associated with pain and respiratory distress or not. Lump in abdomen followed by distension of abdomen gives suspicion about *development of ascites, huge enlargement of the malignant growth, presence of metastatic growth to the omentum or other abdominal organs.*
- Query should be made about early symptoms that are associated with epithelial ovarian cancer such as:
  - History of bloating, dyspepsia
  - Difficulty in eating or feeling full
  - Urinary urgency or frequency
  - Abdominal or pelvic pain.

Woman who present with recent onset of abdominal or pelvic symptoms, i.e. bloating, increased abdominal size, urinary frequency or urgency, difficulty in eating or feeling full and abdominal or pelvic pain, ovarian cancer should be considered in differential diagnosis. Particularly in ovarian cancer, these symptoms are more common and are more severe and have shorter duration:

- *History of weight loss:* In malignant disease, weight reduction may occur rapidly.
- *History of nausea, vomiting, diarrhea, passage of blood with stool:* These symptoms are suspicious of primary colonic cancer metastatic to ovary.
- *Dyspnea, chest pain* may be the presenting complain, due to presence of pleural effusion or metastasis to lungs in advanced stage of the disease.
- *Family history of any malignancy:* Family history of ovarian or breast cancer increases the chance of developing ovarian cancer.
- *History of use of oral contraceptives in reproductive life:* Long continued use of oral contraceptives are protective for development of ovarian cancer.

Next the patient should be examined thoroughly.

Examination

General Examination

- Appearance
- Body built (patient may be cachexic due to the weight loss)
- Decubitus (there may be difficulty in lying down due to presence of ascites)
- Anemia
- Lymph modes (supraclavicular lymph nodes may be enlarged)
- Edema (in advanced ovarian malignancy edema may be present due to lymphatic and venous blockage)
- Pulse and blood pressure
- Examination of lungs and heart
- Thyroid gland and breast examination.

Abdominal Examination

- Lump should be assessed in terms of:
  - Size
  - Surface smooth or nodular
  - Margin regular or irregular
  - Consistency cystic or solid and firm
  - Tenderness present or not
  - Mobile or fixed.
- Fluid thrill and shifting dullness, if ascites present

Vaginal Examination

- *Per speculum examination to inspect cervix:* In ovarian tumor cervix looks apparently healthy.
- *Bimanual examination:*
  - Size and position of uterus
  - Any lump felt through fornices.
  - *Mobility:* Whether lump moves with the movement of the cervix. Uterine lump will move along with movement of the cervix, but not in ovarian tumors. Whether any cleft between uterus and lower pole of the tumor can be felt. If the ovarian tumor is small in size and is pelvic organ a definite cleft will be felt between uterus and lower pole of the tumor. A clear cleft exclude the uterine growth.
  - Pulsatile uterine vessel felt through one of lateral fornix indicates uterine growth.

- Nodularity in the Pouch of Douglas indicates malignant deposit.
- *Rectovaginal examination:* The examination helps to evaluate the extension in the parametrium and exclude rectal mass.

> From the history and examination you elicited that she is 60-year-old and mother of four children. Her abdominal lump was growing slowly followed by rapid enlargement. Abdomen became distended for last 2 months. There is anorexia, weight loss, but no history of vaginal bleeding and dyspnea. On examination, she is cachexic, and anemic. Ascites is present with shifting dullness and a lump of 12 × 10 cm is present in right iliac fossa and extending to lumber and umbilical region, which is partly solid and partly cystic with irregular surface and ill-defined margin. Lump is tender and restricted in mobility. Per vaginal examination revealed an irregular firm lump with restricted mobility, which cannot be separated from the uterus, but is not fixed to pelvic bones and rectum. Posterior and right fornixes are full and nodules felt in the posterior fornix. Breasts are normal and no supraclavicular lymph nodes are palpated.
>
> On the basis of above findings what is your probable diagnosis

Most probable diagnosis is malignant ovarian tumor.

RELATED INFORMATION

Incidence

The ovaries are the ninth most common site of cancer in women and accounting for approximately 3% of all new cases. Around the world more than 200,000 women are estimated to develop ovarian cancer every year and almost 100,000 die from the disease. Epithelial ovarian cancer is more common in white women of industrialized countries and least common in Asia and India. According to American Cancer Society report, ovarian cancer declined at a rate of 2.4% annually and death rate from ovarian cancer has been stable since 1998.

Etiology of Ovarian Cancer

The precise cause of ovarian tumor is unknown. There are certain risk factors for development of ovarian tumor. Risk factors are given below:

A. Reproductive Factors

- *Length of reproductive life:* Early menarche and late menopause are risk factors for developing epithelial ovarian cancer. Risk related to number of ovulation in whole reproductive period.
  - During ovulation repeated ovarian epithelial trauma caused by follicular rupture and subsequent epithelial repair results in genetic alterations within the surface epithelium.
    The probability that ovarian cancer development will depend on function of total number of ovulatory cycles, together with a genetic predisposition and probably an environmental factor (Casagrandle, 1979).
  - Long continued stimulation of the ovaries by gonadotropins along with local effects of endogenous hormones, increases mitotic activity and proliferation of the surface epithelium. Under excessive gonadotropin stimulation and resulting estrogenic stimulation surface epithelium is entrapped in inclusion cysts where it proliferates and undergoes malignant transformation (Choi, 2007).
- *Parity:* Nulliparous women are more risky for development of ovarian tumor as ovaries get regular stimulation by gonadotropins and regular ovulation causes regular tear and ware of surface epithelium of ovaries leading to genetic mutation. Multiparous women remained anovulatory during pregnancy and lactational period, so there is no damage and repair and proliferation of surface epithelium. There is 50% reduced risk of ovarian cancer in multiparous women and there is 13–19% risk reduction per pregnancy. So repeated pregnancies and oral contraceptive are protective phenomenon and decrease the risk of ovarian cancer. Women who use oral contraceptives for 5 years or more the risk of epithelial ovarian cancer decreases by 50%.

B. Genetic Factors

- Family history has a strong association with development of ovarian cancer. The life time risk of ovarian cancer is 1.6%, but risk increased to 4–5% when first-degree family member is affected and to 7% when 2 are affected. Overall 5–10% of epithelial ovarian cancer results from hereditary predisposition. At least two distinct clinical syndromes of hereditary genes are identified for ovarian cancer. The most common disorder of genes is associated with breast cancer called hereditary breast ovarian cancer (HBOC), which accounts for 85–90% of all hereditary cancer cases. It is associated with *BRCA1* and *BRCA2* gene. The lifetime risk of ovarian cancer is 28–44% in women carrying *BRCA1* gene, while 27% with *BACA2* gene (Frank, 1998). HBOC syndrome is associated with early onset of breast or epithelial ovarian cancer.

The second syndrome is hereditary non-polyposis colorectal cancer (HNPCC) syndrome (also known as Lynch syndrome), (Lynch, 1992), which involves mutation of *hMSH2* and *hMLH1* genes. There is higher risk of ovarian and endometrial cancer in women with this syndrome.

- Chromosomal abnormalities are commonly associated with ovarian malignancies. Patients with Turner's syndrome (45 XO) are at increased risk of dysgerminoma and gonadoblastoma.

C. Use of Fertility Drugs and Hormone Replacement Therapy

Both fertility drugs and hormone replacement therapy (HRT) are associated with a small increase in overall risk.

A Danish study showed that the risk for ovarian cancer is increased with HRT regardless of duration of use, formulation, dose of estrogen, type of progesterone and route of administration (Morch, 2009). Several other studies have established an association between hormone replacement therapy and risk of ovarian cancer. A study in the United States confirmed an association with estrogen alone (Lacey, 2002).

Some fertility drugs act through releasing endogenous gonadotropin and in other situation direct gonadotropins are used. In both the situations gonadotropin theory might have some role in producing tumor. Use of clomiphene citrate for >12 ovulatory cycles causes 2–3 fold increased risk of ovarian cancer. But a large pooled analysis of 5,207 women with cancer and 7,705 controls did not find any association of increased risk of fertility drugs (Ness et al. 2002). Another pooled study showed no convincing association between use of fertility drugs such as gonadotropins, clomiphene, human chorionic gonadotropin or gonadotropin releasing hormone and risk of ovarian cancer (Jensen, 2009). Rather infertility or nulliparity itself has a higher risk of ovarian cancer compared to multiparity. Infertility longer than 5 years carries higher risk.

D. Endometriosis

Epidemiologic evidence from large cohort studies suggests that endometriosis is an independent risk factor for epithelial ovarian cancer. The risk of malignant transformation of ovarian endometriosis has estimated at 2.5%. Endometriosis associated ovarian cancer appears to occur in younger and nulliparous patients, these tumors are well differentiated, low stage carcinomas that result in better survival (Orezzoli, 2008). Though, recent studies showed that removal of chocolate cysts in endometriosis reduces the chance of ovarian malignancy.

E. Cigarette Smoking

Current smoking or past smoking appears to increase the risk of mucinous ovarian cancer, but not other types of epithelial ovarian cancer (Jordan, 2006).

F. Other Factors

Use of talcum powder on the vulva and perineum and consumption of lactose may by associated with increased risk of ovarian cancer.

Protection

- *High parity:* Multiparity provides protection against ovarian cancer through anovulation in pregnancy and lactation. Women who were even pregnant have 30–60% less risk of ovarian cancer than nulliparous women.

- *Breastfeeding:* Breastfeed women are a lower risk of developing ovarian cancer than women who have never breastfed their babies.
- *Oral contraceptive pills (OCP):* Use of OCP for 6 years or more reduces 30–60% risk of developing epithelial ovarian cancer. The protective effect is exerted by: (a) Reducing in ovulation. (b) Independent protective effect of progesterone causing apoptosis on surface epithelium.
- *Fenretinide:* It is a synthetic retinoid, which is given to breast cancer patients to reduce the risk of developing new breast cancer. It has shown to have protective effect on ovarian cancer.
- *Prophylactic oophorectomy:* Women who are at high risk for developing familial ovarian cancer syndrome with *BRCA1* or *BRCA2* gene are found to be protective against ovarian cancer, if prophylactic oophorectomy is done at age 35 years or after child bearing is completed. But they must be counseled that the risk of peritoneal carcinomatosis still persists after oophorectomy.
- *Prophylactic salpingectomy:* American College of Obstetricians and Gynecologists practice committee opined recently that prophylactic salpingectomy might prevent ovarian cancer in some patients. Salpingectomy at the time of hysterectomy or as a means of tubal sterilization appears to be safe, without an increase in complications compared with hysterectomy alone or tubal ligation (ACOG practice committee, 2015).

Types of Malignant Ovarian Tumor

Common Types

- Epithelial ovarian cancer accounts for 85–95% of all ovarian cancer in US. These occur most commonly in women over 50 years of age. They are classified as serous or mucinous cystadenocarcinoma, endometroid, undifferentiated or clear cell carcinoma.
- Cancer of low malignant potential accounts for 15% of all epithelial ovarian cancers. Features are benign to intermediate and occur more frequently in younger population with average age incidence is 40.
- Germ cell tumors are derived from primitive germ cells of embryonic gonad accounts for 20% of all ovarian tumor. Occurs mostly in second and third decades of life.

Rare Types

- Immature malignant teratoma accounts for less than 1% of ovarian teratomas.
- Embryonal carcinoma a highly malignant tumor accounts for 4% of malignant ovarian tumor. Mean age of presentation is 15 years with abdominal or pelvic lump. The tumor produces hCG.
- Nongestational choriocarcinoma occurs in children and young adults secretes hCG.
- Polyembryoma a highly malignant rare tumor.

Pathology

Serous Cystadenocarcinoma

Serous tumors are mostly benign, about 25% are malignant, which comprises 75% of epithelial cancer. They are fairly large and in 50% cases are bilateral. Mostly (about 70%) are semisolid in nature, 25% purely cystic and very small portion are purely solid. Malignant tumors are usually adherent with bowel, pelvic wall and organs and there may be widespread deposit in peritoneum and omentum, if papillae are present on the outer surface. Cut section shows area of hemorrhage and necrosis and cystic fluid becomes blood stained. Until and unless external surface is eroded it is difficult to distinguish between benign, malignant or borderline malignant. Frozen section biopsy can confirm the diagnosis, which shows typical features of malignancy with a wide variety of patterns such as, papillary, adenopapillary or diffuse in well-differentiated cases and mixed patterns of differentiation in others.

Mucinous Cystadenocarcinoma

About 23% mucinous cystadenocarcinoma are primary ovarian malignancy and most of them arises from a benign or borderline tumor and only 5–10% are *de novo* (Seidman et al. 2003). Primary ovarian carcinoma are usually unilateral, having expansile pattern of invasion, complex papillary pattern, size >10 cm, smooth external surface, microscopic cystic glands, necrotic luminal debris, mural nodules and accompanying teratoma, adenofibroma, endometriosis or Brenner tumor (Lee and Young, 2003). Expansile tumors are usually stage I, but behave as benign. Infiltrative type of invasive tumors are poor prognostic and cause death even, if stage I (Rodriguez and Part, 2002). Distant metastasis of mucinous tumors is rare. Stromal invasion, disorderly penetration of stroma by neoplastic glands, more solid growth, atypia, stratification, papillae, loss of glandular architecture, necrosis (resembles colon carcinoma), greater complexity of glands are typical features of malignancy. Glands are almost always intestinal type. Rarely has signet ring cells, but differs from Krukenberg tumor (McCluggage and Young, 2008).

Endometroid Adenocarcinoma

Benign tumor is rare. Almost, all are malignant and comprises 2% of epithelial cancer. These are the primary ovarian malignancy develop either from ovarian endometriosis or from surface epithelium of the ovary through a process of metaplasia along endometrial lines.

They are usually large about 10–25 cm in diameter. Usually surface is smooth, but sometimes there are papillary outgrowths. On cut section tumors may be partly solid, cystic or wholly cystic. There may be abundant papillary growth in cystic variety and area contains clear, mucoid and hemorrhagic fluid. Histologically, it resembles adenocarcinoma of endometrium, but stroma resembles that of ovary rather than that of endometrium. They are formed of cuboidal and columnar cells arranged in a glandular or acinar pattern having papillary form in some places. They also contain mucinous or serous elements, having squamous metaplasia and clear and vacuolated cytoplasm, may be confused with mesonephroid adenocarcinoma. There is an association of endometrial adenocarcinoma with endometroid adenocarcinoma of the ovary creates problem in diagnosis whether the tumor is primary or secondary. Most of the tumors are well differentiated.

Clear Cell (Mesonephroid) Carcinoma of the Ovary

Almost all are malignant. Histologically, they have to be distinguished from the endodermal sinus tumor, endometroid carcinoma, papillary serous cystadenocarcinoma and the lipoid cell tumor.

Presentation of Malignant Ovarian Tumor

Epithelial ovarian cancer present with a wide variety of vague and nonspecific symptoms. At its initial stage an ovarian tumor may present as an adnexal mass. When the tumor grows, then it rises above the pelvic brim and becomes an abdominal organ. Sometimes it may occupy almost whole of the abdominal cavity. Usual complaints are:
- Bloating (abdominal distension and discomfort)
- Pressure effects on the bladder and rectum (frequency of micturition and dysuria)
- Early satiety (loss of appetite)
- Constipation
- Indigestion
- Acid reflux
- Shortness of breath
- Tiredness and weight loss
- Abdominal mass with distension.

Pelvic pain, abdominal pain, increased abdominal size, bloating, difficulty in eating or feeling of full is commonly associated with ovarian cancer. Abdominal distension, anorexia, nausea, vomiting, constipation, diarrhea, early satiety or other digestive disorders due to the presence of malignant ascites and omental or bowel metastases and dyspnea due to pleural effusion are associated with advanced stage of the disease (Eitan and Levine, 2005). Swelling of leg due to venous thrombosis may occur at late stage of the disease.

Physical Examination

Per Abdominal Examination

The usual tendency of an ovarian tumor is to grow towards midline and rest against the anterior abdominal wall. In doing so, a tumor arising from one-sided ovary may come to lie to the other side of pelvic cavity or abdomen crossing the midline. So by abdominal or pelvic examination, it is not possible to determine the origin site of tumor. Ovarian tumor may occupy the midline extending laterally to the iliac region and lumbar region or it may be in the lateral part of abdominal cavity and extending towards midline. The size of ovarian tumor should be expressed in centimeter.

In case of malignant ovarian tumor, there may be bilateral distribution. Presence of upper abdominal mass is suggestive of omental cake (metastases to the omentum). Malignant ovarian tumors are usually hard, partly cystic and partly solid with irregular nodular surface, ill-defined margins and fixity to adjacent organs and/or pelvic bones. Ovarian tumor is always dull to percussion, as it grows towards midline displacing the intestines laterally. So the percussion note is dull in the midline over the tumor resonant at the flanks.

Ascites may be present along with ovarian tumor. The presence of ascites is determined by eliciting the finding of either fluid thrill or shifting dullness (depending upon the volume of ascitic fluid in the peritoneal cavity):

- If ascites is not associated with ovarian tumor then percussion note will be resonant at the centre (as air-filled intestines float on fluid at the centre) and dull at flank (due to presence of fluid at flanks).
- If ovarian tumor is associated with ascites the percussion note will be dull at the center due to the presence of ovarian tumor at the center and the percussion note will be resonant at the flank (due to presence of fluid, with intestines float on fluid at the flanks).

Note:
- Benign ovarian tumors are usually (80%) cystic, non-tendar, smooth with well-defined margins and mobile in all directions. So the lower limit of the ovarian tumor can be reached.
- Malignant ovarian tumors at early stage may also be mobile before forming any adhesion.
- Benign ovarian tumors may have restricted mobility, if it is large and occupy the whole of the abdominal cavity or adherent with uterus after torsion.

Bimanual Examination

- The lower pole of the lump may be felt through the posterolateral fornix, which may be separated from the uterus by a sharp cleft. The lump may be fixed to the lateral pelvic bone. The cervix will not move, with the movement of the lump in the abdomen.
- There may be nodular growth felt through the posterior fornix, rectal mucosa will be free. Nodularity in posterior fornix also may be present in chronic pelvic inflammatory disease (PID) tuberculosis and endometriosis.
- Palpation of an asymptomatic adnexal mass during a pelvic examination is the usual reason for initiating a diagnosis for ovarian cancer.

The presence of a solid, irregular fixed pelvic mass on pelvic examination is highly suggestive of an ovarian malignancy. The diagnosis of malignancy is almost certain, if there is presence of an upper abdominal mass or ascites.

Rectovaginal Examination

Rectovaginal examination is done to assess the fixity of the solid mass to other organs and pelvic bones and its extension in the pelvis and to exclude rectal mass.

Note:
- Edometriomas are benign lesions that may be fixed, irregular and tender there may be associated fixed retroverted uterus and nodular thickening of the uterosacral ligament and rectovaginal septum. The age of the patient and relevant history of endometriosis will differentiate the case from ovarian malignancy.
- The PID with ovarian mass may produce irregular, soft to firm tender, fixed lump in the pelvis, usually adherent to the uterus. Uterine manipulation will be painful. There will be relevant history.

> What may be the differential diagnosis of this case?

Adnexal masses present a diagnostic dilemma. The differential diagnosis is extensive, with most masses representing benign masses. In this

postmenopausal woman other malignant causes may be considered such as:
- Metastatic lesions from breast
- Malignant gastric tumor
- Rectal cancer
- Colon cancer
- Ascites due to other cause
- Fallopian tube carcinoma
- Retroperitoneal growth.

Nonmalignant Etiologies

- Cyst adenoma
- Leiomyoma.

> What are the differential diagnosis of malignant ovarian tumors in young girls and perimenopausal women?

Differential diagnosis of malignant ovarian tumor differs according to age.

Young Girls

- Physiologic cysts
- Benign cystic teratoma
- Par ovarian cyst
- Hematometra due to imperforate hymen
- Noncommunicating uterine horn
- Ectopic pregnancy
- Appendicular abscess.

Premenopausal Women

- Functional cyst
- Ectopic pregnancy
- Hydrosalpings
- Pyosalpings
- Endometrioma
- Leiomyoma (degenerated)
- Inflammatory ovarian mass/ovarian abscess
- Benign ovarian neoplasms
- Ovarian torsion
- Paraovarian cyst
- Pelvic kidney
- Peritoneal cyst
- Pelvic inflammatory disease
- Gastric, rectal and colonic cancer
- Uterine anomaly
- Pelvic abscess.

> What relevant investigations do you want to do for preoperative evaluation of Mrs Aklima?

Investigations needed for preoperative evaluation are:
- Complete blood counts
- Liver function test
- Renal function test
- Blood sugar
- USG of the whole abdomen
- Chest X-ray
- Estimation of tumor markers such as CA-125, C19-9
- Abdominopelvic computerized tomography (CT) scan or magnetic resonance imaging (MRI), if USG cannot give satisfactory interpretation.

Note: Though diagnosis can be confirmed only pathologically by removing the ovaries and when disease is advanced, by sampling tissue or ascetic fluid.

RELATED INFORMATION

Role of Ultrasonography in Malignant Ovarian Tumor

Ultrasonography (USG) is an important aid in the evaluation of ovarian tumor. It is considered as initial imaging modality of choice for characterizing an ovarian mass as benign or malignant.

Transvaginal ultrasonography may have a somewhat better soft tissue resolution than transabdominal ultrasonography for adnexal mass specially confined to the pelvis. Transabdominal USG is complementary to TVS when a large field of view is required such as mass has extended out of the pelvis. Evaluation of associated findings such as ascites, peritoneal implants, hydroureter, hydrosalpings is better delineated through this approach.

Features associated with malignant as revealed by USG are:
- Mass with thick irregular border
- Multiple echogenic patterns due to solid element with papillary projections
- Multiple irregular septa
- Bilateral tumors
- Ascitis

- Neovascularization (increased number of tortuous blood vessels with arteriovenous shunt) of Doppler evaluation.

The USG has 95–99% negative predictive value (NPV) in excluding ovarian malignancy. Combining morphological assessment with Doppler evaluation improves the diagnostic performance of ultrasound examination (Kinkel, 2000).

Role of CT Scan in Ovarian Cancer

Ovary scan is done using CT scan for preoperative evaluation of ovarian cancer, but it is not necessary for diagnosis. It gives more specific information than USG in regards to:
- Size, lobulation, septa, solid with cystic components of the ovarian mass
- Adhesions and infiltrations of surrounding organs uterus, urinary bladder, pelvic ureter, small and large bowels. Whether the intervening fat planes between the ovary and surrounding organs obscured or not are noticed.
- Metastasis in distant sites with sensitivity of 90–100% in liver and 80–86% in peritoneum and greater omentum metastasis. It can also detect metastasis in pelvic and para-aortic lymph nodes, but limitation is it cannot detect nodules or implants or metastatic deposits, which are <1 cm in size.
- In situations where neoadjuvant chemotherapy is planned for nonresectable ovarian cancer (advanced stage ovarian cancer) CT scan gives staging informations.

The sensitivity and specificity of CT scan for characterizing malignant ovarian tumor is 92–94%; respectively.

Role of MRI in Ovarian Cancer

The MRI is equivalent to CT scan for characterizing adnexal masses. The relatively high cost of MRI precludes its routine use in evaluating ovarian cancer.

Role of PET Scan in Ovarian Cancer

Positron emission tomography (PET) is suitable for detecting suspected recurrent ovarian disease and thus is helpful to monitor treatment response (Musto, 2011). Fluro-2 deoxy glucose (FDG) is used in PET scan. There is increased uptake of glucose in the metastatic sites and thus these sites can easily be recognized.

Role of imaging to diagnose primary source of tumor metastatic to ovaries: Other radiographic studies may be needed in selected patients depending upon initial physical examination and the presence of patient symptoms:
- Brain and bone scan are indicated in selected cases where patients symptoms suggests metastases to these sites.
- A colonoscopy is indicated in those patients with signs and symptoms suspicious for colon cancer. This should include any patient who has evidence of melena or acute blood in the stool or given a recent history of diarrhea or constipation.
- A gastroscopy is indicated, if there are upper gastrointestinal symptoms such as nausea, vomiting or hematemesis.
- Bilateral mammography is indicated, if there is any breast mass. There is strong association of ovarian cancer with breast cancer in HBOC syndrome where breast cancer may metastasize to ovaries or ovarian cancer may aggravate breast cancer.

Note: Besides imaging patients who have irregular menses or postmenopausal bleeding should have an endometrial biopsy and an endocervical curettage, to exclude the presence of uterine or endocervical cancer metastatic to the ovary.

Role of Tumor Markers in Ovarian Cancer

Tumor markers are substances produced in response to neoplastic proliferation, which indicate the likely presence of cancer. Majority of the markers are tumor associated rather than tumor specific. Therefore, they are not diagnostic, but contribute to differential diagnosis. They have important role to play in screening, determining response to treatment, detecting recurrence and predicting prognosis. In suspected cases of epithelial ovarian malignancy serum CA-125, serum CA 19-9 and serum carcinoembryonic antigen (CEA) is done. They are considered as valuable tool in conjunction with other tests and clinical findings.

Serum CA-125

Serum CA-125 is a glycoprotein and is the most currently available marker for epithelial ovarian cancer. It is of value in differentiating between benign and malignant adnexal masses particularly in postmenopausal women.

The normal CA-125 level is <35 unit/mL, this level rises to >65 units/mL in 50% cases in stage I disease and 80–90% in advanced stage of epithelial ovarian cancer. In serous epithelial variety of ovarian cancer serum CA-125 level is raised and may show a rise of 80–90% in advance staged disease. In mucinous adenocarcinoma of ovary serum CA-125 level can be normal (David, 1986).

In postmenopausal women with asymptomatic pelvic masses, an elevated serum CA-125 (>65 u/mL) had a sensitivity of 97% and a specificity of 78% for ovarian cancer (Niloff, 1985). So raised CA-125 is very significant for postmenopausal women. In contrast, in premenopausal women, there is a higher prevalence of non-malignant conditions that can produce elevated serum CA-125 levels (e.g. pregnancy, endometriosis, adenomyosis, uterine fibroids and PID). CA-125 is not specific for epithelial ovarian cancer and may be elevated in 1% of healthy women (Best, 1983). In postmenopausal women with an adnexal mass, an elevated CA-125 level indicates the need for prompt surgical exploration, whereas in premenopausal woman, additional work-up in needed to exclude ovarian malignancy.

Serum CA-125 as tumor marker reveals greatest importance in monitoring the response to treatment and in follow-up (Jacobs, 1993). Thus, a baseline value is estimated before treatment and the test is repeated during treatment at intervals. A raised value during recurrence demands additional tests for further evaluation.

Serum CA 19-9

The CA 19-9 marker is a Lewis antigen derivative. Normal cut off value is 37 U/mL. Mucinous ovarian cancer express the antigen more frequently than serous tumor. Thus, it is useful in detecting mucinous adenocarcinoma of ovary.

Serum CEA

The CEA is an oncofetal antigen found in small amounts in adult colon. The normal cut off value is 5 mg/L and level increase >5 mg/L in 88% of mucinous variety, but in only 20% in serous variety. Elevated levels are mostly associated with colon and pancreatic carcinoma. But in 25–50% of women with ovarian cancer serum CEA level are elevated. Although, this elevated levels are less satisfactory, it is an indirect reflection of gut involvement.

Spread of EOC

Ovarian epithelial cancer spread primarily by:
- *Exfoliation and implantation:* Exfoliation of malignant cells into the peritoneal cavity occurs when the tumor penetrates through the surface of ovarian epithelium, from there cells follow the normal circulation of peritoneal fluid. Implantation followed by metastasis are typically seen on the posterior cul-de-sac, paracolic gutters, right hemidiaphragm, liver capsule, peritoneal surfaces of intestine and their mesenteries and omentum. The lesion progressively agglutinates the intestinal loops and may cause functional intestinal obstruction. Rarely lesion may invade intestinal lumen.
- *Lymphatic dissemination:* The second mode of spread occurs through retroperitoneal lymphatics that drain the ovaries. These follow:
  - Ovarian blood vessels in the infundibulopelvic ligaments to terminate in the para-aortic lymph nodes.
  - Lymph channels along the broad ligament and parametrium to terminate in the pelvic lymph nodes.

Lymphatic dissemination to the pelvic and para-aortic lymph nodes; Spread may also occur along the round ligament to the inguinal lymph nodes. Spread may also occur through retroperitoneal lymphatics to the supra clavicular nodes. 78% of patients with stage III disease have metastasis to the pelvic lymphnodes, while para-aortic nodes positive for metastasis is 18% in stage I, 20% in stage II, 42% in stage III and 67% in stage IV disease (Burghardt et al. 1991).

- *Hematogenous:* It spreads to lungs and liver parenchyma, bones, cardiovascular system (CVS), etc, but it is uncommon to find at the time of diagnosis.

> What management you will offer for Mrs Aklima?

Clinically, it seems to be a ease of malignant ovarian tumor in advanced stage. Treatment for this case is following:
- Primary cytoreductive surgery followed by
- Systemic chemotherapy.

Surgery includes removal of uterus, both ovaries as much as possible and tubes, removal of infracolic omentum (total hysterectomy, bilateral salpingo-oophorectomy and infracolic omentectomy) and associated metastatic disease.

A vertical medial incision is the best approach for cytoreductive surgery. It allows access to the upper abdomen, which is difficult to visualize through a low transverse incision.

> Why surgical evaluation is needed and what are the points for surgical evaluation in this case?

Surgical evaluation is done for *clinical diagnosis of malignancy* and *staging* of the disease. Ovarian cancer is always surgically staged according to International Federation of Gynecology and Obstetrics (FIGO) guidelines. Surgical evaluation includes:
- Hemorrhagic free fluid
- Adhesion
- Engorged vessels over the growth
- Distribution of growth in the ovary either unilateral or bilateral
- Necrotic or fungatic (rupture of growth) growth
- Exploration of intra-abdominal organ to determine the sites of disease spread.

Immediately after assessing these conditions, comprehensive surgical staging is done, which includes:
- Collection of fluid for cytology, if free fluid is present. If ascites is not there washings are obtained by instilling and removing at least 50–100 mL of saline from pelvic cul-de-sac, each paracolic gutter and beneath each hemidiaphragm.
- Exploration of the intra-abdominal viscera, pelvis, peritoneal surface, diaphragm, omentum and lymph nodes (pelvic and paraaortic).
- Samples for biopsy:
  a. Systematic peritoneal biopsies from:
     - Pelvic cul-de-sac
     - Anterior bladder peritoneum
     - Infundibulopelvic ligament pedicles
     - Bilateral pelvic sidewalls
     - Paracolic gutters bilaterally
     - Hemidiaphragms bilaterally.
  b. Any suspicious area or adhesions on the peritoneal surfaces.
  c. Infracolic omentum (omentectomy)
  d. Pelvic and para-aortic lymph node sampling (lymphadenectomy).

> When comprehensive surgical staging is indicated and why?

Comprehensive surgical staging should always be done in early staged ovarian cancer. Here the initial spread of disease occurs by lymphatics and intraperitoneally when the disease is clinically occult. In 10% patients with early staged ovarian cancer metastasis is found in para-aortic lymph nodes and occult disease identified in peritoneal washing and biopsy from diaphragm and omentum.

Thus comprehensive surgical staging in early staged disease allows accurate staging and plan appropriate adjuvant therapy, which improves progression free interval and overall survival of the patient (Young, 1990).

> What is the benefit of surgical staging?

Thorough surgical staging is needed to determine the extent of disease, plan the treatment and determine the prognosis of the disease. It has been found that 5-year survival rate is better in patients who have been properly surgically staged (Young, 1990).

RELATED INFORMATION

Staging of Ovarian Malignancy

The FIGO staging for primary carcinoma of ovary.

Stage I: The cancer is limited to the ovaries:
- *IA:* Limited to one ovary and the outer ovarian capsule is not ruptured. There is no tumor on the external surface of the ovary and there is no ascites and/or the washings are negative.
- *IB:* Cancer is present in both ovaries, but the outer capsule is intact and there is no tumor on external surface. There is no ascites and the washings are negative.
- *IC:* The cancer is either stage IA or IB level, but the capsule is ruptured or there is tumor on the ovarian surface or malignant cells are present in ascites or washings.

Stage II: Cancer involves one or both ovaries with spread to other pelvic organs or surfaces:
- *IIA:* Extension or implants onto the uterus and/or fallopian tube. The washings are negative washings and there is no ascites.
- *IIB:* Extension or implants onto other pelvic tissues. The washings are negative and there is no ascites.
- *IIC:* Pelvic extension or implants such as Stage IIA or IIB, but with positive pelvic washings.

Stage III: Cancer spread outside the pelvis to the abdominal area, including metastases to liver surface:
- *IIIA:* Tumor is grossly confined to the pelvis, but with microscopic peritoneal metastases beyond pelvis to abdominal peritoneal surfaces or the omentum.
- *IIIB:* Same as IIIA, but with macroscopic peritoneal or omental metastases beyond pelvis <2 cm in size.
- *IIIC:* Same as IIIA, but with peritoneal or omental metastases beyond pelvis, larger than 2 cm or lymph node metastases to inguinal, pelvic or para-aortic areas.

Stage IV: Metastases or spread to the liver or outside the peritoneal cavity to areas such as the chest or brain.

Treatment of Malignant Ovarian Tumor

The treatment of malignant ovarian tumor depends on:
- Stage of the disease
- Histological cell type
- Patient's age and overall condition.

There are basically three forms of treatment for ovarian cancer. They are:
- The primary one is surgery, which aims to completely remove the malignant tissue.
- Chemotherapy is second line modality to kill the cancer cells. There are three forms of chemotherapy:
  - Adjuvant chemotherapy, which is given after surgery to kill the left over cancer cells.
  - Neoadjuvant chemotherapy, which is given before surgery in non-resectable ovarian cancer.
  - Induction chemotherapy.
- Radiation therapy is third line modality for certain instances to kill cancer cells by high energy X-rays.

Surgery

Meticulous surgery to remove as much cancer tissue as possible is the key point for survival for the patient. So, it must be performed by gynecologic oncologists, who are specially trained in the management of gynecologic malignancy.

Type of surgery according to staging of the disease: Ovarian malignancy has been broadly classified as:
A. Early ovarian cancer (Stage I and II)
B. Advanced ovarian cancer (Stage III and IV)

A. Early ovarian cancer (stage I and II)
Primary surgery in this group includes:
- Hysterectomy.
- Bilateral salpingo-oophorectomy.
- Infracolic omentectomy.
- Comprehensive surgical staging (lymphadenectomy). Pelvic and paracolic lymphadenectomy in EOC is thus a mandatory part of comprehensive surgical staging according to FIGO guidelines. It is done to achieve accurate staging and select appropriate adjuvant chemotherapy. The effect of lymphadenectomy on progression free survival (PFS) and overall survival is unclear.

In young women, who want to preserve fertility where one ovary is affected, but other is proved healthy by frozen section biopsy unilateral salpingo-oophorectomy without hysterectomy can be performed. After having birth of the baby those must be removed.

B. **Advanced ovarian cancer (stage III and IV)**
- *Cytoreductive surgery:* In advanced ovarian cancer (AOC), the surgery of choice is cytoreductive or debulking surgery. The goal is to remove all primary cancer and associated metastatic disease. It includes: (i) hysterectomy, bilateral salpingo-oophorectomy, omentectomy, resection of metastatic disease from peritoneum or intestine (rectosigmoid colon, terminal ileum, cecum). The concept is simply to diminish the residual tumor burden to a point at which adjuvant therapy will be optimally effective. Adjuvant therapies are most effective when a minimum tumor burden exists. Removal of large ovarian masses and omental involvement often reduces the tumor burden by 80–90%.
- *Optimum cytoreduction:* If resection of all metastatic disease is not possible, then the goal is to reduce the tumor burden to an optimal status when adjuvant therapy will be maximally effective. The gynecologic oncology group defines optimum cytoreduction as residual tumor that is less than 2 cm in maximum diameter. Patients with AOC whose disease has been optimally cytoreduced has best progress and 60% patients remain free of disease for 5-year. Hacker and Berek showed that patients whose largest residual lesions were greater and equal to 5 mm had a superior survival (Hacker, 1983).

Benefits of cytoreduction
- Cytoreduction offers physiologic benefits, which includes:
  - It improves patient comfort because ascites becomes well controlled and omental cake is removed
  - It alleviates nausea and early satiety with removal of omental cake
  - It improves nutritional status of the patient by removing intestinal metastases and restoring its function
  - These collectively increases patient's ability to tolerate the intensive chemotherapy that is required.
- Cytoreduction enhances the response of remaining tumors to chemotherapy as disease burden is minimum and drugs exert their maximum effects on small tumor that are well perfused and therefore mitotically active. The mechanism involves:

Large tumor masses have relatively poor blood supply. They are composed of large proportion of cells that are in GO phase of cell cycles (low growth fraction). In other words these cells are relatively insensitive to the effects of chemotherapy. Cytoreduction removes tumor with low growth fraction and exposes residual mass with higher growth fraction, which are highly sensitive to chemotherapy. Removal of volume of residual disease after cytoreductive surgery inversely correlates with survival (Bristor, 2002).

Difficulties and complications of surgery

Sometimes, in advanced malignant ovarian tumor there may be extensive adhesion, which make the surgery very difficult. There may be profuse bleeding and injury of adjacent organs. Due to optimal debulking portion of other organs may be sacrificed. Sometimes, the surgeon will need to remove a piece of colon to debulk the cancer properly. In that situation for some cases, the two ends that remain are sewn back together. In other cases, colostomy may be needed. A piece of bladder may also need to be removed. Debulking may also require removing the spleen and/or the gallbladder, as well as part of the stomach, liver, and/or pancreas.

Cytoreductive surgery was done. Surgical staging and histopathological report reveals that Mrs Aklima is suffering from stage IIIC serous papillary adenocarcinoma with grade two tumor.
What will be the treatment for her?

Surgery alone is not curative for women with advanced stage ovarian carcinoma. Adjuvant treatment is needed in this case. Systemic chemotherapy is the standard adjuvant treatment for metastatic epithelial ovarian cancer.

She will be treated by intravenous (IV) paclitaxel (175 mg/m^2) and carboplatin (AUC 7.5) for 6 cycles at 3 weeks interval. IV fluid should be infused for 1 hour before giving injection. Pactitaxel should be given over 3 hours and carboplatin should be given with 100 mL of fluid over 1-hour. Response rate of serous carcinoma is 70–80% with this regimen.

RELATED INFORMATION

Chemotherapy

Chemotherapy is the adjuvant treatment of choice in most cases of ovarian malignancy. The rationale of adding postoperative chemotherapy is to:
- Prolong remission and survival.
- For palliation in advanced and recurrent disease.

Types of Chemotherapy

Single agent chemotherapy
Cisplatinum, carboplatin, cyclophosphamide, paclitaxel and docetaxel are active against epithelial ovarian cancer:
- Cisplatin and carboplatin has the same efficacy, but now-a-days carboplatin has replaced to cisplatin because of less side effects and better tolerability. Carboplatin has less gastrointestinal side effects such as nausea, vomiting and has less neurotoxicity, nephrotoxicity and ototoxicity, but has higher myelosuppression than cisplatin. Absence of nephrotoxicity permits carboplatin administration in an outpatient setting without forced hydration.
- The efficacy of docetaxel is similar to paclitaxel, but docetaxel has less extremity weakness, neurologic effects, arthralgia and myalgia than paclitaxel.

Combination chemotherapy
Combination chemotherapy has proved to be superior to single agent chemotherapy in the treatment of ovarian cancer because:
- It elicits better response rate
- There is improved overall survival.

Combination is selected on the basis of:
- All drugs should be active against the tumor.
- Each drug should have different mode of action to avoid drug resistance.

The preferred standard combination chemotherapy for patients with ovarian cancer is paclitaxel and carboplatin and they are considered as first line chemotherapy. This combination causes significant improvement in both progression free survival and overall survival in both optimally and suboptimally cytoreduced patients (Piccart, 2003). Combination of docetaxel and carboplatin is associated with more myelosuppression and its consequences such as severe infection and prolonged severe neutropenia.

Dose and duration
There is a minimum dose below, which response to treatment is compromised, but unfortunately this dose determination is difficult. Thus, dose of chemotherapy required for a patient is determined on the basis of acceptable toxicity profile. The duration of chemotherapy use is preferably between 5 and 6 cycles. Prospective randomized trial have failed to demonstrate an improved outcome by increasing the dose of drugs per cycle or extending the duration of treatment beyond 5-6 cycles (Cure et al. 2004), though another study showed significant improvement of progression free survival after 12 cycles of single agent (Pacletaxel) chemotherapy (Markman et al. 2009).

Route of administration
Mostly for EOC chemotherapy is given intravenously. The role of intraperitoneal (IP) chemotherapy is still controversial. But Cochrane review and meta-analysis has concluded that IP chemotherapy is associated with better outcomes in regards to progression free survival and overall survival in AOC who is optimally debulked (Hess et al. 2007). But there is more catheter related complications, which introduced into abdominal cavity for IP.

Role of intermittent therapy
Combination chemotherapy is given at an interval of 3 weeks for:
- Maximum killing of tumor cells
- Minimizing prolonged immunosuppression.

Criteria for selection of patient for adjuvant therapy

This depends upon the stage of the disease and certain prognostic variables. The general principle is to provide adjuvant chemotherapy to patients who belong to:
- Early stage ovarian cancer with prognostically unfavorable category. These are:
  - Stage IA, IB–Gd3
  - Stage IC
  - Stage II
  - Tumors on external surface or ruptured capsule
  - Ascites or positive peritoneal washing.

There is 20% relapse rate. Adjuvant therapy improves progression free interval and overall survival.

- Advanced stage ovarian cancer.

Note: Stages IA, IB, G1 and G2 are prognostically favorable category of early staged ovarian cancer. They do not need adjuvant therapy and 5-year survival rate is 90%.

Monitoring of Patients During Chemotherapy

Patients are monitored during chemotherapy for two purposes:
- Monitoring for response
- Monitoring for toxicity.

Monitoring of response

Evaluation for monitoring of response during chemotherapy is done on the basis of response evaluation criteria in solid tumors (RECIST), through history, physical examination, USG or CT scan and tumor markers.

The RECIST definition of response:
- *Complete response (CR):* Disappearance of all target lesions.
- *Partial response (PR):* About 30–50% decrease in size of target lesion.

It is difficult to define partial response. When there is 30–50% reduction in the size of the tumor with subjective improvement and absence of new lesion during treatment, then it is said to be partial.

Progressive disease (PD): At least 20% increase in tumor diameter or appearance of one or more new lesions during treatment is called progressive disease.

Stable disease (SD): No significant shrinkage in tumor diameter to qualify for PR nor sufficient increase to qualify for PD.

Monitoring of toxicities

Toxicities of chemotherapy is evaluated by history, physical examination and laboratory investigations such as:
- Blood for CBC
- Renal function tests
- Liver function tests.

If the following parameters are evident, the schedule for next chemotherapy should be postponed:
- *WBC count:* <2,000/mm^3
- *Platelet count:* <50,000/mm^3
- *Renal function test parameters:* Double than normal
- *Hepatic function test parameters:* Double than normal.

Toxicities those might occur are following:
- Bone marrow toxicity is the most common side effect associated with cytotoxic drugs. Neutropenia is the most common manifestation of bone marrow toxicity and occurs about 7–14 days after the initiation of treatment. Thrombocytopenia is less common than neutropenia and is associated with more frequent and wider use of carboplatin. Moderate degrees of anemia are common in cancer patients receiving chemotherapy.
- Gastrointestinal toxicity comprising of nausea, vomiting and anorexia are associated with most chemotherapeutic agents. Mucositis in lower GI tract is associated with diarrhea.
- Skin toxicities occurring during chemotherapy are usually drug specific and self-limiting. These toxicities include allergic reactions, skin hyper pigmentation, photosensitivity and local extravasation necrosis.
- Scalp alopecia associated with chemotherapy is almost always reversible. Total scalp alopecia is common with paclitaxel and doxorubicin and partial alopecia with cisplatin, carboplatin, cyclophosphamide and 5-fluorouracil.

- Neurotoxicity in the form of peripheral neuropathy is associated with cisplatin, paclitaxel and docetaxel. Neurotoxicity due to carboplatin is less common than cisplatin.
- Renal toxicity is an important side effects of cisplatin. Carboplatin is associated with a lower toxicity.
- Hemorrhagic cyst is a troublesome side effect of cyclophosphamide and ifosfamide.

Hypersensitivity Reaction

Paclitaxel is associated with hypersensitivity reaction, which usually occurs during either first or second cycle of drug administration and can usually be managed with prophylactic medicine (corticosteroids, antihistamines H1/H2/blocked).

Carboplatin is associated with late allergic reactions, which are not readily prevented with prophylactic medication. Patients receiving a second course of carboplatin-based therapy should be closely monitored for early signs of hypersensitivity to avoid more serious reactions.

> Suppose Mrs Aklima's condition is not fit for general anesthesia for surgery. She developed pleural effusion and dyspnea along with huge ascites.
> What should be her treatment option?

Patient should be treated by neoadjuvant chemotherapy. After therapy she will recover from pleural effusion, dyspnea and ascites, tumor bulk will reduce significantly then interval cytoreductive surgery will be done.

RELATED INFORMATION

Neoadjuvant Chemotherapy

Neoadjuvant chemotherapy (NACT) is a type of chemotherapy prescribed to patients before surgery. It is an alternative strategy for selected number of patients with advanced ovarian cancer in whom primary cytoreductive surgery is not possible.
- Ovarian malignancy, which are felt to be optimally unresectable by experienced ovarian cancer surgical team. Optimal debulking may expose the patient to unacceptable morbidities.
- Patients with advanced ovarian cancer that are at high risk of operative morbidity and mortality due to bulky disease, large pleural effusion, liver parenchymal metastases, lung metastases and poor performance status.

Before prescribing NACT diagnosis of presumed ovarian cancer must be established either by biopsy or FNAC from the ovarian mass. Patients are subjected to 2–3 cycles of chemotherapy preferably paclitaxel and carboplatin and then reassessment for interval cytoreductive surgery is done. If the patient has a response to chemotherapy and becomes more appropriate surgical candidate, then interval cytoreductive surgery may be considered after initial chemotherapy.

The NACT reduces tumor bulk, ascites and pleural effusion, and facilitates:
- Maximum cytoreduction
- Decreased blood loss.

But primary cytoreduction should always be considered the standard of care for most patients as many studies have demonstrated survival outcome achievable with NACT is inferior to primary cytoreduction.

Note: Surgery, which is done in between chemotherapies is known an interval cytoreductive surgery.

Radiotherapy

An alternative to first-line combination chemotherapy, whole abdomen radiotherapy is not used now-a-days. The principal problem associated with this approach is the development of acute and chronic intestinal morbidity. About 30% of patients treated with whole abdomen radiation therapy develop intestinal obstruction that may had exploratory surgery. Radiation therapy as a palliative modality may be useful for symptomatic relief in patients having localized tumor. For example a fixed pelvic mass eroding the vaginal mucosa causing bleeding, pain bowel or bladder dysfunction without obvious disseminated symptomatic peritoneal disease. Symptomatic relief with tumor regression can often be obtained in these situations from local irradiation. Palliative irradiation may also be useful for extra-abdominal disease, particularly supraclavicular or inguinal node masses and bone or brain metastases.

> How will you do post-treatment follow-up for Mrs Aklima?

According to consensus based guideline for post-treatment follow-up recommended by society of Gynecologic Oncologists the follow-up schedule for Mrs Aklima will be:
- Review of symptoms and physical examinations every 3 months for the first 2 years, every 4–6 months during 3rd year, every 6 months for years 3–5 then annually.
- The CA-125 testing at each visit
- The CT and/or PET is recommended for clinically suspected recurrence (Salanic, 2011).

Post-treatment surveillance performed at regular interval is designed to detect recurrent or persistent epithelial ovarian cancer. Serum levels of the tumor marker CA-125 correspond to disease activity in about 90% of patients and rising serum level of CA-125 may predict progression of the disease.

Prognosis/Survival

Prognosis and survival depends upon a number of factors:
- *Tumor stage:* The 5-year survival of patients with epithelial ovarian cancer is directly correlated with the tumor stage. Peroperative spillage or rupture do not worsen the prognosis, but tumors found already ruptured bears poor prognosis.
- *Volume of residual disease:* It is followed by primary surgery and is directly correlated with survival.
- *Histological features and grading:* Poorly undifferentiated cells are poor prognostic. Clear cell carcinomas are associated with poor prognosis than other histologic type.
- *Biologic factors:* Amplification or expression of genetic loci of proto-oncogens have relationship with the development and progression of ovarian cancer. The ovarian cancer, which bears mutated p53 tumor suppressor gene bear poor prognosis. Almost half of all epithelial ovarian cancers have evidence of mutated p53 in the tumor.
- *CA-125 levels:* An elevated level of CA-125 is an indicator of progression of disease following completion of chemotherapy.

The 5-year survival rate for carefully staged patients in different stages of ovarian tumor are as follows (**Table 13.1**): (Heintz, 2006)

Table 13.1 The 5-year survival rate in different stages of ovarian cancer

Protocol	Monitoring
Stage 1A	89.6%
Stage 1B	86.1%
Stage 1C	83.4%
Stage 11A	70.7%
Stage 11B	65.5%
Stage 11C	71.4%
Stage 111A	46.7%
Stage 111B	41.5%
Stage 111C	32.5%
Stage 1V	18.6%

> Mrs Aklima responded to treatment and cured after chemotherapy. During follow-up after 12 months you found that she developed symptoms and on examination a small pelvic lump felt through the vault. Serum CA-125 value was also rising. For confirm diagnosis you did CT scan and found a small lump of about 3 x 2.5 cm arising in iliac fossa.
>
> How will you manage her?

This is a case of recurrence of the disease.

Patient was cured by combined platinum and pecletaxel. So she is platinum sensitive and again she should be treated with the same regime.

RELATED INFORMATION

Recurrent Ovarian Epithelial Cancer

Second-line Chemotherapy

When cancer developed after surgery or chemotherapy is called recurrent disease. Eighty percent of women with advanced stage ovarian cancer who completely respond to first line chemotherapy will ultimately relapse. These patients are offered further chemotherapy to:
- Improve disease-related relapse
- Improve quality of life
- Delay time to progression
- Prolong survival.

This chemotherapy is called second-line chemotherapy.

The recurrent disease usually fall under one of three categories:
1. Patients who showed good response to initial therapy and disease recur later than 6 months of the completion of therapy are platinum-sensitive group are good prognostic and show the best response to retreatment with paclitaxel and carboplatin.
2. Women who relapse within 6 months of completing first line chemotherapy are classified as platinum resistant and have 10–30% likelihood of responding to chemotherapy. They are usually intermediate prognostic.
3. Patients are resistant to primary therapy and have shown tumor growth during treatment. They are refractory to the drug or platinum resistant and have <20% chance of response to chemotherapy. They should be treated by non-cross resistant chemotherapies or biological therapies. Their prognosis is bad.

Response to salvage chemotherapy markedly dependent upon the:
- Types of previous chemotherapy regimen such as third and fourth line chemotherapies are of limited benefit. Cancer relapses after primary treatment using a single agent have less resistant to treatment than cancer that relapses after primary treatment using multi-agent treatment.
- Size of the tumor, number, sites and histological type are also independent predictors of response to salvage chemotherapy.

Treatment of primary treatment sensitive recurrent cancer: Chemotherapy sensitive recurrent disease should be treated with primary chemotherapy. For low-volume disease, intraperitoneal chemo or radiotherapy can be considered. If relapse occurs more than 18 months after previous chemotherapy having up to 94% chance of response to subsequent platinum-based therapy. Whereas response is only 10% when those relapsing within 6 months of last platinum therapy.

Treatment of primary treatment resistant recurrent cancer: These groups of patients will not be benefited with rechallenge with conventional platinum regime. These patients appear to be benefit from single agent secondary chemotherapy drugs. These are, topotecan, single agent etoposide, docetaxel, gemcitabine, oxaliplatin, liposomal doxorubicin, 5-FU and leucovorin.

This platinum-resistant group of patients should strongly consider for phase II and some phase I clinical trials. The trial regime increases the dose density and dose intensity of platinum to overcome platinum resistance. With double dose of platinum weekly for 6 cycles achieved 46% response rate in comparison to 10–20% with conventional monotherapy and much higher response than primary platinum dose response <10%.

Role of second-look surgery: Second look surgery was previously a standard practice, done after a prescribed course of chemotherapy to determine the response to therapy. With the improvement in surgery and advancement in chemotherapy there is no evidence of disease at completion of treatment in 30% patients. Thus second look operation is seldom performed. Moreover, following chemotherapy, physical examination, serum CA-125 and CT scan and/or PET scan easily assess the response of therapy (though CT scan cannot image the tumors smaller than 2 cm). There is no difference in relapse free survival after second look surgery versus no surgery (Chu and Rubin, 2001). So second look surgery is now been replaced by secondary cytoreduction, where attempts at resection of macroscopic disease are done in recurrent cases.

The patients who are benefited with secondary cytoreduction are:
- Patients who develop recurrence (macroscopic disease) after a disease free interval of 12–24 months and whose disease is resectable.
- Patients whose recurrent disease is resectable regardless of disease free interval.

Role of Laparoscopy

There is no role in primary surgery, but it can be used for:
- Second-look surgery to assess response to treatments
- Secondary cytoreduction
- To administer intraperitoneal chemotherapy.

Case scenario: *Halima a 19-year-old unmarried girl presents to you with abdominal lump associated with abdominal pain, fullness, early satiety, urinary frequency and dysuria for the last 1 month. She is feeling that lump is growing very fast. Abdominal examination revealed a solid tender tumor with restricted mobility in the lower abdomen extending up to the umbilical region. There is no ascites. Her menstrual function is normal. USG of the whole abdomen reveals solid mass of about 15/12 cm in size arising from left adnexa. The right ovary and the uterus are normal.*

What is the probable diagnosis? What further investigations you want to suggest for diagnosis?

Age of patient, rapidity of growth, associated pain and undisturbed menstrual function suggests ovarian tumor, most probably germ cell tumor.

Suggestive investigations, which aid in diagnosis are:
- Tumor marker alpha-fetoprotein (AFP), hCG, lactic dehydrogenase (LDH) and placental alkaline phosphatase
- The CT scan of whole abdomen
- Chest X-ray
- Karyotyping.

Many germ cell tumors produce biologic marker that can be detected in serum. Serial measurement of circulating marker aid the diagnosis and more importantly are useful for monitoring response to treatment and detection of subclinical recurrences:
- The LDH and placental alkaline phosphatase (PLAP) are produced by as many as 95% of dysgerminomas.
- Embryonal carcinoma synthesizes both hCG and AFP.
- Endodermal sinus tumor produces AFP. Non-gestational choriocarcinoma produces hCG.
- Immature teratoma is devoid of secretion of marker.
- Germ cell tumors may be mixed cell types, produce more than one type of marker.
- CA-125 may be elevated in some patients with ovarian germ cell tumors, but this is nonspecific.

After laparotomy and careful exploration of the abdomino–pelvic cavity you found that the tumor is confined to one ovary and its capsule is intact and there is no adhesion. The other ovary is normal in size and appearance. There is no ascites.

How will you proceed?

Age and rapidity of growth and benign like feature on examination is suggestive of dysgerminoma. As almost all dysgerminoma are malignant frozen section biopsy of affected ovary and collection of peritoneal washing for cytology are to be done.

The histopathological report of frozen section shown features of dysgerminoma with evidence of malignancy. Cytology report is normal.

What steps do you want to take?

Surgical staging is to be done. Here the disease is confined to one ovary with intact capsule without any adhesion and there is no evidence of metastasis then we can consider it as stage IA disease. As patient is very young, tumor capsule is intact, no adhesion and cytology report normal, which indicates that there is no spillage and it is stage IA then conservative surgery is to be done such as:
- Unilateral salpingo-oophorectomy with preservation of the opposite ovary, tube and uterus
- Ipsilateral pelvic and bilateral para-aortic lympadenectomy
- Infracolic omentectomy
- Peritoneal biopsies.

For stage IA:
- No need of further follow-up
- No adjuvant chemotherapy is needed.

Note:
- Frozen section biopsy of healthy ovary is not recommended by some authors for two reasons:
  i. As dysgerminomas are highly responsive to both chemotherapy and radiotherapy so treatment of recurrent disease is very successful.
  ii. Biopsy of normal ovary may diminish fertility potential as a result of adhesion formation following biopsy, where fertility preservation is the only reason for conservation of ovary.
- After completion of her family the preserved ovary tube and uterus must be removed.

Suppose metastatic cancer cells found in the peritoneal fluid. What will be next step?

As patient needs to preserve reproductive function, even in the presence of metastatic disease, the contralateral ovary, fallopian tube and uterus should be preserved because of the sensitivity of the tumor to chemotherapy. Dysgerminoma is highly sensitive to both chemotherapy and radiotherapy.

Adjuvant chemotherapy is needed. The drugs of choice are Bleomycin 30,000 for 10 weeks for a total of 12 weeks, Etoposide 100 mg/m^2/day for 5 days every 3 weeks and cisplatin 20 mg/m^2/day for 5 days every 3 weeks [Bleomycin, Etoposide, Cisplatin (BEP regimen)].

After completion of family the preserved ovary, tube and uterus must be removed.

> If there is bilateral ovarian dysgerminoma in a patient who desires to preserve fertility what treatment option you can offer her?

There are no data regarding the ability of chemotherapy to eradicate a primary ovarian tumor, moreover, it could increase the risk for recurrence in these selected case.

So decision to preserve an involved ovary is difficult. With the advent of assisted reproductive technologies involving donor oocyte and hormonal support, it is potentially possible that a women without ovaries could sustain a normal intrauterine pregnancy, though not her own biological one.

So bilateral salpingo-oophorectomy with preservation of uterus can be considered in this case.

> **Case scenario:** Mrs Laila, a 36-year-old lady, mother of two children came to you with ovarian tumor. Tumor marker estimation revealed raised LDH level. At laparotomy, frozen section reveals dysgerminoma.
> What is your plan of treatment?

As Mrs Laila has two children and family is complete, she will undergo:
- Surgery:
  - Exploratory laparotomy
  - Pelvic washing
  - Total abdominal hysterectomy
  - Bilateral salpingo-oophorectomy
  - Ipsilateral pelvic and bilateral para-aortic lymphadenectomy
  - Infracolic omentectomy
  - Peritoneal biopsies
- Surgery should be followed by systemic chemotherapy.

> How will you follow-up the patient of dysgerminoma?

Follow-up care depends upon the stages of the disease. Ovarian dysgerminomas tend to recur most often within first 2–3 years of initial treatment. So follow-up observation and a physical examination should be done every 3–4 months for first 3 years, every 6 months during the 4th–5th year and annually for rest of the life:
- If tumor markers are negative during diagnosis CT imaging is to be considered during 6th and 12th months
- If tumor markers positive during diagnosis only LDH is to be done
- If tumor markers unknown then LDH, AFP and beta-hCG are to be done
- Increasing trend in tumor markers warrant repeat imaging and surgical exploration, if necessary
- If AFP and beta-hCG raised pregnancy should be ruled out in patient who underwent fertility sparing surgery
- Tumor markers begins to rise several months before the diagnosis of clinical recurrence.

> What is the prognosis of the disease?

In patients with stage IA disease, unilateral salpingo-oophorectomy alone results in 5-year disease free survival rate of greater than 95%. In patients with advanced disease surgery followed by chemotherapy (BEP), cure rate is about 90–100% (Williams, 1991). Ten year survival rates comparing conservative surgery alone versus surgery along with radiation are 92 and 85%, respectively.

RELATED INFORMATION

Germ cell tumors comprise approximately 20–25% of ovarian neoplasms overall, but account for only about 5% of all malignant ovarian neoplasms. These tumors arise primarily in young women between 10 and 30 years of age and about 70% of ovarian tumors in this age group is germ cell in origin (Zalel, 1996).

Ovarian germ cell tumors (OGCTs) grow rapidly and are associated with abdominal pain, which may be due to capsular stretching, hemorrhages and necrosis in the tumor. As a result most of the patients (65%) present with stage IA disease. This picture is unlikely with epithelial tumors, which grow slowly and produce symptom when the tumor has already spread in the peritoneal cavity.

So, about 75% of patients with malignant epithelial ovarian tumor present with advanced stage disease. Majority of the germ cell tumors present as unilateral ovarian masses except benign cystic teratoma, dysgerminoma and a tumor with components of dysgerminoma, which have bilateral distribution in 10–12% of cases.

Germ Cell Tumors of Extraembryonic Origin

Dysgerminoma

Dysgerminoma is the most common ovarian malignant germ cell tumor. About 20% of the patients with gonadal dysgenesis develop dysgerminoma and patients have stage 1 disease at diagnosis. These patients can be treated with unilateral salpingo-oophorectomy and if fertility is an issue, they can be observed carefully with regular pelvic exams, abdominal CT scan and tumor marker LDH. 15–25% of patients treated with conservative surgery recur and will require chemotherapy. In patients with more advanced disease, the risk of recurrence is significant enough and need adjuvant chemotherapy. Approximately 75% of recurrences occur within the 1st year after initial treatment and the most common sites being the peritoneal cavity and the retroperitoneal lymph nodes. Radiation therapy may be used for any stages Ib-III. The field of exposure extends from T11 to L5, with shielding of the contralateral ovary and the femur head.

Dysgerminoma in patients with karyotypic abnormality: Dysgerminoma may be associated with karyotypic abnormalities such as 46 XY (testicular feminizing syndrome), 45 XO (gonadal dysgenesis), 45 XO/46 XY (mixed gonadal dysgenesis). As they bear streak gonads and are usually sterile, both dysgerminoma and contralateral streak gonad must be removed to prevent gonadoblastoma formation. Individual with Y chromosome require delayed gonadectomy after puberty to allow the development of secondary sexual characteristics.

Endodermal Sinus Tumor (Yolk Sac Tumor)

These tumors derive from the primitive yolk sac. Approximately one third of the patients are premenopausal at time of presentation. Abdominal and pelvic pain is the most frequent presenting symptom in about 75% of patients.

Surgical treatment includes unilateral salpingo-oophorectomy, surgical staging and frozen section for diagnosis. Patients with all stages of disease needs adjuvant chemotherapy with conservative surgery and fertility can be preserved as other germ cell tumor. Before the routine use of combination chemotherapy for this disease the 2–3 years survival rate was 25%. Currently treatment with BEP regimen, the chance of cure approaches 100% for early stage patients and 75% for more advanced stage patients (Fujta, 1993).

Choriocarcinoma (Nongestational)

Choriocarcinoma usually arises from trophoblastic tissue of placenta. But here it arises from germ cell and associated with other malignant germ cell component and form a mixed tumor. It secretes beta-hCG, as trophoblastic tissue does. They are usually variable in size and nodular. Histological feature is identical to those of a gestational choriocarcinoma with both malignant cytotropoblast and syncytiotrophoblast. Diagnosis is difficult sometimes in reproductive age than postmenopausal women and prepubertal girls. But in an unmarried girl of reproductive age it might cause social problem. The prognosis is very poor. It rapidly spreads by invasion to other pelvic and abdominal organs. It also disseminated by blood and lymph. Chemotherapeutic response is not as good as gestational uterine choriocarcinoma due to its mixed germ cell component.

Germ Cell Tumors of Embryonic Origin

Immature Teratoma

Immature teratomas are the third most common form of malignant ovarian germ cell tumors. The immature elements almost always consists of immature neural tissue. Malignant transformation of a mature teratoma is reported to be between 0.5% and 2% of teratomas, usually in postmenopausal patients. These are rapidly developing, solid mass consisting of haphazard mass without formation of tissue. These are found in childhood and adolescent period and are highly malignant and fatal.

> **Case scenario:** Mrs Anisa, a 33-year-old lady is carrying for 16 weeks. She is a mother of two children. She developed lower abdominal pain for which she underwent USG and found a complex mass of 10 x 14 cm in left adnexal region. Tumor marker LDH is raised.
>
> How will you manage her?

Most likely, tumor may be dysgerminoma. These are usually malignant. So immediate surgery is indicated. Under general anesthesia a vertical incision is to be given because ovary will be placed higher than usual due to enlarging uterus.

Frozen section biopsy is to be done. If comes malignant total abdominal hysterectomy, bilateral salpingo-oophorectomy and infracolic omentectomy are to be done irrespective of fetal outcome. Because by the time of gaining fetal maturity the tumor may be metastasise. Lymphadenectomy is avoided as uterus obstructs pelvic sidewalls or para-aortic regions. Adjuvant chemotherapy is to be given after surgery.

> If patient is at or near term then what will be the management?

At or near term cesarean section is to be done first. Then rest procedure will be same as mentioned before.

Note: Same is true for all malignant ovarian tumors in pregnancy.

> **Case scenario:** Mrs Rodela, 22-year-old lady has been suffering from abdominal pain, bloating, loss of appetite and abdominal distension for few days. On examination irregular lump felt occupying whole of the lower abdomen, which seems bilateral ovarian mass. Due to fullness of the abdomen lump could not be moved freely. Bimanual examination revealed that irregular lump arises from both ovaries, which are free from adhesion.
>
> Contd...

> Contd...
>
> No deposit found in the posterior fornix. Exploratory laparotomy was done, bilateral ovarian lump of about 12 x 12 cm each were found, nodular, firm in consistency, capsule intact and free from adhesion. Ascites present and there is an irregular growth present in the under surface of the stomach.
>
> What is your diagnosis? What will be your plan of surgery?

- Most likely diagnosis is secondary malignant tumor of the ovary called Krukenbergs **(Fig. 13.1)** tumor with primary source in the stomach
- Frozen section biopsy is to be done to confirm the growth of the stomach
- Total abdominal hysterectomy, bilateral salpingo-oophorectomy, infracolic omentectomy, total gastrectomy, and esophagojejunostomy are to be done
- Adjuvant chemotherapy is to be given afterwards.

RELATED INFORMATION

Secondary malignant ovarian tumor occurs in 5% ovarian malignancies. Spread from primary sites that takes place via blood vessels and lymphatics by the mechanism of embolism and permeation.

Krukenberg tumors account for only 1–2% of all ovarian tumors (Fazzari et al. 2008; Al-Agha O and Nicastri, 2006). These tumors primarily originate from carcinomas of the GI tract and less commonly from the breast, gallbladder, colon, appendix or pancreas. Most common primary is the stomach and most generally follow a scirrhous type of carcinoma.

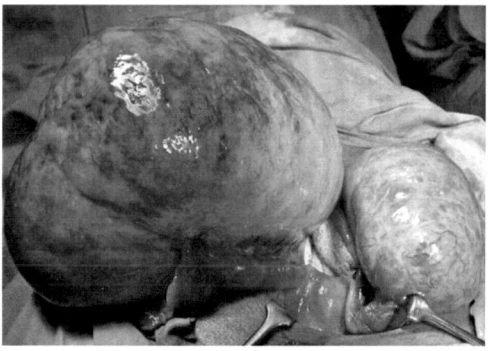

Fig. 13.1 Krukenberg's tumor (bilateral)
(For color version, see Plate 2)

In all cases of GI malignancy in the female, ovaries should be explored at the time of operation in addition to the exploration of the liver, mesenteric and retrogastric glands. In all solid tumors of the ovary, the stomach and intestines should be explored.

Microscopically, these tumors are characterized by mucin-secreting signet ring cells in the ovarian tissue and in the primary tumor site (Young and Scully, 1994; Mandai et al. 2001).

Patients with a Krukenberg tumor have a poor prognosis, with most patients averaging 2 years life expectancy, with a median survival time of 14 months (Benaaboud et al. 2002). The prognosis is poor when the primary tumor is identified after metastasis of the cancer to the ovaries.

> **Case scenario:** *A 30-year-old nulliparous lady had USG of pelvic organs as a part of infertility evaluation. Incidentally, a cyst of 10 x 9 cm was found in left ovary, which is partly cystic, partly solid and multilocular. CA-125 was done, which is 1,200 IU/L. On examination cyst is smooth, mobile, nontender with regular outline. On the basis of ultrasonographic findings and CA-125 it is suspected as malignant ovarian tumor. So exploratory laparotomy is planned. After laparotomy tumor was found intact, free from adhesion. Frozen section biopsy shows well-differentiated serous cystadenocarcinoma, peritoneal washing cytology was negative. Patient is very eager to preserve her fertility status.*
> *What surgical procedure do you like to perform on her?*

This is a case of stage IA serous cystadenocarcinoma. As patient wants to preserve her fertility status conservative surgery is to be done in the form of:
- Unilateral salpino-oophorectomy with preservation of the opposite ovary, tube and uterus
- Ipsilateral pelvic and bilateral para-aortic lymphadenectomy
- Infracolic omentectomy
- Peritoneal biopsies.

RELATED INFORMATION

Fertility Sparing Surgery of Malignant Ovarian Tumor

In more than two thirds of the cases epithelial ovarian cancers have an advanced disease during diagnosis as patients are symptomless until metastasis. Due to health consciousness and use of ultrasonography and other imaging tools in many situations early detection of ovarian cancer has increased. If it can be diagnosed at stage I conservative surgery to preserve fertility can be done.

The standard management of EOC even in stage I includes hysterectomy and bilateral salpingo-oophorectomy with peritoneal sampling-peritoneal washing, infracolic omentectomy, multiple peritoneal biopsies, and the removal of peritoneal implants with lymph node biopsy.

Mode of Surgery

In fertility preserving surgery for stage I disease a complete staging operation should be performed with preservation of the healthy ovary tube and uterus. Because lymph node metastasis were reported in patients with clinically apparent stage I ovarian carcinoma (Piver et al. 1978; Chen and Lee, 1983; Burghardt et al. 1991; Cass et al. 2001).

Adjuvant Therapy

Adjuvant chemotherapy in patients with stage I epithelial ovarian cancer is necessary in situations including:
- Unfavorable cell types (clear cell)
- Poor histologic differentiation
- Stage IC.

A number of studies have concluded that the use of adjuvant chemotherapy offers no survival advantage to patients with well-differentiated stage IA epithelial ovarian cancers (Young et al. 1990; Le et al. 1999).

Effect of Chemotherapy in Fertility

The recent regimens of chemotherapy include paclitaxel and carboplatin, cytotoxic effects of which have not been proven. In a small study, with using platinum-based cyclophosphamide there was no evidence of cytotoxic effects in the fertility compared to patients without adjuvant chemotherapy.

Treatment Afterwards

Complete surgery is to be done after completion of family. But time should be reasonable. For quick completion of family help of ART may be needed.

Alternative Treatment

Alternate treatment for fertility, if someone worried to keep other ovary or if there is fear of effect of chemotherapy in preserved ovary:

- The ultimate aim of fertility-preserving treatment in patients with early EOC is childbearing and delivery of a healthy infant. So it is not necessary that ovary must be preserved. By using advanced ART technology following can be preserved for future use in preserved uterus:
  - For unmarried girls/women oocyte and ovarian tissue can be preserved.
  - For married women oocyte, embryo and ovarian tissue can be preserved.

Can Oocyte Depletion be Prevented during Chemotherapy?

The ovarian toxicity of chemotherapeutic agents varies and depends on the patient's age, ovarian function before chemotherapy, the number of treatment cycles and the dose of the drug (Posada et al. 2001).

Concomitant use of gonadotropin—releasing hormone agonists (GnRHa) with chemotherapy may be beneficial in preserving future fertility in women treated with chemotherapeutic agents. GnRHa can reduce follicular loss in patients of different ages. Chemotherapeutic drugs are active against mitotically active cells (Clowse et al. 2009). It is believed that when ovaries are suppressed by GnRHa:

- Follicles are more resistant because they remain in an inactive state
- Suppression results in a reduction in ovarian blood flow, and therefore the chemotherapeutic agents do not reach the ovary in high concentrations
- The GnRHa may have direct ovarian effects that could limit the toxic effect of chemotherapy.

Each of these mechanisms might explain the potential benefits of adjuvant GnRHa treatment.

The long-acting GnRHa in pituitary-gonadal axis suppression is more lasting and stable. Generally, GnRHa adjuvant therapy should be maintained to the end of chemotherapy due to the metabolism of chemotherapeutic drugs. Therefore, 2 months after the completion of chemotherapy and generally at 6, 12 and 18 months follow-up, one should reassess the ovarian function.

BIBLIOGRAPHY

American College of Obstetricians and Gynecologists. Committee Opinion No. 620. Salpingectomy for ovarian cancer prevention. Obstet Gynecol. 2015; 125:279-81.

Al-Agha O, Nicastri AD. An in-depth look at Krukenberg tumor. Arch Pathol Lab Med. 2006;130:1725-30.

Benaaboud I, Ghazli M, Kerroumi M, Mansouri A. Krukenberg tumor: 9 cases report. J Gynecol Obstet Biol Reprod. 2002;31:365-70.

Best RL Jr, Klug TL, St John, et al. A radioimmunoassay using a monoclonal antibody to monitor the cause of epithelial ovarian cancer. N Ergl J Med. 1983;309(15):883-7.

Bristor RE, Tomacruz RS, Armstrong DK, et al. Survival effects of maximal cytoreductive surgery for advanced ovarian carcinoma during the platinum era: a meta-analysis; J Clini Oncol. 2002;20(5):1248-59.

Burghardt E, Girardi F, Lahousen M, et al. Patterns of pelvic and para and aortic lymph node involvement in ovarian cancer. Gynecol Oncol. 1991;40(2):103-6.

Casagrandle JT, Louie EW, Pike MC, et al. Incessant ovulation and ovarian cancer. Lancet. 1979;2:170-3.

Cass I, Li AJ, Runowicz CD, et al. Pattern of lymph node metastases in clinically unilateral stage I invasive epithelial ovarian carcinomas. Gynecol Oncol. 2001;80:56-61.

Chen SS, Lee L. Incidence of para-aortic and pelvic lymph node metastases in epithelial carcinoma of the ovary. Gynecol Oncol. 1983;16(1):95-100.

Choi JH, Wong AS, Huang HF, et al. Gonadotropin and ovarian cancer. Endor Rev. 2007;28:440-61.

Chu CS, Rubin SC. Second-look laparotomy for epithelial ovarian cancer: a reappraisal. Curr Oncol Rep. 2001;3(1):11-8.

Clowse ME, Behera MA, Anders CK, et al. Ovarian preservation by GnRH agonists during chemotherapy: a meta-analysis. J Womens Health (Larchmt). 2009;18:311-9.

Cure H, Battista C, Guastalla JP, et al. Phase III randomized trial of high-dose chemotherapy and peripheral blood stem cell support as consolidation in patients with advance ovarian cancer: Five-year follow-up of GINECO/FNCLCC/FGM-TC. Study (abstract) Proc Am Soc Clin Oncol, 23:449A, Abstract 5006;2004

David HM, Zurawski VR, Bast RC, et al. Characterization of the CA125 antigen associated with human epithelial ovarian carcinomas. Cancer Res. 1986;46:6143-8.

Eitan R, Levine DA, Abu-Rustum N, et al. The clinical significance of malignant pleural effusions in patients with optimally debulked ovarian carcinoma. Cancer 2005;103(7):1397-401.

Fazzari C, Fedele F, Pizzi G, et al. Krukenberg tumor of the ovary: a case report with light microscopy, immunohistochemistry and electron microscopy study. Anticancer Res. 2008;28:1417-20.

Frank TS, Manley SA, Olopade OL, et al. Sequence analysis of BRCA 1 and BRCA2: correction of mutations with family history and ovarian cancer risk. J Clin Oncol. 1998;16(7):2417-25.

Fujta M, Inove M, Tanizawa O, et al. Retrospective review of 41 patients with endodermal sinus tumor of the ovary. Int J Gynecol cancer. 1993;3(5):329-35.

Hacker NF, Berek JS, Lagasse D, et al. Primary cytoreductive surgery for epithelial ovarian cancer. Obstet Gynecol. 1983;61(4):413-20.

Heintz AP, Odicino F, Maisonneuve P, et al. Carcinoma of the ovary. FIGO 26th Annual Report on the results of treatment in gynecological cancer. Int J Gynecol Obstet. 2006;95(Supple 1):s161-92.

Hess LM, Benham-Hutchins M, Herzog TJ, et al. A meta-analysis of the efficacy of intraperitoneal cisplatin for the front-line treatment of ovarian cancer. Int J Gynecol Cancer. 2007;17(3):561-70.

Jacobs I, Davies AP, Bridges J, et al. Prevalence screening for ovarian cancer in postmenopausal women by CA125 measurements and ultrasonography in screening for ovarian cancer. BMJ. 1993;306(6884):1030-4.

Jensen A, Sharif H, Frederiksen K, Kjaer SK. Use of fertility drugs and risk of ovarian cancer: Danish Population Based Cohort Study. BMJ. 2009;338:b249.

Jordan SJ, Whiteman DC, Purdie DM, et al. Does smoking increase risk of ovarian cancer? A systematic review. Gynecol Oncol. 2006;103(3):1122-9.

Kinkel K, Hricak H, Lu Y, et al. US characterization of ovarian masses: a meta-analysis. Radiology. 2000;217(3):803-11.

Lacey JV Jr, Mink PJ, Lubin JH, et al. Menopausal hormone replacement therapy and risk of ovarian cancer. JAMA. 2002;288(3):334-41.

Le T, Krepart GV, Lotocki RJ, et al. Clinically apparent early stage invasive epithelial ovarian carcinoma: should all be treated similarly? Gynecol Oncol. 1999;74(2):252-4.

Lee KR, Young RH. The distinction between primary and metastatic mucinous carcinomas of the ovary: gross and histologic findings in 50 cases. Am J Surg Pathol. 2003;27(3):281-92.

Lynch HT, Cavalieri RJ, Lynch JF, et al. Gynecologic cancer clues to Lynch syndrome II diagnosis: a family report. Gynaecol Oncol. 1992;44(2):198-203.

Mandai M, Konishi I, Tsuruta Y, et al. Krukenberg tumor from an occult appendiceal adenocarcinoid: a case report and review of the literature. Eur J Obstet Gynecol Reprod Biol. 2001;97:90-5.

Markman M, Liu PY, Moon J, et al. Impact on survival of 12 versus 3 monthly cycles of paclitaxel (175 mg/m^2) administered to patients with advanced ovarian cancer who attained a complete response to primary platinum-paclitaxel: follow-up of a southwest oncology group and gynecologic oncology group phases 3 trial. Gynaecol Oncol. 2009;114(2):195-8.

McCluggage WG1, Young RH. Primary ovarian mucinous tumors with signet ring cells: report of 3 cases with discussion of so-called primary. Am J Surg Pathol. 2008;32(9):1373-9.

Mørch LS, Løkkegaard E, Andreasen AH, et al. Hormone therapy and ovarian cancer. JAMA.2009;302(3):298-305.

Musto A, Rampin L, Nanni C, Marzola MC, et al. Present and future of PET and PET/CT in gynaecologic malignancies. Eur J Radiol. 2011;78(1):12-20.

Ness RB, Carmer DW, Goodman MT, et al. Infertility, fertility drugs, and ovarian cancer: a pooled analysis of case-control studies. Am J Epidemiol. 2002;155(3):217-24.

Niloff JM, Bast RC Jr, Schaetzl, et al. Predictive value of CA-125 antigen level in second-look procedure for ovarian cancer. Am J Obstet Gynecol. 1985;151(7):981-6.

Orezzoli JP, Russell AH, Oliva E, et al. Prognostic implication of endometriosis in clean cell carcinoma of the ovary. Gynaecol oncol. 2008;110(3):336-44.

Piccart MJ, Bertelsen K, Stuart G, et al. Long-term follow-up confirms a survival advantage of the paclitaxel-cisplatin regimen over the cyclophosphamide cisplatin-combination in advanced ovarian cancer. Int J Gynecol Cancer. 2003;13(2):144-8.

Piver MS, Barlow JJ, Lele SB. Incidence of subclinical metastasis in stage I and II ovarian carcinoma. Obstet Gynecol. 1978;52(1):100-4.

Posada MN, Kolp L, García JE. Fertility options for female cancer patients: facts and fiction. Fertil Steril. 2001;75(4):647-53.

Rodriguez IM, Part J. Mucinous tumors of the ovary: a clinicopathologic analysis of 75 borderline tumors (of intestinal type) and carcinomas. Am J Surg Pathol. 2002;26(2):139-52.

Salanic R, Backes FJ, Fung MF, et al. Post-treatment surveillance diagnosis of recurrences in women with gynecologic malignancies: Society of Gynecologic Oncologists recommendations. Am Obstet Gynecol. 2011;204(16):466-78.

Seidman JD, Kurman RJ, Ronnett BM, Seidman JD, et al. Primary and metastatic mucinous adenocarcinomas in the ovary: incidence in routine practice with a new approach to improve intraoperative diagnosis. Am J Surg Pathol. 2003;27(7):985-93.

Williams SD, Blessing JA, Hatch KD, et al. Chemotherapy of advanced dysgerminoma: trials of the Gynecologic Oncology Group. J Clin Oncol. 1991;9(11):1950-5.

Young RC, Walton LA, Ellenberg SS, et al. Adjuvant therapy in stage I and stage II epithelial ovarian cancer: Results of two prospective randomized trials. N Engl J Med. 1990;322(15):1021-7.

Young RH, Scully RE. Metastatic tumors of the ovary. In: Kurman RJ (Ed). Blaustein's pathology of the female genital tract, 4th edn. New Delhi: Springer; 1994.pp.939-74.

Zalel Y, Piura B, Elchalal U, et al. Diagnosis and management of malignant germ cell ovarian tumors in young females. Int. Gynecol Obstet. 1996;55(1):1-10.

CHAPTER 14

Cervical Cancer

Farhat Hossain, Rashida Begum

INTRODUCTION

Cervical cancer is the second most common cancer in women worldwide and the most common female cancer in many developing countries. Annual global estimates for the year 2002 were 493,000 new cases and 274,000 deaths. Eighty three percent of these cancers occur in developing countries where risk before age 65 is 1.5% while in developed countries it accounts for only 3.6% of new cancers; with a cumulative risk (age 0–64) is 0.8% (Ferlay et al. 2004). The annual number of new cancer cases in Bangladesh is 12931 while the mortality from the disease is 6561 each year. Both the incidence and mortality rates are likely to be underestimated, because of poor registry reporting. In recent years, a causal relationship between persistent infection with high-risk human papilloma virus (HPV) and cervical cancer has been established (Walboomers et al. 1999). This causal relationship has led to the promise of global cervical cancer prevention using both primary prevention through vaccination against HPV and secondary prevention by screening directly (Schiffman and Castle 2005). Scientists are now exploring the cost-effectiveness of vaccination and screening strategies in the prevention of cervical cancer.

> **Case scenario:** Mrs Kulsum Begum, a 38-year-old multiparous woman of lower social class has come to you with the complaints of irregular pervaginal bleeding for four months.
> How will you proceed to make a diagnosis?

Detailed History

Age

Age should be taken into consideration. At this age dysfunctional uterine bleeding (DUB), pregnancy-related irregular bleeding may occur. Carcinoma cervix may also occur at this age. It has two peaks of age incidence, one is around 35 years and other is about 50–55 years.

Nature of Bleeding

- *Amount of bleeding*
- *Type of bleeding:* Cyclical or acyclical? Acyclical bleeding or metrorrhagia occurs due to surface lesion. As there is irregular bleeding it may be due to infected endometrial polyp, endometrial carcinoma, myomatous polyp, cervical polyp and cervical carcinoma.
- *History of preceding postcoital bleeding:* Occurs in cervical lesion.
- *History of preceding excessive vaginal discharge:* Presence of excessive vaginal discharge creamy or white or dirty brown in color, associated with foul smell is feature of cancer cervix. The offensive odor is caused by infection of necrotic tissue with saprophytes. Ninety percent patients of endometrial cancer also present with abnormal vaginal discharge.

About Menstrual Cycle

Menstrual cycle: Before 4 months how was her menstrual pattern? Before starting of irregular bleeding whether she had amenorrhea?

(in reproductive age, abortion-related bleeding need to be excluded)

About Parity

- *Number of children and age of last child:* More number of children has an association with carcinoma cervix.
- *Age of marriage:* Early marriage has an association with carcinoma cervix.
- *Pelvic pain:* It is a feature of cervical cancer in its advanced stage.
- *History of taking any drugs:* Irregular use of hormones (estrogen, progesterone) causes irregular bleeding.
- *History of diabetes mellitus (DM) and hypertension:* Obesity, DM and hypertension are risk factors for endometrial cancer. Women, who are overweight, have 3-10 fold increased risk of developing endometrial cancer because of increased peripheral conversion of androstenedione to estrone by aromatization in fat.

Physical Examination

- General examination:
  - Body built
  - Anemia.
- Per abdominal examination.
- Per vaginal examination.
- Per rectal examination.

> On enquiry, it was elicited that she was a regularly menstruating woman before 4 months. She had history of postcoital bleeding for long time before starting the irregular bleeding. She also gave history of profuse vaginal discharge before irregular per vaginal (PV) bleeding. She got married when she was 14 years old and she gave birth to eight children.
>
> On examination, she is average weighted, looking sick, anemic. On per abdominal examination no abnormality was detected. Per vaginal (PV) examination: On inspection foul smelled dirty bleeding present. On speculum test, a small fungating growth is present in the anterior lip of the cervix. It was friable and bleeds on touch. Bimanual examination revealed normal-sized uterus and thickened right lateral fornix. Rectovaginal examination revealed bilateral free parametrium.
>
> On the basis of these findings what is your diagnosis?

On the basis of history and examination findings most likely diagnosis is carcinoma cervix.

> *For confirmation, which test do you like to do?*

Histopathology of tissue from growth will give confirm diagnosis.

> *Is there any role of Pap smear here?*

No. Pap smear is a screening test. Here, growth is obvious so only biopsy will be done here. Moreover, Pap becomes negative as active cancer cells lie in deep of the lesion and superficial desquamated cells give false result.

> *Is there any role of tumor markers in diagnosis of carcinoma cervix or extent of the disease?*

No. Squamous cell carcinoma antigen (SCCA) is present in normal squamous cervical epithelium and its expression is increased in cervical squamous cell cancer, but is insufficiently reliable for diagnosing the disease and identifying the risk of having extension and metastasis.

RELATED INFORMATION

Types of Growth

According to site of the growth it is one of the following types:

1. *Squamous cell carcinoma (70-75%):* It arises at squamocolumnar junction or transformation zone of the cervix. Cells are large cell keratinizing (Grade-1 or well-differentiated tumor), large cell non-keratinizing (Grade-2 or moderately differentiated tumor), small non-keratinizing (Grade-3 or poorly differentiated tumor). Growth may be only.
   - *Eroding:* Very early stage can simulate erosion. May be microinvasive or invasive.
   - *Ulcerative:* Usually infiltrative and invasive.
   - *Hypertrophic or exophytic:* Cauliflower-like fungating growth, definitely invasive.
2. *Adenocarcinoma (20-25%):* When growth arises from columnar cells of the endocervix. Hence, the name is adenocarcinoma. It is usually *ulcerative* and *infiltrative* type. Cervix becomes hard, indurated and barrel shaped.

At early stage, it remains hidden and patient remains symptomless. So, diagnosis is usually delayed in case of adenocarcinoma.
3. *Adenosquamous (1–2%)*: When adenocarcinoma extends to exocervix then forms adenosquamous growth where both squamous and columnar cells are present. On rare occasion, synchronous adenocarcinoma and squamous carcinoma may develop and may invade each other called collision tumors.
4. *Other rare types are*:
   - Adenoma malignum
   - Verrucous carcinoma
   - Adenoid cystic carcinoma
   - Neuroendocrine carcinoma
   - Small cell carcinoma
   - Undifferentiated carcinoma.

Symptoms

Symptoms are evident when there is surface ulceration on the cervix. In the early stage of the disease it remained symptomless.
- *Postcoital bleeding*: Earliest symptom is postcoital bleeding. So, history of any postcoital bleeding must need evaluation to exclude carcinoma cervix.
- *Perimenopausal or postmenopausal bleeding*: The first episode of bleeding commonly follows coitus or straining at stool. Later the bleeding becomes heavy. In perimenopausal patients, the usual menstrual bleeding either normal or heavy but in addition there is intermenstural bleeding. With progression, in both cases (perimenopausal or postmenopausal) the patient experiences continuous per vaginal bleeding.
- *Per vaginal discharge*: Purulent and non-pruritic discharge is frequently present. This is at first creamy or white, but subsequently resembles dirty brown water. It becomes offensive with characteristic odor when there is infection of necrotic tissue with saprophytes.

Symptoms Related to Advanced Cancer

- *Loss of weight and weakness* at late stage of the disease.
- *Pelvic pain* particularly in the lumbosacral or gluteal area indicates possibility of iliac or para-aortic lymph node involvement with extension into lumbosacral nerve roots or hydronephrosis.
- *Hematuria/rectal bleeding* suggests invasion of bladder or rectum.
- *Hemoptysis* and persistent cough suggests lung metastasis.
- *Incontinence:* Vaginal passage of urine or feces is suggestive of vesicovaginal and rectovaginal fistula.

Physical Examination Findings

- *General examination:*
  - Anemia: In chronic bleeding or prolonged heavy bleeding, anemia is a common manifestation.
  - Palpable liver, supraclavicular and groin nodes due to metastasis in these regions.
- *Speculum examination*:
  - Eroding or ulcerative lesion can be visualized **(Fig. 14.1A)**.
  - In exophytic lesion, the growth is cauliflower, ulcerative or polypoidal and is well visualized **(Figs 14.1B and 1C)**.
  - In endophytic lesion, the growth is hidden from view in the endocervical canal. The ectocervix appears normal macroscopically. Extension of growth into the vagina can be visualized.
  - May bleed due to touch of speculum.
- *Bimanual examination*: This examination gives an assessment of the size of the uterus, involvement of vaginal fornices and diameter of the growth. The feeling of growth is usually irregular, hard or firm in consistency, friable, fix and growth bleeds on examination. Cervix may be fixed due to thickening of uterosacral and cardinal ligament by extensive parametrial involvement by infiltrative lesion. Fixation occurs relatively early in endophytic growth and the cervix feels big, broad and barrel shaped.
- *Rectovaginal examination*: Extension of the disease into the parametrium and uterosacral ligament is best evaluated by rectovaginal examination. Thus this examination carries significant importance for clinical staging of the disease. Rectal mucosa becomes fixed and indurated if growth extends to bowel.

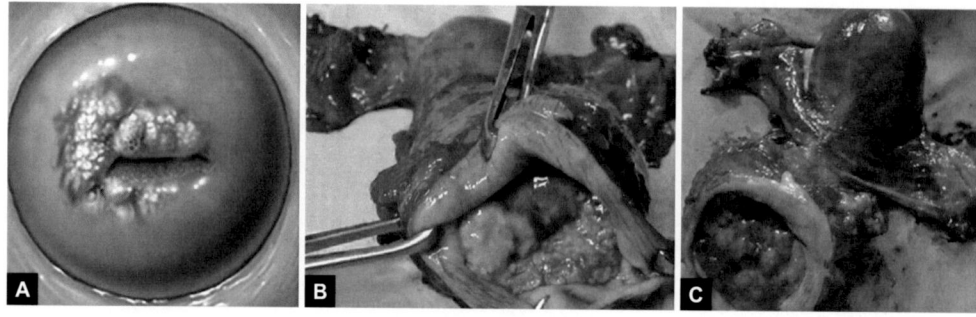

Figs 14.1A to C (A) Ulcerative growth; (B) Exophytic growth; (C) Cauliflower growth
(For color version, see Plate 3)

Which of the growth is more dangerous?

- *Exophytic versus endophytic growth*: Endophytic growths are diagnosed relatively late and it spreads to the broad ligaments and lymph nodes relatively early-thus carries bad prognosis in comparison to exophytic growth.
- *Adenocarcinoma versus squamous cell carcinoma*: Adenocarcinoma bears poor prognosis than squamous cell carcinoma, because they are usually diagnosed in advanced stage. Patients are usually young. They are usually endocervical in type. Moreover, adenocarcinomas are assumed to be less radiosensitive, because they are bulky tumors and thus are predominantly made of hypoxic cells.

Factors Playing Role in Developing Carcinoma Cervix (Etiology)

A. Predominant factor

Human papilloma virus (HPV): It is a necessary cause of cervical cancer [Walboomers, 1999]. The eight most common HPV types detected in descending order of frequency are HPV 16, 18, 45, 31, 33, 52, 58 and 35 and these are responsible for about 90% of all cervical cancers worldwide. Presence of HPV is demonstrated in more than 75–95% of all cervical intraepithelial neoplasia (CIN) lesions and in 95–100% of all invasive cancers (Bosch et al. 1995; Jacobs et al. 1997). HPV 16 is the most prevalent in squamous cell carcinoma and HPV 18 is the most prevalent in adenocarcinoma. HPV is epitheliotropic. Once it invades epithelium acutely it turns into one of following three stages:

1. It may remain latent asymptomatic.
2. It replicates with active infection, but not integrated into the genome of human and is responsible for development of CIN I and condyloma.
3. It replicates with integration into the human genome causing *immortalization of cell* and undergoes malignant transformation.

Almost 90% of squamous cell carcinoma of the cervix develops from intraepithelial layer.

B. Potential cofactor

1. *Established cofactors*
   - *Smoking*: Smoking is directly related to squamous cell carcinoma (SCC) of cervix. Cigarette smoking and HPV infection has synergistic effect on the development of CIN and smoking is associated with 2-4 fold increase in the relative risk for development of carcinoma cervix. The smoke carcinogens accumulate in the cervical mucus, but mechanism of carcinogenesis is poorly understood. The probable mechanism involved in carcinogenesis includes:
     - Reduction of immune response in the cervix
     - Direct genetic damage caused by tobacco related carcinogens.

     Cigarette smokers are found to have increased risk of SCC and the risk is directly related to the number of cigarettes smoked per day.
   - *Long-term oral contraceptive use*: Combined oral contraceptive pill has been categorized as carcinogenic to the cervix by International Agency for Research on Cancer (IARC) (Cogliano, 2005). The

risk increases with increasing duration of use. Ten years use is associated with the doubling in risk of cancer. Estrogen or progesterone enhances HPV gene-expression in the cervix via progesterone receptor.
- *Co-infection with HIV:* HIV infection is an immonocompromised state and such conditions are at increased risk of cervical cancer.
- *High parity:*
  - High parity causes transformation zone to be exposed on the exocervix for many years, which facilitates its exposure to HPV infection.
  - Hormonal changes during pregnancy possibly making women more susceptible to HPV infection and cancer growth.
  - Pregnant women might have weaker immune system allowing for HPV infection and cancer growth.

2. *Probable cofactors*:
   - *Co-infection with Chlamydia trachomatis and herpes simplex virus-2 (HSV-2)*: Increased risk associated with CT and HSV-2 is due to inflammatory response, which generates free radicals and causes genetic instability.
   - *Early age of sexual debut*: Early sexual debut is associated with cervical cancer, because of the following mechanisms:
     - Cervical immaturity
     - Inadequate production of protective cervical mucus
     - Increased cervical ectopy.

   All these make an individual susceptible to HPV infection.
   - *Multiple sexual partners*: In multiple sexual partner relationship, there is increased likelihood of exposure to HPV infected partners and partners who have sexual exposure to someone with cervical neoplasia.

Differential Diagnosis of Carcinoma Cervix

- Chronic cervicitis
- Cervical tuberculosis
- Condyloma acuminata
- Cervical ectropion
- Cervical erosion
- Ulceration due to syphilis, granuloma inguinale
- Lymphogranuloma venereum and chancroid
- Vaginal growth
- Cervical polyp
- Myomatous polyp.

> You received Mrs Kulsum's biopsy report, which shows invasive and moderately differentiated squamous cell carcinoma.
> What will be the next action?

Clinical staging is to be done by examining the patient under general anesthesia along with some investigative aid:
- Thorough clinical evaluation includes per speculum examination, bimanual examination and rectovaginal examination.
- Investigations needed for staging are:
  - Cervical biopsy
  - Endocervical curettage (ECC)
  - Colposcopy—when the lesion is not visualized in cervix in naked eye
  - Cystoscopy
  - Proctoscopy
  - Intravenous urography (IVU)
  - Chest X-ray
  - In suspected cases of bladder or rectal involvement, biopsy from these particular sites and histopathological evidence are needed.

RELATED INFORMATION

Staging of Cervical Cancer (Table 14.1)

Table 14.1 FIGO staging of cervical cancer

FIGO stage	Description
Stage 0	Carcinoma in situ (confined within the epithelium)
Stage I	Cervical carcinoma confined to the cervix
• Stage IA	Invasive cervical cancer diagnosed by microscope only
– Stage IA$_1$	Stromal invasion no deeper than 3 mm, no wider than 7 mm in horizontal spread

Contd...

Contd...

FIGO stage	Description
– Stage IA$_2$	Stromal invasion greater than 3 but less than 5 mm and no wider than 7 mm in horizontal spread
• Stage IB	Clinically visible lesion confined to the cervix or microscopic disease greater than stage 1A
– Stage IB$_1$	Lesion not greater than 4 cm
– Stage IB$_2$	Lesion greater than 4 cm
Stage II	Tumor extends beyond uterus, but not to pelvic side wall or lower third of vagina
• Stage IIA	Vaginal involvement without parametrial involvement (**Fig. 14.2A**)
• Stage IIB	Parametrial involvement (**Fig. 14.2B**)
Stage III	Tumor extends to pelvic side wall and/or causes hydronephrosis and/or extends to lower third of vagina
• Stage III A	Involvement of lower third of vagina with no extension to side wall
• Stage III B	Extension to pelvic side wall and or hydronephrosis
Stage IV	Extension beyond the true pelvis or into mucosa of rectum or bladder
• Stage IVA	Extension into adjacent organ
• Stage IVB	Distant metastasis

(*Adopted from* FIGO Annual Report on the results of treatment in gynaecologic cancer 1998)

Note:
- The clinical staging must not be changed, because of subsequent finding. In cases treated by surgical procedures, the pathologist's findings in the removed tissues should not be allowed to change the clinical staging. They can be recorded as pathological staging, which determines exactly the extent of disease.
- If pelvic examination shows uterus in normal size with free fornices and rectovaginal examination reveals bilateral free parametrium, but the X-ray chest reveals metastasis in the lung or there is bilateral hydronephrosis in IVU, the accurate clinical staging will be cancer cervix stage IVB or cancer cervix stage IIIB respectively regardless of pelvic findings.

Thus, *primary clinical staging must include the essential investigations required in addition to clinical evaluation.*

Accuracy Rate in Clinical Staging

Clinical staging is often inaccurate in defining the extent of disease. Inaccuracy is observed as much as 24% for stage IB and 67% for stage IVA. Most patients are upstaged following surgical exploration.

Importance of Staging

Staging is done to plan appropriate therapy:
- It determines the prognosis of the disease
- It allows comparison of results of therapy from various centers.

Spread of the Disease

Lymphatic Spread

Lymphatic spread occurs by embolism or permeation. Earliest spread occurs at the base of broad ligament and uterosacral ligament. Commonly involved nodes are obturator, external iliac and bifurcation of common iliac, internal iliac, sacral and para-aortic. In early stromal invasion up to a depth of 3 mm chance of lymphatic spread is less. When penetration increased >3 mm lymphatic involvement is likely and tumor cells are carried to the regional lymph nodes. Early

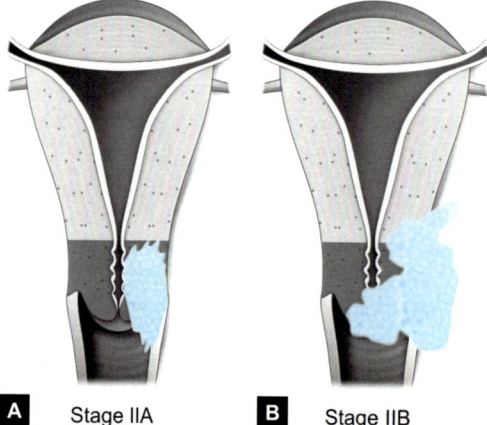

A Stage IIA **B** Stage IIB

Figs 14.2A and B (A) Malignant cells involved vagina only (Stage IIA); (B) Malignant cells involved vagina and parametrium (Stage IIB)

invasion <1 mm is associated with risk of lymph node involvement only 0.02%, 1-<3 mm and 3-5 mm invasion are associated with risk of involvement of 0.6% and 6.5% respectively.

Direct Extension

The growth due to increment of size gradually spreads around directly. According to direction of expansion of growth it extends to the adjacent organs. Usually extends to body of the uterus, the vaginal wall, the bladder and the cellular tissue of the broad and uterosacral ligaments. Due to deep pouch of Douglas direct invasion to the rectum is delayed and rare. It may cause hydronephrosis by creating pressure on the lower end of the ureter by broad ligament growth. It may also cause sciatic pain by irritating sacral plexus by expanding growth though nerves or sheaths are not involved.

Bloodstream Spread

Bloodstream spread takes the cancer cells to any part of the body called distant metastasis. The liver and lungs are the most common sites of distant metastasis followed by brain, bones, bowels, adrenal glands, spleen and pancreas. Involvement of ovaries is rare 0.5% in case of squamous cell carcinoma and 1.7% in adenocarcinoma. The more advanced the local disease, greater the chance of distant metastasis.

> Mrs Kulsum's clinical staging shows cancer cervix stage IIA.
> What will be your approach for pretreatment evaluation?

Pretreatment Evaluation for Cancer Cervix

- Thorough history
- Physical examination
- Ultrasonography of pelvic organs
- Cervical biopsy
- Conization if needed
- Complete blood count (CBC)
- Liver function tests (LFTs)
- Renal function test (RFTs)
- Chest X-ray
- Intravenous urography (IVU)
- Magnetic resonance imaging (MRI) or
- Computed tomography (CT) scan or
- Positron emission tomography (PET) scan.

RELATED INFORMATION

Radiological Staging

International Federation of Gynecology and Obstetrics (FIGO) staging does not consider the result of radiological assessment. Radiological assessment of the patients with obvious visible cancer of cervix is essential part in determining the most appropriate management of patients both for primary disease, relapsed disease and complications of treatment. Thus, it is helpful in treatment planning.

Three options are available:
1. Magnetic resonance imaging (MRI).
2. Computer tomography (CT) scan.
3. Positron emission tomography (PET) scan.

Magnetic Resonance Imaging

Magnetic resonance imaging (MRI) is considered as a valuable tool in pretreatment evaluation of cancer cervix. It is the best imaging modality because of improved soft tissue resolution. It has the ability to determine accurately.

- Tumor diameter (93% accuracy)
- Depth of stromal invasion (78% accuracy)
- Parametrial extension (90% accuracy)
- Lymph node involvement (60% sensitivity)
- Bladder involvement (75% sensitivity)
- Rectal involvement (71% sensitivity)
- Corpus extension.

Advantages of MRI over CT Scan

- Magnetic resonance imaging (MRI) is more accurate in primary tumor assessment of Ca Cx than CT scan (40–97% accuracy) and both modalities are more accurate than clinical staging, though tumor diameter less than 5–10 mm cannot be reliably imaged by either modality. MRI is also superior to CT scan in assessment of vaginal invasion (78–94% accuracy), parametrial invasion (75–90% accuracy) and bladder and rectal invasion.
- The MRI is superior to CT in detecting lymph nodes in cancer cervix. MRI can detect the

lymph node sized <1 cm which the CT cannot rectify. But no one can differentiate between metastatic and non-metastatic enlargement of lymph node.

Disadvantages of MRI over CT Scan

- Magnetic resonance imaging cannot be used in patients with pacemakers or metallic implants
- Intervention procedures cannot be performed simultaneously
- It is costly
- More time is required (30–60 minutes).

Note: CT scan is more appropriate than MRI in above-mentioned case as well as for women with clinically apparent stage IVA or IVB disease, postcontrast spiral or multi-slice scan of chest, abdomen and pelvis.

Positron Emission Tomography

Positron emission tomography (PET) is more accurate than CT and MRI in detecting metastatic lymphadenopathy, which can significantly change the patient management and survival. PET is a new imaging modality that depends on metabolic alteration for detection of cancer cervix. PET can detect sites of malignancy by identifying sites of increased glycolysis. Fluoro-2-deoxy–D-glucose (FDG) is used. Because cancer cells are users of glucose, there is uptake of glucose and PET can easily recognize those sites. Thus, PET scan has the potential to determine more accurately the extent of disease, particularly in pelvic lymph node that are not enlarged and in distant sites that are not detectable by conventional imaging studies.

> What will be the treatment option for Mrs Kulsum?

The treatment option in such a case would be *"radical hysterectomy (RH) with pelvic lymphadenectomy"* followed by *adjuvant therapy*.

RELATED INFORMATION

Surgical Treatment of Cancer Cervix

Primary surgery is applicable for only stage I and early stage II cases. Though radiotherapy is equally effective in these cases, but advantages of primary surgery are:

- It has the advantage of removing the primary disease and allowing accurate surgical staging, thereby allowing adjuvant therapy to be more accurately targeted
- It allows resection of bulky positive lymph nodes, which cannot be sterilized by radiation only, thereby improving the prognosis significantly
- In young women, primary surgery has the advantage of preserving the ovarian function
- It also gives a sense of relief to the patient that the disease organ has been removed
- It overcomes the difficulties of introduction of radium in narrow vagina or in endocervical tumor.
- It is applicable in Ca Cx associated with pregnancy.

Radical Hysterectomy with Lymphadenectomy

Radical hysterectomy with pelvic lymphadenectomy was previously called Wertheim's hysterectomy as Wertheim first described this procedure. In Wertheim's original operation selectively only enlarged lymph nodes were removed. Subsequently much modification was done in the procedure with extensive tissue dissection and removal of lymph nodes. Some modification was done to keep the nerve intact to reduce the incidence of bladder and bowel dysfunction and to decrease the rate of ureteric fistula formation.

Currently 5 classes of hysterectomy are described for carcinoma cervix

Type I: Extrafascial hysterectomy with removal of all cervical tissue. It is done in IA$_1$ disease.

Type II: Modified radical hysterectomy:
- Uterine artery is ligated medial to ureter
- Uterosacral ligaments are resected midway between the uterus and their sacral attachments
- Medial half of the cardinal ligaments are removed
- The upper one third (1/3rd) of vagina is resected.

Type III: Classical Meigs' radical hysterectomy:
- The uterine artery is ligated at its origin from internal iliac artery
- Uterosacral ligaments are resected at their sacral attachments
- Cardinal ligaments are resected at the pelvic wall
- The uterosacral and cardinal ligaments are divided at their attachment to sacrum and pelvic sidewall
- The upper half (1/2) of vagina is resected.

Type IV:
- The ureter is completely dissected from the vesicouterine ligament
- The superior vesical artery is sacrificed
- Three fourth (3/4th) of vagina is resected

Type V:
- Additional resection of portion of bladder
- Resection of lower part of ureter
- Reimplantation of ureter into the bladder

Stage-wise Surgical Options

Surgery for Microinvasive Carcinoma

Microinvasive carcinoma is defined as a lesion that invades to a depth of 3–5 mm below the basement membrane and the horizontal spread is less than 7 mm.

Stage IA$_1$

Option 1: Extrafascial or type I radical hysterectomy. No need of pelvic lymph node dissection as the prevalence of lymph node metastasis is low (0.8–2.6%).

Option 2 (fertility preserving surgery if patient desires child):
Conization is the only acceptable treatment, provided:
- Depth of invasion is 3 mm or less
- Surgical margins are negative
- No evidence of lymphovascular space invasion (LVSI)
- Endocervical curettage is negative.

Note: If cone margin or endocervical curettage (ECC) reveals high-grade dysplasia or microinvasive carcinoma *repeat conization* should be done to rule out invasive disease.

Stage IA$_2$

Option 1: Modified radical hysterectomy with pelvic lymph node dissection. Prevalence of lymph node metastasis is high, 3.4% (<7 mm horizontal spread) and 9.1% (>7 mm horizontal spread).

Option 2 (fertility preserving surgery if patient desires child):
Conization or radical trachelectomy and extraperitoneal or laparoscopic pelvic lymph node dissection.

Note: *Fertility preserving surgery* is only applicable where possibility of adequate and regular follow-up by cytology and colposcopy can be ensured.

Surgery for Stage IB and IIA

Patients with *stage IB and stage IIA* are universally regarded as being ideal candidates for radical hysterectomy *RH and pelvic lymphadenectomy*, although equal cure rates may be obtained with primary radiation therapy.

Procedure Involved in Radical Hysterectomy

The most commonly performed operation is a *combination of type II and type III radical hysterectomy* where anatomic nerve supply to the bladder is not threatened:
- Structures removed are:
  - Uterus
  - Fallopian tubes and sometimes ovaries
  - Upper one-third of vagina
  - Medial half of cardinal ligament
  - Proximal half of uterosacral ligament.
- The uterine artery is ligated at its origin from internal iliac artery or superior vesicle artery.
- Anterior leaf of the ureteric tunnel is cut and ligated.

Pelvic Lymphadenectomy

Pelvic lymphadenectomy includes dissection of all fatty lymph node bearing tissue anterior, lateral and posterior to common, external and internal iliac vessels and anterior to obturator nerve.

Obturator lymph node is the first and most common site of tumor metastasis followed by internal iliac lymph node. It is called sentinel nodes.

Guidelines to be Followed for Dissection of Pelvic Lymph Nodes

Pelvic lymphadenectomy for cancer cervix includes systemic en-block removal of pelvic lymph nodes. Removal must be confined within the boundary as follows:

Proximal : Bifurcation of common iliac blood vessels
Distal : Lateral circumflex iliac vein
Lateral : Genitofemoral nerve on psoas muscle
Medial : Internal iliac artery
Inferior : Obturator nerve

Importance of Pelvic Lymphadenectomy in Radical Hysterectomy

Pelvic lymphadenectomy is an essential component of RH. Pelvic lymph nodes are the most important independent determinant of survival in cancer cervix. Thus pelvic lymphadenectomy has diagnostic, therapeutic and prognostic value in cancer cervix.
- Pelvic lymphadenectomy helps to differentiate between metastatic and nonmetastatic lymph node and thereby accurately target adjuvant therapy.
- It determines the prognosis of the disease.
- External beam radiotherapy (EBRT) is incapable of sterilizing bulky metastatic lymph nodes. Removal of such lymph nodes helps to achieve better tumor control by adjuvant radiation and thus provide survival benefit.
- Pelvic lymphadenectomy is a simple procedure in the hands of expert with less time consumption (25 minutes) with minimum blood loss (25 mL) and minimum morbidity.

Route of Surgery

- *Abdominal*: Commonly done.
- *Vaginal*: Less extensive RH can be carried out by vaginal route (Schauta's or Schauta-Amreich's operation) where lymph node dissection cannot be carried out. To correct this deficiency two separate abdominal incisions can be given for bilateral extraperitoneal lymphadenectomy. Alternatively laparoscopic lymphadenectomy can be done.
- *Laparoscopy*: Laparoscopic radical hysterectomy and pelvic lymphadenectomy can be done. It needs expertise. It reduces the operative morbidity and hospital stay in comparison to abdominal route.

Complications of Radical Hysterectomy

- **Intraoperative:**
  - *Blood loss:* Average blood loss is between 500 mL and 1,500 mL.
  - *Injuries:* Intraoperative injuries occasionally occur to pelvic blood vessels, ureter, bladder, rectum and obturator nerve.
- **Postoperative:**
  - *Early:*
    - Urinary tract infection (UTI)
    - Wound infection
    - Paralytic ileus/Lymphocyst formation
    - Venous thrombosis
    - Ureterovaginal fistula (due to direct injury or ischemic injury or both)
    - Vesicovaginal fistula (due to direct injury or ischemic injury or both)
  - *Late:*
    - Bladder dysfunction
    - Sexual dysfunction
    - Lymphedema—onset of lymphedema occurs within 3 months in 53% of patients, within 6 months in 71% and 12 months in 84% of patients. Postoperative radiation further enhances the risk of lymphedema.

> Mrs Kulsum's histopathology report shows the metastasis in two pelvic lymph nodes. The vaginal cuff is free of tumor and there was no parametrial involvement in clinical examination.
> On this ground which adjuvant therapy will be selected for her?

The most important prognostic factor in cervical cancer is the status of pelvic lymph nodes. The patient falls in high-risk group and should be treated by *concurrent chemoradiation following surgery*. *Chemoradiation* improves pelvic control, higher disease-free survival and overall survival.

RELATED INFORMATION
Postoperative Adjuvant Therapy

The decision for postoperative adjuvant therapy is taken on grounds of risk factors, which predisposes to pelvic recurrence and distant recurrences. Thus, the disease-free survival and overall survival of the patient is greatly affected. Factors predicting high failure rate includes:
- **High risk factors**
  - Positive pelvic lymph nodes
  - Positive parametrial disease
  - Positive surgical margin.
- **Intermediate risk factors**
  - Bulky tumor (>4 cm)
  - Depth of stromal invasion (>⅓)
  - Lymphovascular space invasion (LVSI)
  - Histologic cell type (small cell carcinoma and adenocarcinoma are reported as poor prognostic factors).

Modalities of Adjuvant Therapy

They are:
- Radiotherapy (RT)
- Concurrent chemoradiation.

Radiotherapy
There are two main modalities of irradiation in cancer cervix:
- External irradiation or external beam radiotherapy (EBRT) or teletherapy.
- Intracavitary radiotherapy or brachytherapy.

Radiotherapy is the treatment of choice in majority of cases of cancer cervix and is applicable in all stages of disease. It is solely the gold standard of treatment for advanced disease. Patients with intermediate risk factors should receive EBRT (pelvic radiation). Brachytherapy should be added to the regime if there are positive surgical margins. In patients having high-risk factors, concurrent chemoradiation is the preferred adjuvant treatment.

Its aim is to deliver cancericidal dose of 70–80 Gy to the cervix, which is distributed in point A and point B:

- Point A is situated 2 cm above the mucosa of lateral vaginal fornix and 2 cm lateral to central uterine canal and represents cervix and paracervix.
- Point B is 3 cm lateral to point A and represents parametrium and pelvic lymph nodes.

Mechanism of Action of Radiation

Gamma rays act on the targeted cancer cells both directly and indirectly.

Directly: It directly kills cancer cells by breaking the DNA strands of the cells. It accounts for 1/3rd damage of target cells.

Indirectly: It kills cancer cells by interacting with H_2O of tissue, liberating OH radical, which diffuses to DNA of cells and causes damage. It accounts for 2/3rd damage of target cell.

Radiation induced cell death eventually occurs either by cell necrosis or apoptosis.

Techniques of Delivery of Radiotherapy

1. **External irradiation or external beam radiotherapy (EBRT) or teletherapy:** EBRT preferably from a linear accelerator is given in short daily treatment (180–200 #) over a period of 5 weeks (Sunday to Thursday basis) (5 × 5 = 25 days). A total of 50 Gy is given covering the *parametrium* and *pelvic lymph nodes*, which are the target organs of coverage for EBRT. This fractionation of the total dose required is much more effective than single dose.

Portals Used

Four-field technique is adopted in EBRT. This is:
a. Anteroposterior beam (AP beam).
b. Posteroanterior beam (PA beam).
c. Two lateral beams.

The use of lateral beams allows significant protection of small bowels.

Extended Field Radiotherapy

Extended field radiotherapy (EFRT) is beneficial for patients with proven positive para-aortic lymph node metastasis, but this technique delivers a high dose of radiation to surrounding organs such as spinal cord, kidneys and small intestine, which is beyond their tolerance. Thus, its use is controversial. Moreover, majority of patients with para-aortic nodal metastases have systemic disease, which do not achieve benefit with EFRT in terms of survival.

Various techniques are now utilized to deliver EFRT. Intense modulating radiation technique (IMRT) is one such technique where high doses of RT can be delivered to target organ, while maintaining acceptable doses to surrounding tissues.

For patients without proven para-aortic nodal disease study demonstrated that pelvic radiation plus concurrent chemotherapy was superior to prophylactic extended field radiation without chemotherapy (Morris, 1999). Radioactive isotopes currently being used are cesium and cobalt-60.

2. **Intracavitary radiotherapy or brachytherapy:** Brachytherapy or intracavitary therapy is very effective in cervical cancer, because high dose can be given centrally within the tolerance level of adjacent normal tissues. Brachytherapy is always given after EBRT, as tumor geometry must be corrected beforehand for effective application of applicators. The target organ of coverage by brachytherapy is the cervix and paracervical tissue.

Afterload Technique

This is the technique adopted for brachytherapy. Intrauterine tandem and paired vaginal colpostats or ovoids are inserted in the lateral fornix under general anesthesia (GA), but sources are introduced later by remote control. Thus, medical and nursing staffs are protected from radiation. High dose rate (HDR), delivery system is adopted here. To reduce the dose of radiation to adjacent bladder and rectum, vaginal packing is used to increase the distance between them and source of radiation.

Several isotopes are available for brachytherapy:
- *Low dose rate (LDR) system*: LDR therapy is the oldest system, which requires fewer sessions and hospitalization. The dose of radiation is delivered slowly in 27–30 hours in Stockholm technique or 72 hours in Manchester technique and patient remains isolated. Cesium (Cs) 137 is the most popular radioisotope used in LDR system.
- *High dose rate (HDR) system*: HDR therapy involves delivery of high dose of radiation over a shorter period of time (15–30 minutes). It can be done on outpatient basis. It has less morbidity and is more cost effective, but the equipment is more expensive. Iridium (Ir) 192 is used for HDR system.

Dose and Duration

In each brachytherapy application 6–7 Gy is given at an interval of 10 days to 2 weeks. In early stages, brachytherapy is recommended. In advanced disease, a total of 5 brachytherapy applications are proposed, while in postoperative cases only 2–3 applications are given.

When both EBRT and brachytherapy are used, the dose is adjusted as follows:
- EBRT = 40–45 Gy
- Brachytherapy = 30–35 Gy

Stage Wise Management by Radiotherapy

Stage IB and early IIA (Operable cases)

Step 1: Radical hysterectomy with pelvic lymphadenectomy followed by:

Step 2:
- Node negative and low-risk group → Observation
- Node negative and high-risk group → Small field radiotherapy
- Multiple positive or bulky positive nodes → Extended-field radiotherapy.

Stage IIB–IV (Non-operable cases):

Step 1: Advanced investigations:
- CT scans of the chest, pelvis and abdomen
- Position emission tomography (PET) scans.

Step 2:
- PET negative para-aortic node → Pelvic chemoradiation
- PET positive para-aortic node → Extended field chemoradiation
- Pelvic or para-aortic nodes and adnexal mass →
  - Resection of adnexal mass
  - Extraperitoneal resection of bulky nodes

- Extended-field chemoradiation if para-aortic nodes positive.
- Systemic metastasis → Palliative pelvic radiation.

Complications of Radiotherapy

The morbidity resulting from radiotherapy is minimal provided it is given properly. Major complications are caused by over dosage or technical errors:
1. *Complications during treatment*:
   a. *Gastrointestinal complications:* The small intestine has the lowest tolerance to radiation. Thus, the bowel mucosa are affected after administration of 20–30 Gy of radiation causing:
      - Diarrhea
      - Abdominal cramps
      - Nausea
      - Bleeding from bowel occasionally.

      The bowel symptoms usually settle down with appropriate treatment within few weeks of completion of treatment, but some minor change in bowel habit persists for long time.
   b. Cystitis uncommon.
   c. Moist desquamation of skin.
   d. Perforation of uterus at the time of insertion of uterine tandem in advanced disease.
2. *Late complications*: It occurs in 5–10% of patients due to continued arteritis and fibrosis in the small and large bowel and occasionally in the bladder:
   - Radiation proctitis causing blood loss from pelvic colon. This complain occurs usually one and half year after radiation and resolves with measures such as keeping feces soft and using prednisolone suppositories.
   - Suprapubic subcutaneous fibrosis. This develops 4–6 months after radiation.
   - Fibrotic and vascular changes in the bowel may cause serious complication in the form of impaired function and narrowing of the bowel with subacute or acute obstruction.
- Necrosis may also lead to perforation of bowel and fistula formation.
- Radiation cystitis. Episodes of hematuria may occur due to superimposed infection.
- Vesicovaginal fistula (VVF), rectovaginal fistula (RVF) (1–2%).
- Menopausal symptoms due to loss of ovarian function.
- Narrowing and shortening of the vagina causing coital difficulties and is aggravated by fixation of tissues following treatment.

Chemoradiation

Chemoradiation is application of chemotherapy in a patient, who is already getting radiotherapy. Chemotherapy during pelvic radiation therapy improves long-term progression-free survival (PFS) and overall survival (OS) among locally advanced cervical cancer patients collectively and for stage IIB and III disease individually without developing any increased toxicity. The rationale of adding chemotherapy with radiation is of two fold:
1. To increase the sensitivity of the tumor to the effects of radiation.
2. To eradicate microscopic systemic disease.

Regime of chemotherapy
Cisplatin weekly: 40 mg/m^2/week during EBRT is widely used. It is more effective and tolerable than any other single or combination therapy, as concomitant chemoradiation has been proved by different clinical trials.

Cisplatin is given on the 1st day of week followed by radiation on the rest 5 days of the week. Thus, cisplatin is given for a total of 5 days in 5 weeks.

> Mrs Kulsum has completed her treatment with concurrent chemoradiation followed by brachytherapy.
> How will you monitor her following treatment?

The *post-treatment surveillance* of Mrs Kulsum will be as follows:

Schedule

- She should be monitored monthly for the first 3 months
- Then every 3 months until 2 years

- Every 6 months until 5 years
- Every year life-long.

Process of Follow-up

- *History*: At each visit patient should be questioned for symptoms.
- *Physical examination includes*:
  - Assessment of supraclavicular and inguinal lymph nodes
  - Abdominal examination
  - Bimanual examination
  - Rectovaginal examination.
- *Investigations*:
  - Blood for complete blood count (CBC)
  - Serum creatinine
  - Blood for liver function test (LFT)
  - USG of whole abdomen
  - Pap's smear.

Use of Pap smear is controversial. If the patient is exposed to radiation, radiation-induced atypia is the likely findings in the report. This may arise confusion whether the atypia is due to recurrence or radiation induced. As a general rule, cytology is done in women when there is return of symptoms to pelvic organs after a symptom-free period.

The PET scan has a sensitivity of 96% and specificity of 84.4% to detect recurrent disease, but its high cost has limited its use for patients, who have clinical findings suspicious for recurrence.

> What are the factors which determine the prognosis of cancer cervix?

Irrespective of the type of treatment, the prognosis depends on the following:

- *Stage of disease*: The extent of disease at the time of treatment is the single most important prognostic factor. Since staging does not account nodal status and is indirectly related to tumor volume, its prognostic importance is not similar to that of lymph node status and tumor volume.
- *Tumor volume*: Tumor volume is the powerful prognostic variable. Bulky tumors are associated with greater incidence of pelvic recurrence, distant metastasis and overall reduced disease-free survival.
- *Lymph node status*: The most important prognostic factor is the status of lymph nodes. Survival data for patients with positive nodes show decreasing 5-year survival rates. Positive pelvic lymph nodes more than two and positive para-aortic lymph nodes are adverse prognostic factors.
- *Lymphovascular space invasion (LVSI) and depth of stromal invasion*: LVSI and depth of stromal invasion correlates significantly with nodal metastasis and pelvic recurrence. This has been proved in many surgicopathologic studies. Disease-free survival is thus affected in patients with LVSI and stromal invasion.
- *Histologic cell type*: The prognostic significance of adenocarcinoma and adenosquamous carcinoma of cervix is controversial. There is no difference in survival between squamous and adenocarcinoma of cervix if properly matched. The same applies for adenosquamous carcinoma. But in adenocarcinoma relatively unfavorable factors may precipitate inferior salvage rate of patients. The factors are:
  - Most of the cancers are endocervical, thus diagnosed late in the advanced stage
  - Endocervical tumors cause barrel-shaped cervix with predominant hypoxic cells. As a result the tumor is said to be less radiosensitive.

Small cell carcinoma of cervix has poor prognosis because of aggressive tumor behavior.

- *Parametrial invasion and close vaginal margin*: Both of these variables are evaluated in patients undergoing radical hysterectomy. Close vaginal margin and parametrial extension, regardless of lymph node status has a shorter disease-free survival.

> **Case scenario:** Mrs Mahmuda, aged 67 years reports with foul smelling vaginal discharge for 2 months. She feels pain in the lower abdomen for the same duration. On speculum examination, there was a cauliflower growth in the cervix. Bimanual examination revealed uterus is normal sized, but both fornices were thick and involved. Rectovaginal examination explored that both parametrium are involved with tumor and fixed to left pelvic wall.
>
> What is your diagnosis? What will be the treatment option after confirmation of diagnosis?

The diagnosis is cancer cervix stage IIIB. After confirmation of the diagnosis by cervical biopsy and clinical staging the treatment option for the patient will be concurrent chemoradiation followed by brachytherapy.

> *Does she need any intervention before the commencement of radiation therapy?*

Since in Mrs Mahmuda's case the tumor was fixed to left lateral pelvic sidewall, we should carefully exclude left-sided hydronephrosis by CT scan or IVU.

If there is left-sided hydronephrosis due to left ureter obstruction below the pelvic brim, elective ureteral stenting of left ureter should be considered before the commencement of radiation therapy. This has proven to improve the progression free survival (PFS) and overall survival (OS) of the patients.

Note: Patients with bilateral hydronephrosis and creatinine clearance <50 mL/min should be considered for elective ureteral stenting before the commencement of radiation therapy.

> *What are the criteria for diagnosis of stage IIIB cervical cancer?*

There are two criteria, i.e. tumor fixation to pelvic side wall and presence of hydronephrosis.

> *Suppose stage IIIB cancer cervix is diagnosed on the basis of hydronephrosis and there is no pelvic sidewall fixation.*
> *What is the likely explanation of hydronephrosis and what treatment option is the most appropriate?*

The cause of hydronephrosis in such a case is due to ureteric obstruction above the main tumor mass as a result of external ureteric compression from enlarged pelvic or para-aortic lymph nodes.

These patients are best treated by resection of bulky pelvic lymph nodes via extraperitoneal approach before radiation therapy. This treatment option has proved to improve the survival of the patient.

Special Modalities of Treatment

- *Adjuvant hysterectomy after radiation therapy:* Bulky endocervical tumors (barrel-shaped cervix) or patients with stage IB_2 cervical cancer have a higher incidence of central recurrence, pelvic and para-aortic lymph node metastasis and distant dissemination whatever primary modality of treatment is chosen. These recurrences anticipated to be reduced by the addition of extrafascial hysterectomy 3-6 weeks after primary pelvic radiation. There is good evidence to suggest that patients with tumor size of 4, 5 and 6 cm may have an improved PFS with combined therapy and a significant improvement in survival. Thus, each case must be judged individually (Keys 2003).
- *Neoadjuvant chemotherapy followed by surgery:* Results of randomized trials and meta-analysis of neoadjuvant chemotherapy (NACT) for patients with bulky stage IB cervical cancer reveals favorable outcome. There is significant improvement in the progression free interval and overall survival of patients with bulky stage IB cervical cancer, who received 3 cycles of NACT followed by RH. This favorable outcome is achieved because of decrease in locoregional failures (pelvic recurrences) (Neoadjuvant Chemotherapy for cervical cancer meta analysis collaboration, 2003). The chemotherapy regime and dose has been differently given in different trials. The chemotherapy consisted of combination of vincristine, bleomycin and cisplatin (VBP), given at 10–14 days interval.

> **Case scenario:** Mrs Nuzhat, 42-year-old underwent total abdominal hysterectomy for fibroid uterus 10 days back. The histopathology of the specimen reveals invasive adenocarcinoma of cervix.
> *What will be the treatment option for this patient?*

When invasive cervical cancer is discovered after simple hysterectomy, the treatment option includes:
- Radical surgery consisting of radical parametrectomy, upper vaginectomy and pelvic lymphadenectomy.
- Full pelvic radiation
- Concurrent chemoradiation to the pelvis.

The choice of treatment options depend upon the presence or absence of:
- High-risk factors in the hysterectomy specimen.
- Metastatic disease elsewhere.
- Histologic cell type.

Factors determining the choice of treatment are:
- Macroscopic or microscopic residual disease at the resected margin.
- Positive pelvic lymph nodes.
- Lymphovascular space invasion.
- Deep stromal invasion.
- Evidence of metastatic disease elsewhere.
- Histologic grading adenocarcinoma.
  - In absence of high-risk factors, the preferred treatment is radical surgery. The operation is considerably more difficult than a RH, the main difficulty being the identification of the bladder, which is usually adherent over the vaginal vault. Thus, higher complication rate is anticipated.
  - When high-risk factors are present, EBRT with or without brachytherapy is the treatment of choice. Brachytherapy should be added to EBRT if there is evidence of residual disease in the resected margin. The radiation should be administered immediately after recovery from operation, as prognosis worsens if therapy is delayed.
  - The option of concurrent chemoradiation is widely considered in patients following simple hysterectomy in whom the following are present:
    - Gross residual disease
    - Positive surgical margin
    - Positive pelvic lymph nodes
    - Histologic grading of adenocarcinoma.

> How will you evaluate this patient after simple hysterectomy to determine the high-risk factors?

Evaluation

The evaluation includes:
- Some sophisticated investigations
- Details of histopathologic evaluation of hysterectomy specimen.

Investigations

The investigations are:
- X-ray or CT scan of chest to exclude lung metastasis, and
- CT scan or MRI of abdomen to exclude pelvic lymph node metastasis, or
- PET scan of whole body to exclude metastasis

Histopathology

Histopathologic evaluation of hysterectomy specimen includes:
- Histologic type of tumor
- Surgical margin (whether free of disease or not)
- LVSI
- Deep stromal invasion.

> **Case scenario:** Mrs Monira, 55-year-old has been treated by radical hysterectomy followed by EBRT 5 years back for cancer cervix stage IIA. Now she develops central pelvic recurrence of 2 cm size involving the vault as confirmed by vault biopsy.
> How will you treat her?

Monira had central pelvic recurrence of small volume (2 cm), which had developed after completion of definitive surgery and adjuvant radiotherapy and disease-free interval of 5 year. The ideal option for her is pelvic exenteration provided PET scan excludes the contraindications of laparotomy. But since such radical surgery is associated with high morbidity and mortality and substantial loss of structure and function of pelvic organs, most patients refuse such surgery.

Re-irradiation is better tolerated, has little operative morbidity and preserves structure and function of pelvic organs. Intracavitary radiation will be the feasible curative intent therapy for Monira with anticipated higher survival rate.

RELATED INFORMATION

Therapeutic Options

Therapeutic options for recurrent disease include:
- Surgery (salvage)
- Chemoradiation
- Palliative treatment only.

Decision for treatment of recurrent disease should be made on an individual basis and depends on:
- Patient's wish
- Patient's general health
- Stage of the disease
- Previous treatment
- Probable efficacy of current treatment options
- Probable treatment related morbidity.

Salvage Therapy

Salvage therapy is any therapy that is done in an attempt to cure cancer following the failure of an initial treatment. Salvage therapy, also known as rescue therapy.

Options of salvage therapy in recurrent cervical cancer and assessment of success of therapy: Patients with recurrent disease confined to the pelvis following definitive therapy, whether that therapy is surgery or RT, are potentially curable. Salvage options for patients with central recurrence depends upon the primary therapy:
- If the primary therapy is surgery alone, patients are managed with EBRT with or without brachytherapy. Concurrent chemotherapy is also recommended in such cases.
- If primary therapy is definitive with adjuvant RT, radical surgery in the form of pelvic exenteration is recommended when there is no evidence of metastasis in selected patients. As an alternative, re-irradiation using interstitial implants or highly conformal EBRT can also be given with chemotherapy for meaningful palliation.

The success of salvage therapy is determined by:
- Site of recurrence
- Extent of recurrent disease at presentation
- Disease-free interval
- Performance status
- Comorbidities.

Patients with small volume central recurrence having long disease-free interval and good performance status and minimum comorbidities have higher complete response rate following salvage therapy and there is no evidence of disease for a longer period of time.

Surgery

Total pelvic exenteration

Pelvic exenteration is mainly done for:
- Central recurrence of Ca Cx after primary treatment, that involves bladder and rectum.
- Sometimes as primary therapy for advanced pelvic cancers of all kinds.

It relieves pain, discharge and incontinence and sometimes can cause complete cure. A multi-disciplinary team should carryout the operation.

Total pelvic exenteration includes excision of all the pelvic viscera, fascia and lymphatics and the women are left with a separate colostomy and ileal loop bladder.

In anterior exenteration, rectum and in posterior exenteration bladder is not removed. But it is not possible to remove potential lymphatic spread without removing rectum, bladder and ureters. So, total exenteration is the preferred option.

Selection of the patient
- Total pelvic exenteration should be reserved as salvage surgery in recurrent central pelvis cancer after failed previous surgery and chemoradiation.
- *Physical examination to exclude pelvic sidewall involvement*: A clinical diagnosis of pelvic sidewall involvement can almost always be made in the presence of a triad of sciatic pain, leg edema and hydronephrosis.
- A whole body PET or PET–CT scan is to be done for selection of operable patients and eliminate unnecessary morbidity associated with salvage procedures in unsuitable patients. Extra-pelvic metastasis, pelvic lymph node metastasis, intraperitoneal disease or malignant ascites contraindicates pelvic exenteration.
- CT or MRI is required to assess resectability.

Pelvic exenteration is accompanied by substantial functional loss so it is always followed by vaginal and perineal reconstruction to restore vulvovaginal functions. Reported postoperative morbidity and recurrence rate is 35.7% and 50% respectively. 5 year survival rate is less than 50%. A dedicated multiprofessional team can reduce both morbidity and mortality.

Palliative Treatment

Palliative treatment is designed to relieve symptoms and improve the quality of life. It can be used at any stage of an illness if there are troubling symptoms, such as pain or sickness. Palliative care begins at diagnosis and continues during cancer treatment and beyond. It also includes the treatment of side effects of cancer treatments. In advanced cancer, palliative treatment may help someone to live longer and to live comfortably, even if they cannot be cured. The goal of comprehensive palliative care is to address the full range of problems associated with a serious illness, from physical symptoms to emotional anxiety and even spiritual concerns.

Palliative care is different from hospice care, although they share the same principles of comfort and support. In hospice care only care is given but not for cure. The care is given at the end of the life to improve the quality of life.

Treatment of Common Complications

- Pain control:
  - Analgesics
  - Nerve blockade.
- Deep venous thrombosis (DVT):
  - Leg elevation
  - Early ambulation after surgery
  - Low-molecular-weight heparin (LMWH)
  - Compression garments.
- Minor hemorrhage:
  - Systemic causes should be excluded
  - Drugs that may cause bleeding should be discontinued
  - Antibiotics for infection
  - Oral tranexamic acid or aminocaproic acid
  - Local tranexamic acid to superficial fungating wound
  - Rectal or bladder instillation of tranexamic acid
  - A single fraction of radiotherapy.
- Major hemorrhage:
  When hemorrhage is profuse and life-threatening
  - Midazolam for anxiolytic effect (10 mg subcutaneous or buccal route)
  - Blood transfusion
  - If bleeding due to erosion of a major artery, local pressure and adequate packing should be applied.

> **Case scenario:** Mrs Rahima, a 70-year-old lady is suffering from Ca Cx stage IIIB with pyometra. The size of the uterus corresponds to 14 weeks size of pregnancy.
>
> What is the preferred treatment for her and why? What precaution should be adopted for her before starting the treatment?

Radiation is the Preferred Treatment

The coexistent pyometra or hematometra must be drained using ultrasonic guidance if necessary before radiation. Ultrasonic evidence of further collection demands repeated dilatation of cervix every 2–3 days interval. Broad-spectrum antibiotic should be used to cover bacteroids, anaerobic streptococci and aerobic coliforms. Active infection decreases the response to radiation and may be exacerbated into a systemic infection if brachytherapy rods are packed into the uterus.

> **Case scenario:** Mrs Saleha, a 62-year-old menopausal lady had subtotal hysterectomy 17 years back. Now she complaints of postmenopausal bleeding and foul-smelling vaginal discharge. On evaluation, it was found that there is advanced squamous cell carcinoma of cervical stumps.
>
> How will you treat her?

Since the disease is advanced, the only option of treatment is radiation. If the length of cervical canal is 2 cm, adequate dose of radiation can be given by both EBRT and brachytherapy. Great precautions are needed to give radiation particularly brachytherapy as bladder and rectum are at the top of the stump and the dose is limited to 2–3 applications at an interval of 1–2 weeks.

> What is the prognosis of stump carcinoma?

Stump carcinoma of cervix carries less favorable prognosis because:
- Peritoneal cavity, the bladder and the rectum are all at the top of the stump. So, they become invaded early.
- High intrauterine dose of radiotherapy cannot be allowed, because of close proximity of the bladder and rectum over the stump.
- Radical trachelectomy becomes difficult, because of disturbed anatomy and need of careful dissection of the bladder which is likely to be adherent to the stump.

Although with the advancement in the radiotherapeutic techniques, 5-year survival rates are comparable to those in patients with an intact uterus, the complication rates are higher.

Cervical Cancer

> **Case scenario:** Mrs Sharmin, 26-year-old lady married for 2 years is diagnosed as a case of Ca Cx stage IB. The tumor is exophytic and less than 2 cm in size. Since Sharmin does not have any issue she wants to spare the uterus and reproductive function. Radiotherapy will destroy ovarian function. So, conservative surgery can preserve reproductive function.
>
> What surgical approach can be adopted for her and what structures are removed in that surgery? What will be the preoperative evaluation of Mrs Sharmin?

Radical abdominal trachelectomy is the fertility preserving surgery that can be offered to Mrs Sharmin where good clearance of tumor, parametrium and pelvic lymph nodes can be achieved. The operation intends to resect the cervix, 1–2 cm of vagina, parametrium and upper paracolpos sparing the uterine fundus or corpus through abdominal approach.

The preoperative evaluation includes:
- MRI abdomen to exclude involvement of parametrium, upper endocervix and lower uterine segment.
- CT scan or PET scans of the abdomen to exclude disease outside the cervix.
- Preoperative counseling for informed consent on:
    - Oncologic safety of operation.
    - Complications of the procedure.
    - Risk of infertility as a result of loss of cervix and cervical mucus.
    - Early pregnancy loss and preterm delivery.
    - The need of cesarean section.

RELATED INFORMATION

Indications of Radical Trachelectomy

This operation is offered to young patients of cervical cancer, who desires to preserve fertility and who meets the following criteria:
- *Early stage disease*: Stage IA_1 with LVSI, stage IA_2, stage IB_1.
- Adenocarcinoma or squamous cell carcinoma (SSC).
- Exophytic tumor.
- Tumor less than 2 cm in size.
- No evidence of disease outside the cervix-parametrium, upper endocervix or lower uterine segment, pelvic lymph node.

Complications

Post-trachelectomy stenosis leading to hematometra formation.

Outcomes of Surgery

- *Oncologic safety*: Radical trachelectomy is highly successful operation with recurrence rate similar to traditional radical hysterectomy (RH) as the patients are highly selected.
- *Obstetric outcome*:
    a. Chances of conception is 50% following surgery. These are double than that of → general population and are related to decreased cervical length, alteration in cervical mucus, presence of cervical suture leading to ascending infection and premature rupture of membrane.
    b. Second trimester loss (11%).
    c. Preterm birth (18%).
    d. Increased operative interference in the form of cesarean section due to cervical dystocia secondary to scar tissue in the cervix.

Carcinoma of Cervix and Pregnancy

Invasive cancer of cervix diagnosed during pregnancy are usually stage I or stage II in developed countries where organized screening with Pap's smear is available. If Pap's smear is strongly suggestive of invasive cancer, colposcopy directed biopsy or diagnostic conization is done for confirmation in the second trimester to avoid the risk of abortion.

The prognosis of invasive cancer in pregnancy is similar to that of nonpregnant patients when matched for stage, tumor type and tumor volume. There is no evidence that pregnancy accelerates the natural history of cervical cancer and the fetus is also not affected by maternal disease (Hopkins, 1992, Zemlickis, 1991).

Though under following circumstances due to delayed treatment prognosis may be unfavorable:
- Diagnosis may be missed at early stage as bleeding for Ca Cx may be confused with pregnancy-related bleeding.
- Might delay in starting treatment for getting a mature baby.

- Hormonal and vascular changes in late pregnancy may encourage rapid growth.

Treatment depends on the stage of disease, period of gestation and wishes of the patient. Women who want to continue the pregnancy or when gestation is near viability, pregnancy can be continued after careful and clear discussion regarding the maternal risk.

Management of Carcinoma of Cervix in Pregnancy (Stage IA and Stage IB)

Stage IA_1 with no LVSI

- Delivery vaginally at term (vaginal delivery is possible in noninvasive cases)

Six weeks later.
- Total abdominal hysterectomy (TAH) if no childbearing is required.
- Conization if further childbearing is required.

Stage IA_1 with LVSI and Stage IA_2

- Cesarean section (CS) (at term) and modified radical hysterectomy with pelvic node dissection (in invasive cases always cesarean section is advocated to avoid hemorrhage and cervical dystocia).

Note: *Troublesome hemorrhage is anticipated during hysterectomy and pelvic lymph node dissection (PLND).*

Stage IB

- Cesarean section (at 32 weeks) and radical hysterectomy (RH) with PLND.
- In early cases of diagnosis, cesarean section can be delayed to a maximum of 4 weeks for fetal lung maturity (FLM) followed by RH and PLND.

Management of Carcinoma of Cervix in Pregnancy (Stage II–IV)

- *First trimester*: EBRT→Abortion takes place. Subsequent doses are given later.
- *Second trimester*: EBRT, Patient's wishes and available facilities must be taken into consideration. In two ways it can be done
  i. Hysterotomy followed by radiotherapy.
  ii. Radiotherapy and awaiting spontaneous expulsion, continue radiotherapy.
- *Third trimester*: Cesarean section when FLM is achieved. 4–21 days after delivery EBRT followed by brachytherapy.

BIBLIOGRAPHY

Bosch FX, Manos MM, Munoz N, et al. Prevalence of human papillomavirus in cervical cancer: a worldwide perspective. International biological study on cervical cancer (IBSCC) Study Group. J Natl Cancer Inst. 1995;87(11):796-802.

Cogliano V, Grosse Y, Baan R, et al. Carcinogenecity of combined estrogen progestagen contraceptives and menopausal treatment. Lancet Oncol. 2005;6: 552-3.

Ferlay J, Bray F, Pisani P, et al. GLOBOCAN 2002 cancer incidence. Mortality and Prevalence worldwide. IARC cancer Base No. 5 version 2-0 Lyon: IARC Press. 2004.

Hopkins MP, Morley GW. The prognosis and management of cervical cancer associated with pregnancy. Obstet Gynecol 1992;80:9-13.

Jacobs MV, Snijders PJ, van den Brule AJ, et al. A general primer GP5+/GP6 (+)-mediated PCR-enzyme immunoassay method for rapid detection of 14 high-risk and 6 low-risk human papillomavirus genotypes in cervical scrapings. J Clin Microbiol. 1997;35(3): 791-5.

Keys HM, Bundy BN, Stehman FB, Okagaki T, et al. For the Gynecology Oncology Group. Radiation therapy with and without extra fascias hysterectomy for bulky stage IB cervical cancer: a randomized trial of GOG, Gynecol Oncol. 2003;89:343-53.

Morris M, Eifel PJ, Lu J, et al. Pelvic radiation with concurrent chemotherapy compared with pelvic and para-aortic radiation for high-risk cervical cancer. N Engl J Med. 1999;340:1137-43.

Neoadjuvant Chemotherapy for cervical cancer meta analysis collaboration. Neoadjuvant chemotherapy for locally advanced cervical cancer: a systematic review and meta analysis of individual patient data from 21 randomized trials. Euro J Cancer 2003;39:2470-86.

Schiffman M, Castle PE. The promise of global cervical cancer prevention. J Pathol. 2005;353:2101-4.

Walboomers JM, Jacobs MV, Manos MM, et al. Human Papillomavirus is a necessary cause of invasive cervical cancer worldwide. J Pathol. 1999;189: 12-9.

Zemlickis D, Lishner M, Degendorfer P, et al. Maternal and fetal outcome after invasive cervical cancer in pregnancy. Clin Oncol. 1991;9:1956-61.

CHAPTER 15

Precancerous Disease of Cervix and its Prevention

Farhat Hossain

INTRODUCTION

The effort to eliminate cervical cancer began over 50 years ago with the introduction of the Pap test. Cytology-based screening has reduced the incidence of cervical cancer by up to 75% in countries that have been able to implement and sustain centralized quality controlled screening programs. The next significant milestone in cervical cancer prevention came in the 1980 with the discovery of a link between cervical cancer and human papillomavirus (HPV) (Zur, 1994). During the following 20 years, epidemiologic studies clearly demonstrated that persistent infection with 'high-risk' or 'carcinogenic' types of HPV is essential for the development of cervical cancer (Bosch, 2003). Today, 12–18 types of HPV are classified as 'known human carcinogens' (IARC monographs). This invention has further led to the development of sensitive molecular methods for detecting HPV, which are responsible for high-grade cervical cancer precursor lesions. HPV-DNA testing is now a clinically validated and FDA approved test after Pap test for secondary prevention of cancer cervix. More importantly, the link between cervical cancer and HPV also provided the basis for vaccination-based strategies for the primary prevention of cervical cancer. Now HPV vaccine cancer prevention efforts protection against cervical cancer and precancerous cervical lesions.

Case scenario: *Mrs Rahela, a multiparous woman has come to you with the complaints of pervaginal discharge, which is not associated with any itching. She has four children and got married when she was 13. She has come from a low socioeconomic class. On examination, you found presence of discharge, but no visible abnormality. Bimanual examination and transvaginal examination show normal findings.*
What investigations do you want to do?

- A high vaginal swab and intracervical swab is to be taken for gram staining, culture and sensitivity.
- A smear is taken for cytology (Pap smear).

Why Pap smear is taken? What is its significance?

Pap smear is taken for screening of cervical precancerous lesion. Vaginal discharge occurs in early lesion of the cervix. Importance of screening is to prevent carcinoma cervix by detecting and managing precancerous lesion. Most of the cervical cancers start with precancerous changes in the cervix. There are different risk factors for developing carcinoma cervix like high parity, sexual contact at early age, multiple sexual partner, HPV infection, long-term use of oral contraceptive and smoking. So, eliminating the risk factors can prevent the precancerous changes and identifying the changes if occurs at earliest stage can prevent the development of cervical cancer.

RELATED INFORMATION

It is now well-established fact that cervical cancer prevention needs coordinated efforts for wide coverage and creating awareness of the need for:
- Primary prevention through vaccination
- Secondary prevention through screening.
  Even after vaccination, programs have been instituted and reasonable levels of coverage obtained, cervical cancer screening programs need to be continued side by side, because vaccination will not protect against the HPV types not included in the vaccines.

Primary Prevention

Prevention of precancers in the first place.
1. HPV vaccination

2. Avoid contact with human papilloma virus
3. Avoidance of smoking

HPV Vaccination

Vaccination offers primary prevention against cervical cancer. In other words, vaccination protects an individual against acquiring HPV infection, which leads to cervical cancer, i.e. vaccination is effective against the etiological agent.

Vaccination induces the development of high level of antibodies in the serum, which transudates to the site of infection, i.e. cervix. When a new HPV infection occurs, these antibodies are ready to neutralize the virus and prevent its entry into the cervical epithelial cells. The success of HPV vaccines are based on a good understanding of natural history and transmission dynamic of genital HPV infection.

Types of Vaccination

There are mainly two types of vaccination against cancer cervix:
1. **Cervarix:** It is a bivalent vaccine, which is composed of HPV 16 and 18 antigens in the form of virus-like particles (VLPs) combined with a novel adjuvant system called AS04. This AS04 induces stronger and longer lasting antibody titers and higher memory B-cell responses against both HPV 16 and 18 than any other adjuvant used in vaccine.

   This vaccine gives protection against cervical cancer caused by HPV 16 and 18. This vaccine is produced by GlaxoSmithKline and is available in Bangladesh since February 2009.
2. **Gardasil:** It is a quadrivalent vaccine, which is composed of HPV 6, 11, 16 combined with aluminum hydroxide as adjuvant. This vaccine is produced by Merck. Gardasil gives protection against cervical cancer caused by HPV 16 and 18. It also gives protection against genital warts, anal, vaginal and vulval cancer caused by HPV 6 and 11.

Efficacy of cervarix: Follow-up data suggests that cervarix is capable of reducing HPV 16 or 18 associated cervical intraepithelial neoplasia II (CIN II) and III by 100% and it also provides cross–protection against infection with HPV 45 and 31 (Harper, 2006).

Duration of protection: With cervarix immunogenicity, study has shown antibody levels against both HPV 16 and 18 to stay consistently high (≥ 10 fold high than after natural infection) for a period of 9.4 years till date (Roteli–Martins, 2012). Further, mathematical models predict that these antibodies are likely to persist for at least 20 years, (David et al. 2008).

Safety: Both vaccines were studied in thousands of people from 9 through 26 years old and found to be safe and effective for these ages. Pregnant women are not included in the recommendation of HPV vaccination.

Side effects
- The most common side effects are:
   - Short-term redness
   - Swelling
   - Soreness of injection site
   - Rarely faintness shortly after injection.
- *Major side effects from Gardasil*:
   - Long-term pain
   - Numbness
   - Infertility and
   - Paralysis.

The only reported symptoms are pain, redness and swelling at the injection site. It is found to be well tolerated and acceptable.

Optimal Age for Vaccination

Human papillomavirus (HPV) vaccines offer the best protection to girls, who receive complete doses and have time to develop an immune response *before being sexually active*. But, sexually active women also continue to remain at risk of acquiring an HPV infection throughout their lives. Therefore, all women from 9 year onwards can benefit from vaccination. Hence, the vaccine is licensed for use in women from 9-year of age onwards.

The explanation for giving vaccination in women who are already sexually active is as follows:
- A previous HPV infection by sexual contact does not protect individuals against future infections with the same or different HPV

types. This is also applicable for women who are in a monogamous relationship.

- Thus, vaccination in these individuals protect them from acquiring new infections with the same and even other HPV types which might lead to cervical cancer in the future regardless of an ongoing infection (Anne Szarewski, 2010).

What is the Schedule of Vaccine?

Both vaccines are given as a series of three injections within 6 months period. According to centers for disease control and prevention (CDC) recommendation, the second dose is to be given 1–2 months after the first, and the third dose is to be given 6 months after the first dose. So, it is to be administered in 3 doses (0, 1 and 6 months) via intramuscular injection into the deltoid area.

Note: Vaccination is always followed by screening.

Vaccination along with regular screening offers the best possible protection against cervical cancer, because it ensures that an infection caused by a non-vaccine HPV type does not progress to invasive cancer. Thus, screening after vaccination is essential. On the other hand, screening is not recommended before vaccination, as screening will not protect against new infections leading to lesions.

Avoid Contact with Human Papilloma Virus

Human papilloma virus is a sexually transmitted disease (STD), but is a transient infection about 90% of which clears up spontaneously within 6–9 months. It is the persistent infection of the cervix with oncogenic HPV, which causes cervical cancer. The major steps in cervical carcinogenesis include infection of the metaplastic epithelium of cervical transformation zone with one or more carcinogenic HPV type, viral persistence, clonal progression of persistently infected epithelium to cervical precancer, which then progresses to invasive cervical cancer **(Fig. 15.1)**.

It is thus clear from the Figure, that the most critical steps in cervical carcinogenesis is not the acquisition of HPV infection, but the progression of disease to clinically important precursor lesions (i.e. CIN III). In between HPV positivity and CIN III progression, there is an intermediate step of HPV persistence and there are cofactors identified, which influences HPV persistence and neoplastic progression.

More than 75–95% CIN and 95–100% invasive cervical carcinoma shows the presence of HPV (Bosch et al. 2003). So, *avoidance of contact of HPV virus can prevent a vast majority of Ca Cx.* Contact of HPV can be avoided by avoiding:

i. Multiple sexual partner.
ii. Early sexual activity.
iii. High-risk sexual partner (history of multiple sexual partners, HPV infection, lower genital tract neoplasia, prior exposure to someone with cervical neoplasia).

Note: Condom is not a protective mechanism like other STDs, as transmission can occur from labial-scrotal contact.

Secondary Prevention

To find out and treat the precancers before they become true cancer.

Secondary prevention of cervical cancer is offered through screening, which intends to reduce the incidence of cancer and mortality from the disease by identifying women with precancerous cervical lesions and early invasive cancers and treating these women appropriately. In other words, screening enables the identification of

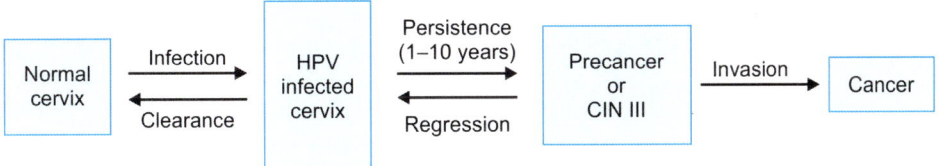

Fig. 15.1 Steps in cervical carcinogenesis

unrecognized disease by the application of tests or examination in order to permit timely intervention.

In Bangladesh, where vaccination cannot be generalized, screening has got tremendous role to prevent carcinoma cervix.

Cervical cancer is an important public health problem that can be successfully screened. The points in favor of screening are:
- The accessibility of uterine cervix.
- The propensity of cells to exfoliate from precancerous lesions.
- Apparently prolonged natural history of the disease.
- Existence of a spectrum of histologic changes from mild atypia through premalignant lesion to frank malignancy.
- Presence of a valid and acceptable screening test.
- Earlier and efficient diagnosis of the disease.
- Effective therapy against detectable disease.

Implementation of an organized screening program for cervical cancer requires the following:
- A national policy that defines the screening age (target population) and interval.
- Availability of a cheap and easily performable screening test.
- Sufficient political and financial investment to run the program.
- Training of healthcare providers in:
  a. Carrying out the screening test.
  b. Interpretation of data.
  c. Patient counseling.
- Setting up health infrastructure for smooth performance of screening test.
- Ensuring high quality laboratory services.
- Establishing a referral pathway for treatment of patients, i.e.:
  a. Training of people at local level
  b. Referral for more advanced cases needing specialized treatment.
- Developing the capacity to offer treatment.
- Setting up national monitoring system.
- Education of the population to ensure participation in the screening program.

The process of screening of cancer cervix identifies:
- A test negative group for whom no further action is needed
- A test positive group, who are again grouped into two categories:
  a. One group is subjected to specific diagnostic tests and categorized as true positive. They are referred immediately for treatment.
  b. Another group are those for whom surveillance and repeat testing is recommended.

Screening Tests

The *primary screening* tools for cancer cervix are:
- Cervical cytology.
- Visual inspection with acetic acid (VIA).
- HPV–DNA testing.

The *secondary screening* tool for cancer cervix is colposcopy:
- Colposcopy: It is considered as a secondary screening tool for cancer cervix and is used to evaluate women, who have abnormal cytology or whose VIA test is positive.

Primary Screening Tools

Cervical cytology

Cytology-based screening program was the mainstay of cervical cancer prevention in early 90s and involves collection of exfoliated cells from the cervix and microscopic examination of these cells after staining.

This concept of utilizing exfoliated cytology to identify women with cervical cancer was introduced by Papanicolaou and Babes in 1920s (Papanicolaou 1928), subsequently. Papanicolaou refined the technique and demonstrated that conventional cytology could be used to identify precancerous lesions of the cervix (Papanicolaou, 1954) and from then onwards cervical cytology began to be widely used in many developed countries for cervical cancer prevention.

Preparation for cervical cytology: The best time to collect Pap smear is 2 weeks after the first day of last menstrual period. In postpartum women, it should be 8 weeks postpartum. The precautions are:
- Avoid sexual intercourse and douching for 24–48 hours before collection.

- Women should not use any intravaginal medicine for several days before the smear is taken.
- Women with cervicitis or vaginitis as indicated by significant cervical or vaginal discharge should be appropriately treated before cytology specimen is collected, otherwise inflammatory exudates or mildly reactive cells may be misinterpreted as cytological abnormality.

Cervical cytological test can be done by any one of the two methods:
1. Conventional cytology
2. Liquid-based cytology.

Conventional cytology: Equipment for convention cervical cytology—For collection of cervical cytology, the equipment required are:
- Bivalved self-retaining Cusco's speculum
- A light source
- Collection devise
  - Wooden Aye's spatula
  - Endocervical brush
- Glass slide
- Fixative, e.g. alcohol or spray fixative.

Procedure of Pap smear
The steps involved are:
- Filling of requisition form with required informations such as:
  - Name and indication.
  - Date of birth or age.
  - Menstrual status (date of LMP, whether the woman is pregnant, postpartum, on hormone replacement therapy or has had hysterectomy).
- Labeling of slide with woman's identification number.
- Procedure—The woman is placed in dorsolithotomy position. Appropriate size speculum is inserted into the vagina to allow complete visualization of cervix and transformation zone.

Note: Smear must be obtained before bimanual examination. The cervix should not be subjected to bimanual examination with lubricant or water-soluble gel that may obscure the smear. Excess mucus or discharge from the cervix can be removed with cotton for better quality smear.

Specimen collection
The spatula is placed against the ectocervix with the long projection extending into the endocervical canal and is rotated 360° around the portio to cover the entire squamocolumnar junction. Rotation of spatula can be done twice or thrice if needed provided it is gentle and is not provoking bleeding. The cellular materials are then transferred onto the glass slides from both sides of the spatula.

The endocervical canal is then sampled using a conical cervical brush, which is placed in the endocervical canal so that the last few bristles remain visible. The brush is then rotated gently 90° once. One rotation will adequately sample the endocervical canal, which is spread onto the slide.

Cell fixation
Cell fixation should be done within few seconds of specimen collection in order to prevent air-drying, which obscure cellular details and hinders interpretation. This can be done either by immersing the slide in alcohol or spraying it with spray fixative. The fixative should be liberally applied such that the slide appears most over the entire surface. With immersion fixation, the slide is either immersed in alcohol in Koplin's jar and transferred to the laboratory or allowed to fix for 20–30 minutes in the alcohol, removed and allowed to air-dry.

Sensitivity and specificity of conventional cervical cytology: A recent large cervical cancer screening study shows the sensitivity of Pap smear ranges from 40 to 65%, while specificity ranges from 92 to 96%. The low performance of Pap smear is attributable, because of following reasons:
- Failure to capture the entire squamocolumnar junction as most of the cells collected are left behind on the sampling device.
- Inadequate fixation of the smear occurs due to damage and degeneration of some cells on contact with dry slide before fixation.
- Abnormal cells are obscured by blood and inflammatory debris.
- Most of the time, the smear prepared on the slide is thick, i.e. poor quality of smear is produced.

Satisfactory for Evaluation

In conventional cervical cytology, a well-prepared slide is said to be '*Satisfactory for Evaluation*' when if fulfills the following criteria:
- The slide must be properly labeled with patients identifying number.
- Adequate number (8,000–12,000) of both squamous and endocervical cells must be present on the slide.
- There must be five clusters of epithelial cells in one high power field and each cluster must contain at least one endocervical cells.
- About 25–30% of epithelial cells should be free from being obscured by inflammation, blood or poor preservation.

Liquid-based cytology: To improve the sensitivity of Paps smear, liquid-based cytology (LBC) was introduced in mid-1990.
- Here, the exfoliated cells after collection is directly immersed in a liquid preservation where the clumps of cells and mucus are broken up by mechanical agitation to produce a homogeneous sample.
- The homogeneous sample is then filtered through a membrane filter, which traps epithelial cells while allowing contaminated red cells and inflammatory cells to pass through.
- The epithelial cells collected on the membrane filter are then transferred onto a glass slide and stained. This produces a relatively thin, monolayer-type preparation.

The above technique of LBC is called ThinPrep method and is approved by FDA in USA. ThinPrep-3000 processor allows up to 80 samples to be processed at a time.

Advantages of LBC over conventional cervical cytology
- There is more representative transfer of cells from the collection device to the glass slide.
- There is reduction in the number of unsatisfactory cytology specimen.
- The overall performance of LBC is better than Pap smear.
- LBC is associated with shorter interpretation time than required for conventional cytology.
- Residual cellular material is available for HPV testing or making additional glass slides.

Disadvantages of liquid-based cytology: Only drawback is that it is more expensive than usual Pap test.

Reporting

With the advancement of knowledge and understanding of the role of HPV in the pathogenesis of cervical cancer, Bethesda system terminology is introduced for interpretation of Pap smear. It was modified twice in 1991 and in 2001. Now, The Bethesda system in widely used in many countries of the world for reporting (**Table 15.1**).

Table 15.1 Comparison of different terminologies used for cytologic reporting

Bethesda system	CIN*	World Health Organization (WHO)
Within normal limit		
Benign cellular changes		
ASCUS[+]		
ASC–H[#]		
Low-grade SIL	CIN I	Mild dysplasia (dysplastic cells involve only lower one-third)
	CIN II	Moderate dysplasia (dysplastic cells involve only lower two-thirds)
High-grade SIL	CIN III	Severe dysplasia (dysplastic cells involve more than two-thirds but not whole thickness)
		Carcinoma in situ (dysplastic cells involve whole thickness)
Invasive carcinoma	Invasive carcinoma	Invasive carcinoma

*CIN, cervical intraepithelial neoplasia; [+]ASCUS, atypical squamous cell of undetermined significance; [#]ASC–H, high-grade lesion cannot be excluded; SIL; squamous intraepithelial lesion.

The interpretation/result of the 2001 Bethesda system includes the following:
- Negative for intraepithelial lesion or malignancy.
- Epithelial abnormalities.

Squamous cell
- Atypical squamous cell of undetermined significance (ASCUS).
- ASC-H (high grade lesion cannot be excluded).
- Low-grades squamous intraepithelial lesion (LSIL).
- High-grade squamous intraepithelial lesion (HSIL).
- Squamous cell carcinoma.

Glandular cell
- Atypical glandular cells (AGC).
- Atypical glandular cell, which favor neoplasia.
- Endocervical adenocarcinoma in situ.
- Adenocarcinoma.

Limitations of cytology-based screening:
- Cytology has low sensitivity for detection of precancerous lesions and treatable cancers. A meta-analysis found that cytology has a sensitivity of 51% (range 30–87%) for histologically confirmed CIN II/III (Nandak et al. 2000). Thus, repeated cytology over short intervals are used to achieve program efficacy.
- Cytology is poorly reproducible. It is a subjective test and in programs without quality control/quality assurance it is impossible to achieve and maintain the clinical performance.
- Cytology is labor intensive. It is refractory to automated screening.
- Despite of the low cost of consumables and because of above three reasons, high quality cytology is expensive.
- Three visit approach is needed for an intervention, i.e. cytology, colposcopy and treatment.

Visual inspection with acetic acid

Because of the failure of cytology-based screening programs to be developed and sustained in low resource settings, alternative method of screening test has been developed which is called visual inspection with acetic acid (VIA). VIA involves examination of the cervix with naked eye under light after application of 3–5% dilute acetic acid for minute. Appearance of well-defined acetowhite area close to squamocolumnar junction (SCJ) indicates a positive test.

Why acetowhitening occurs?

Acetowhitening occurs due to reversible coagulation of intracellular proteins following application of acetic acid (AA). In CIN or neoplasia, there is high concentration of proteins in the atypical cells, which appears as well-demarcated intensely opaque acetowhite lesion following application of AA. This lesion is located in the transformation zone. Acetowhitening can also occur in:
- Immature squamous metaplasia.
- Inflamed cervix (chronic cervicitis).
- Regenerating cervical epithelium in a previous scar.

Acetowhite lesion is said to be positive when it is dense white with sharp border and one of the borders is abutting the squamocolumnar junction.

Note: *If positive acetowhite lesion is identified, the patient is referred to a higher center where confirmatory test, i.e. colposcopy can be carried out.*

Advantages of VIA
- It yields an immediate result. Thus, immediate referral for confirmatory test can be done or screen and treat approach can be adopted.
- The method is inexpensive and can be carried out using widely available consumables without the need for a laboratory infrastructure.
- Health personnel, such as doctors, nurses, midwives and paramedics can be trained in 5–10 days time.
- The sensitivity of VIA for identifying women with HSIL as proved in various studies is equivalent to Pap smear.

Limitations of VIA
- Visual inspection with acetic acid is provider dependent-screening method. It has low specificity with high false positive results. Thus, over treatment may cause burden to the healthcare system, increase cost and cause unnecessary tension.
- VIA is less effective in postmenopausal women, because SCJ recedes into the cervical os making identification of lesions difficult.

- The accuracy of VIA is disturbed if there is prevalence of STD, which may increase the level of inflammation and render visual inspection difficult to assess.
- The specificity of VIA is relatively low, as such high rate of over treatment is expected if 'screen and treat' approach is adopted.

HPV-DNA testing
After the establishment of the causal role of HPV in the genesis of cervical neoplasia, attention was focused on the potential clinical utility of HPV testing for identifying cervical cancer precursors since 1990s.

It is done as a primary screening test, solely or in combination with cytology to detect cervical cancer precursors. HPV testing can be done by:
- Second generation Hybrid Capture 2 (HC2) system, which is approved by US FDA.
- Polymerase chain reaction.

HPV testing by HC2
A conical brush is introduced into the cervical canal and rotated three times to collect both ecto- and endocervical cells, which is retrieved and inserted into the STM in the vial. The tip is broken and vial is closed.

Advantages
- HC2 assay is easy to perform in clinical practice and amenable to automation, which makes it attractive for high volume screening use.
- Since it is based on signal, HC2 is less prone to cross specimen contamination, thus obviating the need for special laboratory facilities to avoid cross-contamination.
- Probe B (high-risk probe) is used for cervical lesion screening, which reduces the time and cost to perform the test.

HPV testing by polymerase chain reaction
Polymerase chain reaction (PCR) has lower threshold of molecular detection for HPV DNA than HC assay. Cross-contamination is a major problem in application of PCR in HPV testing. PCR, thus gives better result when applied in research studies to detect specific type of HPV.

Clinical applications of HPV testing
- In combination with Pap test in women 30 years or older. Below this age the infection goes away on its own so result of this test is not significant rather it is confusing. So, it is not recommended before the age of 30.
- As a triage test in women with minor cytological abnormalities in Pap test such as atypical squamous cells of undetermined significance (ASCUS), low-grade squamous intraepithelial lesions (LSIL). This helps to select women, who really need referral for diagnosis and treatment.
- Following LSIL, HPV testing done after 6 and 18 months is safe and cost effective. This reduces the need for colposcopy allowing time for viral clearance.
- As a follow-up test for women treated for high-grade intraepithelial lesion with local ablative or excisional therapy. HPV testing picks up residual disease quicker and with higher sensitivity and similar specificity compared to follow-up cytology. Combined cytology and HPV testing has been proposed at 6 months and 24 months after treatment. If previous results are negative, patient is referred to 5 years cytology screening.

Note:
- If Pap test result is negative, but HPV DNA is positive.
  Co-testing (Pap + HPV) is to be repeated within 1 year.
  If test is positive for HPV type 16 or 18 colposcopy is recommended.
- If both Pap test and HPV DNA positive colposcopy is recommended.

Sensitivity and Specificity of HPV Testing
HPV test by HC2 for high-risk HPV types is more sensitive than cytology for CIN II and CIN III, but it has lower specificity. HPV testing has a sensitivity of 95% for detecting CIN II or CIN III compared with 75% for cytology in detecting ASCUS and 70% in detecting LSIL. The specificity improves if HPV testing is done in women over 30 years of age. The specificity is 93% for CIN II or CIN III compared with 95% and 98% specificity for cytology in detecting ASCUS and LSIL respectively in women over 30 years age. For younger women, both tests have poorer specificity.

HPV testing as a triage test: Triage is a second test performed only if the first test is neither

Precancerous Disease of Cervix and its Prevention

completely normal nor definitely indicative of need for treatment. In other words, triage is an additional test done in between screening and diagnosis to further stratify women with positive primary screening results according to cancer risk. In cervical cancer, screening triage test is of value, because cytology has low specificity and diagnostic procedure is expensive or is limited. Thus, triage test reduces over treatment, patient anxiety and inconvenience as well as overall management cost without compromising sensitivity for detection of disease.

Note: HPV DNA testing is not recommended
- As a routine screening in women younger than 30 years
- In women with ASC-H, LSIL or HSIL cytology. Exception postmenopausal women with LSIL, HPV DNA testing may be used.
- Alone for screening. It should not replace other effective cervical cancer screening methods.

Further testing for abnormal Pap tests: All abnormal Pap smear require, further evaluation by visualization of cervix, repeat cytology, HPV DNA testing, Schiller test, colposcopy, colposcopy directed biopsy, endocervical and endometrial curettage for biopsy and diagnostic conization.

According to American Cancer Society following are the recommended further testing for abnormal Pap test:
- For ASC-US:
  - If the Pap test shows AUS-CUS then any one of the two is recommended:
    i. *Repeat Pap test:* Repeated every 6 months till two consecutive normal smears. Before testing antimicrobials and hormones are given for infection and atrophic vaginitis respectively.
    ii. HPV DNA testing is recommended.
       - If HPV is detected, colposcopy is recommended
       - If HPV is not detected, co-testing is to be repeated after 3 years.
       - If result labeled ASC-H, high grade SIL is suspected and colposcopy is recommended.
- For LSIL further testing is dependent upon HPV testing
  - If HPV testing is negative, co-testing after one year is recommended.
  - If HPV testing is positive, colposcopy is recommended
  - If no HPV testing is done and woman is 25 years old, colposcopy is recommended, if woman is under 25 repeat Pap test in one year is recommended.
  - Pregnant woman with LSIL should have colposcopy
- For HSIL:
  - For women of age 25 or older, colposcopy or loop electrosurgical procedure is recommended.
  - For women under 25 colposcopy is recommended
- For atypical glandular cells or adenocarcinoma:
  - Colposcopy with biopsy of endocervical curettage.
  - Biopsy of endometrial curettage.

Secondary Screening Tool

Colposcopy

Colposcopy is a screening tool, which involves systemic evaluation of low genital tract by magnified illumination. It is an accepted procedure for verification of cytologic finding. Hinselmann first described colposcopy in 1925.

Objective of Colposcopy

To rule out invasive cancer by identifying the most severe lesion and perform directed biopsy.

Targeted Structure to be Examined

Transformation zone of cervix which includes:
- Superficial epithelium
- Blood vessel of underlying connective tissue stroma.

Indications of Colposcopy

- Abnormal cervical cytology:
  - HSIL – CIN II, CIN III
  - LSIL in developing countries

- LSIL in developed countries. Repeat cytology at 6 months internal for 2 years is done.

  If persistent or progressive abnormalities: Referred to colposcopy
- Suspicious looking cervix with normal cytology
- Leukoplakia of cervix (obscures lesion and interferes in adequate cytological sampling)
- Postcoital bleeding
- VIA + VIAM +
- VILI +
- History of diethylstilbestrol (DES) exposure.

Instruments for Colposcopy
- Colposcope.
- Bivalved cusco speculum.
- Punch biopsy forcep.
- Endocervical curette.
- Endocervical speculum.
- Skin or cervical hook.
- Vaginal side wall retractor.

Parts of Colposcope

An optical colposcope consists of:
- Optics carrier.
- Colposcopic stand.
- Floor pedestals with wheels.
- Light source (in built).

Optic Carrier

Optic carrier consists of:
a. Objective lens.
b. Two ocular lenses or eye pieces.
c. Green filter.

Magnification

Fixed magnification: Less expensive microscope. Changeable low, medium and high magnification:
- Low power magnification for examination of vulva and male genitalia.
- Medium power magnification for examination of vulva, vagina and cervix.
- High power magnification for details of vascular patterns.

Light Source

- May be tungsten, xenon or halogen.
- Halogen light provides a brighter light that is excellent for photography.

Modern Colposcope: Video Colposcope

- Video colposcopy provides magnification and illumination without use of binocular eyepieces
- The system includes video colposcope and a high resolution video monitor
- One of the main criticism of video colposcope is that the colposcopic image on the video monitor is a two dimensional rather than a three dimensional image, making assessment of the contour and density of the lesion more difficult.

Supplies for colposcopy
- Normal saline
- 3–5% acetic acid
- Lugol's iodine.
- Monsel's solution or silver nitrate solution.

Application of normal saline
To study the subepithelial vascular architecture normal saline is used. Green filter can be used here to see the vessels more clearly.

Application of 3–5% acetic acid
Normal findings of cervix under colposcope
- In ectocervix the healthy squamous epithelium is seen in between original squamocolumnar junction and mucocutaneous junction of vulvovagina. The overall effect is light pink color (squamocolumnar junction is the junction between the stratified squamous epithelium of ectocervix and columnar epithelium of endocervical canal).
- Endocervix consists of single layer of columnar cells. Superficial capillaries are directly beneath the single layer. The overall effect is dark pink to red coloration.
- The transformation zone (metaplastic squamous epithelium) is seen between original and active squamocolumnar junction. The area will appear more white than surrounding

pink ectocervix or red endocervix. The capillaries are seen as fine punctation (closely applied).

Squamous metaplasia is a dynamic and reversible process. It shifts at different stages of life depending on the hormonal and environmental influences. In reproductive life estrogenic influence brings it down toward ectocervix and oral contraceptive pills and pregnancy further draw it down towards ectocervix. Due to lack of estrogen, it shifts towards endocervix and in postmenopausal women, it lies within the endocervical canal.

Cervical neoplasia almost invariably originates within the transformation zone. In satisfactory colposcopy transformation zone must be entirely visualized.

- The columnar epithelium of endocervical canal is seen.

Abnormal findings of cervix under colposcope

Acetic acid causes a reversible coagulation or precipitation of the nuclear proteins and cytokeratins.

- An area of white and thickened epithelium called leukoplakia or hyperkeratosis is seen before application of acetic acid which indicates underlying neoplasia.
- After application of acetic acid acetowhite epithelium is seen which indicates dysplasia.
  - As a result of coagulation, the subepithelial vessel pattern is obliterated and the epithelium appears white. This reaction is termed as acetowhitening. Acetowhitening appears quickly and persist for >1 min.
  - In low grade CIN, AA must penetrate into the lower one-third of epithelium. Acetowhiteness is less intense and delayed.
  - In high grade CIN, dysplastic cells are in the superficial layer and there is higher concentration of nuclear protein due to large number of dysplastic cells, the area becomes densely white and opaque with well-demarcated margins.
  - In severe lesion, abnormal large and coarse vascular pattern of surface capillaries give the appearance of *mosaicism* and *punctation*.
  - Atypical vessels with bizarre capillaries with corkscrew, comma shaped or spaghetti-like configuration is seen in early stromal invasion.
  - Nonvisualization of transformation zone. Evaluation of these cases need endocervical canal curettage (ECC).

Note: Acetowhiteness is also seen in other situations such as in leukoplakia, condylomata and in inflammation. In these situations, acetowhiteness is less pale, patchily distributed without well-defined margins, distributed widely outside transformation zone and disappear, quickly.

Principles of Schiller's (Lugol's) I_2 test

The widely use of colposcopy dimmed the use of *Schiller test* nowadays. It is done by applying Lugol's iodine on the surface to observe the change of color of the tissue. Normal cells contain glycogen, which mixed with iodine turn into a deep mehogany-brown color. If it does not take the color, it indicates that epithelial cells are abnormal due to scarring, cyst formation, metaplasia and constitutes a positive Schiller test. Biopsy can be taken from this unhealthy area.

Monsel's solution/silver nitrate

Monsel's solution or silver nitrate is applied after colposcopic biopsy to achieve hemostasis. Both will interfere in the interpretation of biopsy. So, should be applied when all biopsy samples are collected.

Colposcopic Features Guiding Provisional Diagnosis

Low grade CIN
- Moderately dense shiny AW lesion
- Well-demarcated irregular or angular or geographic margins
- Flat, smooth surface
- Fine punctation or mosaicism
- No iodine uptake.

High grade CIN
- Dull, dense, grayish white or oyster white lesion
- Well-demarcated, regular margins, sometimes raised or peeled out

- Irregular or nodular surfaces
- Coarse punctation or mosaicism
- No iodine uptake.

Preclinical Invasive Cancer

- Chalky white, thick, opaque lesion
- Well-demarcated, raised and rolled out margins
- Irregular nodular or mountains and valley pattern
- Coarse mosaicism or punctation, atypical blood vessels seen
- No iodine uptake.

Note: *In all these abnormal situations, colposcopy-guided biopsy is taken for histopathological examination.*

RELATED INFORMATION

Types of Biopsy

- Punch biopsy
- Cone biopsy.

Diagnostic conization (Cone biopsy)
After colposcopy, diagnostic conization or cone biopsy is done under the following circumstances:
- If colposcopy is unsatisfactory and lesion extends beyond view.
- If there is dysplasia in ECC.
- If there is significant discrepancy between the histologic and cytological tests.
- If microinvasive carcinoma is suspected.
- If adenocarcinoma is suspected.

A cone biopsy removes the whole of the squamocolumnar junction and also a considerable part of endocervix. Hemorrhage may occur after cone biopsy, which is controlled by packing or suturing the cervix laterally. Bleeding should not be controlled by cauterization as it may destroy the tissue, which may need study if hysterectomy is done subsequently.

Interpretation of biopsy result
The abnormal cells are described as abnormal differentiation or undifferentiated, pleomorphic and hyperchromatic nuclei and abnormal number of chromosome with active mitosis. The lesion is classified according to involvement of epithelium by abnormal cells:
- When only basal third or less of the epithelium is occupied by the undifferentiated cells, the lesion is classified as CIN I, LSIL or LSIL (mild dysplasia).
- When between one-third and two-thirds epithelium is occupied by undifferentiated cells, the lesion is classified as CIN II or HSIL (moderate dysplasia).
- When the undifferentiated cells occupy more than two-thirds of the epithelium, but full thickness is not involved, the lesion is classified as CIN III or HSIL (severe dysplasia).
- In the most severe form of CIN III atypical disorderly and disoriented closely packed cells occupy whole thickness of the epithelium sparing the basement membrane is called carcinoma in situ.
- When cells of CIN III breaks the basement membrane and involve the stromal of less than 3 mm from the base of the epithelium is called microinvasive carcinoma.
- When invasion is more than 3 mm it is called invasive carcinoma.

Screening Schedule

According to American Cancer Society (ACS); American Society for Colposcopy and Cervical Pathology (ASCCP); The American Society for Clinical Pathology (ASCP) (Saslow et al. 2012); United States Preventive Services Task Force (USPSTF) [Moyer, 2012]; American College of Obstetricians and Gynecologists the schedule for cervical cancer screening is as follows [ACOG Practice Bulletin Number 131, 2012]:
- All women should begin screening at the age of 21 years. Women aged 21–29 years should have a Pap test every 3 years. HPV testing is not needed at this age group except as a part of follow-up in abnormal Pap test.
- Beginning at age of the 30 screening with a Pap test along with HPV test (cotesting) is preferable. Repeat this cotesting every 5 years and should continue till 65 years.
- If only Pap test is used for screening between 30 and 65 years, test is to be repeated every 3 years.

- Women who are at high risk of cervical cancer, because of suppressed immune response due to HIV infection, organ transplantation and long-term use of steroids or because of exposed to DES in utero need more frequent testing usually annually.
- Women over 65 years with negative findings in the previous 10 years should stop further testing, but with history of CIN II or CIN III should continue testing every 3 years for at least 20 years after the abnormality was found.
- Women who have had hysterectomy for indication other than cervical precancer or cancer, should stop screening testing.
- Women should continue to be screened if they have had a total hysterectomy and have a history of CIN II or higher in the past 20 years or cervical cancer ever.
- Women who have hysterectomy without removal of cervix for indication other than cervical precancer or cancer should continue cervical cancer screening according to usual guideline.
- Women who have vaccinated against HPV should still follow the screening as usual guidelines for their age group.

Note: Abnormal screening results may need to have a follow-up Pap test sometimes with HPV test within a year.

> **Case scenario:** Mrs Fatema, aged 32 years, having a son of 8 years and a daughter of 5 years old came worried with a biopsy report of CIN II. Fatema was having excessive vaginal discharge and on speculum examination cervix was found to be unhealthy. She was subjected to Pap smear, which revealed HGIL. Then her doctor referred her to colposcopy. Colposcopy was satisfactory with acetowhite opaque lesion in the transformation zone of the cervix. Biopsy was taken from that area, which revealed CIN II.
>
> What will be the management of CIN II for Fatema?

There are two modalities of treatment for CIN II:
1. Conservative for young patients who did not complete her family in the form of:
   - Ablation
   - Surgical excision.
2. Hysterectomy for women who are elderly and completed her family.

Since Fatema is young, though her family is complete, the best choice of treatment will be either:
- Ablative therapy which can be done by:
  - Cryosurgery.
  - CO_2 laser therapy.
- Surgical excision by loop electrosurgical excision procedure (LEEP).

> Why colposcopy was done in this case?

Colposcopy was done here to:
- Determine the best site from where cervical biopsy should be taken.
- Determine the extent of lesion, i.e. whether the lesion is confined to the ectocervix or has extended to endocervix.

> In this scenario, it was evident that the lesion was confined to ectocervix on the basis of satisfactory colposcopy.
>
> If the colposcopy would have been unsatisfactory, would there be any change in the evaluation?

Yes, unsatisfactory colposcopy demands ECC to rule out invasion in the endocervix.

> How Fatema will be followed up?

Fatema will be followed up by:
- Cytology alone 6 monthly or
- Combined cytology and colposcopy 6 monthly.

If two consecutive reports are negative, Fatema will enter routine screening for next 20 years.

RELATED INFORMATION

Cervical Intraepithelial Neoplasia

Cervical intraepithelial neoplasia is a range of intraepithelial abnormalities of varying degree, which begins in the squamocolumnar junction in the cervical epithelium of the transformation zone. It is a single disease, which follows a continuous process, but it is difficult to predict the natural history of disease. The etiological factors involved are same as for carcinoma of cervix.

Pathological Grading

Cervical intraepithelial neoplasia is graded according to the proportion of epithelium occupied by undifferentiated cells. Accordingly they are graded as CIN I, CIN II and CIN III.

CIN I (Fig. 15.2A): When only basal one-third or less cervical epithelium is occupied by undifferentiated cells it is called CIN I. Genuine regression to normal occurs with CIN I and it is difficult to distinguish in this grade true CIN from inflammatory changes including HPV infection, but one-fourth of the cases progress to severe lesion.

CIN II (Fig. 15.2B): When undifferentiated cells occupy between one-third and two-thirds of cervical epithelium it is called CIN II. There is considerable heterogenecity in the microscopic diagnosis, biology and clinical behavior of CIN II. Some are produced by noncarcinogenic HPV types with a severe microscopic appearance and are destined to regress. But others are incipient precancer and will persist and progress to cancer. One quarter of the cases if left untreated will progress to more severe lesion **(Table 15.2)**.

CIN III (Fig. 15.2C): When more than two-thirds of cervical epithelium thickness is occupied by undifferentiated cells it is called CIN III. *In the most severe form of CIN III, atypical cells occupy the full thickness of cervical epithelium it is called carcinoma in situ.* Histologically CIN III is clearly established as a cancer precursor, but separating CIN II from CIN III is sometimes difficult. Over a half of the untreated cases of CIN III will eventually develop invasive carcinoma **(Table 15.2)**.

The main histological criteria of CIN III are:
- Disorderly and disoriented arrangement of closely packed cells throughout the epidermis with loss of stratification.
- Intact basement membrane with absence of rete ridges.
- Variation in shape and size of cells.
- Variation in shape, size and staining characteristics of nuclei with few mitosis.

Treatment

CIN I

CIN I can be kept under observation and monitored by cytology and colposcopy 6 monthly for 1 year, provided the colposcopy is satisfactory and endocervical sampling is negative.

If CIN I persists after 1 year and is preceded by HSIL, diagnostic excisional procedure is done.

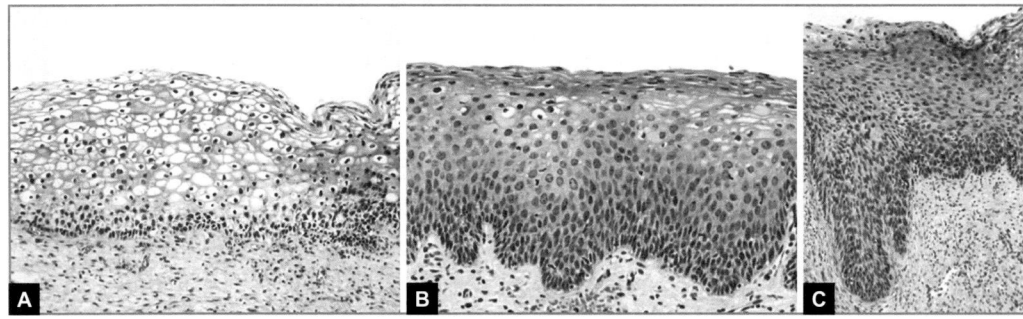

Figs 15.2A to C (A) CIN I; (B) CIN II; (C) CIN III
(For color version, see Plate 3)

Table 15.2 Natural history of different grades of cervical intraepithelial neoplasia

Grades	Regression	Persistence	Progression to severe lesion	Progression to invasive cancer
CIN I	57%	32%	11%	1%
CIN II	43%	35%	22%	1.5%
CIN III	32%	32%	56%	12%

If preceded by ASCUS, ASC-H or LSIL further observation can be done for one more year by cytology and colposcopy at 6 months intervals.

CIN II and CIN III

- Patients with lesion confined to ectocervix with satisfactory colposcopy and negative ECC, any one of the following treatment can be adopted though each one has got its advantage and disadvantage:
  - Cryotherapy
  - Carbondioxide laser
  - LEEP.
- Patients with endocervical lesion or positive ECC or unsatisfactory colposcopy or when there is discrepancy between cytology and colposcopy, the stepwise approach is cold knife conization and ECC to rule out invasion. The subsequent management depends upon the final histopathology report.
- Elderly patients who have completed their family, hysterectomy can also be an option of treatment.

Cervical Adenocarcinoma In Situ

Hysterectomy is the preferred treatment for women, who is histologically diagnosed as adenocarcinoma in situ (AIS).

Because of the extension of the disease to within the endocervical canal and presence of multifocal 'skip lesion', hysterectomy is preferred.

If fertility is desired, conservative excisional procedure can be done, but the patient need to be closely followed-up using a combination of cytology, colposcopy, HPV DNA testing and endocervical sampling at 6 monthly interval.

Post-treatment Follow-up

The treatment failure rate following treatment of CIN is around 10% if evaluated for 2 years. The risk of recurrence is high in women older than 50 years. There is no consensus regarding the duration of post-treatment surveillance. Follow-up data shows that these women are at risk up to 10 years, but some propose that they should be followed-up for 20 years:
- Cytology 6 monthly.
- Combined cytology and colposcopy 6 monthly.

- HPV DNA testing at 6–12 months.
  - If HPV DNA test is negative or two consecutive cytology reports are negative, the women will enter routine screening:
    - Annually for 5 years then
    - 3 yearly for the next 15 years
    - If repeat cytology shows ASCUS or HPV DNA test is positive, colposcopy and endocervical sampling is recommended.

Treatment Procedure

Cryosurgery

Cryosurgery is a simple, effective, inexpensive and relatively easy therapeutic option for treating CIN. It is most effective for small lesion confined to the ectocervix. In other words, LSIL without extension to endocervical canal are the most effective indications for cryosurgery.

Equipment
- Cryogun with a probe. The probe must cover the lesion and entire transformation zone.
- Cylinder with compressed refrigerant gas such as N_2O or CO_2. N_2O is mostly used.

Principles of cryosurgery

Compressed N_2O is allowed to expand through a small jet producing an ice ball at the surface of metal probe, which remains in contact with the lesion and the transformation zone. Crystallization of intracellular water occurs resulting in cell death and this occurs when the temperature ranges between 20° and 30°C. Crystallization begins on the probe and proceeds until the ice ball is seen to extend 7 mm laterally beyond the edge of the probe. This visual landmark ensures that the depth of freezing is 5 mm and this is needed in order to extend the freezing beyond the depth of crypts of glands.

Technique adapted

A freeze-thaw-freeze technique is commonly used. Two sequential freeze thaw cycle causes effective freezing. Each cycle consists of 3 minutes of freezing followed by 5 minutes of thawing monitored by stop watch. The minimum working pressure shown on the gauze should be 40 kg/cm^2.

Success

For CIN lesions, cryosurgery provides more than 90% cure rate. But larger the lesion, lower is the cure rate. Endocervical lesion also increases the failure rate.

Complications

Complications are rare. The patient experiences blood stained watery discharge for 3-4 weeks.

Limitations
- There is no specimen to evaluate histopathologically.
- It cannot treat lesion that extends into the endocervix.
- It cannot destroy tissue where the lesion has extended deep to the crypts, i.e. to a depth of 7 mm.

Carbondioxide Laser Ablation

Carbondioxide laser ablation is an alternative to cryotherapy performed under local anesthesia, which destroys tissue to a precisely determined depth. But the procedure is expensive and needs training to perform. The electric current should be adjusted between 25 and 60 watt to minimize thermal injury of tissue.

Advantages

- Carbondioxide laser ablation is able to destroy cervical tissue to a depth of 7 mm, which is sometimes needed when the deepest crypts of glands are involved in CIN III or carcinoma in situ.
- There is minimum lateral thermal injury.
- Post-treatment vaginal discharge is less than cryosurgery.

Complications

Cervical stenosis and cervical incompetence rarely occurs.

Success

The primary cure rate is 95% in CIN with minimum morbidity.

Loop Electrosurgical Excision Procedure

Loop electrosurgical excision procedure (LEEP) is a widely used and valuable therapeutic option management of CIN. It is done under local anesthesia. It is applicable for lesions in the transformation zone (TZ), which has extended into the endocervix, but distal limit do not extend beyond 1 cm.

Equipment

- Plastic-coated speculum with suction attached
- Electrosurgical system which consists of:
  - Loop electrode. Large loop electrode is 1-2 mm in width and 0.7-1.5 cm in depth for excision of entire TZ usually in a single pass.
  - Ball electrode 5 mm in size for fulguration of tissue.
  - Electrosurgical generator where appropriate power is set for the size of loop. Usually, 35-55 w of either pure cutting or blended current is required, for the procedure.
  - Grounding pad is attached to patients thigh.
  - Smoke evacuator is attached to the anterior blade of insulated speculum to remove the smoke that is generated during electrical cutting, thus ensuring clean operative field.

Principles of LEEP

The CIN lesion in the cervix is excised in appropriated width and depth by electric current mostly by single pass followed by fulguration of the base to achieve hemostasis.

Note:
- The lesion that is excised by electric current must have 2-3 mm healthy margin around the lesion and a depth of 5-7 mm.
- An endocervical curettage should be performed if one has not done previously.

Advantages

- The procedure is quicker and easier.
- Histological assessment of entire excised tissue is possible.
- 'See and tract' approach at one visit can be adopted in low resource setting and that has brought the procedure the extra popularity.

Complications

- Postoperative bleeding occurs in 2–5% patients.
- Cervical stenosis and cervical incompetence is rare.

Success

The primary cure rate is more than 95% in CIN and is comparable with those achieved with CO_2 laser procedure.

Cervical Intraepithelial Neoplasia CIN in Pregnancy

Abnormal epithelium in cervical cytology in early prenatal visit:
- Colposcopy.
- Colposcopy directed biopsy from ectocervix only if there is strong suspicion.
- If dysplasia diagnosed, patient should be carefully followed-up with colposcopy and cervical cytology.
- Repeat biopsy is only performed in progressive lesion.
- *No endocervical curettage:* There is a potential risk of infection and hemorrhage.

Treatment

- Treatment is deferred in pregnancy and in postpartum period. Even high-grade lesion has a high rate of regression during postpartum period.
- Conization is indicated only if early invasive disease is suspected.

Complications

Conization may cause:
- Abortion
- Hemorrhage
- Infection
- Premature labor due to cervical incompetence
- Difficult labor due to cervical dystocia.

BIBLIOGRAPHY

ACOG Practice Bulletin Number 131: Screening for cervical cancer. Obstet Gynecol. 2012;120(5):1222-38.

Anne Szarewski. HPV Vaccine: Cervarix. Expert Opin Biol Ther. 2010;10(3):477-8.

Bosch Fx, de Sanjores. Human papilloma virus and cervical cancer-burden and assessment of causality. J Natl. Cancer Inst Monograph. 2003;(31):3-13.

David MP, Hardt K, Tibaldi F, et al. Modeling of long-term persistence of Anti-HPV-16 and Anti-HPV-18 antibodies induced by an ASO4-adjuvanted cervical cancer vaccine. Eurogin, Nice, France, 2008.

Harper DM, France El, et al. Sustained efficacy up to 4.5 years of a bivalent L, VLP vaccine against HPV 16 & 18: follow-up from a randomized controlled trial. Obstet Gynecol. 2006;107(1):18-27.

Moyer VA. Screening for cervical cancer: US Preventive Services Task Force recommendation statement. Ann Intern Med. 2012;156:880.

Nandak, McCrory DC, et al. Accuracy of Papanicolaou test in screening for and follow-up of cytologic abnormalities a systematic review. Ann Intern Med. 2000;132(10):810-9.

Papanicolaou, GN. Proceedings of the Third Race Betterment Conference January. New cancer diagnosis. Battle Creek, Michigan Race Betterment Foundation; 1928.pp.528-34.

Papanicolaou, GN: Atlas of Exfoliative Cytology. Cambridge Mass. Harvard University Press; 1954.p.9.

Roteli-Martins CM, Naud P, Borba PD, Teixera JC, Carvalho NSD, Zahaf T, et al. Sustained immuno-genicity and efficacy of the HPH-16/18 ASO4-adjuvanted vaccine. Human Vaccines and immuno-therapeutics. 2012;8(3):390-97.

Saslow D, Solomon D, Lawson H, et al. American Cancer Society, American Society for Colposcopy and Cervical Pathology, and American Society for Clinical Pathology screening guidelines for the prevention and early detection of cervical cancer. Am J Clin Pathol. 2012;137(4):516-42.

Zur Hausen H. Molecular pathogenesis of cancer of cervix and its causation by specific human papillomavirus types. Curr Top. Microbiol. Immunlol. 1994;186: 131-56.

CHAPTER 16

Endometriosis

Rashida Begum

INTRODUCTION

Endometriosis is defined as the presence of endometrial glands and stroma in extrauterine locations. Most often it is located in the posterior cul-de-sac and in the ovaries, but it has been diagnosed in the pleural cavity, liver, brain and incisional lines. Endometriosis occurs in about 8–10% in reproductive aged women (Pritts, 2003). It is more frequently found among infertile women. About 20–70% endometriotic women are infertile. Association of endometriosis and infertility is not very clear, but management of endometriosis has become a component of infertility evaluation and treatment (Pritts, 2003; Olive and Pritts, 2001; D'Hooghe, 2003). The disease occurs most commonly between the ages of 30 and 40 years, but may occur any time between menarche and menopause. The risk of development of the disease is 7 times more in first-degree relatives. It is more common in highly civilized communities and their well to do members. That is why it is called a disease of the rich.

> **Case scenario:** Mrs Salma aged 32 years has come to you with the complaints of severe pain during menstruation. Her cycle is regular and blood loss is excessive with 5–6 days duration. She has also complaints of painful coitus.
>
> How will you proceed to establish your diagnosis?

More information is to be taken by history.

History

Dysmenorrhea, dyspareunia and menorrhagia are the typical features of endometriosis, adenomyosis and pelvic inflammatory disease (PID). But there are some differences in pattern of dysmenorrhea. So *detailed* history is to be taken to isolate these three conditions:

- Duration of the symptoms
- Pattern of pain
- About bleeding
- About parity
- Contraceptive history
- Treatment history

Duration of the Symptoms

How long she has been suffering from these symptoms?

Pattern of Pain

- Whether it increases or decreases with flow of menstruation. Whether pain subsides with painkillers or not?
    - In endometriosis pain starts slowly before onset of menstruation due to congestion of endometriotic focus, becomes severe during menstruation as bleeding takes place in a closed space and reach a maximum at the end of menstruation due to creation of tension by accumulating blood. There is progressive dysmenorrhea. But pain usually subsides with painkillers.
    - In PID due to pelvic congestion pain starts before menstruation and begins to decline with menstrual flow. Pain usually subsides with pain killers.
    - In adenomyosis dysmenorrhea is severe in nature continued throughout the

cycle even beyond, and patient becomes crippled and pain does not subside with ordinary painkillers.
- Whether there is any intermenstrual pain?
  – Intermenstrual pain is also common in PID endometriosis and adenomyosis, but more common in PID.
- Pain is deep-seated and there is pain during defecation due to rectal involvement in endometriosis.

About Bleeding

Menorrhagia may be due to fibroid, dysfunctional uterine bleeding (DUB), endometriosis, PID, adenomyosis use of intrauterine contraceptive devices (IUCDs)

Things to be enquired:
- How much bleeding does take place? Whether there is passage of any clotted blood?
  – In fibroid bleeding becomes more on 2nd and 3rd day and menorrhagia is progressive in nature.

About Parity

- Endometriosis, adenomyosis, fibroid and PID are associated with infertility or low parity.
- In PID there may be history of childbirth, abortion, MR and dilatation and curettage (D&C) following abortion.

Contraceptive History

- The IUCD use is associated with dysmenorrhea and menorrhagia.
- History of vaginal discharge and sexually transmitted diseases (STD) is associated with PID.

Treatment History and Response to Treatment

- Whether she received any treatment or not?
- If received whether it did work or not?

Physical Examination

Per abdominal and per vaginal examination is to be done.

> On enquiry, you elicited that she has two children with ALC of 8 years, her husband is using condom for contraceptive, pain increases with flow of blood and becomes more at the end of menstruation. Bleeding is heavy but she does not pass any clot. Pain usually subsides with painkillers. Dyspareunia is deep seated. She has been suffering for 2 years from these symptoms and did not visit any doctor for this. On abdominal examination there is no lump present, but there is tenderness in the pelvis on deep palpation. Per vaginal examination revealed that cervical motion tenderness is present, uterine mobility is restricted, and fornices are tender.
>
> What might be your diagnosis?

Most likely diagnosis is endometriosis.

RELATED INFORMATION

Diagnostic features of endometriosis are given below:

Symptoms

- Secondary dysmenorrhea: Pain starts before menstruation because endometrial implants are stimulated by estrogen and progesterone during menstrual cycle and grow in the same way as the uterine endometrium. The implant enlarge undergo secretory changes causes bleeding in closed space. Due to surrounding adhesions it prevents expansion and due to accumulation of blood in the closed space it causes pain. Pain is also produced by pressure and inflammation within and around the lesion, by traction on adhesions. Severity of pain depends on number of implants and their proximity to nerves and other sensitive organs and pressure by large masses. Degree of pain also depends on depth of invasion. Deeply infiltrating lesions causes more pain.

Repeated cycle increases the amount of pain for further progression of sequel of disease. That is why dysmenorrhea is progressive in nature.

Note: Many patients with severe endometriosis have no pain and it is common observation that most of the time the occurrence and severity of pain from endometriosis bears little relationship to the amount and extension of disease. With small lesion there may be

maximum symptoms and minimum symptoms with extensive and large lesions.
- Deep dyspareunia when pouch of Douglas and rectovaginal septum are affected and when uterus is fixed retroverted.
- Menorrhagia: Excessive bleeding is due to associated endometrial hyperplasia, which is present in about 60% of cases of pelvic endometriosis. Due to ovarian involvement and vascular upset polymenorrhea and polymenorrhagia may occur.
- Sacral backache, worse during menstruation.
- Infertility.
- Painful defecation and hematuria due to involvement of rectosigmoid and bladder.
- Lump formation due to chocolate cyst and adhesions.
- Abdominal pain.
- Progressive constipation, tenesmus and obstruction due to bowel involvement.

Signs

- Cervical motion tenderness
- Restricted uterine mobility
- Fixed retroverted uterus
- Posterior vaginal fornix becomes shallow with thickening of the tissues
- Uterosacral ligaments become tender, nodular and thickened
- Nodularity in pouch of Douglas
- Painful ovarian palpation
- Adnexal mass (ovarian endometrioma).

How will you confirm the diagnosis?

Making diagnosis on the basis of symptoms is difficult as clinical presentations are very variable. Following aids can make diagnosis.

Ultrasonography

With classical history and physical examination ultrasonography may provide supporting evidence by demonstrating the presence of ovarian cyst. Routine ultrasonography does not have significant role in the diagnosis of endometriosis in the absence of pelvic mass or other obvious pelvic abnormality (Friedman et al. 1985). It is useful in differentiating endometriomata from other ovarian cysts by internal echogenicity. Chocolate cysts give hypoechoic appearance. In absence of cyst formation early endometriosis sometimes can be diagnosed by observing adhesion of both ovaries behind the uterus giving the appearance called 'kissing ovaries' **(Figs 16.1A and B)**.

Laparoscopy

A confirm diagnosis can be made after direct visualization by laparoscopy and can be reconfirmed by histological examination. It is the gold standard diagnostic tool for endometriosis.

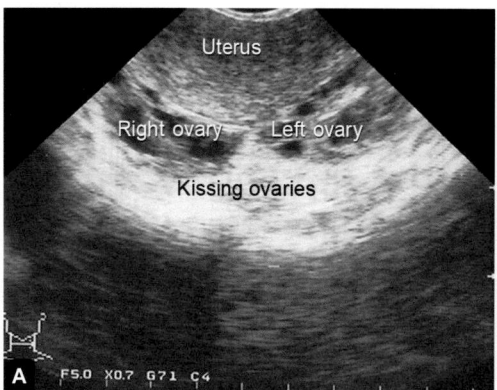 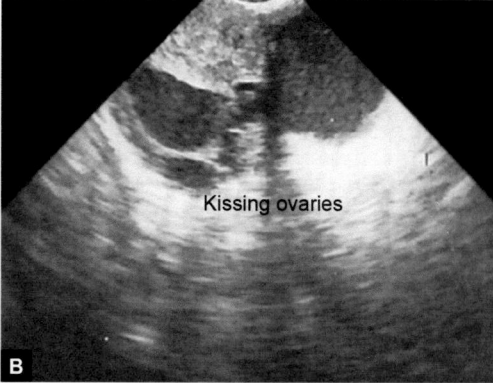

Figs 16.1A and B (A) Kissing ovaries without cyst; (B) Kissing ovaries with cyst

Magnetic Resonance Imaging

Magnetic resonance imaging (MRI) is a noninvasive tool can demonstrate endometriotic implants in the cul-de-sac (Hricak et al. 1985) but unable to demonstrate superficial lesions (Arrive et al. 1989) and cannot be used as a substitute for laparoscopy in the definitive diagnosis or staging of endometriosis. It can be used to monitor treatment response in place of laparoscopy once a diagnosis is firmly established.

Biochemical Test Like CA 125

CA 125 is raised in endometriosis, but it is not confirmatory as it increases in other ovarian tumor. So it is not recommended to do the test for diagnosis of endometriosis.

> What are the bases of diagnosis by laparoscopy?

There are multiple and varied appearance of endometriotic lesions at laparoscopy ranging from typical scarred black lesions to subtle lesions. In general, there are three broad groups of endometriotic lesions.

Subtle Lesions

Small fluid-filled vesicles are found either pigmented red petechial or nonpigmented lesions on the peritoneal surface. They represent early foci of disease from implanted endometriotic cells on the peritoneal surface.

Gunshot or Powder-burn Lesions

They are recognized as classical pigmented endometriotic deposits. They occupy a large surface area and penetrate to a greater depth. Due to accumulation of menstrual blood within the lesion it becomes cystic, dark brown, dark blue or black appearance. The surrounding peritoneal surface becomes thickened and scarred. These powder burn implants attain a size of 5–10 mm. With progression of disease the number and size of the lesion increase causing extensive adhesions. In the ovary cysts enlarged to several centimeters called endometrioma or chocolate cysts.

Deeply Infiltrating Lesions

These are significant degree of penetration from peritoneal surface down to the subperitoneal fat layer >5 mm (Cornillie et al. 1990; Martin et al. 1989). Lesions erode into underlying tissues and distort the remaining organs with extensive adhesions and involve the uterosacral ligaments, vagina, bowel, bladder and ureters.

Other Variety of Lesions

In addition to these classical features lesions can have other variety of nonclassical presentations like clear vesicles, white or yellow spots or nodules, circular folds of peritoneum.

> How does this ectopic endometrium develop?

Numbers of theories have been put forward, but no single theory adequately explains the pathogenesis of this disease.

Transplant Theory

Most frequently cited theory is Sampson's endometrial spill theory, which occurs due to retrograde spillage of viable endometrium during menstruation (Sampson, 1987). Endometrial cells within the fallopian tube and peritoneal cavity are viable and capable of implantation (Noble et al. 1996). But this theory does not explain why endometriosis develops in only 5–10% women in spite of documented menstrual efflux in 70–90% women (Liu and Hitchcock, 1986) and why does it occur in müllerian agenesis, hysterectomized and postmenopausal women?

Serosal Cell Metaplasia

Differentiation of embryonic cells into müllerian tissue in and around the pelvic peritoneum or on the surface of the ovary. Adult cells of these sites may retain the potential to differentiate into endometrium and myometrium. This theory explains the occurrence of endometriosis in women with müllerian agenesis, hysterectomized and in postmenopausal women (Olive and Henderson, 1987) and at distant and unusual sites.

Lymphatic and Vascular Embolism

Viable endometrium may enter into blood vessels and lymphatic, and transported to distant site and get implanted. This theory explains the development of endometriosis in lungs, brain incisional line and so on.

Immunological

It has been suggested that abnormal cellular and humoral immune mechanisms aid the attachment of spilled endometrial cells on the peritoneal surface various cytokines and growth factors could then maintain the presence of these endometrial cells (Startseva, 1980). This theory explains that due to this immune dysfunction spilled endometrium gets implanted in these women only.

Genetic Predisposition

There may be association of genetic predisposition with endometriosis. Because first degree female relatives have a 6–9% occurrence rate versus 1% rate for nonrelated controls (Simpson et al. 1984).

So the etiology of endometriosis is multifaceted. No single factor is responsible for the disease.

> In recent years many theories have emerged regarding development of endometrioma. What are those?

Sampson thought endometriomas are from corpus luteum, which was proved by Nezhat et al. (Nezhat et al. 1992). Nezhat et al. further developed theory regarding origin of endometriomas. According to their theory there are two types of endometriomas.

Type I or Primary Endometriomas

They inverted or invaginated from cortex of the ovary into interior of the ovary. These endometriomas when submitted to the pathologist always come back as endometrial glands and stroma. Clinically they are slow developing and very hard to remove the capsule. The capsule is very fibrotic and often should be piecemealed at the time of the removal. They usually develop by small endometrial glands sitting on the surface and gradually into the ovary. They hardly ever get more than 5 or 6 cm.

Type II or Secondary Endometriomas

These usually can get very large. They attain a size even up to 25 cm. These are the ones that Sampson referred to. The origin of all these endometriomas is somehow functional cysts. They could be corpus luteum or any other functional cyst. They are type II A and B.

1. Type II A is when the cyst looks exactly like a chocolate cyst and contains concentrated blood. During removal it comes off easily except when superficial endometriosis is invading. Pathology reports almost always come back as corpus luteum unless the pathologist is looking at the small segment of the cyst that has been invaded by endometriosis.
2. Type II B again looks exactly like a chocolate cyst having wall with endometrial glands and stroma. During dissection luteal cells are found in the cyst wall (Nezhat et al. 1995)

> What are the common sites of development of endometriosis?

Ovary
Most common site is ovary, involved in 30–40% cases. Lesions are ranging from burn match head spots to large chocolate cyst with varying degrees adhesions.

Pelvic peritoneum, uterovesical pouch, pouch of Douglas
Second most common site of endometriosis. Puckering and thickening of peritoneum manifest lesions, small tarry cysts with dense adhesion behind the uterus occluding the uterorectal pouch and making the uterus fixed retroverted.

Round ligaments, uterosacral ligaments and rectovaginal septum
Uterosacral ligaments are commonly affected becomes tough and shorter.

Outer coat of uterus
Endometriosis of the ovary, pelvic peritoneum and ligaments when adherent to the uterus sometimes invade its outer coat.

Fallopian tubes
Outer surface of the tubes affected get adherent with surrounding structures, but remains patent.

Intestine
Rectum and pelvic colon are most commonly affected parts of the gut. The lesions from peritoneum and ovaries invade them. Rarely lesions penetrate the rectal mucosa causing rectal bleeding and pain during defecation. Ileum, cecum, appendix and other parts may also be affected causing thickening, puckering of the outer coat of the bowel leads to stricture formation and adhesion, which can cause intestinal obstruction.

Bladder and ureters
Surrounding lesions can invade bladder and ureters.

Vagina, vulva
On rare occasion lesion can be seen in scars of the vagina and perineum. Sometimes lesions infiltrated from pouch of Douglas and rectovaginal septum into posterior fornix. Lesions appear as multiple small blue cysts. When it is indurate and ulcerated can be mistaken as carcinoma.

Abdominal wall
Endometriosis occurs in umbilicus, inguinal canal and incisional lines without any intrapelvic lesions. It appears as blue lesions causes swelling, which becomes bigger and more painful during menstruation and sometimes it discharges blood during menstruation. It occurs following cesarean section and gynecological operations.

Lungs, pleura
Though it is extremely rare, endometriosis can occur in lungs and pleura, more commonly in pleura. Cyclical development of pleuritic pain, hemothorax and hemoptysis with menstrual period is characteristic feature.

Brain
Very rarely it involves the brain.

> Are there any risk factors for development of endometriosis?

There are certain risk factors:
- Increasing age
- Shorter menstrual cycle (less than 27 days)
- Longer duration of menstrual flow (greater than 7 days)
- Heavy menstrual flow
- Delayed child birth
- Low or no parity
- First degree relatives (mother, sister, daughter) with endometriosis.

> What is the most common condition simulate endometriosis?

Pelvic inflammatory disease (PID). Confirm diagnosis can be made by laparoscopy or laparotomy.

> How can you categorize the severity of the disease?

"The Revised American Society for Reproductive Medicine Classification of Endometriosis" evaluates the extent of the disease, location and laterality. Staging is determined during surgery. Four stages are considered according to extent of the disease **(Table 16.1)**. Stages I and II are considered as mild or early stage of the disease, and stages III and IV are considered as severe stage of disease (The American Fertility Society, 1997).

> Ultrasonography shows cystic ovaries seemed to be adherent with posterior surface of the uterus. Cysts are multiple with maximum size is 3 × 2.8 cm. She does not want any more children. She wants to get relieve from these symptoms as early as possible. She will be happy to conserve her uterus.
>
> What management would you like to offer her?

Here the symptom is severe with moderate to severe degree of disease assuming by clinical examination. Surgical treatment in the form of total abdominal hysterectomy with bilateral salpingo-oophorectomy would be the best option

Table 16.1 Stages of endometriosis

Stage I: Minimal	Few or superficial implants are evident in the early stage of disease
Stage II: Mild	More implants with deeper involvement
Stage III: Moderate	More implants with ovarian involvements with surrounding adhesions
Stage IV: Severe	Along with features of stage III multiple and more dense adhesions present

for this patient as the disease is noncurable and it is recurrent. But here patient is young and radical surgery will produce iatrogenic menopause at this early age. Moreover, the patient wants to conserve the uterus.

So after proper counseling about the recurrence of the symptom medical treatment can be offered to this patient in the form of GnRHa for 6 months to keep the patient amenorrheic. Add back therapy in the form of OCP or norethindrone plus conjugated equine estrogen or tibolone is to be added after 6 weeks of starting of the therapy to relieve menopausal symptoms.

RELATED INFORMATION

Treatment Modalities

There are four modalities of treatment for endometriosis like:
1. Expectant treatment, wait and see approach with a few analgesics, which is feasible only in mild endometriosis.
2. Medical treatment.
3. Surgical treatment.
4. Combined medical and surgical treatment.

Which can be judged according to:
- Age of the patient
- Desire for pregnancy
- Severity of symptoms
- Stage of her disease
- Prior response to treatment if any.

Aim of the Treatment

Aim of the treatment is to:
- Provide symptomatic relief
- Permit satisfactory coitus
- Control abnormal bleeding
- Promote possibility of pregnancy if desired.

Surgery in the form of total abdominal hysterectomy and bilateral salpingo-oophorectomy is the definitive treatment for endometriosis as it is a recurrent disease. So if patient is elderly and has completed family this is the ideal option.

> GnRHa is expensive. There are other cheaper drugs to keep the patient amenorrheic. Why did you choose GnRHa?

As patient's symptom is severe GnRHa will be effective than other drugs such as oral contraceptive pill (OCP) or danazol.

RELATED INFORMATION

Treatment

Medical treatment can be given in the form of:
- *Analgesics*: Aspirin and other nonsteroidal anti-inflammatory drugs (NSAIDs) can be used to relieve mild to moderate pain in endometriosis. The NSAIDs block the synthesis of prostaglandins, which contribute to pain and inflammation in endometriosis. The NSAIDs are effective for pain relief in endometriosis-associated dysmenorrhea in as many as 80% of women (Milsom and Andersch, 1984).
- *Hormones*: Medical treatment with hormone is given to interrupt the cycles of stimulation and bleeding of endometriotic tissue. The goal of therapy is to induce either a pseudopregnancy (oral contraceptives, progestins) or a menopausal state (GnRHa) to inhibit or delay progression. Hormone therapy is generally most effective when the implants are small. Hormonal therapy is not a cure for endometriosis. Once treatment is stopped, the disease is likely to recur until a woman reaches menopause. For majority of women hormonal treatment has been shown to be beneficial in relieving symptoms, regressing lesions and suppressing disease progression.

Drugs Used

Oral contraceptive pills (OCPs):
Mechanism of action: Continuous exposure to oral contraceptive pills (OCPs) results in decidual changes in endometrial glands followed in several months by atrophy, which reduces the swelling, bleeding and inflammation of endometriotic lesions (Andrews and Andrews, 1959).

Dose and duration: For minimal and mild disease cyclical or continuous use of OCPs for 9-12 months has been shown to be effective in reducing dysmenorrhea and progression of endometriosis.

Efficacy: The drug is cost-effective with mild adverse effect and can be taken for long time. The effects of OCPs on pelvic pain and dysmenorrhea have demonstrated improvement in up to 89% of patients (Schmidt, 1985). If the patient fails to experience relief of symptoms within 3 months of initiating OCPs a more aggressive medical modality is needed.

Progestins

Mechanism of action: Progesterones can be given to inhibit endometriotic tissue growth by causing decidualization and atrophy at high doses progestins will also inhibit gonadotropin secretion and ovarian hormone production inducing an amenorrheic state.

Dose, duration and efficacy: It can be given in the form of:
- Oral medroxyprogesterone acetate at a dose of 50 mg daily for 6 months improves symptoms in 80% cases (Luciano et al. 1988)
- Norethisterone acetate 5 mg daily for 6 months
- Megestrol acetate 40 mg daily for 6 months gives similar response
- Parenteral medroxyprogesterone acetate depot may also be given at a dose 150 mg IM every 3 months for 6 months. It effectively reduces the cyst and pain but significant drawback is the prolonged interval to resumption of ovulation after cessation of therapy.
- Levonorgestrel-releasing intrauterine device has been shown to relieve dysmenorrhea and pelvic pain.
- Dienogest—A fourth generation selective progestin without androgenic, glucocorticoid or mineralocorticoid activity. It can be given 2 mg orally for 3–52 weeks according to response and requirement. 2 mg daily for 24 weeks demonstrated equivalent efficacy to GnRH agonists for relieving pain of endometriosis [Harada et al 2009; Strowitzki et al 2010].

Side effects: Weight gain, fluid retention, headaches and depression, breakthrough bleeding are associated side effects and all of these effects resolve after discontinuation of therapy. Vaginal bleeding, headache, constipation nausea, hot flush and slight reduction of bone mass after 24-52 weeks of treatment was observed after dienogest therapy. Recurrence rate is almost 50% after 2 years of therapy.

Gestrinone: Gestrinone is an anti-progestational steroid used for the treatment of endometriosis. Mechanism of action includes a progestational withdrawal effect at the endometrial cellular level and inhibition of ovarian steroidogenesis. It can reduces the pain effectively at a dose of 2.5–5 mg orally twice in a week. As the tablets are taken twice in a week there are problems of compliance as medication could easily be forgotten.

Side effects: Relate to both androgenic and antiestrogenic effects.

Danazol:

Mechanism of action: Danazol is 19-nortestosterone derivatives with progestin like effects. It acts via several mechanisms like:
- It acts at hypothalamic pituitary level to inhibit gonadotropin release, inhibits midcycle surge of LH and FSH hormone
- It inhibits steroidogenic enzymes in the ovary responsible for estrogen production
- It directly causes atrophy of endometriotic implants
- It reduces sex hormone binding globulin (SHBG) resulting elevated free testosterone level.

By all of these mechanisms it produces a hypoestrogenic hyperandrogenic environment that is unfavorable for the growth of endometriotic lesion.

Dose, duration and efficacy: It can be given orally at a dose of 400–800 mg daily in a divided dose for 6 months. Pain relief is achieved in up to 90% and pregnancy rates reported in the range of 30–72% of patients taking danazol (Barbieri et al. 1982; Dmowski and Cohen, 1975; Dmowski and Cohen, 1978).

Side effects: Weight gain, hot flush, mood change, depression, muscle cramp, acne, deepening of voice, decreased HDL levels and increased liver enzyme are associated with danazol therapy. Most changes are reversible upon cessation of therapy, but deepening of voice may not. Recurrence of symptoms is almost 50% within 4–12 months of discontinuation of therapy.

GnRH agonist

Mechanism of action: The development of GnRHa created a breakthrough in the management of endometriosis. Continuous administration of GnRHa causes pituitary suppression and inhibits synthesis of gonadotropins, resulting in elimination of ovarian steroidogenesis and suppression of endometrial implants.

Dose and duration and efficacy
It can be given in the form of:
- Leuprolide acetate depot or Decapeptyl depot 3.75 mg intramuscularly monthly
- Goserelin depot 3.6 mg subcutaneously monthly
- Nafarelin intranasally 400–800 mg daily
Effectively relieves pain. Completely relieved in most cases by the 2nd or 3rd month of therapy. Any one of these can be used for 6 months only because of adverse effects associated with drug. May recur after 2 years of therapy. After discontinuation of GnRHa if symptoms recur second course of GnRHa therapy is not recommended.

Side effects: Hypoestrogenic states such as, hot flush, vaginal dryness, insomnia, headache, depression, loss of libido, fatigue and loss of bone mineral density. Providing add-back therapy can minimize these side effects.

Add-back therapy

It should be added 6 weeks after starting of GnRHa and need to be continued for 2 years to recover the bone loss.
It can be given in the form of:
- Norethindrone 2.5 mg or conjugated equine estrogen 0.625 mg with medroxyprogesterone 5 mg daily
- Norethindrone 5 mg alone or in conjunction with low dose conjugated equine estrogen
- Tibolone.

Aromatase inhibitors

Mechanism of action: Aromatase inhibitor (AI) inhibits the action of enzyme aromatase, which converts androgens to estrogens. As a result estrogen synthesis reduced and suppresses the growth of endometrial plants.

Dose and duration: Anastrozole 1 mg daily or letrozole 2.5 mg daily can be used continuously for 9–12 months. The drug has not been studied extensively and adverse effects on bone mass limit their use.

Efficacy: It is very much effective when used with GnRHa. GnRHa cannot suppress the extragonadal estrogen synthesis. So complete remission of the disease does not occur. AI stops extragonadal as well as gonadal estrogen synthesis. Edometriotic implants contain large number of aromatase receptors and produce significant estrogens, which can be prevented by AI rather than GnRHa.

Side effects: Hypoestrogenic symptoms.

Other Treatments under Investigation

Medical treatment options for endometriosis, which under investigation are RU486 (mifepristone), selective progesterone receptor modulators, selective estrogen receptor modulators, GnRH antagonists, pentoxifylline and agents that effect tumor necrosis factor (TNF-α), matrix metalloproteinase and angiogenesis.

> *Suppose Mrs Salma's USG shows a big chocolate cyst of about 8 × 9 cm along with other symptoms. She wants to conserve her uterus.*
> *What do you like to do?*

As size of the cyst is bigger only medical treatment will not be effective. So surgery in the form of cystectomy and adhesiolysis as much as possible followed by medical treatment can be done. Patient may remain asymptomatic for a reasonable period or for a long time. If cyst and symptom recurs radical surgery is to be done followed by HRT.

Alternatively USG-guided aspiration of cyst and sclerotherapy followed by medical treatment can be done. Again patient may remain symptom free for a reasonable period or for a long time. If cyst and symptom recurs radical surgery is to be done followed by HRT.

Unfortunately even after definitive surgery endometriosis may recur, though risk is very low about 3%.

RELATED INFORMATION

Surgery

Surgery can be done by laparoscopy or laparotomy. Laparoscopic surgery has gained much popularity due to its advantages over laparotomy that is minimum damage to the healthy tissue, faster postoperative recovery, short hospital stay, better cosmetic results and less morbidity. But very dense or widespread adhesions or some bowel lesions may require laparotomy in some cases. In both the situations in extensive endometriosis surgical intervention requires extreme care and is best attempted by experienced and skilled surgeons. So results of the surgery are very much dependent on the expertise of the surgeon. The main advantage of surgery is that its effects are immediate and if pregnancy desired it is not necessary to wait for a period of time before trying for pregnancy. Disadvantages are risk of anesthesia and surgery itself. Postoperative adhesion in new form may lead to further impairment of fertility.

Modalities of Surgery

A. Conservative surgery

The goal of conservative surgery is to remove as much visible endometriosis and adhesion as possible:
- To relieve pain
- To restore normal pelvic anatomy
- To preserve and enhance fertility.

About 80% patients got relieved from pain with mild to moderate disease and 90% remained symptom free up to 1 year (Sutton et al. 1997). Conservative surgery cannot eradicate the microscopic lesion that is why disease recurs afterwards. In case of infertile patients up to 80% patients got pregnant after conservative surgery (Forbes, 1987). Pregnancy again found to delay the recurrence of endometriosis. Laser surgery appears to have advantages over cautery because it allows for precise vaporization and incision of tissues without damaging underlying structures. Coagulation effect of KTP and argon laser is significantly higher and a greater degree of hemostasis can be achieved.

Conservative surgeries in the form of:
- *Adhesiolysis.*
- *Excision of lesion or cystectomy:* When cyst size is >5 cm and patient wants to restore her fertility status.
- *Vaporization by CO_2 laser.*
- *Diathermy coagulation or fulguration:* When cyst walls are very small and firm to remove then walls are cauterized. Small peritoneal implants are also cauterized.
- *Drainage or aspiration of cyst (USG guided)*:
  - When cyst size is <5 cm
  - Any size where repeat cystectomy is risky in terms of injury of surrounding organs and reducing ovarian reserve
  - Any size before ART
  - Multiparous woman who does not want extensive surgery or definitive surgery.

  Drainage is usually followed by medical treatment in the form of OCP, progesterone, danazole and GnRHa to prevent recurrence. Sclerotherapy can be given for permanent destruction of the cyst wall.

Sclerotherapy

Sclerotherapy is instillation of 5% tetracycline or 95% ethanol in cyst cavity after aspiration of cyst. Those act as sclerosing agent to induce inflammation and adhesion formation so that cyst cannot reactivate. It is safe and effective.

Usually done:
- In recurrent endometrioma before ART
- In-patient who has completed her family, but patient is very young and does not want to go for major surgery.

Due to risk of infection this procedure is not very popular to all.

Note: Care should be taken to prevent infection and abscess formation.

B. Definitive
- Total abdominal hysterectomy and bilateral salpingo-oophorectomy (BSO). In women with severe endometriosis for whom the disease invades vital organs or causes incapacitating or prolonged pain that seriously impairs quality of life, the only treatment is the total abdominal hysterectomy with BSO.

> **Case scenario:** *Mrs Munmun, mother of three children aged 41 years has come to you with the complaints of severe dysmenorrhea, menorrhagia and dyspareunia. On examination, you found uterus is firm and bulky with restricted mobility, fornixes are tender. USG shows bilateral cystic ovaries and bulky uterus with foci of adenomyoma.*
>
> *How will you manage this case? Justify your answer*

Total abdominal hysterectomy with bilateral salpingo-oophorectomy is the choice of treatment. She is a case of endometriosis and adenomyosis. As patient is multiparous and elderly definitive treatment is indicated.

> What care should be taken during surgery in case of endometriosis?

Endometriosis is an invasive disease and occasionally infiltrates deeply in the surrounding structure:
- So care should be taken during adhesiolysis not to injure the gut, great vessels and ureters
- During conservative surgery care should be taken to minimize the tissue damage so that after surgery ovarian reserve is not exhausted
- To prevent re-adhesion antiadhesive (intercede) can be used to cover raw areas.

> **Case scenario:** Miss Naila, a 16 years old unmarried girl has come with the complaints of dysmenorrhea for 2 years. Her USG report shows bilateral chocolate cysts of 14 × 12 cm in right ovary and 14 × 14 cm in left ovary.
> How will you manage her?

As cysts are big and bilateral she needs surgery. Laparoscopic cystectomy would be the logical option for her following the best surgical approach. During surgery care should be taken to protect the ovarian tissue as much as possible. Significant amount of follicle lost due to cystectomy, which reduces the ovarian reserve. Chocolate cyst itself is responsible for reduction of ovarian reserve. Surgery can lead to a further reduction in ovarian reserve by three main mechanisms:
- Excessive stripping of the ovarian cortex,
- The use of coagulation to stop bleeding and
- The presence of surgery-induced inflammation.

So to protect ovarian reserve laparoscopy must be done at skilled hand. Chance of ovarian failure after bilateral ovarian chocolate cystectomy is 2.4% [Busacca et al 2006]. After surgery to prevent recurrence suppressive therapy is to be given by either combined oral contraceptive pills or tab dienogest off and on with ultrasonographic follow up.

> Suppose she has dysmenorrhea and a cyst of about 5 × 4 cm in size in left ovary.
> What should be the management?

As cyst is small she should be treated medically either by combined oral contraceptive pills or tab dienogest for 6–9 months, even 1 year or till subsidence of cyst and pain. Alternatively GnRHa monthly depo can be given for 3–6 doses. Though side effects of GnRHa limit its use. Then she should be followed up at regular interval by ultrasonogram to restart suppressive therapy if needed.

> **Case scenario:** Mrs Nadira aged 28 years married for 5 years has come to you with the complaints of childlessness for 4 years. After taking detail history, after performing physical examination and doing investigations of both partner it is found that husband is quite normal, but Nadira has mild endometriosis with a small chocolate cyst of 2.5 × 3 cm in size. Her cycle is regular and she ovulates regularly. They have been living together with the intention of having baby.
> How will you proceed for fertility treatment?

In spite of normal semen parameters and regular ovulation the couple did not conceive within last 4 years. So in spite of mild disease there is no scope of expectant treatment for this couple. Right at this moment laparoscopic evaluation and management would be the best option for this couple.

> Why not medical treatment for regression of the cyst?

Medical treatment will further delay fertility. Moreover, medical treatment does not improve fertility over expectant management.

> After laparoscopy it was found that ovaries were adherent with posterior surface of the uterus and there was flimsy adhesions with tubes and surroundings. Adhesiolysis was done. Small chocolate cysts were fulgurated. Tubes were found patent and normal anatomy restored.
> What will be their next option of treatment?

After laparoscopy disease is found as moderate and laparoscopic management was done. So the couple can try another 6 months naturally. If no pregnancy controlled ovarian hyperstimulation (COH) and intrauterine insemination (IUI) can be tried. After 3–4 cycles of IUI if pregnancy does not occur *in vitro* fertilization (IVF) is the option of treatment as endometriosis is a recurrent disease and repeated surgery exhaust ovarian reserve dramatically. Repeated surgery fell the patient in real danger of infertility.

> Suppose initially sonographically it was found bilateral chocolate cysts of about 10 cm each. On laparoscopic evaluation it was found that there was dense adhesion with cysts, gut, pelvic walls and POD was obliterated.
> What should be your approach of management?

Adhesiolysis and cystectomy will be attempted to restore anatomy as much as normal. If tubes found patent and anatomy can be restored 6 months natural trial is to be advised. After 3-4 cycles of COH and IUI if pregnancy does not occur IVF is the option of treatment for the same reason as mentioned above.

> Suppose a lady of 38 years has come with such advanced stage of disease.
> What would be the treatment option for her?

First of all ovarian reserve is to be tested. If reserve is good surgery followed by COH and IUI if tubes found patent or ART if tubes found blocked or damaged. As patient is elderly IUI only for 3 cycles will be offered after surgery to shortened the treatment time. If no pregnancy with IUI, ART will be offered.

If ovarian reserve is poor laparoscopic surgery is better to be avoided, as surgery will further reduce the ovarian reserve due to tissue damage during cystectomy, adhesiolysis and cauterization. In that case cyst aspiration followed by down regulation and ART is to be advised. If cyst size is smaller than 5 cm long down regulation and ART is to be advised.

Note: To learn about ovarian reserves go to chapter infertility.

> Is there any role of medical treatment in such a case?

GnRHa can be given as pretreatment of surgery to make the surgical approach easier.

RELATED INFORMATION

Endometriosis Associated Infertility

Endometriosis may induce infertility because of anatomic distortion caused by invasive growth and adhesions. Following are the mechanisms for affecting fertility in endometriosis:

- Defective ovum pick up and transportation in spite of patent tubes:
  - Anatomic distortion and compression of tubes by the lesion
  - Loss of tubo-ovarian relationship due to adhesion
  - Altered tubal mobility
  - Abnormal tubal epithelium.
- Anovulation:
  - Ovulatory dysfunction
  - Luteinized unrupture follicle syndrome (LUFS).
- Impairs fertilization:
  - Chemotaxis and binding of sperms to tubal epithelium, so free sperms reduced for fertilization.
  - Abnormal sperm motility by substance released from endometriotic implants, impairs fertilization.
- Increased cell-mediated gamete injury.

Management of Endometriosis Associated Infertility

- For women with mild or minimal endometriosis who wish to become pregnant a trial period of unprotected coitus for 6 months to 1 year may be recommended. Because pregnancy rates following expectant management have been reported to be similar to those women who have been treated with hormonal therapy or conservative surgery to remove endometrial implants (Badway et al. 1988; Federici et al. 1988; Hull ME, 1987).
- So far fertility is concerned medical treatment by any form delay conception, with no increase in the fertility rate (Vercellini et al. 1999; Parazzini et al. 1994).
- Laparoscopy is the gold standard treatment for endometriosis.
  - Surgical treatment in early stage endometriosis improves pregnancy rates. Average pregnancy rate after laparoscopic treatment has been reported to be in the range of 34–80% (Forbes, 1987).
  - Surgical treatment of advanced endometriosis improves pregnancy rates when tubal patency is restored.

- In women with advanced endometriosis combined medical and surgical treatment may offer many advantages:
  - Patients with severe or extensive endometriosis who are potentially risky for surgical treatment can be treated medically prior to surgery.
  - Preoperative use of danazol or GnRHa can decrease the extent of endometriosis, decreases the size of endometrioma, causes atrophy of ectopic endometrium, making it easier to achieve complete resection of endometriotic implants by laparoscopy (Wheeler et al. 1992).

> **Case scenario 3:** Mrs Nujhat has been suffering from primary subfertility for 10 years due to endometriosis. She underwent laparoscopic chocolate cystectomy from right ovary 3 years ago. Now again she developed a big (10 cm) cyst in her left ovary and a small cyst (4 cm) in her right ovary. Now she is 35 years old and her ovarian reserve is poor. Her husband is normospermic.
>
> How will you manage the case?

Aspiration of cyst **(Fig. 16.2)** with or without sclerotherapy followed by long down regulation and ART will be the ideal treatment for this patient. Because patient has history of long infertility. She did not conceive after first surgery. She is elderly with poor ovarian reserve. Ovarian reserve may reduce due to previous surgery. So she should go for ART straight way without delay. Before ART cyst should be removed. But repeat surgery will be difficult and there is potential risk of surgical injuries due to adhesion formation by endometriosis itself and previous surgery. Moreover, there will be further reduction of ovarian reserve due to inadvertent tissue damage during cystectomy, cauterization and compromised blood supply (Biacchiardi et al. 2011; Celik et al. 2012). So less invasive USG-guided aspiration can be done to protect the ovarian tissue from surgical damage.

> **Case scenario:** Mrs Monowara, a 25 years lady has come to you with the complaints of childlessness for 5 years. She has a big chocolate cyst of about 12/13 cm. She suffers from severe dysmenorrhea. Her husband's semen parameters are very poor. Count is 2–3 million/mL on repeated occasion.
>
> How will you manage this couple?

Here the couple has combined problem. Male partner has severe oligospermia for which they need ART in the form of ICSI.

But the female partner has endometriosis and a big chocolate cyst with severe dysmenorrhea. For which she needs surgery irrespective of her husband's semen parameter. Moreover, surgery will optimize pelvic condition by removing the cysts and adhesions. After 6–8 weeks of surgery they will have to go for ICSI. Usually 4–6 weeks is needed to subside inflammation.

> Suppose Mrs Monowara's husband's semen parameter is normal then what to do?

As patient has pain and cyst is big surgery is to be done in the form of cystectomy adopting the best surgical approach. As she is young after cystectomy if tubes found patent and healthy and ovarian reserve is satisfactory, step by step treatment is to be given. Natural trial for 6 months, then ovulation induction for 6 months, then COH and IUI for 3 cycles and finally ART.

Note: To learn about semen parameters and male infertility go to chapter infertility.

RELATED INFORMATION

For surgical treatment of endometriosis following points are to be considered
- Age and symptom of the patient.
- Size of endometrioma, severity, number, laterality.

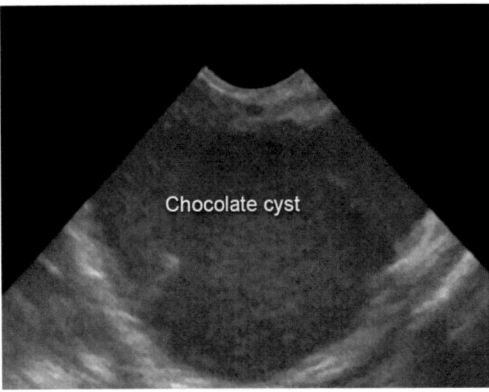

Fig. 16.2 Chocolate cyst

- Choosing the best surgical techniques
- Avoiding unnecessary ovarian surgery.
- Measuring ovarian reserve (OR) before surgery.
- Prevention of adhesion
- Using cryopreservation techniques
- Avoiding repeat surgery in favour of ART.
- Other indications of ART

Choosing the best Surgical Techniques

Surgeons' expertise and skills, differences in the surgical techniques, extent of the disease, laterality of endometrioma and number of surgery have effect on residual ovarian reserve

Three-stage Technique Cystectomy

Donnez et al first described the three-stage technique consists of laparoscopic cyst drainage followed by gonadotropin-releasing hormone (GnRH) agonist treatment for 3 months to reduce cyst diameter, and then a second laparoscopic procedure for vaporization of the cyst wall by CO2 [Donnez et al 1996]. Based on this a study conducted by Tsolakidis et al and found that reduction of AMH is less (.50 pg/mL) in three stage surgery in comparison to traditional one (1 pg/mL) [Tsolakidis et al, 2010].

Combined Ablation and Cystectomy

A surgical technique that combines cystectomy and CO_2 ablation. A surgeon removes 80–90% of the cyst with the cystectomy technique and uses the laser to ablate the remaining cyst wall. This technique reduces the risk associated with cystectomy and recurrence associated with ablation alone. The benefit of this surgery over traditional laparoscopic procedures is that recurrence rates are low. The volume of the ovary after the combined technique was similar to that of the contralateral normal ovary, as well as to that observed in infertile women without endometriosis. The AFC on day 2–5 showed the same number of antral follicles in all subgroups. [Donnez et al, 2010]

Cystectomy with Vasopressin

Vasopressin is injected into the cyst to reduce the amount of bipolar coagulation needed for hemostasis and the amount of healthy tissue that is accidentally removed, since the injection of vasopressin improves the view of the plane of cleavage between the cyst and the ovary. Researchers reported a significant reduction of use of coagulation to achieve hemostasis. They recommended vasopressin as a beneficial technique in treating endometriomas to reduce the potential loss of ovarian reserve. [Saeki et al, 2010].

BIBLIOGRAPHY

Andrews MC, Andrews WC, Strauss AF. Effects of progestin-induced pseudopregnancy on endometriosis: clinical and microscopic studies. Am J Obstet Gynecol. 1959;78:776-83.

Arrive L, Hricak H, Martin MC. Pelvic endometriosis. MR imaging. Radiology. 1989;171(3):687-92.

Badawy SZ, El Bakry MM, Samuel F, et al. Cumulative pregnancy rates in infertile women with endometriosis. J Reported. 1988;33:757-60.

Barbieri RL, Evans S, Kistner RW. Danazol in the treatment of endometriosis: analysis of 100 cases with a 4-year follow-up. Fertil Steril. 1982;37:737-46.

Biacchiardi CP, Piane LD, Camanni M, et al. Laparoscopic stripping of endometrioma negatively affects ovarian follicular reserve even if performed by experienced surgeons. Reprod Biomed Online. 2011;23(6):740-6.

Busacca M, Riparini J, Somigliana E, Oggioni G, Izzo S, Vignali M, Candiani M. Postsurgical ovarian failure after laparoscopic excision of bilateral endometriomas. Am J Obstet Gynecol 2006;195:421-25.

Celik HG, Dogan E, Okyay E, et al. Effects of laparoscopic excision of endometriomas on ovarian reserve: serial changes in the serum antimullerian hormone levels. Fertil Steril. 2012;97(6):1472-8.

Cornillie FJ, Oosterlynck D, Lauweryns JM, et al. Deeply infiltrating pelvic endometriosis: histology and clinical significance. Fertil Steril. 1990;53:978-3.

D'Hooghe TM, Debrock S, Hill JA, et al. Endometriosis and subfertility: is the relationship resolved? Semen Reprod Med. 2003;21:243-54.

Dmowski WP, Cohen MR. Antigonadotropin (danazol) in the treatment of endometriosis. Evaluation of post treatment fertility and three-year follow-up data. Am J Obstet Gynecol. 1978;130:41-8.

Dmowski WP, Cohen MR. Treatment of endometriosis with an antigonadotropin, danazol. A laparoscopic and histologic evaluation. Obstet Gynecol. 1975: 46;147-54.

Donnez J, Nisolle M, Gillet N, Smets M, Bassil S, Casanas-Roux F. Large ovarian endometriomas. Hum. Reprod. 1996;11(3):641-6.

Donnez J, Lousse JC, Jadoul P, Donnez O, Squifflet J. Laparoscopic management of endometriomas using a combined technique of excisional (cystectomy) and ablative surgery. Fertil Steril 2010;94: 28-32.

Federici D, Conti E, Costantini W, et al. Endometriosis and infertility: our experience over five years. Hum Reprod. 1988;3:109-11.

Forbes KL. Endometriosis and infertility: treatment is always necessary. Clin Reprod Fertil. 1987;5:153-66.

Friedman H, Vogelzang RL, Mendelson EB, et al. Endometriosis detection by USG with laparoscopic correlation. Radiology. 1985;157:217-20.

Harada T, Momoeda M, Taketani Y et al. Dienogest is as effective as intranasal buserelin acetate for the relief of pain symptoms associated with endometriosis-a randomized, double-blind, multicenter, controlled trial. Fertil Steril 2009;91;675-81.

Hricak H, Lacey C, Schriock E, et al. Gynecologic masses: value of magnetic resonance imaging. Am J Obstet Gynecol. 1985;153:31-7.

Hull ME, Moghissi KS, Magyar DF, et al. Comparison of different treatment modalities of endometriosis in infertile women. Fertil Steril. 1987;47:40-4.

Liu DTY, Hitchcock A. Endometriosis: Its association with retrograde menstruation, dysmenorrhea and tubal pathology. Br J Obstet Gynecol. 1986;93:859.

Luciano AA, Turksoy RN, Carleo J. Evaluation of oral medoxy progesterone acetate in the treatment of endometriosis. Obstet Gynaecol. 1988;72:323.

Martin Dc, Hubert GD, Levy BS. Depth of infiltration of endometriosis. J Gynecol Surg. 1989;5:55-60.

Milsom I, Andersch B. Effect of ibuprofen, naproxen sodium and paracetamol on intrauterine pressure and menstrual pain in dysmenorrhea. Br J Obstet Gynecol. 1984;91:1129-35.

Nezhat C, Berger GS, Nezhat F, et al. Endometriosis, advanced management and surgical techniques. New York: Springer; 1995.

Nezhat F, Nezhat C, Allen CJ, et al. Clinical and histologic classification of endometriomas. Implications for a mechanism of pathogenesis. J Reprod Med. 1992; 37:771-6.

Noble LS, Simpson ER, John A, et al. Aromatase expression in endometriosis. J Clin Endocrinol Metab. 1996;81:174.

Olive DL, Henderson DY. Endometriosis and mullerian anomalies. Obstet Gynaecol. 1987;69:412.

Olive DL, Pritts EA. Treatment of endometriosis. N Engl J Med. 2001;345:266-75.

Parazzini F, Fedele L, Busacca M, et al. Postsurgical medical treatment of advanced endometriosis: results of a randomized clinical trial. Am J Obstet Gynecol. 1994;171:1205-7.

Pritts EA, Taylor RN. An evidence-based evaluation of endometriosis-associated infertility. Endocrinol Metab Clin North Am. 2003;32:653-67.

Saeki A, Matsumoto T, Ikuma K et al. The vasopressin injection technique for laparoscopic excision of ovarian endometrioma: a technique to reduce the use of coagulation. J. Minim. Invasive Gynecol. 2010;17(2):176-79.

Sampson JA. Peritoneal endometriosis due to menstrual dissemination of endometrial tissue into the peritoneal cavity. Am J Obstet Gynecol. 1987;14:422.

Schmidt CL. Endometriosis: a reappraisal of pathogenesis and treatment. Fertil Steril. 1985;44:157-73.

Simpson JL, Malinak LR, Elias S et al. HLA association in endometriosis. Am J Obstet Gynecol. 1984;148:395.

Startseva NV. Clinical immunological aspects of genital endometriosis. Akush Gineko (Mosk). 1980;3:23-6.

Strowitzki T, Marr J, Gerlinger C, et al. Dienogest is as effective as leuprolide acetate in treating the painful symptoms of endometriosis: a 24 week, randomized, multicenter, open-laben trial. Hum Reprod 2010; 25:633-41

Sutton CJ, Pooley AS, Ewen SP, et al. Follow-up report on a randomized controlled trial of laser laparoscopy in the treatment of pelvic pain associated with minimal to moderate endometriosis. Fertil Steril. 1997;68:1070-4.

Tsolakidis D, Pados G, Vavilis D, et al. The impact on ovarian reserve after laparoscopic ovarian cystectomy versus three-stage management in patients with endometriomas: a prospective randomized study. Fertil. Steril. 2010;94(1):71-77.

The American Fertility Society. Revised American Fertility Society classification of edometriosis. Fertil Steril. 1997;43:351-2.

Vercellini P, Crosignani PG, Padini R, et al. A gonadotropin-releasing hormone agonist compared with expectant management after conservative surgery for symptomatic endometriosis. Br J Obstet Gynecol. 1999;106:672-7.

Wheeler JM, Knittle VD, Miller JD. Depot leuprolide versus danazol in treatment of women with symptomatic endometriosis. Efficacy results. Am J Obstet Gynecol. 1992;167:1367-71.

CHAPTER 17

Infertility

Rashida Begum

INTRODUCTION

Infertility is a condition when a couple failed to conceive within 1 year of unprotected coitus. Every one in 6 couples is facing the problem for getting pregnancy. Both male and female may be responsible for infertility. Usually 40% infertility is due to male factor, 40% due to female factor and 20% combined factors and unexplained. About 80% couples usually become pregnant within 1st year of trial. About 20% take another 1 year to become pregnant. Rest 10% needs some help for getting pregnancy. It is of two types—*Primary infertility* when the woman never conceived and *secondary infertility* when the woman conceived and end up with delivery of a full term or premature child either dead or alive, abortion, ectopic pregnancy, molar pregnancy or menstrual regulation (MR).

> **Case scenario:** Mrs Ayesa has come to you with the complaints of childlessness and she has been trying for babies for 2 years.
> How will you proceed for infertility evaluation?

For evaluation of infertility, both partners are to be evaluated. First of all, detailed history is to be taken:

- Age: Particularly important for female partner—Reproductive potential of female begins to decline after 30 years, decline is more pronounced after 35 years, there is a dramatic fall after 40 years and virtually nil after 45 years
- Duration of marriage
- Duration of infertility
- Occupation of husband
- Occupation of wife
- Knowledge about fertile period
- Use of fertile period
- Frequency of coitus
- Whether they are living together or not
- Any coital problem of husband such as impotency or erectile dysfunction
- Any coital problem of wife such as vaginismus, tight hymen.
- Whether ever conceived or not
- If yes, fate of that pregnancy:
  - Full-term baby, alive or dead
  - Premature baby, alive or dead
  - Abortion
  - Ectopic pregnancy
  - Molar pregnancy
  - Menstrual regulation.
- History of any previous marriage of husband and wife
- If yes, history of any children from that marriage
- Contraceptive history: Type of contraceptives and duration of use
- Menstrual history of wife:
  - Cycle
  - Duration
  - Amount
  - Dysmenorrhea
  - Last menstrual period (LMP)
- Any medical disorder of husband or wife such as diabetes mellitus (DM), tuberculosis, hypo- and hyperthyroidism, hyperprolactinemia, pelvic inflammatory disease (PID) (wife), etc.
- History of any surgery of husband such as vasectomy and herniorrhaphy
- History of any surgery of wife such as appendicectomy and other pelvic surgery, which interferes tubal function
- Family history of any diseases and infertility.

After taking history, a thorough physical examination of female partner is to be performed with particular emphasis on body built and weight, hair distribution, thyroid gland and breast. As irregular cycles are related to polycystic ovary syndrome (PCOS), hypothyroidism and hyperprolactinemia.

> On enquiry, you found that her menstrual cycle is irregular 40–60 days. Duration and amount is normal. They are married for 5 years. Couple has got no coital problem. They are living together. They used barrier method for contraception for first 3 years of marriage. On examination, it is found that her BMI is 30, excessive hair growth in face and other places. Thyroid and breasts are normal. PV findings are normal. Her male partner has no complaints.
>
> What investigations do you suggest for this couple?

For female partner:
- USG preferably transvaginal sonography (TVS) to see the condition of the:
  - Uterus whether normal or presence of any myoma, adenomyoma, septum, polyp, bicornuate uterus, etc.
  - Ovaries whether normal or enlarged and polycystic or presence of any cyst or adhesion, etc.
  - Tubes whether visible in case of hydrosalpinx or pyosalpinx.
- Blood for:
  - CBC, GTT as patient is obese, rubella antibody, *Chlamydia* antibody, VDRL.
  - Hormones: Thyroid-stimulating hormone (TSH), FT4, prolactin, follicle-stimulating hormone (FSH), luteinizing hormone (LH), E2, dehydroepiandrosterone sulfate (DHEAS). If DHEAS is raised then 17-OH-progesterone to exclude adrenal disorder.

(**Note:** Other tests for ovarian reserve assessment are not mandatory for this patient, as she is young).

For male partner:
- Semen analysis: It is *must* and *first test* of male partner. It is the cornerstone of evaluation of male infertility. It must be done though the man has history of previous child birth. A fertile man may become infertile with passage of time. Primary or secondary infertility is not applicable for women only.
- Blood sugar 2 hours after 75 g glucose.
- VDRL.

RELATED INFORMATION

Semen Analysis Procedure and Interpretation

A semen analysis comprises a set of discipline measurements of spermatozoa and seminal fluid parameters that help to estimate semen quality. A semen analysis cannot be interpreted unless certain basic facts are known.

The following instructions for sample collection and delivery should be provided with appropriate and clearly written and oral instructions:
- The sample should be collected by masturbation after proper cleaning of genitalia into a clean wide-mouthed glass or plastic container. The container should be warm to minimize the risk of cold shock.
- Coitus interruptus (causes contamination) and collection in a condom (has toxic effect to sperm) is not acceptable.
- Sample should be collected after 2–7 days abstinence. Sperm motility decline if abstinence is more than 7 days (Comhaire, 1995). Sperm concentration may be reduced if duration of abstinence is <48 hours.
- Incomplete sample should be discarded if the first few drops of the ejaculate spill. It contains most of the spermatozoa and count may come as severe oligospermia.
- Ideally it should be collected in laboratory premises. If not possible, sample should be protected from extreme of temperature (between 20°C and 40°C). It should be carried within 10–15 minutes.
- In the laboratory, sample should be examined immediately after liquefaction and certainly within 1 hour of ejaculation.

Normal Semen Parameters

According to WHO manual (2010, 5th edition), normal semen parameters are given in **Table 17.1**.

Progressive motility (PR): Spermatozoa move actively, either linearly or in a large circle, regardless of speed.

Non-progressive motility (NP): All other patterns of motility with an absence of progression or forward movement.

Table 17.1 Normal semen parameter (WHO, 2010)

Semen parameter	Lower reference limit
Volume (mL)	1.5
Sperm concentration (10^6/mL)	15
Total sperm number (10^6/ejaculate)	39
Motility % rapid progressive (PR) + non-progressive (NP)	40
PR	32
Morphology %	04
Vitality %	58
	Lower threshold value for normal activity of sperm
PH	7.2
Peroxidase-positive WBC (10^6/mL)	<1
Immunobead test (motile spermatozoa with bound bead %)	<50
Mixed agglutination reaction (MAR) test (motile spermatozoa with bound particles %)	<50

Note: *Lower threshold value*—where consensus cannot be made for lower limit of normal for fertile men. But fertility impaired significantly if white blood cell (WBC) <1 and 50% or more motile sperms bound to bead or particles.

Abnormal Semen Parameters

- *Oligospermia*: When sperm count is less than 15 million/mL. Count below 15 million/mL has got significance for fertility. Fertility potential is significantly impaired when count falls below 15 million/mL. Low count may be due to:
  - Pretesticular:
    - Aging
    - Hypogonadism due to various causes
    - Endocrine problem
    - Diabetes, renal and hepatic disease
    - Drugs (mentioned later on), alcohol, smoking
    - Strenuous riding (bicycle riding, horseback riding)
    - Immunological variation.
  - Testicular factors:
    - Genetic defects on the Y chromosome
    - Y chromosome microdeletions
    - Abnormal set of chromosomes *Klinefelter syndrome*
    - Neoplasm, e.g. seminoma
    - Cryptorchidism
    - Varicocele
    - Trauma
    - Hydrocele
    - Mumps
    - Malaria
    - Sexually transmitted diseases (STDs), tuberculosis
    - Surgery
    - Chemo and radiotherapy.
  - Post-testicular:
    - Unilateral or partial obstruction of vas deferens
    - Unilateral or partial obstruction of epididymis.
  - Idiopathic: Most (90%) of the oligospermia are idiopathic.
  - Collection and examination error:
    - Inappropriate sample collection
    - Wrong dilution
    - Short abstinence.
- *Asthenospermia*: When sperm motility is <40% (PR + NP) or <32% (PR).
  Causes of low motility are:
  - Most of the asthenospermia are associated with oligospermia and causes are interrelated. Most (90%) are idiopathic.
  - Increased local temperature of the scrotum due to any cause.
  - Immotile cilia syndrome (Kartagener syndrome)
  - Inappropriate sample collection and examination:
    - Cytotoxicity of collection vessel
    - Contamination
    - Wrong dilution
    - Delay in analysis
    - Poor temperature control
    - Inappropriate chamber depth.
- *Necrospermia*: When all sperms are immotile or dead. Causes are same as asthenospermia.
- *Teratospermia*: When <4% sperms with normal morphology.

- *OATS*: Combination of oligoastheno-teratospermia.
- *Azoospermia*: When no spermatozoa is found in the ejaculate. It is of two types:
    - Nonobstructive azoospermia (NOA): Causes are same as oligospermia.
    - Obstructive azoospermia (OA) due to:
        - Bilateral block of vas deference
        - Congenital bilateral absence of vas deferens (CBAVD). May associated with bilateral absence of seminal vesicle. Usually occurs in cystic fibrosis.
- *Hypospermia:* When semen volume is <1.5 mL. It is the result of:
    - Infection or abnormalities of accessory sexual glands.
    - Obstruction of genital tract due to previous infection.
    - Absence of seminal vesicle and vas deferens.
- *Hyperspermia:* When semen volume is >5.5 mL. It is the result of:
    - Long period of abstinence.
    - Inflammation of seminal vesicle.
    - Varicocele.
- *Aspermia:* When there is no semen volume. It is the result of:
    - Retrograde ejaculation: Due to bladder neck problem, semen enters into urinary bladder. It occurs due to:
    - Excessive drug use
    - Prostatic surgery
    - Severe infection of accessory glands
    - Ejaculatory duct obstruction.

> Investigation reports of Mrs Ayesha and her husband as follows:
>
> On TVS ovaries are bigger than normal and polycystic, TSH, prolactin normal, FSH, E_2 normal and LH high. DHEAS increased and 17OH progesterone is normal. Glucose tolerance test (GTT) is altered.
>
> Husband's semen analysis and other reports are normal.
>
> What may be the cause of infertility for this couple?

Anovulation. Cause of anovulation is polycystic ovary syndrome (PCOS).

> What are the causes of female infertility?

Main factors responsible for female infertility are either isolated or in combination:

- Problem of ovaries (ovarian dysfunction)
- Problem of tubes
- Problem of uterus
- Coital problem
- Unexplained: When no definite cause can be identified.

Main causes are:
a. Ovulatory dysfunction:
   - Anovulation (20–25%).
   - Luteal phase defect (ovulation with inappropriate follicular development).

Basically there are three main causes of anovulation:
- Failure to develop the mature follicles
- Premature luteinization of the follicles
- Luteinized unruptured follicle syndrome (LUFS).

These three situations occur through any of the following diseases:
   i. *Hypogonadotropic hypogonadism:* WHO type I anovulation due to hypothalamic pituitary failure—not very common
      - Anorexia nervosa
      - Kallmann's syndrome
      - Sheehan's syndrome.
   ii. *PCOS:* WHO type II anovulation due to hypothalamic-pituitary dysfunction and the *most common one*. About 90% of all anovulatory causes. Others type II are:
      - Congenital adrenal hyperplasia (CAH)
      - Adrenal tumors
      - Androgen producing ovarian tumors.
   iii. *Ovarian failure:* WHO type III anovulation:
      - Turner syndrome
      - Autoimmune disorder
      - Infection: Mumps
      - Radiotherapy
      - Chemotherapy
      - Genetic
   iv. *Hyperprolactinemia*
   v. *Hypothyroidism:* Both clinically evident and subclinical. TSH level between 1 and 4 mIU/L is optimum for good ovulation. According to ESHRE guideline for recurrent pregnancy loss 2017 TSH level ≤2.5 mIU/L is ideal for ovulation and pregnancy [ESHRE Guideline, Recurrent Pregnancy Loss 2017]
   vi. *Hyperthyroidism.*

b. Endometriosis (20%).
c. Tubal factors (15%):
   - Bilateral tubal block
   - Bilateral salpingectomy
   - Bilateral tubal damage.
d. Uterine factors:
   - Myoma
   - Adenomyoma
   - Asherman's syndrome
   - Thin endometrium.
e. Cervical factor or cervical hostility (5%).
f. Unable to perform coitus due to tough or imperforate hymen.
g. Use of lubricants, which are spermicidal.
h. Unexplained.

> How will you ascertain whether a woman is ovulating or not?

Diagnosis of Ovulation

Whether a woman is ovulating or not can be diagnosed by certain signs and symptoms and tests.

Signs and symptoms

Regular cyclical menstruation: Regular menstruation is a strong evidence of ovulation. Though in certain situations cyclical bleeding may takes place without ovulation. It is not very common.

Midcycle pain (Mittelschmerz pain): During discharge of ovum with follicular fluid there may be peritoneal irritation and pain. Some women feel this pain around ovulation in the middle of each cycle.

Ovulation cascade: Due to estrogenic effect of mature follicle, cervical mucus becomes thin and comes as profuse watery vaginal discharge. Some women complaint of this discharge, which is a sign of follicular maturity and subsequent ovulation.

Premenstrual mastalgia: Postovulatory progesterone release from luteinized corpus luteum causes congestion of the breast. As a result there is pain and tenderness of the breast, which indicates ovulation.

Painful menstruation: Lower abdominal pain during menstruation is called dysmenorrhea occurs in ovulatory cycles. Though may not severe, some forms of cramping pain are experienced by some women during menstruation due to synthesis of prostaglandins from postovulatory (progestational) endometrium.

Basal body temperature (BBT): Due to postovulatory progestational effect, body temperature remains 0.2–0.5°C higher than follicular phase until menstruation. If temperature is recorded daily in a basal condition just before rising from bed there will be a biphasic change in the chart, which is an indicator of ovulation. This is very cumbersome for women to record daily temperature at a fixed time. Moreover, it needs intelligence and precision for gathering correct information. So this parameter is *no longer considered* as evaluation for ovulation as many other alternative signs and tests are available now-a-days.

Tests

- Hormone assay
  - *Serum estradiol:* E_2 level increased in midcycle than basal level. It is an indicator of development of follicles. One mature follicle secretes 100 pg/mL or more estrogen. Most widely used hormone during monitoring of cycles in assisted reproductive technique (ART).
  - *Detection of preovulatory LH surge:* Both serum and urinary LH can be tested to detect LH surge. This test can be done by commercially available LH kit to observe the changes of color of kit by urine containing high LH 36–40 hours before rupture of the follicle. It is not so popular as it needs to do the test repeatedly starting from D10 of the cycle to detect the LH surge.
  - *D21 or midluteal phase progesterone:* A minimum of 4 ng/mL is considered as indication of ovulation. Though 10 ng/mL or more is indicator of good quality follicle and ovum (Magyar, 1979). Morning sample is good predictive as in the evening there is 50% rise of the value due to diurnal variation. Average of three samples is the best predictive competent luteal phase.
- *Vaginal smear test:* This test is not done now-a-days.

- *Cervical mucus test*: Fern test of cervical mucus is observed due to different effects of estrogen and progesterone. Not used now-a-days.
- *Endometrial biopsy during luteal phase*: Subnuclear vacuolation observed due to secretory activity of the postovulatory endometrium. This test is *no longer exists* as it is invasive and other alternative tests are available.
- *Ultrasonogram*: Availability of transvaginal ultrasonogram (TVS) made it the most popular method of test for diagnosis of ovulation. It is widely used to monitor the stimulatory cycles to observe the response of the treatment. Advantages of TVS are:
  - Avoidance of full bladder
  - Bypasses the problems of obesity-associated attenuation and artifacts
  - Higher frequency, hence better resolution
  - Better visualization of pelvic organs as nearer the target
  - Serial ultrasonogram from D10 to D18 of the cycle can detect both the development and rupture of follicles. It needs two to three TVS to assess the condition.
- *Laparoscopy*: Direct observation by laparoscopy or laparotomy can detect corpus luteum in the ovary as well as visualization of corrugation of ovary is indicative of previous ovulation. *It is not used for diagnosis of ovulation*, but it can give retrospective information of ovulation.

So for practical purpose serial TVS, midcycle serum estrogen and midluteal progesterone are good guide for assessment of ovulation and quality of ovum.

> What are the diagnostic criteria of PCOS?

Rotterdam criteria 2004, a consensus developed from joint meeting of American Society of Reproductive Medicine (ASRM) and European Society of Human Reproduction and Embryology (ESHRE). According to that consensus any two out of following three criteria are diagnostic for PCOS (Rotterdam ESHRE/ASRM consensus, 2004):
1. Oligo-ovulation or anovulation
2. Hyperandrogenism
3. Ultrasonographically polycystic ovaries.

A raised LH/FSH ratio *is no longer a diagnostic criteria* for PCOS due to inconsistent level (Cho, 2005).

> For Mrs Ayesa do you like to do the tests for ovulation such as serum progesterone or endometrial biopsy in second half of cycle?

No. By history (oligomenorrhea), physical examination (sign of hyperandrogenism) and ultrasonography, it is evident that the patient has PCOS and she is anovulatory.

> For investigation of female partner, ovarian reserve testing is very important.
> What is it? Who are the candidates for ovarian reserve testing?
> Does Mrs Ayesa need it?

Ovarian reserve (OR) testing is done to assess the quantity of follicles are retained in her ovaries. By which one can assess the duration of reproductive life. If reserve is poor, then it indicates her reproductive life becomes shorter. If reserve is good, then longer time will be available for reproduction.

Ovarian reserve testing is to be done:
- For all women of 30 or more
- At any age:
  - When previous response of stimulation is not satisfactory
  - History of unilateral or bilateral ovarian cystectomy
  - History of one oophorectomy
  - History of unilateral or bilateral salpingectomy
  - History of repeated pelvic surgery
  - History of chemo or radiotherapy
  - Small ovaries on ultrasonogram.

Ovarian reserve test includes:
- Ovarian volume: Normal—$5C^3$–$10C^3$
- Antral follicle count (AFC) by TVS on D2/D3 of the cycle. 8–10 follicles of 7 mm size in each ovary is normal
- FSH and E2 on D1–D3 of the cycle. FSH should be <10 IU/L and E2 should be <100 pg/mL.
- Anti-müllerian hormone (AMH), anytime of the cycle.

≥3 ng/mL is very good, 1–3 ng/mL is optimum, <1 ng/mL is poor.
- Inhibin B: Should be 180 pg/mL or more.

Note: All tests are not necessary at the same time. *Antral follicle* count and *AMH* are the best predictors for ovarian reserve. So these two are enough for OR assessment.

This patient is young with polycystic ovaries with lots of antral follicles. So for practical purpose, this patient does not need other testing for ovarian reserve assessment.

> What management do you like to offer to this couple?

As anovulation is the apparent cause of infertility for this couple, so treatment is to be directed to female partner:
- *Lifestyle modification:* It is the first-line management of PCOS-related infertility particularly if patient is overweight and obese. It is to be done in the form of *caloric restriction* and *exercise*. Obesity causes anovulation. Only 7% reduction of body weight can restore ovulation and menstruation (Franks et al. 1991).
- *Induction of ovulation.*

> What are the drugs can be used for induction of ovulation in PCOS?

There are a number of drugs for ovulation induction.
Commonly used drugs are:
- Antiestrogens:
  - Clomiphene citrate
  - Tamoxifen
  - Letrozole.
- Gonadotropins.

Less commonly used drugs are:
- Gonadotropin-releasing hormone agonist (GnRHa)
- GnRH antagonist.

Adjuvant Therapy

- *Insulin sensitizer:* Metformin to correct hyperinsulinemia.
- *Corticosteroid:* To combat adrenal androgen production.
- *Bromocriptine:* If there is associated hyperprolactinemia.
- *Thyroxin:* If there is associated hypothyroidism
- *D-Chiro-Inositol:* To reduce androgen level.

Note: Before induction of ovulation endocrine problems such as hypothyroidism, hyperprolactinemia, diabetes and other medical diseases such as tuberculosis should be corrected.

RELATED INFORMATION

Chronic anovulation is the most common feature of PCOS. About 85–90% of patients of anovulatory infertility are due to PCOS. High ovarian androgen level prevents normal ovulation leading to infertility. The induction of ovulation is the main treatment for PCOS is a complex issue, which requires a thorough understanding of the syndrome and a careful, and individual assessment of each patient. Different pharmacological agents are used to make the women ovulatory. Some are causing ovulation by increasing production of pituitary gonadotropins, some directly stimulates the ovaries and some reduces the androgen production and make the ovaries sensitive to stimulating agents.

What is induction?

Ovulation induction is a treatment for infertility designed to bring about ovulation in women who are otherwise anovulatory. The aim of induction is to induce one or at the most two mature follicles (>17 mm).

What is stimulation?

Ovarian stimulation is the treatment for infertility to bring about more follicles in women who are already ovulating regularly, but who are nonetheless undergoing stimulation with exogenous hormones/gonadotropins to increase their chances of conceiving.

The aim of stimulation is intended to schedule ovulation at a desired time.

Ovulation Inducing Agents

Ovulation inducing agents are:
- Clomiphene citrate
- Tamoxifen
- Aromatase inhibits
- Low-dose gonadotropins

Clomiphene Citrate

Clomiphene citrate (CC) alone or in combination with weight loss continues to be the first-line of treatment for anovulatory infertility associated with polycystic ovary syndrome. Clomiphene citrate is widely available and relatively well-accepted in terms of safety, simplicity, side effects and cost.

Mechanism of action
- Clomiphene citrate acts predominantly as an antiestrogen. By binding to the hypothalamic estrogen receptors, CC displaces endogenous estrogen from the receptors, leading to a decrease in the negative feedback exerted by endogenous estrogen.
- As a result gonadotropin releasing hormone (GnRH) secretion appears to increase.
- This increased GnRH stimulates pituitary to release gonadotropins, FSH and LH.
- Follicle-stimulating hormone stimulates the development of follicles in the ovaries.
- The developing follicles begin to secrete estrogens.
- This rising estradiol levels then appear to trigger the midcycle LH surge and ovulation.

Dose and administration
The recommended starting dose is 50 mg/day (1 tablet) as almost half of the pregnancies are achieved with this dose (Gysler et al. 1982). The tablets are usually given for 5 days following the onset of a spontaneous or a progesterone-induced period. Administration of clomiphene citrate can start at any time from D2 to D5 of the cycle as there is no difference in the outcome between these time-points (Wu and Winkel, 1989). Until normal ovulation occurs the dose should be increased in each of the next cycles by 50 mg/day up to a maximum dose of 150 mg/day. Maximum recommended dose is 150 mg/day as there is no clear evidence of efficacy at higher doses.

Monitoring
A baseline ultrasound before starting the treatment is needed to exclude any pre-existing cysts. During stimulation, monitoring by ultrasound is not mandatory to ensure good outcome, but it is helpful to monitor the first cycle to allow adjustment of the dose in subsequent cycles based on the observed response.

Monitoring of the response of drug can be done by:
- Serial follicular phase TVS. It determines:
  - The development of follicles. A mature follicle attains the size of 18 mm or more.
  - The development of endometrium. A triple line endometrium of 8 mm or more indicates optimum response.
  - Ovulation: Indicated by—
    - Absence of pre-existent follicle.
    - Reduction of size of the follicle by 5 mm from previous one.
    - Collapsing of the follicle.
    - Fluid in the pouch of Douglas.
- Serum estradiol in midcycle. A mature follicle secretes 80–100 pg/mL or more estradiol.
- Serum progesterone in luteal phase (D21). A level 4 ng/mL indicates ovulation though good quality follicle and ovum is indicated by 10 ng/mL or more progesterone (Magyar, 1979).

Efficacy
Approximately 75–80% of patients with PCOS ovulate after CC administration (Homburg R, 1999) but only about 20–25% of those conceive (Gysler et al. 1982).

This discrepancy is due to the following facts:
- It causes cervical hostility by making mucus thick
- It causes reduced thickness of endometrium due to antiestrogenic effect
- Out-of-phase preimplantation endometrium
- In 33% cases, it is associated with luteinized unruptured follicle syndrome (LUFS). So there is no ovulation
- It is associated with luteal phase defect (LPD)
- There is reduced uterine blood flow
- It has detrimental effects on oocyte.

Duration of treatment
Treatment generally should be limited to six ovulatory cycles. Further cycles (maximum 12 in total) may be considered on an individual basis after discussion with the patient. Cumulative live birth rates vary between 50% and 60% for up to six cycles (Kousta et al. 1997).

Adverse effects
Hot flushes, headaches and visual complaints are well-recognized side effects during CC treatment,

but the drug is generally well tolerated. The multiple pregnancy rate is less than 10% and ovarian hyperstimulation syndrome (OHSS) is rare. Antiestrogenic effects on endometrium and cervical mucus may occur, but appear to represent an idiosyncratic response.

Effect of long-term use
In long-term use, it may cause endometrial insensitivity. Chance of ovarian malignancy is 2.3 times more than normal population if used for long time. Use of CC less than 1 year was not associated with an increased risk. But it increased when CC used more than 1 year (Rossing, 1994). But a Danish population-based cohort study among 54362 women and US-based case control study found no association between use of fertility drugs and risk of ovarian cancer after adjusting known confounding factors (Jensen et al. 2009; Kurta et al. 2012).

Clomiphene failure
As the goal of treatment is the induction of ovulation and pregnancy, CC failure must be subclassified into those who fail to ovulate (*ovulation failure*) and those who ovulate, but fail to conceive (*conception failure*). While considerable overlap exists between these two subgroups, the distinction is important, as the clinical management of the two problems may be quite different.

Ovulation failure
Women who fail to ovulate after maximum dose of CC are considered as clomiphene resistant (Nestler et al. 2002). In women with PCOS, the rates of CC resistance are around 10–30% (Hughes et al. 2000). Several investigators have identified a relationship between CC dose and body weight, BMI or ponderal index (Shepard et al. 1979; Nestler et al. 2002). There is also a strong relationship between CC resistant and insulin resistant.

Conception failure
In spite of ovulation with CC when patients fail to conceive, it is called clomiphene failure or conception failure. Among those who do not conceive within six ovulatory cycles are couples with other infertility factors or PCOS-related factors, which may account for these continuing infertility. The antiestrogenic actions of CC may adversely affect vaginal cornification, cervical mucus, and endometrial thickness, thus potentially affecting sperm transport, sperm survival and early implantation.

Tamoxifen

Tamoxifen appears to be as effective as CC for induction of ovulation. It can be considered as an alternative to CC in women who suffer intolerable side effects such as hot flushes.

Dose and administration: Oral tablet 10 mg twice daily from D3 to D7. Maximum dose is 40 mg/day. Can start any day between D2 and D5.

Mechanism of action and monitoring: Same as CC.

Aromatase Inhibitors

Aromatase inhibitors are also antiestrogenic agents. It has been widely used to treat estrogen sensitive Ca breast where it reduces the synthesis of estrogen. It is not approved for the treatment of infertility. It is used in most countries as off-label drug after appropriate discussion of risks and benefits. There is no scientific basis for not using this drug. Only reason is that it is still not Food and Drug Administration (FDA) approved.

Mechanism of action
It inhibits the enzyme aromatase, which is responsible for conversion of androgen to estrogen. So there is reduced synthesis of estrogen leading to a decrease in the negative feedback exerted by endogenous estrogen. Rests are same as the action of CC.

Dose and duration of treatment
Starting dose is 2.5 mg (1 tablet) per/day from D3 to D7. As CC, it also can be started any day from D2 to D5. Gradually, dose can be increased up to 10 mg/day according to response. No fixed higher dose is scheduled till today. Once ovulation is ensured, six ovulatory cycles are to be used.

Monitoring
Same as CC.

Efficacy
The reported success of aromatase inhibitor in inducing ovulation in women with PCOS are 75% (Mitwally and Casper, 2001), 77.9% (Sammour et al. 2001) and 40.63% in CC resistant PCOS

(Begum, 2009). Other studies also proved the efficacy of aromatase inhibitor in ovulation induction (Mitwally and Casper, 2001; Mitwally and Casper, 2000; Heasley et al. 1987). Initial preliminary study suggests that letrozole appears to be as effective as CC for induction of ovulation.

Adverse Effects

Commonly used AI is letrozole for ovulation induction. Others are anastrozole and exemestane. Most side effects are anastrozole related.

Common side effects
- Hot flashes and night sweats
- Joint and muscle pain
- Loss of bone mineral density.

Uncommon or rare side effects
- Carpal tunnel syndrome
- Hair thinning
- Heart problems
- Increased blood pressure
- Increased cholesterol
- Mood swings and depression.

Advantage of Aromatase Inhibitors over Clomiphene Citrate

- *No antiestrogenic effect in AI*: Antiestrogenic effect of CC includes long-lasting estrogen receptor (ER) blockage as CC accumulates in the body for long time because of long half-life (15 days) leading to negative effect on endometrial development and quality, and quantity of cervical mucus. But half-life of aromatase inhibitor is only 45 hours, so there is no profound antiestrogenic effect on endometrial or cervical mucus (Mitwally and Casper, 2000).
- *Monofollicular development is more in AI*: Due to long half-life of CC there is continuous stimulation to the pituitary to release more and more FSH. As a result multiple follicles get chance to grow. On the other hand due to short half-life of AI, negative feedback effect begins to work as soon as there is a growing follicle. So there is no continuous release of FSH for growth of multiple follicles. As a result monofollicular development is more pronounced in AI.

Low Dose Gonadotropins

For anovulatory patients who do not respond to other ovulation inducing agents, gonadotropin is the supreme drug for induction of ovulation. For PCOS, gonadotropin should be given with caution to avoid clinical hyperstimulation. In the first treatment cycle, a very low dose of hMG (FSH and LH) or pure rFSH should be given daily or alternate day till the development of follicles.

Advantage of using gonadotropin is chance of ovulation is more precise.

Disadvantages
- It requires meticulous judgment for application
- Dose is very much individualized
- Expensive
- Chance of ovarian hyperstimulation syndrome (OHSS) (sometimes fatal) is more, so needs meticulous monitoring
- Chance of multiple pregnancies is also more.

Currently, two low-dose regimens are used:
1. *Step-up regimens:* Step-up regimens are based upon the principle of a stepwise increase in FSH supply to determine the FSH threshold for follicular development. After commencement of gonadotropin administration, if follicle development is not observed on ultrasound after 1 week, an increase in the dose is recommended. Once follicle growth is observed, the same FSH dose is maintained until follicular selection is achieved.
2. *Step-down regimens:* This regimen is designed to achieve the FSH threshold through a loading dose of FSH with a subsequent stepwise reduction as soon as follicular development is observed on ultrasound.

Monitoring

- *Monitoring is mandatory* if induction is given by gonadotropins.
- Ultrasound assessment of the ovary can be performed at baseline before the initiation of each cycle. Serial ovarian ultrasound is an excellent method of determining follicle growth and development in response to gonadotropin stimulation. Before ovulation

induction with gonadotropins, it is mandatory to counsel the patient about the risks associated with higher-order multiple pregnancies after polyovulation and risk of ovarian hyperstimulation syndrome.

Efficacy

Overall, low-dose regimens result in a monofollicular ovulation rate of approximately 70%, a pregnancy rate of 20%, and a multiple live birth rate of 5.7% (Homburg et al. 1999).

Adverse Effect

Ovarian hyperstimulation syndrome is the most common and grave complication of gonadotropin stimulation. There is growth of multiple follicles and subsequently development of ascites, renal failure, coagulation disorder may leads to death.

> Suppose Mrs Ayesa received CC up to 150 mg/day without any response. Then you tried with AI up to dose of 10 mg/day. You found that follicle developed up to the size of 14 mm by day 16.
> What can you do for further improvement?

This patient may be insulin resistant (IR). Insulin resistant patients usually do not respond to CC or AI even to highest dose. Investigation can be done to detect insulin resistance, but therapeutic failure is enough for assessing insulin resistance. By assessing homeostatic model assessment (HOMA) it is found that all CC resistant patients were insulin resistant (Begum, 2013). Considering this fact metformin at a dose of 500 mg thrice daily can be added to this patient along with AI.

RELATED INFORMATION

Effect of Insulin Resistance in Ovulation

The patients who are insulin resistant are genetically determined. Insulin cannot act to utilize blood glucose. So increased blood glucose stimulate pancreas to release more insulin. There is a positive vicious cycle, which increases blood insulin level causing hyperinsulinemia. There is a strong association between hyperinsulinemia and hyperandrogenism. Increased insulin stimulates both adrenal glands and ovaries to synthesis androgens. This hyperandrogenism causes folli-

Table 17.2 Diagnosis of insulin resistance (IR)

Parameters	Normal value	IR value
Basal fasting insulin level	<12 mU/mL	>12 mU/mL
Fasting glucose and insulin ratio	>6.4	<6.4
Homeostatic model assessment (HOMA) test	<47	>47
Quantitative insulin-sensitivity check index (QUICKI)	>0.333	<0.333

cular atresia and anovulation. Before complete atresia the underdeveloped follicles come as small cyst producing polycystic ovaries. Diagnosis of IR can be made by measuring fasting blood glucose and fasting insulin **(Table 17.2)**.

Calculation of HOMA

$$\text{HOMA} = \frac{\text{Fasting insulin } \mu\text{IU/mL} \times \text{Fasting glucose mmol/L} \times 18}{22.5}$$

> How to revert this hyperinsulinemia?

Exercise

Exercise independently can reduce insulin level. Exercise can help to use glucose by mobilizing a protein called GluT4, which opens the channel for glucose entry. So glucose can be utilized without the help of insulin. As blood glucose comes down, pancreatic stimulation withdrawn and insulin secretion decreased. Finally androgen concentration also lowered.

Insulin Sensitizing Agents

There is a number of insulin sensitizing agents, but commonly used drug is metformin. Others are rosiglitazone, pioglitazone, troglitazone are not used due to adverse effects. None of the insulin-sensitizing drugs has FDA approval for use in PCOS. Nonetheless the scientific evidence supporting their salutary effects in PCOS is substantial and progressively mounting and their use for this purpose by clinicians is already established.

Metformin

Metformin is a biguanide antihyperglycemic that is approved for the management of type 2 diabetes mellitus. The mechanism by which metformin enhance insulin sensitivity are not fully characterized.

Metformin reduces blood glucose level, which in turn reduces insulin level and finally hyperandrogenemia. As a result there is resumption of ovulation or increased sensitivity to ovulation inducing drugs.

Mechanism of Reduction of Blood Glucose

Metformin appears to:
- Suppress hepatic glucose output
- Decreased intestinal absorption of glucose
- Increased insulin-mediated glucose utilization in peripheral tissues
- Has an antilipolytic affect on fatty acid concentration reducing gluconeogenesis (Bailey et al. 1996).

It does not produce hypoglycemia in either normal subjects or patients with type 2 diabetes.

Dose and Duration of Treatment

In insulin-resistant patient if there is no response to CC/AI, metformin is to be started according to BMI of the patient. It takes 12 weeks to revert the metabolic derangement. So after 12 weeks of metformin therapy, ovulation inducing agent is to be restarted. It is available in a generic form as 500 mg, 850 mg and 1,000 mg tablets. The target dose of metformin is in the range of 1,500–2,550 mg/day according to BMI (Patance et al. 2,000). Daily dose is 1,500 mg for BMI up to 30, 2,000 mg/day up to BMI 34 and 2,500 mg/day for BMI more than 34. Metformin is given with meals and is to be started with small dose with weekly increment of dose till desired level to reduce the gastrointestinal side effects. Drug is to be continued till conception. It also can be continued till delivery as it reduces both abortion and GDM (Glueck et al. 2001; 2002; Begum et al. 2009). It is category B drug and no teratogenicity is reported.

Efficacy

A large number of studies evaluated and proved the efficacy of the drug in resuming ovulation, menstruation and reverting metabolic changes (Nestler et al. 1996; Moghetti et al. 2000; Heard et al. 2002; Kocak et al. 2002).

Side Effects

The most common side effects of metformin are diarrhea, nausea, vomiting, flatulence, indigestion and abdominal discomfort. The gastrointestinal side effects may be caused by high intestinal metformin concentration that causes build up of lactic acid in the bowel. A rare problem caused by metformin is lactic acidosis, which is fatal in as many as 30–50% of cases. Chance of lactic acidosis is increased when patients have renal insufficiency. It is rapidly absorbed from the small intestine and without metabolism largely excreted in the urine. So it should not be prescribed if serum creatinine level is greater than 1 mg/dL. Liver disease, congestive heart failure and previous history of lactic acidosis are other contraindications of metformin therapy. Metformin should be temporarily suspended for all major surgical procedures that involve restriction of fluid intake. It also should be discontinued 48 hours before any radiologic procedure that involves intravenous administration of iodinated contrast material.

> After adding metformin, you gave same stimulating drugs. This time you found that the patient developed follicles of 20 × 20 mm sized with a very good triple lined endometrium (12 mm). But by serial TVS it is recognized that follicle did not rupture. There was a single follicle, estrogen level was 180 pg/mL and D21 serum progesterone was 25 ng/mL.
>
> What might be the problem and how it can be corrected?

This is a case of *luteinized unruptured follicle syndrome* (LUFS). Estrogen and progesterone level indicates that it is a mature follicle and ovum trapped into the follicle.

In subsequent cycles ovulation is to be triggered by injection human chorionic gonadotropin (hCG) to release the egg.

RELATED INFORMATION

Luteinized Unruptured Follicle Syndrome

The LUFS is a condition in which the follicle fails to rupture and expel the oocyte within 48 hours of LH surge. As a result no ovum is available for fertilization and pregnancy resulting infertility. Ovulation associated with significant hormonal changes, and it takes place after final maturation of oocyte by LH. Prostaglandins and proteolytic enzymes weaken the wall of the follicle, resulting in its rupture. The granulosa cells of the dominant follicle luteinize and the ruptured follicle forms the corpus luteum. But in certain situations follicle gets mature, but fails to rupture and granulosa cells become luteinized.

Causes

Exact cause is not known. But the factors, which make the follicular wall tough are responsible for this condition. Use of nonsteroidal anti-inflammatory drugs (NSAIDs) in midcycle interferes ovulation by inhibiting prostaglandin synthesis.

Frequency

It is found in 11% of cycles of normal women and almost 50% in unexplained infertility (Kerin et al. 1983). Higher incidence also found in PCOS (37.5%), endometriosis (35%), pelvic adhesions, PID and after pelvic operation (26.2%) (Toda, 1990).

Diagnosis

All features of ovulation are present in this condition. Changes of basal body temperature (BBT), changes in cervical mucus, midcycle estrogen level, LH surge, luteal phase progesterone level and secretory changes (subuclear vacuolation) in endometrial biopsy. So diagnosis only can be made by follicular tracking by serial ultrasonogram.

Treatment

Ovulation can be triggered by hormone when follicle gets matured (18–20 mm). Human chorionic gonadotropin (hCG) in doses of 5,000–10,000 IU intramuscularly, or, recombinant LH 250 µg subcutaneously, can be administered to induce ovulation. It takes about 36–40 hours for the oocyte to be released after the injection. Ultrasound can be used to document ovulation.

Luteal Phase Defect

Corpus luteum deficiency that leads to a defect in endometrial maturation or short luteal phase is called LPD. It causes infertility due to defective endometrial preparation and recurrent pregnancy loss due to short luteal phase.

Causes

- Decreased FSH production at the follicular phase
- Abnormal pattern of LH secretion
  - Leads to poor quality follicle and oocyte formation
  - Leads to poor corpus luteum production and decreased progesterone production by poor corpus luteum
- Poor response of endometrium to progesterone also may be the cause.

Frequency

The reported incidence of LPD is 8.1–17.5% depending upon author's definition and sample size (Rosenberg, 1980; Witten and Martin, 1985).

Diagnosis

- Midluteal serum progesterone level <10 ng/mL
- Out of phase defect, 2 days or more in 2 subsequent endometrial biopsy.

Treatment

- Ovulation induction
- Progesterone supplementation.
  - Vaginal suppository 100 mg twice daily
  - Intramuscular injection 50 mg daily
  - Oral micronized progesterone 100 mg two to three times daily.
- Bromocriptine or cabergoline if associated hyperprolactinemia present.

> Mrs Ayesa responded to letrozole 10 mg/day along with metformin 500 mg thrice daily. On D12 you found that a follicle, sized 20/22 mm developed in right ovary with a very good (10 mm) triple-lined endometrium. On D16 you confirmed by TVS that ovulation took place.
>
> How long do you want to give this treatment?

Treatment should be continued for 6 cycles. Implantation is critical and fertilized embryo does not implant in each cycle. Only 35% of fertilized embryo implants in each cycle (Wilcox et al. 1988). So at least 6 cycles are to be given to get the optimum result. Metformin should be continued till pregnancy.

> After 6 cycles, she did not get pregnant. You stopped stimulation for 4 months and kept the patient only on metformin to get the benefit of rebound ovulation and spontaneous pregnancy. But it also did not work. Cycle became irregular again.
> What should be your next action?

At this point, her tuboperitoneal factor needs to be evaluated. For this patient, laparoscopy is the ideal test to see tubal patency as laparoscopic ovarian drilling (LOD) will be possible at the same time.

> Suppose patient did not response even after addition of metformin, then you added injection gonadotropin with meticulous monitoring. Even after addition of gonadotropin she did not response.
> What to do?

- Laparoscopic ovarian drilling and tubal patency test is to be done.

As optimum medical treatment failed to ovulate, surgical treatment is indicated. Surgical treatments are:
- *Laparoscopic ovarian drilling:* Electrocauterization by multiple puncturing of ovaries.
- *Wedge resection of ovaries:* Ovarian tissue is removed by giving a wedge incision. But it causes much postsurgical adhesion. This procedure is abandoned now-a-days.

So LOD would be the logical option for this patient. Tubal patency should be tested at the same time.

> What are the indications of LOD?

Indications of LOD in PCOS patients are:
- When medical treatment with gonadotropin failed to ovulate.
- When laparoscopy is done due to other reason.
- When patient lives far away and is unable to come for monitoring.

> Usually how many punctures should be done?

The LOD is usually done under general anesthesia (G/A). By using unipolar coagulating current ovarian tissue is coagulated. Usually 4 punctures in each ovary are to be done with 40 watts for 4 seconds at a depth of 4 mm and 1 cm apart. But there is no agreement on the optimum dose of diathermy to apply. Number of punctures should be individualized. If any patient ovulates with minimum dose of first-line drug then for this patient 4 punctures will be enough for resumption of spontaneous ovulation. But if someone is very resistant to drug even to gonadotropin then number of punctures will be more and will depend on the size of the ovary. More is the size of the ovary more punctures will be needed. But not more than 10 punctures in each ovary. Aggressive puncture may lead to premature ovarian failure (POF). All punctures should be done away from hilum and mesovarium to protect against damage to the ovarian blood supply.

> What are the other situations where drilling may cause POF?

Improper selection of cases such as:
- Irregular cycle but patient has no PCOS (hypogonadotropic hypogonadism)
- Multicystic ovaries, but patient has no PCOS.

> What is the difference between multicystic and polycystic ovaries?

Sometimes multiple cysts are present in ovaries of some patients without the evidence of PCOS. In 25% cases, ovaries are multicystic due to inappropriate gonadotropin stimulation. Those patients can be identified by certain parameters.

Multifollicular ovaries are seen in various physiological and even pathological situations such as:
- Delayed normal puberty
- Central precocious puberty
- Hypothalamic anovulation
- Hyperprolactinemia
- Early normal follicular predominant phase.

According to Adam et al. the multifollicular ovaries are different from PCOS by following characteristics (Adam et al. 1985):
- Follicles are larger
- Stromal echodensity is less
- Ovarian volume is normal
- Usually a dominant follicle is seen.

How does LOD revert metabolic derangement?

Various theories are proposed in favor of mechanism of action of LOD:
- Drilling of follicles release androgen-rich follicular fluid and also decreases the androgen producing stroma. So as to decrease circulating androgens.
- There is transient reduction in inhibin and precipitous fall in LH, which results in increased secretion of FSH and its expression.
- Crowding of cortex decreases, which allows progress of normal follicles to the surface resulting in resumption of normal ovulation.
- Due to damage of ovarian tissue, ovarian androgen and LH synthesis reduced. So ovaries become more responsive and less ovulation inducing drugs are needed.

You did laparoscopy and LOD on Mrs Ayesa. Both tubes are healthy and patent. Pelvis is clear. What will you suggest her?

She will be advised to try for pregnancy for 6 months to 1 year. As OD overcome insulin resistant and resume ovulation, so ovulation and pregnancy can be expected after OD.

How much it is effective?

Reported ovulation rate ranging from 64% to 92% and pregnancy rate 41–80% (Li, 1998; Kriplani, 2001; Abdel, 1993; Keckstein, 1989).

Efficacy

Efficacy depends on:
- *Age:* More age less response
- *BMI:* More BMI less response, thin PCOS responds well
- *Testosterone level:* High testosterone level less response.

In an unpublished data of 450 PCOS patients we observed that patient who ovulates with CC or letrozole usually ovulates spontaneously after LOD. But who were nonresponsive to CC, letrozole and even to gonadotropin did not resume spontaneous ovulation after LOD. These patients needed ovulation inducing drugs after LOD. Only advantage was that after LOD response to the drug increased and gonadotropin requirement reduced. Farquhar also reported that 20–30% of women with PCOS failed to respond to LOD (Farquhar, 2004).

Advantages

Advantages of LOD over gonadotropin are:
- Less expensive in comparison to gonadotropin
- No need of monitoring
- No chances of OHSS
- No chance of multiple pregnancy
- Abortion rate is significantly lower.

Disadvantages

Disadvantages of LOD over gonadotropin are:
- It is invasive procedure needs general anesthesia and has the potential risk of surgical *complications* such as injury to bowel, bladder, ureter and postoperative complications such as:
  - Bleeding from drilling site causing postoperative adhesion and may interfere future fertility
  - Laceration of ovarian ligament and the use of cauterization may effect ovarian circulation through uterine vessels
  - Aggressive cauterization destroys large number of follicles and reduces ovarian reserve
  - Deep penetration of electrode into the ovary may destroy hillar blood vessels, resulting in POF caused by necrosis.
- It is expensive
- It needs surgical skill.

Mrs Ayesa did not get pregnant, rather she developed irregular menstruation after 6 months of natural trial. What do you want to do now?

As her menstruation became irregular, again she will need drug for ovulation. She received OI drug previously for several cycles. So now along with ovulation induction (OI), intrauterine insemination (IUI) will be logical option for her. At this age 4–6 cycles IUI can be done if patient desires. Even then if she does not get pregnant *in vitro* fertilization and embryo transfer (IVF and ET) can be done.

> After 6 months of LOD, why her menstrual cycle became irregular?

The effect of LOD does not persist for long. It was reported that the beneficial effect of LOD is of limited duration, in most studies up to 1 year (Buttram, 1975; Keckstein, 1989). Though Amer and co-workers reported that 50% of the total study group continued regular menstruation 7 years later (Amer, 2002).

> After 1 year of OD, if patient again becomes anovulatory do you recommend 2nd time ovarian drilling?

No. Redrilling is not indicated in any way in the fear of POF.

> **Case scenario:** Mrs Rabeya, aged 32 years has complaints of irregular menstrual cycle. Ultrasonography shows normal uterus and very smaller ovaries with 1 tiny antral follicle in each ovary. FSH is 58 IU/L, LH 35 IU/mL and E2 is <20, which is done for the first time. She took OI for last 5 years from different clinicians, but did not get pregnant. Her response of induction was never assessed. Her husband is quite OK.
>
> What treatment do you like to offer this couple for pregnancy?

This patient is a case of premature ovarian failure (POF). She will not produce any egg after induction. Patient will be counseled and another test will be done to confirm the hormone level. After 2nd testing she will be declared as POF. It is recommended that at least two tests at different cycle should be done to declare failure.

Treatment will be:
- IVF with donor egg
- Adoption.

RELATED INFORMATION

Premature Ovarian Failure

Premature ovarian failure occurs when onset of menopausal symptoms appears before the age of 40. It occurs due to exhaustion of all eggs in 1% of women and 0.1% of women younger than 30 years of age. One may have no or few eggs. Depending on the cause, premature ovarian failure may develop as early as the teen years, or the problem may have been present from birth.

Causes

Although the exact cause of premature ovarian failure is not known. Suggestive causes are:
- Genetic factors
- Autoimmunity
- Repeated pelvic surgery
- Bilateral ovarian cystectomy (particularly in chocolate cyst)
- Chemotherapy
- Radiotherapy.

Symptoms

- Oligomenorrhea: Long menstrual cycle irregular or no periods
- Secondary amenorrhea
- Infertility
- Menopausal symptoms:
  - Hot flashes
  - Night sweats
  - Irritability
  - Poor concentration
  - Decreased interest in sex
  - Pain during sex
  - Dryness of the vagina.

Diagnosis

- High FSH >30 IU/L, high LH >20 IU/L, low estrogen <20 pg/mL
- No progesterone withdrawal bleeding
- Low AMH and inhibin B
- On biopsy of ovarian tissue no primordial follicles exist in the ovary.

Treatment

- Treatment for fertility:
  - ART with donor egg
  - Sometimes estrogen treatment for several days followed by gonadotropin causes gonadal activity to resume at least temporarily where complete follicular depletion does not occur.
- General treatment:
  - *HRT:* Conjugated equino estrogen 0.625 mg daily from D1 to D21 with progesterone 5 mg daily from D16 to D25. It reduces the symptoms and prevents bone loss.

Resistant Ovary Syndrome

When ovaries are not responsive to gonadotropins. It is one sort of POF where ovaries contain reasonable number of primordial follicles, but those are not responsive to gonadotropins.

Symptoms

Symptoms are same as before.

Causes

- Autoimmune reaction with antibody formation against FSH receptors
- Mutation in FSH receptor gene.

Diagnosis

- High FSH >30 IU/L, high LH >20 IU/L, low estrogen <20 pg/mL
- No progesterone withdrawal bleeding
- Normal AMH and inhibin B
- On biopsy ovarian tissue contains reasonable primordial follicles.

Treatment

A. Treatment for fertility
   - ART with donor egg
B. General treatment: Same as before.

> **Case scenario**: Mrs Khadija, aged 29 years has undergone HSG after 1 year of medical treatment. It shows bilateral tubal block. Her husband's semen analysis report is normal.
> What will you offer for her?

Her tubal condition should be rechecked by laparoscopy. HSG may show both false-positive and false-negative result. So it must be checked by laparoscopy.

> Laparoscopy also shows bilateral tubal block.
> What do you want to do?

There are two modalities of treatment for bilateral tubal block:
1. Reconstructive microsurgery
2. Assisted reproductive technique.

As the patient is young, tubal reconstructive surgery that is end-to-end anastomosis can be done. But criteria of the surgery should be the following:
- There should be single block in each tube
- Tubal length should be in a state that after reconstruction, the repaired tubal length must be at least 4 cm
- In properly selected cases pregnancy rate is 20–25%
- After tubal anastomosis, couple will be observed for at least 1–2 years
- If patient does not get pregnant within this period, ART will be done.

> Suppose her age is 38 years. On laparoscopy, it is diagnosed bilateral tubal block.
> What is your decision?

In this case, ART will be logical option. Patient is elderly so there is not enough time for reproduction. After reconstructive surgery at least 1 year time should be allowed for pregnancy. By this time OR may be reduced and scope of ART might lost. So ART is ideal treatment for this patient.

Note: At any age if OR is poor and bilateral tubal block is diagnosed, ART will be logical option for the same reason. There is no role of microsurgery even the patient is very young.

RELATED INFORMATION

Assessment of Tubal/Tuboperitoneal Factors

Indications of tubal and tuboperitoneal factor assessment:

A. It is indicated when patients fail to get pregnant after 6 ovulatory cycles.
B. But in certain situations, tuboperitoneal factor assessment should come as primary investigation or after 2–3 cycles of OI.

These are following:
- Patient more than 35 years of age and infertility more than 3 years.
- Patient of any age with poor ovarian reserve where quick treatment is needed.
- History of chronic pelvic pain, PID, childbirth, abortions, MR, dilatation and curettage (D&C), salpingectomy after ectopic pregnancy, endometriosis, sonographically presence of cysts, myomectomy, adenomyomectomy, ovarian cystectomy and other pelvic surgery.

Tests for tubal/tuboperitoneal factor assessment:

- *Hysterosalpingogram (HSG)*: Introduction of water- or oil-based radiopaque dye through cervical os, which passes through uterus and tubes into the pelvis. During this passage of dye, X-ray is taken to see whether dye has passed or not into peritoneal cavity.
- *Saline sonosalpingogram*: A self-retaining catheter is introduced through Cx and balloon is inflated. Normal saline is introduced during transvaginal sonographic procedure to observe whether fluid is passing through the tubes or not.
- *Laparoscopy*: Invasive surgical procedure to observe interior of the pelvis and for chromopertubation. A camera is introduced through umbilicus to visualize the abdominal cavity:
  - *Chromopertubation* is the procedure in which methylene blue dye is introduced through cervical os to pass through the uterus and tubes into peritoneal cavity. By laparoscopy spillage of dye through tubes into peritoneal cavity can be visualized (Fig. 17.1).
  - *Assessment of tubal condition and tubo-ovarian relationship:*
    - Tubal length, normal or short
    - Caliber whether dilated or not, any constriction, diverticula formation, kinking, cord like, etc.

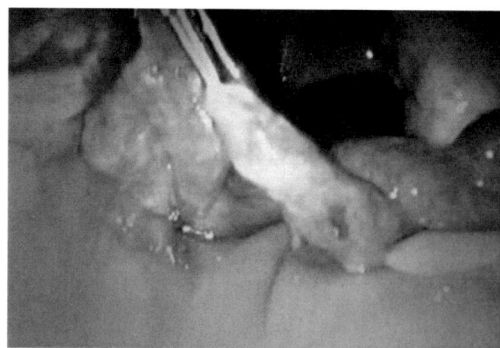

Fig. 17.1 Laparoscopic dye test showing positive dye test *(For color version, see Plate 4)*

- Condition of the fimbria, free or coagulated
- Relation with ovaries, whether normal or away from ovaries due to adhesion with surroundings.

Selection of Test for Tuboperitoneal Factor Assessment

- Laparoscopy is the ideal test for tuboperitoneal factor assessment for patients mentioned in group B of indication of tubal and tuboperitoneal factor assessment.
- In other situations, HSG or sonosalpingogram can be done.

Advantages of laparoscopy
- It gives detailed information about anatomy of tubes, ovaries and uterus.
- It can identify tubo-ovarian relationship. If there is any misplacement of tubes due to adhesion, it can be diagnosed and corrected at the same time.
- Uterine and ovarian adhesion can be released and anatomy can be restored.
  - These are the *advantages of laparoscopy* and all these factors optimize pregnancy.

Disadvantages of laparoscopy
- It is invasive procedure needs general anesthesia and has the potential risk of surgical *complications* such as injury to bowel, bladder, ureter and postoperative complications
- It is expensive
- It needs surgical skill.

Advantages of HSG
- It is cheaper, easily available
- No need of surgical skill
- Information about interior of the uterus can obtained.

Disadvantages of HSG
- It is very painful as it is usually done without anesthesia
- Radiopaque dye is used, which causes pain and may cause hypersensitive reaction may leads to shock
- It cannot give detailed information of the interior of the pelvis
- False positive test report is not uncommon as patent tubes may remain adherent with lateral pelvic wall or in other direction from where ovum pickup is impossible
- False negative report of cornual block is more in HSG due to smooth muscle spasm.

Advantages of saline sonosalpingogram
- It is done by ultrasonogram, which is widely available, easy-to-use and less expensive than other imaging methods
- Less painful than HSG as normal saline is used in this procedure instead of oil-based dye
- Sonosalpingography is a simple, minimally invasive procedure that is well tolerated by patients and has very few complications
- Ultrasound imaging uses no ionizing radiation
- Ultrasound scanning gives a clear picture of soft tissues that do not show up well on X-ray images
- Ultrasound causes no health problems and may be repeated as often as is necessary
- Many uterine abnormalities that may not be seen adequately with routine transvaginal ultrasound may be viewed in detail with hysterosonosalpingography.

Disadvantages of saline sonosalpingogram
It also cannot give detailed information about interior of the pelvis.

Timing of the Tests

All three tests are to be done in the proliferative phase of the cycle preferably on D9 or D10. It excludes pregnancy so there is no chance of destroying the most expected undiagnosed valuable pregnancies. If these tests are done during bleeding there is chance of dissemination of endometrial tissue through blood vessel.

> **Case scenario:** Mrs Rahima, aged 30 years has complaints of childlessness for 3 years. Her husband's semen report is normal. On USG it is found that there is a myoma of 5 × 4 cm at the top of fundus. Endometrial cavity is clear. Menstrual history is normal. About 2 months back HSG was done. Tubes are patent. Patient is very anxious about the myoma.
>
> What will be your decision about myoma?

No need of doing anything with this fibroid right at this moment as:
- Myoma is subserous and fundal, and not disturbing endometrial cavity. So it is not responsible for infertility.
- It is not producing any symptom such as menorrhagia or pain.
- Chance of malignancy is very low.

So it should be kept as it is, as postmyomectomy adhesion may disturb tuboperitoneal factors.

RELATED INFORMATION

Uterine Factor Infertility

Causes

A. Poor development of endometrium due to:
   - *End organ damage:* The basal endometrium is permanently damaged:
     - Repeated infection of the uterine lining; endometritis following septic delivery and abortion
     - Tuberculosis
     - Following repeated or over aggressive D&C and MR
     - Following uterine surgery that causes excessive endometrial scarring.
   - *Low estrogen due to poor quality follicle.*
   - *Resistant to estrogen* due to:
     - Prolonged use of CC
     - Prolonged use of oral contraceptive pills (OCP)
     - Prolonged use of progesterone
     - Intrauterine exposure to diethylstilbestrol (DES).
   - *Reduced blood flow to the basal endometrium* due to

- Extensive uterine surgery
- Asherman's syndrome (uterine synechiae)
- Multiple uterine fibroids (submucus)
- Adenomyosis.
  - *Overexposure to ovarian testosterone.*
  - *Radiation damage*
B. Pathological condition of uterus:
  - Infection
  - Asherman's syndrome
  - Polyps
  - Myoma
  - Adenomyoma.
C. Developmental defect: Septate and subseptate uterus may cause infertility, as embryo cannot implant over relatively poor vascular septum. Unicornuate uterus sometimes delayed pregnancy as one tube is working.
D. Absence uterus:
  - *Congenital*
  - *Iatrogenic:* Hysterectomy due to any cause.
E. Cervical hostility.

Diagnosis

- USG preferably 3D transvaginal USG, which can diagnose septum and bicornuate uterus, any growth in the uterus, hyper- and hypoplastic endometrium, irregular endometrium due to adhesion.
- Color Doppler USD to assess subendometrial vascularity.
- Application of estrogen and progesterone to see the response of the endometrium.
- FSH, LH, E2 if there is amenorrhea.
- HSG can identify space occupying lesions, adhesion.
- Saline hysterosonography can identify space occupying lesions and adhesion.
- Hysteroscopy to view in details of the interior of the uterus. Hysteroscopy can replace HSG and saline hysterosonography.

Treatment

- Treatment of thin endometrium:
  - *Exercise:* Increases uterine circulation.
  - *Hysteroscopy*: Hysteroscopy and correction of adhesions and introduction of IUD + estrogen and progesterone application.
  - *Estrogen:* Helps in proliferation of endometrial tissue.
  - *Low dose aspirin:* 75 mg daily to increase subendometrial vascularity by making blood thin.
  - *Sildenafil (Viagra):* Vaginal pessary causes vasodilatation and increases blood circulation.
  - *Endometrial injury:* Hysteroscopic injury to endometrium increases NO_2 and growth factors and helps development of endometrium.
  - *Transvaginal endometrial perfusion with granulocyte colony-stimulating factor (G-CSF):* Same as endometrial injury.
  - *Protein rich platelet (PRP):* Intrauterine transfusion of PRP can improve endometrial development.
  - *Stem cell therapy:* Under investigation.
- Treatment of polyp, myoma, adenomyoma: It includes *surgical treatment*, i.e. polypectomy, myomectomy and adenomyomectomy.

Indications of myomectomy
- Intracavitary myoma of any size.
- Submucous and intramural myoma, which distort the cavity.
- Submucous myoma did not distort the cavity, but size is >3 cm.
- Multiple myomas, which occlude the endometrial cavity.

Indications of adenomyomectomy: Severe dysmenorrhea with:
- Big adenomyoma occupying whole uterus or whole of the posterior wall of the uterus.
- Any size compressing the uterine cavity.

Indications of medical treatment for adenomyoma:
- For focal and small adenomyoma, GnRHa or levonorgestrel (LNG) intrauterine system for 6 months can relieve the symptom and reduce the size of the mass to an extent that pregnancy can possible.
- Before adenomyomectomy of big adenomyoma GnRHa or LNG intrauterine system for 4–6 months can be used to reduce the size of the tumor, as a result to minimize bleeding during operation. Moreover, it converts discrete adenomyoma to identifiable mass.

- Where whole uterus is replaced by adenomyoma in those cases surgery may destroy the uterus then only medical treatment is indicated whatever may be the chance of pregnancy.
- Treatment of septum and subseptum: Hysteroscopic septal resection.
- Treatment of Asherman's syndrome: Discussed later on.
- Treatment of noncorrectable factors and absent uterus either congenital or iatrogenic:
  1. Surrogacy.
  2. Uterine transplantation.

  These are:
  - Nonresponding endometrium
  - Congenital or iatrogenic absence of uterus
  - Nonfunctioning distorted uterus due to massive adenomyoma and after surgery of multiple myomas and adenomyoma.

Asherman's Syndrome

Partial or complete obliteration of endometrial cavity due to destruction of endometrial layer is called uterine synechiae and when associated with scanty menstruation and amenorrhea is called Asherman's syndrome (AS).

Symptoms

- Sudden reduction of menstrual flow, amenorrhea mostly secondary
- Pain or cramping at the time of menstruation with little or no blood
- Infertility, mostly secondary
- Recurrent pregnancy loss
- Morbid adhesion of placenta.

Causes

- Vigorous curettage, repeated curettage and curettage in presence of infection destroy basal layer of endometrium. It has been reported that 88% of AS cases occur after a D&C is performed on a recently pregnant uterus, following a missed or incomplete miscarriage, birth, or during an elective termination (abortion) to remove retained products of conception.
- Infection, which destroys the endometrial layer. Most common is tuberculosis. Uterine packing due to control of massive postpartum hemorrhage (PPH) may cause infection and AS. Rarely infection following cesarean section may cause AS.
- Extensive myomectomy and adenomyomectomy may cause adhesion.
- Pelvic irradiation.
- Manual removal of placenta.
- Uterine artery embolization.
- Endometrial ablation (intentionally created for treatment of abnormal uterine bleeding).

Diagnosis

- FSH, LH, E2 in case of amenorrhea to exclude ovarian failure
- Estrogen and progesterone challenge test if ovarian failure is excluded
- USG to assess endometrial development during follicular phase of menstrual cycle
- Hysteroscopy
- HSG or saline hysterosonogram where hysteroscopy facility is not available.

Treatment

- Hysteroscopy-guided adhesiolysis or dilatation and adhesiolysis by Hegar's dilator where hysteroscopy facility is not available followed by:
  - Introduction of CU T to keep endometrial cavity apart
  - Application of conjugated equino estrogen 0.625 mg daily from D5 to D25 and progesterone 5 mg daily from D16 to D25 for development of endometrium. It is to be continued for at least three cycles
  - PRP
  - Stem cell therapy

Prognosis

- If subsequent endometrial development is satisfactory, outcome is also satisfactory
- If endometrium still is not responding surrogacy is the option
- If endometrial development is satisfactory, but still no pregnancy tubal factor assessment is considered as there is association between uterine synechiae and tubal block

- If pregnancy occurs there is:
  - Risk of abortion
  - Risk of morbid adhesion of placenta.

> **Case scenario:** Mrs Selina, aged 35 years has come to you with the complaints of childlessness for 8 years. After taking detailed history, performing physical examination and doing USG, she is found normal. Her husband Mr Rakib's semen analysis shows count 4 million/mL, motility 45% and morphology 38% normal. His previous two reports showed same condition.
>
> What management would you like to offer for this couple?

Here male factor is responsible for infertility as three reports showed severe oligospermia. So male partner is to be evaluated thoroughly.

But female partner is elderly so her basic profile is to be tested to judge the duration of her reproductive prospect. For which:
- Her ovarian reserve is to be tested
- Other basic investigations, which mentioned earlier is to be done.

Evaluation of Male Partner

The male partner is to be evaluated to assess whether his condition is correctable or not.

Detailed history

Detailed history is to be taken focusing:
- *Occupation and environment*:
  - Whether place of work is hot or not. Hot weather effects sperm production and motility by increasing testicular temperature. Workers of mine, foundries and welders, traffic police are exposed to high temperature. For optimum spermatogenesis and good motility scrotal temperature should be 2°C less than body temperature.
  - Increased exposure to synthetic estrogen in working place. Synthetic estrogens are used in the livestock, poultry and dairy industries.
  - Exposure to pesticide.
  - Exposure to heavy metal, like lead and mercury.

  All causes reduces spermatogenesis
- *Lifestyle*:
  - Wearing tight-fitting nonporous synthetic cloths increases scrotal temperature.
  - Habit of taking frequent hot bath, sauna effect sperm production by increasing local temperature of testes.
  - Habit of smoking and alcoholism is to be asked for. Smoking has effect on sperm production and motility. Alcohol intake may cause impotency and reduces frequency of coitus.
  - Food habit: Taking food, which is grown by fertilizers has effect on sperm production. Reduced intake of fruits, vegetables, whole grains, and dietary fibers reduces sperm production. Certain foods, which contain phytoestrogen cause reduced sperm production.
- *History of medical disorder:* Particularly diabetes, which effects motility of the sperm, uncontrolled diabetes causes impotency. Renal disease cannot excrete and liver disease cannot detoxify the estrogen, so level of estrogen increased, which interferes spermatogenesis.
- *History of drug:* Certain drugs such as steroid, cyproterone, spironolactone, sulphasalazine, reserpine, cimetidine, nitrofurantoin, colchicines interfere spermatogenesis. Chlorpromazine, lignocaine, procaine and propranolol impairs sperm motility and nifedipine, allopurinol and nicotine impair the fertilizing capacity.
- *History of chemo and radiotherapy:* Those causes oligo or azoospermia.
- *History of male accessory gland infection (MAGI):* Childhood mumps causes severe oligospermia or azoospermia. *Chlamydia*, gonorrhea tuberculosis can cause block of vas deferens. Other infections cause reduced motility of sperm.
- *History of stress:* Disturbs hypothalamic pituitary axis and spermatogenesis.
- *History of previous surgery:* Herniorrhaphy may cause vassal block.
- *History of accident or exposure to X-ray:* Cause damage to the testes.

Physical examination

Patient's general and local examination is to be done.

Local examination
- *Testes:* Volume and consistency, small and soft testes indicate low or no spermatogenesis.

Undescended testes causes fibrosis of testicular tissue and azoospermia.
- **Epididymis:** Any abnormality. If blocked causes azoospermia.
- **Vas deference:** Presence or absence or any other abnormality like cord-like due to blockage. Absence or block vas deference causes azoospermia.
- **Presence of varicocele:** Causes oligo and asthenospermia.

Investigations
- To exclude diabetes, GTT or glucose challenge test is to be done.
- Hormone such as FSH, LH, testosterone and prolactin are to be assayed.
- Color Doppler USG of external genitalia to diagnose varicocele and presence or absence of accessory glands.
- Transrectal ultrasonogram (TRUS) for better visualization of accessory glands can be done.
- If possible, genetic test is to be done to detect Y chromosomal microdeletion. If deletion present, patients are to be counseled for quick and advanced treatment as any time failure may occur.
- Karyotyping: Abnormal karyotype does not alter treatment, but patient can be counseled before ART that same thing may happen to their male child.

Note: For azoospermia along with above mentioned tests additional tests are to be done:
- *Per epididymal sperm aspiration (PESA):* Aspiration of sperm by syringing from epididymis.

If no sperm found.
- *Testicular sperm aspiration (TESA):* Aspiration of sperm by syringing from testes.

If no sperm found
- *Testicular sperm extraction (TESE):* Incision is given to the testes to extract seminiferous tubules, which minced and observed under microscope to detect spermatozoa. In wet film if no spermatozoa is detected, the tissue is to be sent for histopathology to detect sign of spermatogenesis.

Special Tests for Sperm Function
- *Sperm cervical mucus contact test (SCMCT):* Cervical mucus is tested within 12 hours of coitus under high power microscope to observe sperm binding in the mucus. It is not done now-a-days.
- *Zona free hamster egg penetration test:* It is not done in practical purpose as at this point for both negative and positive result, ART is the treatment.
- *Hypo-osmotic swelling test* (HOST).

> After history taking, physical examination and investigation you found that Mr Rakib has no significant problem except the history of smoking. Her wife's AMH is 1.2.
> What treatment will you offer for them?

- ART intracytoplasmic sperm injection (ICSI) is the treatment of choice
- Smoking should be prohibited.

Why not IUI?
Wife is elderly and her ovarian reserve is poor so quick treatment is needed. Sperm count is too low for IUI. For satisfactory result at least 10 million 50% motile sperm is needed. So that after preparation 5 million 100% motile sperm can be transferred. Here both count and motility are too low for IUI.

RELATED INFORMATION

Causes of Male Infertility
- Abnormal semen parameters
  Discussed in details in page 255
- Coital disorder:
  - Impotence
  - Premature withdrawal.
- Ejaculatory dysfunction:
  - Retrograde ejaculation
  - Premature ejaculation.
- Ductal obstruction:
  - Congenital bilateral absence of vas deference (CBAVD) occurs in cystic fibrosis.
  - Postinfectious obstruction
  - Vasectomy.

- Disorders of accessory glands:
  - Infection
  - Inflammation
  - Absence of seminal vesicles (associated with CBAVD)
  - Antisperm antibodies.

> **Case scenario:** Mr Halim's semen analysis report shows sperm count 10 million/mL, motility 28%, morphology 54% normal. Mr Halim wants some treatment to increase the sperm count. This is his first analysis. His wife is 32 and having no problem.
>
> What treatment do you like to offer them?

A single analysis report is not conclusive. At least two analyses at 4 weeks interval should be considered. If there is any febrile history during first analysis, 8 weeks interval should be given between two tests:

- So Mr Halim's semen analysis will be repeated after 4–8 weeks
- If it remains the same or lower in repeated tests FSH, LH, testosterone and prolactin are to be done to exclude compromised spermatogenesis.

Treatment Options

Options of treatment will be according to test result

Option 1
If FSH and LH increased and testosterone decreased, it indicates compromised spermatogenesis and patient's spermatogenesis may fall to a level of azoospermia at any time
- In that case IUI for 3 cycles is to be done
- If no pregnancy, ART is indicated.

Option 2
If all hormones are normal then after exclusion of all other causes of oligospermia it will be considered as idiopathic.

Idiopathic oligospermia can be treated by:
- Lifestyle changes
- Empiric antibiotics to correct infection of upper genital tract, which cannot be diagnosed by culture and sensitivity (C/S)
- Antioxidants, which help in spermatogenesis and protect from membrane damage
- Repeat analysis after two months of therapy
- If improved, antioxidants should be continued and stimulation is to be given to female partner
- If no improvement, IUI for 3 cycles
- If no pregnancy, ART will be considered.

Note: In about 90% cases there is no specific cause for oligospermia. So in most of the cases after giving some empirical treatment, advanced treatment is to be done. Though spontaneous pregnancy may occur at any time during waiting period. Previously empiric CC 25 mg daily for 3 months (25 days in a month) and letrozole 2.5 mg daily for 3 months were used to nullify estrogenic effect. But they are no more recommended by National Institute for Health and Care Excellence (NICE) guidelines.

> Suppose Mr Halim's hormone report is normal, but color Doppler USG shows bilateral varicocele.
>
> What can be done?

In that case varicocele may responsible for oligoasthenospermia. If there is significant varicocele then varicocelectomy is the treatment of choice.

Varicoceles are enlarged varicose veins that occur in the scrotum. They are not very uncommon and affect 15% of all men and 5% of them become infertile. Overall 40% of men with known infertility have varicocele (ASRM, 2008). Left side is more affected than right side. According to a Cochrane review of 2013, surgical or radiological treatment of varicocele improved semen quality and 14.29% female partners got pregnant (Kroese, 2013).

> **Case scenario:** Mr Khaleque's semen analysis report shows azoospermia. Wife is 22 years and alright.
>
> What do you want to do now?

- If this is first test, it is to be repeated at least one more time and centrifuged semen should be tested at 4 weeks interval. Because after centrifugation if only 1 spermatozoa is found, it will exclude azoospermia.
- If again the same report physical examination is to be done to predict the cause.
- Color Doppler USG of testes is to be done.
- Hormones are to be tested.
  - If FSH and LH high, but testosterone low, it indicates testicular failure or extremely low synthesis of spermatozoa, which cannot come out. It is known as

hypergonadotropic hypogonadism, which causes nonobstructive azoospermia (NOA)
- If FSH, LH and testosterone all low, it indicates hypogonadotropic hypogonadism (NOA).
- If all three hormones are normal, it indicates obstructive azoospermia (OA), where spermatogenesis is normal, but cannot come out due to bilateral obstruction of vas deference or due to congenital bilateral absence of vas deference (CBAVD).
- Karyotyping is to be done.

> Is there any role of hormonal treatment to increase sperm count in azoospermia?

The only indication of hormonal treatment is hypogonadotropic hypogonadism where FSH, LH and testosterone all reduced.

Treatment

- LH 2000 IU thrice in a week till increment of testosterone (8-12 months).
- Once testosterone rises, but no sperm or few sperm.
  - FSH 75 IU thrice in a week till appearance or increment of sperm in semen
  - Continue both LH and FSH in same dose till pregnancy.

Note: No role in normogonadotropic and hypergonadotropic cases.

In these situations use of FSH will drain the money of the patient. Use of testosterone will further reduce spermatogenesis. If FSH and LH are high or normal there is no role of hormonal treatment.

> Suppose on examination, it is found that there is no abnormality in testes. Vas deference seems to be thickened. USG of testes normal. Hormones are normal.
> What is the next action?

This may be a case of obstructive azoospermia:
- PESA is to be done; in obstructive azoospermia usually spermatozoa can be found even plenty
- If found, ICSI is the treatment of choice
- In case of plenty motile spermatozoa, IUI also can be done.

> Suppose after PESA, you found a few motile spermatozoa. He wants correction of block (Vasovasostomy) if possible.
> What will you suggest for him?

The ART is the treatment of choice.
Because sperm count is very low, which itself is an indication for ART.

Following Criteria should be Fulfilled if Someone Wants Surgery

- Where wife is very young with ample of reproductive time at hand. Because after vasovasostomy one should be allowed a reasonable time to get the result.
- In epididymis or behind the block there must be presence of adequate amount of motile spermatozoa for normal pregnancy.

Vasovasostomy is not feasible if:
- Women are elderly where quick treatment is needed
- At any age if OR is poor
- If enough spermatozoa is not found behind the block.

> **Case scenario:** Mr Quasem is azoospermic and on physical examination it is found that testes are smaller in size. FSH is a bit higher and testosterone is a bit lower level.
> What do you want to do?

Most likely this is a case of NOA. Chance of sperm retrieval from PESA is very low or few can be retrieved in some cases.

PESA, TESA and TESE are to be done sequentially. If sperm is found, ICSI is to be done.

> Suppose he is azoospermic and on physical examination it is found that both testes are atrophied. FSH is high-55 IU/L, LH is high-23 IU/L and testosterone is low 50 ng/mL.
> What will you do?

This is a case of testicular failure. So patient is to be counselled that chance of sperm retrieval is nil. Even then a biopsy is needed to declare that this is a case of testicular failure. Option of having bay:
- Donation (use of donor sperm for wife if wants)
- Adoption.

RELATED INFORMATION

Advanced Fertility Treatment

Advanced fertility treatments are:
- Intrauterine insemination
- Assisted reproductive technology.

Intrauterine Insemination

Intrauterine insemination is the method by which a quantity of motile sperm from semen of husband or donor is introduced into the female partner's uterus by means other than sexual intercourse to enhance fertilization.
- When insemination is done from husband's semen then it is called artificial insemination by husband (AIH)
- When insemination is done from donor's semen then it is called artificial insemination by donor (AID)

It is the procedure where sperms are removed from the seminal fluid by processing the semen in the laboratory and they are then injected directly into the uterine cavity.

It is not advisable or in other word it is contraindicated to inject the unprocessed semen into the uterus as it contains prostaglandins and pus cells.

Though IUI is an artificial procedure, it is not called ART as only one gamete, sperm is manipulated here. The procedure where both sperm and ovum are manipulated is called ART.

Indications of IUI
- For male factor:
  - Abnormal semen parameters oligospermia, asthenospermia.
    - Count must be ≥10 million/mL
    - Motility must be 50% or more, because 5 million 100% motile sperm should be retrieved for transfer to get optimum result.
  - Impotence
  - Retrograde ejaculation
  - Antisperm antibody
  - Cryopreserved sperm:
    - Husband preserved for use when he is living abroad
    - Preserved before chemotherapy in malignancy.
- Female factors:
  - Cervical hostility
  - Failure of 6 ovulatory cycles
  - In poor ovarian reserve where quick treatment is indicated: One or two cycles can be done before going to ART.
- Unexplained infertility: Where there is no problem with any partner and received all step-by-step treatment.

Conditions where IUI is not applicable
- Refractory male infertility:
  - *Severe oligospermia:* When count is <10 million/mL
  - *Severe asthenospermia:* When motility is <20
  - OATS.
- Bilateral tubal block or damage: At least one functioning tube must be open.
- High basal FSH or low antimüllerian hormone (AMH) of female partner.

How does it facilitate pregnancy?
- It allows one to by pass the cervix to deposit sperm closer to the tubal ostia, thereby facilitating a large number of motile sperm to reach the fertilization site. In cervical hostility the procedure overcome the barrier.
- Procedure removes the dead and moribund sperms, which generate reactive oxygen species (ROS) that is free oxygen radicals and reduce the functional capacity of intact sperm.
- Procedure removes antisperm antibodies.

Procedure
- The woman is either stimulated and monitored or natural cycle monitored for at least one mature egg
- Selection of appropriate time for insemination
- A semen specimen is produced (after at least 1 day abstinence)
- Semen is processed in the laboratory
- The separated washed highly motile sperm is placed in the uterine cavity using a very thin soft disposable sterile catheter.

Preparation of female partner
- Natural cycle
- Ovulation induction by any drug mentioned before

- Triggering of ovulation by hCG 5,000–10,000 IU when 1–3 mature follicle of ≥18 mm developed (alternatively GnRHa 0.1 mg can be used for triggering)
- Insemination is to be done either when ovulation is imminent or just after, usually 36–40 hours of hCG triggering:
  - If it is done once in a cycle it is better to do between 36 and 40 hours of hCG
  - For two attempts in the same cycle it is done at 24 hours apart within 48 hours of triggering.

Semen Preparation is done by Two Procedures

- *Swim up*
- *Swim down (gradient)*: When semen parameter is very poor then gradient method is suitable.

How many cycles can be done?
There is no specific time frame for this procedure. It should be judged according to couple's reproductive profile.

For patients:
- <35 years maximum 6 cycles or more can be done if couple desire
- 35 and above maximum 4 cycles.

Success
Success rate depends upon:
- Age of the women
- Type of ovarian stimulation
- Cause of infertility
- Number and quality of motile sperm.

  By and large, birth rates per cycle of IUI:
- 15% under the age of 30
- 12% between 30 and 35
- 7–8% between 35 and 39
- <2% over 40
- Cumulative success rate rises up to 60% after 4–6 cycles.

Risk of IUI
- Ovarian hyperstimulation syndrome
- Multiple pregnancy
- Transmission of infection (donor).

Assisted Reproductive Technique

Assisted reproductive technique includes all fertility treatments in which both eggs and sperms are manipulated outside the body. It does not include where only spermatozoa are manipulated such as IUI. It involves surgically removing eggs from a woman's ovary and combining them with sperm in the laboratory or surgically removing sperm from testes of azoospermic man and injection of sperm into the oocyte. Finally returning the resulting embryos to the woman's womb or donating them to another woman. It was first used for infertility in human in 1977 at Bourn Hall in Cambridge, England. As it allows fertilization to occur outside the body in a glass dish, hence the use of Latin words *in vitro* which literally means in glass, hence test tube. Patrick Steptoe and Robert Edwards after their endless trail first announced the birth of Louise Brown in July 1978. Since then millions of babies were born worldwide as a result of ART treatment.

Types of ART
- *In vitro* fertilization and embryo transfer (IVF-ET)
- Gamete intrafallopian transfer (GIFT)
- Zygote intrafallopian transfer (ZIFT)
- Intracytoplasmic sperm injection (ICSI)
- Round spermatid or nucleus injection (ROSNI)
- Partial zona dissection (PZD)
- Subzonal injection (SUZI)
- Zona drilling
- Assisted hatching
- Preimplantation genetic diagnosis (PGD).

Among all IVF, ICSI are widely using and PGD and assisted hatching are practicing in some places now-a-days.

In vitro fertilization and embryo transfer
In vitro fertilization (IVF) is the procedure where sperms are kept with ovum in a dish for fertilization. Usually for one egg 50,000–100,000 motile spermatozoa are needed for fertilization.

Prerequisite for ART:
- One healthy uterus
- Source of sperms
- Source of eggs.

Indications of ART
- Absent fallopian tubes or bilateral tubal block or disease that cannot be treated successfully by surgery
- Endometriosis that has not responded to surgical or medical treatment
- Oligospermia
- Asthenospermia
- Teratospermia
- Oligoasthenoteratospermia
- Azoospermia
- Unexplained infertility that has not responded to other treatment
- Failure of previous all treatment
- Infertility secondary to sperm antibody
- Genetic disease that result in miscarriage or abnormal births
    - Selection of normal embryo by PGD
    - Use of donor egg.

Two common procedures are done IVF and ICSI.

Indications of IVF
All indications of ART except severe male factor infertility such as count <5 million, motility <20%, severe teratospermia, OATS and azoospermia.

Steps of IVF
- Down regulation (pituitary desensitization)
- Ovarian stimulation (super ovulation)
- Oocyte retrieval
- Insemination: Mixing of eggs and sperms after washing and culture in the laboratory
- Transfer of embryos into the womb.

Step 1
Down-regulation: When drug is used to temporarily shut down the function of the pituitary. It is done to prevent LH surge so that ovum can be collected at a desired time.

There are two methods of prevention of LH surge:
1. *GnRHa protocol*: GnRHa is used to inhibit the secretion of LH from pituitary by down regulation. There are four different protocols for GnRHa:
    i. *Long protocol*: GnRHa starts on D2 or D21 of previous cycle. It takes 2–3 weeks for complete desensitization of pituitary. Then the drug is continued along with gonadotropin till the day before hCG.
    ii. *Short protocol*: GnRHa starts on the 1st or 2nd day of cycle. Initially it stimulates the pituitary and serves as an initial stimulation for follicular recruitment. Continues along with gonadotropin and continued till the day of hCG.
    iii. *Ultrashort protocol*: GnRHa used only for 3 days.
    iv. *Stop Lupron protocol*: GnRHa starts on D21 of previous cycle, but stop when stimulation begins.
2. *GnRH antagonist protocol*: Its block the LH receptor. Drug starts on D6 of the cycle (fixed protocol) or when size of the leading follicle becomes 14 mm (flexible protocol) and continues till the day of hCG.

Step II
Ovarian stimulation with monitoring: Drug used are:
- Human menopausal gonadotropin (hMG)
- Recombinant follicle stimulating hormone (rFSH)

    Dose of drug: 150–450 IU depending upon age and OR of the patient. Low OR and more age needs higher dose. It needs 10–12 days to get mature eggs. When at least 3 follicles attain the size of 18 mm ovulation is triggered by hCG 10,000 unit.

Step III
Egg retrieval: After 36 hours of triggering by hCG injection eggs are retrieved by a long needle under deep sedation or GA.

At the end of the retrieval *luteal support* is started and is given by any one of the following:
- Progesterone injection 50 mg daily
- Progesterone vaginal pessary (cyclogest, microgest, gestanon) 300–400 mg daily
- Progesterone gel (crinone gel) 1 tube daily
- Injection hCG 2,000 IU biweekly.

Continued till 12 weeks of pregnancy.

Step IV
Insemination: For 1 egg, 50,000–100,000 sperms are inseminated in the special media in a dish and is kept in the incubator. After 18 hours of incubation, eggs are checked for fertilization. Development of 2 pronucleus (PN) indicates fertilization. On D2 eggs are checked for cleavage or cell division.

On D3 embryos are checked for further development. At this stage 4-8 cells embryo develops. Embryos can be cultured up to D5 for blastocyst development.

Step V
Embryo transfer: Embryos may be transferred at any stage between 2PN to blastocyst stage that is from D1 to D5 of culture. Commonly done on D3 at 8 cells stage **(Fig. 17.2)**. If number of embryos are more then embryos can be cultured up to blastocyst. It is done in an outpatient basis without anesthesia. It takes only a few minutes to perform and patient can go home after hours of rest.

Beta hCG is to be tested 15 days after ET
If test is positive, TVS is to be done after 15 days to diagnose clinical pregnancy.

Intracytoplasmic sperm injection (Fig. 17.3)
Injection of single mature immobilized normal spermatozoa into the cytoplasm of a mature metaphase II oocyte is known as ICSI. In 1991, Palermo et al. first got pregnancy after injection of spermatozoa into the oocyte. Before 1992 severe oligospermic and azoospermic men remained infertile (Palermo et al. 1992). ICSI made possible to treat the whole spectrum of male infertility including OA and NOA.

Indications of ICSI
- After failed previous trials of IVF
- Severe oligospermia: When count is <5 million/mL
- Severe asthenospermia: When motility is <20%
- Severe teratospermia
- Oligoasthenoterato spermia
- ICSI after failed IVF ('rescue' ICSI)
- Azoospermia: OA and NOA
  - Congenital bilateral absence of vas deferens
  - Acquired epididymal or vasal obstruction
- Necrospermia
- Immunologic infertility
- Failed vasectomy reversal
- Abnormal sperm function
- Retrograde ejaculation
- Preimplantation genetic diagnosis.

Steps of ICSI
Same as IVF except insemination. Here instead of keeping the sperms with eggs, one sperm is injected into one egg. In azoospermia, sperms are retrieved by PESA/TESA or TESE.

Results and Safety

Successfulness depends on the female partner's age and cause of infertility. More the age of the patient, less chance of success. The effect of age appears to be due to
- Reduced response to the drugs
- A smaller chance of embryo implanting
- Higher rate of miscarriage.

According to the most recent statistics from the US Centers for Disease Control (CDC), the pregnancy rate after fresh and frozen embryo transfer in different age group are shown in **Table 17.3**.

Treatment of suitable patients gives a pregnancy rate of about 34% per cycle and a

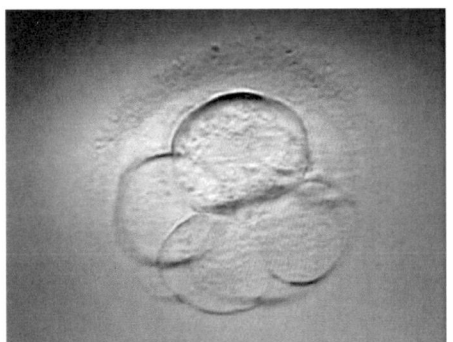

Fig. 17.2 Eight cell grade 1 embryo

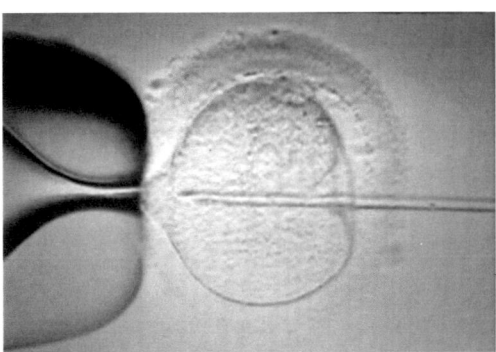

Fig. 17.3 Intracytoplasmic sperm injection

Table 17.3 Pregnancy rate after fresh and frozen embryo transfer (ET) in different age group

Age (Years)	<35	35–37	38–40	41–42	43–44	>44
Percentage of pregnancy after fresh ET	35.6	27.3	17.3	9.4	4.5	1.9
Percentage of pregnancy after frozen ET	30.8	27.9	23.1	18.3	12.5	12

cumulative pregnancy rate approaching 90% (Wright, 2007). The spontaneous abortion rate is 19–22%, which is somewhat higher than for the fertile population (Wood, 1982). There is no increase in the incidence of congenital malformation. The risk of congenital malformation in pregnancies achieved after IVF pregnancies is no higher than in the normal population. One study reported the incidence of anomalies 8.6% in ICSI babies, 9% in IVF babies and 4.2% in babies conceived naturally (Victor, 2005). As majority women come for ART at their late age so age-related anomaly may occur in older age group of patients.

Complications of ART
- Ovarian hyperstimulation syndrome
- Injury to bladder, ureter and internal iliac vessels (rare)
- Multiple pregnancy.

Ovarian hyperstimulation syndrome
Ovarian hyperstimulation syndrome is a rare complication of controlled ovarian hyperstimulation. The incidence is 0.1–6.1% of all controlled ovarian hyperstimulation cycles and severe form is found about 0.4% of cases (AMacLyons et al. 1994).

Risk factors for OHSS
- Young age (<35 years)
- Low BMI
- PCOS
- AMH ->3.36 ng/ml
- High dose of FSH
- Previous OHSS
- Absolute increase or progressively increasing serum E2 (>4,000 pg/mL)
- Multiple follicles (>35)
- Necklace sign
- Pregnancy
- hCG luteal supplementation
- GnRHa protocol.

Types
- Mild
- Moderate
- Severe.

Complications and Fate of OHSS
- Ascites
- Hemoconcentration
- Coagulation disorder
- Renal failure
- Hepatic failure
- Acute respiratory distress syndrome
- Death.

Basic pathology
Increased vascular endothelial growth factors (VEGF) and vasoactive amines triggered by hCG causes increased capillary permeability and fluid shift in extravascular space. As a result there is loss of intravascular albumin and fluid causes ascites and hemoconcentration.

Diagnosis
Symptoms
- Usually history of taking OI drug
- Fullness of abdomen
- Shortness of breath in severe cases.

Investigations
- USG to diagnose ascites and size of the ovaries
- CBC: HB%, WBC count, RBC count and PCV all are increased due to hemoconcentration.

Management
Depends on severity of the disease.
A. *Mild cases*: Outpatient management:
   - Bed rest
   - Plenty of liquid intake
   - Antiemetic/Analgesic.

   Monitoring
   - Clinical symptoms
   - Complete blood count
   - Body weight

- Abdominal girth
- Fluid balance: Strict intake output chart

No improvement: Hospitalization.

B. *Moderate and severe cases*: Hospitalization.

General management:
- Bedrest
- Plenty of liquid intake
- Antiemetic/Analgesic.

Specific management:
- Severe intravascular volume depletion and hemoconcentration indicated by hematocrit and CBC:
  - Parenteral fluid
  - Albumin
  - Heparin if PCV > 40.
- Tense ascites: Paracentesis 1,500–2,000 mL at a time
- Severe complications: ICU management
  - Impaired renal function: Dopamine
  - Thromboembolic phenomenon: Heparin
  - ARDS: Respiratory support
  - In uncontrolled cases, termination of pregnancy may needed
- Other complications like torsion and rupture of the ovaries: Conservative surgery.

Monitoring
- All those are mentioned in mild cases
- Electrolyte
- Total protein/albumin
- Clotting parameters
- Kidney function test
- Liver function test.

Prevention
- Selection of appropriate dose of FSH
- Reduction of dose of FSH
- GnRH antagonist protocol
- Coasting
- Introduction of albumin during OPU
- Reduction of dose of hCG
- Cabergoline
- Cancellation of cycle
- Deferment of ET and cryopreservation of embryos.

BIBLIOGRAPHY

Abdel-Gadir A, Khatim MS, Alnaser HMI, Mowafi RS, Shaw RW. Ovarian electrocautery: responders versus nonresponders. Gynaecol Endocrinol. 1993;7:43-8.

Adams J, Polson DW, Franks S. Prevalence of polycystic ovaries in women with anovulation and idiopathic hirsutism. Br Med J (Clin Res Ed). 1986;293(6543): 355–9.

AMacLyons CA, Wheeler CA, Frishman GN et al. Early and late presentation of the ovarian hyperstimulation syndrome: Two distinct entities with different risk factors. Hum Reprod. 1994;9:792-99.

Amer SA, Gopalan V, Li TC, Ledger WL, Cooke ID. Long term follow-up of patients with polycystic ovarian syndrome after laparoscopic ovarian drilling: Clinical outcome. Hum Reprod. 2002;17:2035-42.

Bailey CJ, Turner R. Metformin. N Eng J Med. 1996; 334(9):574-9.

Begum MR, Akhter S, Ehsan M, et al. Pretreatment and co-administration of oral anti-diabetic agent with clomiphene citrate or rFSH for ovulation induction in clomiphene-citrate-resistant polycystic ovary syndrome. J Obstet Gynaecol Res. 2013;39(5):966-73.

Begum MR, Khanam NN, Quadir E, et al. Prevention of gestational diabetes mellitus by continuing metformin therapy throughout pregnancy in women with polycystic ovary syndrome. J Obstet Gynaecol Res. 2009;35(2):282-6.

Buttram VC, Vaquero C. Post-ovarian wedge resection adhesive disease. Fertil Steril 1975;26;874.

Cho Lw, Jayagopal V, Kilpatric ES. The biological variation of C-reactive protein in polycystic ovarian syndrome. Clin Chem. 2005;51:1905-7.

Comhaire F, Vermeulen L. Human semen analysis. Hum Reprod Update. 1995;1(4):343-62.

ESHRE early pregnancy guideline development group. Guideline of the European Society of Human Reproduction and Embryology for Recurrent Pregnancy Loss; 2017.

Farquhar CM, Williamson K, Brown PM, Garland J. An economic evaluation of laparoscopic ovarian diathermy versus gonadotrophin therapy for women with clomiphene citrate resistant polycystic ovary syndrome. Hum Reprod. 2004;19:1110-5.

Franks S, Kiddy D, Sharp P, et al. Obesity and polycystic ovarian syndrome. Ann N Y Acad Sci.1991;626:201-6.

Glueck CJ, Phillips H, Cameron D, et al. Continuing metformin throughout pregnancy in women with polycystic ovary syndrome appears to safely reduce first-trimester spontaneous abortion: a pilot study. Fertil Steril. 2001;75(1):46-52.

Glueck CJ, Wang P, Kobayashi S, et al. Metformin therapy throughout pregnancy reduces the development of gestational diabetes in women with polycystic ovary syndrome. Fertil Steril. 2002;77(3):520-5.

Gysler M, March CM, Mishell DR, et al. A decade's experience with an individualized clomiphene treatment regimen including its effects on the postcoital test. Fertil Steril. 1982;37(2):161-7.

Heard MJ, Pierce A, Carson SA, et al. Pregnancies following use of metformin for ovulation induction in patients with polycystic ovary syndrome. Fertil Steril. 2002;77(4):669-73.

Heasley RN, Boyle DD, Thompson W. LHRH analogue therapy in infertile women with luteal phase defects. Clinical Reproduction and Fertility. 1987;5(3): 133-7.

Homburg R, Howles CM. Low-dose FSH therapy for anovulatory infertility associated with polycystic ovary syndrome: rationale, results, reflections and refinements. Hum Reprod Update. 1999;5(5): 493-9.

Hughes E, Collins J, Vandekerckhove P. Clomiphene citrate for ovulation induction in women with oligomenorrhoea. Cochrane Database Syst Rev. 2000;2: CD 000056.

Jensen A, Sharif H, Frederiksen K, et al. Use of fertility drugs and risk of ovarian cancer: Danish Population Based Cohort Study. BMJ. 2009;338:b249.

Keckstein J, Tuttlies F, Steiner R. Lasereffekt am Ovar: CO2 versus Nd:YAG versus argon. In: Proceedings of the 4th Jahrestagung der Deutschen Gesellschaft für Lasermedizin, Ulm, Germany, September 1989, 84-88

Kerin JF, Kirby C, Morris D, et al. Incidence of luteinized unruptured follicle phenomenon in cycling women. Fertil Steril. 1983;40(5):620-6.

Kocak M, Caliskan E, Simsir C, Haberal A. Metformin therapy improves ovulatory rates, cervical scores, and pregnancy rates in clomiphene citrate resistant women with polycystic ovary syndrome. Fertil Steril. 2002;77:101-6.

Kousta E, White DM, Franks S. Modern use of clomiphene citrate in induction of ovulation. Hum Reprod Update. 1997;3(4):359-65.

Kriplani A, Manchanda R, Agarwal N, Nayar B. Laparoscopic ovarian drilling in clomiphene citrate-resistant women with polycystic ovary syndrome. J Am Assoc Gynecol Laparosc. 2001;8:511-8.

Kroese AC, de Lange NM, Collins JA, et al. "Varicocele surgery, new evidence". Human Reproduction Update. 2013;19(4):317.

Kurta ML, Moysich KB, Weissfeld JL, et al. Use of fertility drugs and risk of ovarian cancer: results from a US-based case-control study. Cancer Epidemiol Biomarkers Prev. 2012;21(8):1282-92.

Li TC, Saravelos H, Chow MS, Chisabingo R, Cooke ID. Factors affecting the outcome of laparoscopic ovarian drilling for polycystic ovarian syndrome in women with anovulatory infertility. Br J Obstet Gynaecol. 1998;105:338-44.

Lyons CA, Wheeler CA, Frishman GN, et al. Early and late presentation of the ovarian hyperstimulation syndrome: two distinct entities with different risk factors. Hum Reprod. 1994;9(5):792-9.

Magyar DM, Boyers SP, Marshall JR, et al. Regular menstrual cycle and premenstrual molimina as indicators of ovulation. Obstet Gynecol. 1979; 53(4):411.

Mitwally MFM, Casper RF. Use of an AI for induction of ovulation in patients with an inadequate response to clomiphene citrate. Fertil Steril. 2000;75: 305-9.

Mitwally MF, Casper RF. Use of an aromatase inhibitor for induction of ovulation in patients with an inadequate response to clomiphene citrate. Fertil Steril. 2001;75(2):305-9.

Moghetti P, Castello R, Negri C, et al. Metformin effects on clinical features, endocrine and metabolic profiles and insulin sensitivity in polycystic ovary syndrome: a randomized double-blind, placebo-controlled 6-month trial, followed by open long-term clinical evaluation. J Clin Endocrinol Metab. 2000;85(1): 139-46.

Nestler JE, Jakubowicz DJ. Decreases in ovarian cytochrome P450c 17 alpha activity and serum free testosterone after reduction of insulin secretion in polycystic ovary syndrome. N Engl J Med. 1996;335(9):617-23.

Nestler JE, Stovall D, Akhter N, et al. Strategies for the use of insulin-sensitizing drugs to treat infertility in women with polycystic ovary syndrome. Fertil Steril. 2002;77(2):209-15.

Palermo G, Joris H, Devroey P, et al. Pregnancies after intracytoplasmic injection of a single spermatozon into an oocyte. Lancet. 1992;340(8810):17-8.

Patance G, Piro S, Rabuazzo AM, et al. Metformin restores insulin secretion altered by chronic exposure to free fatty acids or high glucose: a direct metformin effect on pancreatic beta-cells. Diabetes. 2000;49(5):735.

Rosenberg SM, Luciano AA, Riddick DH. The luteal phase defect: the relative frequency of and encouraging response to, treatment with vaginal progesterone. Fertil Steril. 1980;34(1):17.

Rossing MA, Daling JR, Weiss NS, et al. Ovarian tumors in a cohort of infertile women. N Eng J Med. 1994;331(12):771-6.

Sammour A, Biljan MM, Tan SL, et al. Prospective randomized trial comparing the effects of letrozole and clomiphene citrate (CC) on follicular development endometrial thickness and pregnancy rate in patients undergoing superovulation prior to intrauterine insemination (IUI). Fertil Steril. 2001;76:S110.

Shepard MK, Balmaceda JP, Leija CG. Relationship of weight to successful induction of ovulation with clomiphene citrate. Fertil Steril. 1979;32(6): 641-5.

The Practice Committee of the American Society for Reproductive Medicine. Report on varicocele and infertility. Fertil Steril. 2008; Vol 90(Issue 5): S247-S249.

Toda T. [Ultrasonographical study on luteinized unruptured follicle]. Nippon Sanka Fujinka Gakkai, Zasshi. 1990;42(9):195-202.

Victor YH Tu. Are there risks in the long term outcome of children born following Assisted Reproductive Technology? J. Arab Neonatal Forum. 2005;2:1-4.

Wilcox AJ, Weinberg CR, O'Connor JF, et al. Incidence of early loss of pregnancy. N Engl J Med. 1988;319(4):189.

Witten BJ, Martin SA. The endometrial biopsy as a guide to the management of luteal phase defect. Fertil Steril. 1985;44(4):460.

Wood C, Trounson A, Leeto JF, et al. Clinical features of eight pregnancies resulting from in vitro fertilization and embryo transfer. Fertil Steril. 1982;38(1):22.

Wright VC, Chang J, Jeng G, et al. Assisted reproductive technology surveillance-United States, 2004. MMWR Surveill Summ. 2007;56(6):1-22.

Wu CH, Winkel CA. The effect of therapy initiation day on clomiphene citrate therapy. Fertil Steril. 1989;52(4):564-8.

Yu V. Are there risks in the long term outcome of children born following assisted reproductive technology? J Arab Neonatal Forum. 2005;2:1-4.

CHAPTER 18

Abnormal Uterine Bleeding

Saria Tasnim, Rashida Begum

INTRODUCTION

Abnormal uterine bleeding (AUB) is defined as any bleeding from the uterus, which is not normal cyclical menstruation. Abnormal uterine bleeding is one of the most common problems encountered by obstetrician and gynecologist (Bayer, 1993). In the United Kingdom, 5% women of reproductive age seek help for this symptom annually (Vessey, 1992). By the end of reproductive life, the risk of hysterectomy (primarily for menstrual disorders) is 20% (Coulter, 1988). AUB is more common at extremes of reproductive years that is in the postmenarche and premenopausal period.

Population studies have shown that excessive menstrual loss is present in 10% of the population (Hallberg, 1996). However, nearly one third of all women consider their menstruation to be excessive (MORI, 1990). This symptom thus creates a significant workload for health services. In most hospitals dysfunctional uterine bleeding (DUB), one of the cause of AUB is common among top ten diseases in gynecology department.

> **Case scenario:** Mrs Faria, 32-year-old lady complaints of excessive menstrual bleeding for 6 months. Initially she ignored it and expected spontaneous correction. But for last 6 months bleeding took place in same pattern. Now she is feeling weak. With these complaints, she has come to you.
> How will you proceed to diagnosis?

Detailed history is to be taken first followed by physical examination.

History

Information gathered from history should include:

Menstrual history
- Age of menarche
- Amount of flow, number of pads soaked a day, passage of clots, soaking of clothes and bedding
- Length of cycle: Whether it is with regular interval or not
- Duration of bleeding
- Whether there is any intermenstrual bleeding
- Pain during menstruation
- Last menstrual period (LMP).

Associated complaints
- Contact bleeding
- Change in general health, e.g. weight gain polycystic ovary syndrome (PCOS), hypothyroidism.
- Feeling of heaviness or lump in lower abdomen
- Weight loss: Anorexia, excessive exercise, stress
- Family history to rule out any familial disease like diabetes mellitus (DM)
- Any bleeding disorder
- Sexual history: Pregnancy and sexually transmitted infection (STI)
- Drug history: Irregular hormone intake can lead to abnormal uterine bleeding (AUB)
- Any drug, which causes rapid metabolism of steroid hormones and decreasing their bioavailability leading to AUB, e.g. Antiseizure drugs [Somen, 2011].

Physical Examination

General examination
- Height and weight to estimate body built
- Sign of hyperandrogenism such as acne or hirsutism

- Acanthosis nigrican in neck is a marker of insulin resistance
- Thyroid gland
- Breast examination: Nipple discharge may be present in hyperprolactinemia
- Hirsutism.

Perabdomen examination
- Presence of any abdominal mass/lump
- If any lump present its size, consistency, surface regularity, mobility and tenderness are to be assessed
- In case of enlarged uterus, whether it is symmetrically enlarged or not.

Pervaginal examination
- Evaluation of external genitalia including urethra and clitoris
- Per speculum examination to inspect the cervix and vagina to be sure that bleeding is not from cervix or vagina
- Bimanual examination to assess size and mobility of the uterus, and condition of fornices.

Per-rectal examination to exclude any abnormality.

RELATED INFORMATION

Mechanism of Abnormal Uterine Bleeding

Abnormal uterine bleeding (AUB) is common in extremes of reproductive life, more commonly associated with anovulatory cycles. The typical menstrual cycle has two phases 'proliferative and secretory'. The proliferative phase is characterized by a predominance of estrogen over progesterone and a buildup of endometrium. The secretory phase begins after ovulation triggers progesterone production. This phase is marked by a reaction to the combination of estrogen and progesterone and stabilization in the thickness of the endometrium (Malhotra, 2008).

Menstrual bleeding occurs after secretion of estrogen and progesterone tapers off. Early during menses, thrombin plugs restrain blood loss, but later, vasoconstriction of the spiral arterioles is responsible for hemostasis. When ovulation does not take place, progesterone levels do not rise; therefore, typical cyclic withdrawal of estrogen and progesterone cannot occur (Malhotra, 2008).

Normally, menstrual bleeding occurs 21–35 days interval and persists for 2–7 days amounting 5–80 mL in each cycle. Deviation of anyone of these parameters such as length of cycle, duration and amount of bleeding referred as abnormal uterine bleeding. These may be in the following pattern:

- *Menorrhagia:* Cyclical bleeding at normal interval, excessive in amount or duration or both or menstrual blood loss of more than 80 mL per cycle. It is generally caused by conditions affecting the uterus and its vascular apparatus. This term is now recommended to be replaced by heavy menstrual bleeding (HMB).
- *Polymenorrhea:* Cyclical bleeding, normal amount, but occur at too frequent interval (< 22 days) and usually result from functional disturbance of ovary.
- *Hypomenorrhea:* Bleeding last 2 days or less and unusually light menstrual flow.
- *Polymenorrhagia*: Cyclical bleeding, which is both excessive and frequent.
- *Metrorrhagia:* Bleeding of any amount, which is acyclical and occur irregularly or continuously and usually feature of abnormal pregnancy state such as abortion and local lesion such as cervical or myomatous polyp and cervical or endometrial cancer.
- *Oligomenorrhea:* Cycle occur longer than 35 days apart.
- *Dysfunctional uterine bleeding:* It is a subset of AUB and is defined as excessive, prolonged or unpatterned bleeding from the endometrium without an organic cause and is frequently used synonymously with anovulatory bleeding (Jeffcoate, 2008).

Causes of Abnormal Uterine Bleeding

The International Federation of Gynecology and Obstetrics (FIGO) has suggested a common classification of the causes of AUB in nongravid women of reproductive age. The proposed classification have nine main categories, which are arranged according to the acronym PALM-COEIN (**Box 18.1**). These are abnormal uterine bleeding associated with the use of exogenous gonadal

Box 18.1 Causes of abnormal uterine bleeding	
• Polyp	• Coagulopathy
• Adenomyosis	• Ovulatory dysfunction
• Leiomyoma	• Endometrial
• Malignancy and hyperplasia	• Iatrogenic
	• Not yet classified

Adopted from FIGO Classification system (PALM-COEIN) for causes of abnormal uterine bleeding in nongravid woman of reproductive age [Munro MG et al. 2011]

steroids, intrauterine systems or devices or other systemic or local agents is classified as 'iatrogenic'.

Generally along with FIGO proposed causes, following are responsible for AUB:
- Besides coagulopathy obesity, thyroid problems and liver disease, renal disease can contribute to abnormal bleeding. In liver disease and renal disease estrogen cannot detoxified and excreted causes irregular uterine bleeding.
- Besides exogenous gonadal steroids and intrauterine devices (IUDs) many other medications including over the counter drugs and herbal remedies, hormones, antipsychotic drugs and anticoagulants can cause abnormal bleeding.
- Developmental defect of the uterus such as uterine didelphys and bicornuate uterus can cause menorrhagia.
- Pregnancy state
- Infections such as pelvic peritonitis, salpingo-oophoritis and cellulitis tend to cause AUB.
- Chronic symmetrical enlargement of the uterus.
- Psychological upsets by influencing hypothalamus and autonomic nervous system, which controls the blood vessels of pelvic organs.
- Active or passive congestion of pelvis causes hypertrophy of the myometrium and endometrium, so that uterus can enlarge from two to six times the normal size.

According to this nomenclature, it is recommended that the term DUB should be abandoned (Fraser, 2007). In general, the components of the PALM group are discrete (structural) entities that can be measured visually with imaging techniques and/or histopathology, whereas the COEIN group is related to entities that are not defined by imaging or histopathology (nonstructural).

> On further enquiry, it is elicited that her cycle is regular 30 days, duration is 8–10 days and passes clotted blood. She has to change 10–12 pads daily in full soaked stage. Bleeding is painless. She did not take any drug for this complaint. She has an average body build, clinically anemic, normotensive. Breast development normal, no hirsutism present. On per-abdominal examination nothing abnormality detected. On pervaginal examination vulva vagina are normal, cervix is healthy, uterus is normal in size, mobile and symmetrical. Fornices are free and nontender.
>
> On the basis of above findings what is your probable diagnosis?

Chronic abnormal uterine bleeding.

> How will you diagnose the cause of excessive bleeding in this case?

Initially, following investigations are needed for this patient:
- Complete blood count
- Thyroid function test
- Coagulation screen especially for von Willebrand disease
- Transvaginal sonography (TVS)
- Cytology (Pap smear).

> Patient's hemoglobin (HB) is 8 g%. TVS shows normal uterus and ovaries. Endometrial thickness is 2.5 mm in menstrual phase. Cavity is free. Pap report is normal. Thyroid function test and coagulation screening is normal.
>
> Do you need to do further investigations to detect structural causes?

As TVS shows normal uterine cavity with thin endometrium so no further test is needed for this patient.

> To identify the cause of AUB, what other tests are done?

- Sonohysterography
- Hysterosalpingography
- Magnetic resonance imaging (MRI)
- Hysteroscopy
- Endometrial sampling for histopathology
- Pregnancy test.

RELATED INFORMATION

The purpose of investigation is to:
- Assess morbidity associated with increased blood loss
- Exclude major intrauterine disease
- Assess coexistent disorders.

Women with AUB may have multiple identifiable factors that may contribute to the genesis of the abnormal bleeding. Consequently, the investigation of women with AUB must be undertaken as diligent and comprehensive fashion as much as practicable in a given clinical situation and the available resources. One has to judge the appropriateness of the investigations considering the advantage and limitation.

Transvaginal Sonography

Transvaginal sonography can exclude pelvic masses and pregnancy complications. TVS is more informative than transabdominal sonography for measurement of the endometrial thickness. TVS measures endometrial thickness, and diagnose polyps and leiomyoma with a sensitivity of 80% and specificity of 90% (Vercellini et al. 1977). Endometrial thickness more than 12 mm in early follicular phase is indicative of hyperplasia. TVS is the preferred procedure of endometrial assessment before going to more invasive one.

Endometrial Sampling

Sampling techniques using small, flexible, disposable devices are adequate for obtaining endometrial tissue. To ensure accuracy, the procedure must be done before any hormonal treatment is given, and multiple areas of the endometrium must be sampled.

Methods

As an outpatient procedure, without general anesthesia. Most common methods of endometrial sampling are:
- Aspiration curettage (Pipelle, Vabra aspirator).
- Dilatation and curettage.
- Hysteroscopy.

The purpose of endometrial sampling is to exclude endometrial hyperplasia and carcinoma.

Indications

Endometrial sampling is recommended:
- In women aged more than 40 years with abnormal bleeding.
- Young patient with abnormal bleeding with risk factors for endometrial carcinoma such as obesity, DM, chronic anovulation and infertility, family history of endometrial and colonic cancer and tamoxifen therapy.
- In younger women, if abnormal bleeding does not resolve with medical treatment.

If endometrial thickness on TVS is more than 12 mm, then endometrial sample should be taken to exclude endometrial hyperplasia (grade A). Failure to obtain sufficient sample for histopathology does not require further investigation, unless the endometrial thickness is more than 12 mm (grade B).

Hysteroscopy

Hysteroscopy is the gold standard for evaluation of endometrial cavity. It provides direct visualization of the cavity. It can be used for both diagnostic and operative purposes for directed biopsies and excision of polyps (Malhotra, 2008).

Aim

- Excellent view of the uterine cavity and diagnosis of polyps, submucous fibroid and hyperplasia.
- Biopsy of the suspected areas.
- Treatment.

Indications

Mandatory after 40 years with AUB:
- Erratic menstrual bleeding.
- Failed medical treatment.
- The TVS suggestive of intrauterine pathology, e.g. polyp, fibroid.

Disadvantages

- Cost of the apparatus.
- Lack of availability or experience.

Saline Infusion Sonography

Saline infusion sonography involves direct extension of uterine cavity with saline to enhance visualization of the endometrial surface. It is a noninvasive method to diagnose endometrial polyp and submucous myoma. Saline sonography is an alternative to office hysteroscopy in selected cases.

Magnetic Resonance Imaging

May be used to distinguish between leiomyoma and adenomyosis, and also for measuring the myometrial extent of submucosal myoma. However, reliance on MRI is not practical because of cost and inaccessibility (Munro, 2010).

Dilatation and Curettage

Dilatation and curettage is primarily diagnostic, it sometimes appear to be curative but is extremely rare to be necessary for adolescents and young women.

> What might be the cause of bleeding in case of Mrs Faria?

Probable cause is endometrial, might be due to defective hemostasis.

RELATED INFORMATION

Chronic AUB is defined as bleeding form the uterine corpus that is abnormal in volume, regularity and/or timing, and has been present for the majority of the past 6 months.

Acute AUB is defined as an episode of heavy bleeding that in the opinion of the clinician, is of sufficient quantity to require immediate intervention to prevent further blood loss (DeVore, 1982; Munro, 2006).

Intermenstrual bleeding (IMB) occurs between clearly defined cyclic and predictable menses. Such bleeding may occur at random times or may manifest in predictable fashion at the same day in each cycle. This designation is designed to replace the word 'metrorrhagia,' which was one of the terms that the group recommended should be abandoned (Munro, 2011).

When AUB occurs in cyclic menstrual bleeding, typical of ovulatory cycles and particularly when no other definable causes are identified the mechanism is probably a primary disorder of the endometrium. There may be a primary disorder of mechanisms regulating local endometrial hemostasis itself. Principal local factors implicated in the pathogenesis of menorrhagia are prostaglandins (PGs) and components of the endometrial fibrinolytic system. The (PGs) produced are $PGF2_\alpha$ (vasoconstrictor and weak platelet aggregator), PGE2 (vasodilator and weak platelet antiaggregator), thromboxane (TXA2) (potential vasoconstrictor and platelet aggregator) and prostocyclin (PGI2) (a vasodilator). In abnormal bleeding, the normal balance is disturbed and a shift in endometrial conversion of endoperoxides from the vasoconstrictor $PGF2_\alpha$ to vasodilator PGE2 take place.

It has also been found that there is an increased fibrinolytic activity in abnormal bleeding (Dockeray, 1987). There is accelerated lysis of endometrial clots because of excessive production of plasminogen activator. Other endometrially derived factor such as cytokines, growth factors and endothelins might have some role in the pathogenesis of abnormal bleeding (Cameron, 1995).

In other places of ovulatory menorrhagia, there may be prolonged bleeding without excessive loss. Endometrial development is poor due to poor development of corpus luteum. So endometrium does not get adequate hormonal support and breakthrough type of bleeding occurs many days before actual flow. Again due to incomplete or slow degeneration of corpus luteum bleeding may prolong for several days after the proper flow.

> How will you treat this patient?

Aim

Aim of the treatment is to:
- Correct anemia
- Minimize the blood loss during menstruation
- Restore endometrial function
  - To correct anemia oral iron supplement is to be given
  - Minimize blood loss first choice for this patient, is medical treatment.

Nonhormonal

As this patient's cycle is regular 30 days, her bleeding is ovular type. Most probable cause of bleeding is altered activities of PGs or increased activities of fibrinolysis. So, first line of treatment for this patient is nonhormonal such as:
- *Prostaglandin synthetase inhibitor:* Mefenamic acid 500 mg bd or tds
  Or
- *Antifibrinolytics:* Tranexamic acid 500 mg qds.

Hormonal

- If bleeding is not controlled by nonhormonal agents hormone is to be added.
  - *Oral contraceptive pill (OCP):* It can be given cyclically for 3 months
    Or
  - *Progesterone:* Medroxyprogesterone 10 mg bd or norethisterone 5 mg tds for 21 days from 5 to 25 days of the cycle or medroxy progesterone 10 mg daily from 14 to 27 days of the cycle for three cycles.
- If medical treatment fails that is after completion of hormonal treatment same complaints recurs in subsequent cycles *surgical treatment* is to be offered. Dilatation and curettage is the choice of surgery for this young patient.
- If same complaint recurs after dilatation and curettage then aggressive surgery is to be needed. As patient's family is complete following surgeries can be done:
  - Endometrial ablation if patient wants to conserve the uterus.
  - Hysterectomy if patient is not willing to conserve the uterus.

Note: For thin endometrium OCP or estrogen and for thick endometrium progesterone are effective drug.

RELATED INFORMATION

Below 20 years, the disturbance is most likely to be functional one with a tendency to spontaneous cure. For other patients one can decide the treatment option according to **Flowchart 18.1**. Usual treatment available are the followings:
- General
  - Menstrual calendar.
  - Treatment of iron deficiency anemia.

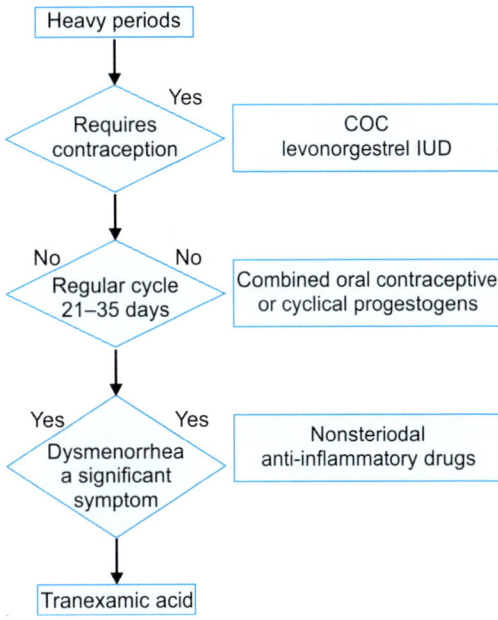

Flowchart 18.1 Algorithm for treatment of AUB

(COC: combined oral contraceptive; IUD: intrauterine device)

- Medical:
  A. *Hormonal:*
     i. Progestogens.
        a. Intrauterine progestogens.
           - Levonorgesterole intrauterine system (Mirena)
           - Progesterone IUS (Progestasert).
        b. Norethisterone.
           - Medroxyprogesterone acetate.
           - Dydrogesterone.
     ii. Estrogen.
     iii. Combined estrogen progesterone (OCP).
     iv. Danazol.
     v. Gonadotropin-releasing hormone agonist (GnRHa).
     vi. Gestrinone.
     vii. Antiprogesterone (RU 486).
  B. *Nonhormonal:*
     i. Prostaglandin synthetase inhibitors (PSI):
        a. *Mefanamic acid*

         b. *Naproxen*
         c. *Ibuprofen*
         d. *Diclofenac.*
   ii. Antifibrinolytics:
         a. *Tranexamic acid*
         b. *Epsilon-aminocaproic acid.*
   iii. Ethamsylate.

Action of Different Drugs in Abnormal Uterine Bleeding

Prostaglandin Synthetase Inhibitor

Mechanism of action: The endometrium is a rich source of PGE2 and PGF2α and its concentrations are greater in menorrhagia. PSI decreases endometrial PG concentrations and reduces endometrial shedding, as a result reduces bleeding.

Dose: Among NSAIDs, mefenamic acid 500 mg three times a day, or Ibuprofen 400 mg three times a day or naproxen 275 every 6 hours has been used most frequently (Munro, 2006; Munro, 2010).

Effect: Nonsteroidal anti-inflammatory drugs reduce menstrual blood loss by 20–50% in about 75% of women.

Side effects: Nausea, vomiting, gastric discomfort, diarrhea and dizziness. Rarely, hemolytic anemia, thrombocytopenia. The degree of reduction of menstrual blood loss (MBL) is not as great as it is with tranexamic acid, but PSI have a lower side effect profile.

Antifibrinolytics

Mechanism of action: The endometrium possess an active fibrinolytic system and the fibrinolytic activity is higher in menorrhagia. Tranexamic acid exerts its antifibrinolytic activity by blocking lysine binding sites on plasminogen and thus prevents fibrin degradation.

Dose: Tranexamic acid 2–4.5 mg/day for 4–7 days.

Effect: Tranexamic acid causes reduction of blood loss of about 50%. Greater reduction of menstrual bleeding than PSI. Tranexamic acid is effective in treating menorrhagia associated with intrauterine contraceptive device (IUCD).

Side effects: Nausea, vomiting, diarrhea and dizziness. Rarely transient color vision disturbance, intracranial thrombosis. But, no evidence that tranexamic acid increases the risk in absence of past or family history of thrombophilia.

Etamsylate

Mechanism of action: Maintain capillary integrity, anti-hyalurunidase activity and inhibitory effect on PG. Cause 20% reduction in MBL.

Dose: 500 mg qid, starting 5 days before anticipated onset of the cycle and continued for 10 days.

Side effects: Headache, rash, nausea.

Progestogens

Norethisterone and medroxyprogesterone acetate commonly used. Norethisterone reduce MBL by 20%.

Mechanism of action: In *ovulatory DUB*, it corrects the luteal phase defect of endometrium in ovulatory cycles, which occurs due to underdeveloped corpus luteum. As a result regular shedding of endometrium takes place.

Progestogens are not effective, if given at low dose for short duration (5–10 days) in the luteal phase. Effective, if norethisterone is given at higher dose (5 mg tds from day 5 to 25).

In anovulatory DUB: It brings the secretory changes in the estrogen primed proliferative endometrium. After withdrawal of drug estrogen progesterone withdrawal bleeding takes place as regular fashion.

Side effects: Weight gain, nausea, bloating, edema, headache, acne, depression, exacerbation of epilepsy and migraine, loss of libido.

Intrauterine Progestogens

Levonorgestrel intrauterine system: The levonorgestrel releasing intrauterine system (e.g. Mirena, projestasert) also have a rational basis for their use. This system consist of a T-shaped intrauterine device sheathed with a reservior of levonorgestrel that is released at the rate of 20 μg daily for 5 years (Prentice, 1999). It exerts effect by preventing endometrial proliferation and consequently reduce both duration of bleeding and amount of menstrual loss.

Effects
- Comparable to endometrial resection for management of DUB.
- Superior to PSI and antifibrinolytics.
- May be an alternative to hysterectomy in some patients.

Side effects
- Break through bleeding in the first cycles.
- In 20% cases, amenorrhea develop within 1 year.
- Functional ovarian cysts.

Special indications
- Intractable bleeding associated with chronic illness.
- Ovulatory heavy bleeding.

Combined Contraceptive Pill

Combined oral contraceptive is an effective contraceptive and may impose an external control of cycle. Reduce MBL by 50%.

Mechanism of action: Combined oral contraceptive pill controls ovarian cycle and causes endometrial glandular atrophy. So bleeding occurs at regular interval and blood losses minimizes by suppressing endometrial function.

Side effects: Headache, migraine, weight gain, breast tenderness, nausea, cholestatic jaundice, hypertension and thrombotic episodes.

Danazol

Synthetic androgen with antiestrogenic and antiprogestagenic activity. In doses of 200–400 mg administered daily for 12 weeks is effective in reducing menstrual blood loss by up to 80% from baseline. More effective than PSI in reduction of MBL at doses more than 400 mg/day.

Mechanism of action: Danazol inhibits the release of pituitary gonadotropins and has direct suppressive effect on the endometrium.

Side effects: Headache, weight gain, acne, rashes, hirsutism, mood and voice changes, flushes, muscle spasm, reduced high-density lipoprotein (HDL), diminished breast size. Rarely, cholestatic jaundice.

GnRH Analogue

Mechanism of action: Gonadotropin-releasing hormone analog downregulates expression of GnRH receptors, which blocks gonadotropin secretion from the anterior pituitary. This leads to ovarian suppression.

Dose: 3.6 mg subcutaneously (SC) or 3.75 mg deep IM on monthly basis for 3–6 months.

Side effects: Hot flushes, sweats, headache, irritability, loss of libido, vaginal dryness, lethargy and reduced bone density.

Gestrinone

Gestrinone is a 19-testosterone derivative, which has antiprogestogenic, antiestrogenic and androgenic activity. It can reduce blood loss in 79% patients with objective menorrhagia.

Side effect: It has androgenic effect.

Antiprogestational Agents

Mifepristone (RU-486) inhibits ovulation, disrupt endometrial integrity and induces amenorrhea. It also reduces size of myoma. Can be used in menorrhagia but adverse effect such as endometrial hyperplasia and availability of other superior drugs limit its use.

Surgeries

Indication for Surgical Treatment (Jeffcoate, 2008)

- Persistent intermenstrual bleeding
- Failed medical treatment
- Age over 40
- Other factors, e.g. associated severe dysmenorrhea.

Surgical treatment includes curettage, endometrial ablation and hysterectomy.

Dilatation and Curettage

Dilatation and curettage can be done:
- To enhance shedding of hyperplastic endometrium in uncontrolled bleeding in spite

of medical treatment. It is effective in reproductive-aged group women. Not effective in elderly women and very restricted use for young adolescent girls.
- To remove endometrial polyps.

Endometrial Ablation

Indications for Endometrial Ablation
- Heavy menstrual loss
- Endometrial atypia excluded
- Uterus less than 12 weeks size
- No pelvic infection
- Completed family or not willing to conserve fertility status
- Fit for surgical procedure
- Willing for hysterectomy, if required.

It is done in the following form:
- Transcervical resection of endometrium (TCRE)
- Endometrial laser resection (ELA)
- Roller ball endometrial ablation (REA)
- Thermal balloons
- Microwave endometrial ablation
- Circulating hot saline
- Cryotherapy.

Transcervical Resection of the Endometrium

Transcervical resection of the endometrium is an alternative to hysterectomy in the younger woman who has no desire for future fertility but wishes to preserve her uterus and in the older woman with obesity or medical contraindications for hysterectomy (Jeffcoate, 2008).

Pretreatment with danazol or GnRH agonists is given for 6 weeks to decrease operative blood loss. The entire endometrium is ablated by electrocautery using a resectoscope, roller ball or a combination of the two, starting with the fundus and proceeding successively to the anterior, lateral and posterior walls, but avoiding the cervix.

Effects: Due to destruction of endometrium, it causes persistent amenorrhea. Presence of adenomyosis is associated with higher failure rate. Subsequent need of hysterectomy is 21% at 6.5 years (Philips G 1998).

Complications

Complications include fluid overload leading to pulmonary edema; uterine perforation and cervical trauma; bleeding; anesthetic complications; electrical/laser injury; infection and air embolism. About 1.3% of patients require emergency hysterectomy because of perforation or injury to the large vessels; about 5–10% need hysterectomy later because of failure of therapy. Thermal injury to the cervix can lead to stenosis, dysmenorrhea and retention of secretions. Hysteroscopic laser photovaporization with the neodymium-doped yttrium aluminum garnet (Nd:YAG) laser has been found to have similar results.

Global Endometrial Ablation Techniques (Jeffcoate, 2008)

Transcervical resection of the endometrium (TCRE) is not universally practiced in spite of its proven efficacy and safety. Several simpler procedures are being developed for the blind ablation of the endometrium. Fluid-filled thermal balloons are placed in the uterus. These use hot water or saline delivered by disposable balloon catheters under sophisticated computer control to regulate temperature, pressure and depth of thermal damage.

Other techniques, which have been tried include radiofrequency thermal balloon, three-dimensional bipolar ablation, microwave endometrial ablation, laser interstitial hyperthermy using an Nd:YAG laser and cryoablation. These methods are still under trial and long-term results are awaited. Here is a figure of thermal ablation **(Fig. 18.1)**.

Abnormal uterine bleeding is a major healthcare problem. The key to the evaluation of abnormal uterine bleeding is a thorough history, physical and pelvic examination governed by the differential diagnosis and the selected use of adjunctive diagnostic tests and procedure. Tranexamic acid as 1st line treatment has found most effective.

Complications
Perforation, hemorrhage in TCRE, fluid overload in laser ablation are common complications.

Abnormal Uterine Bleeding

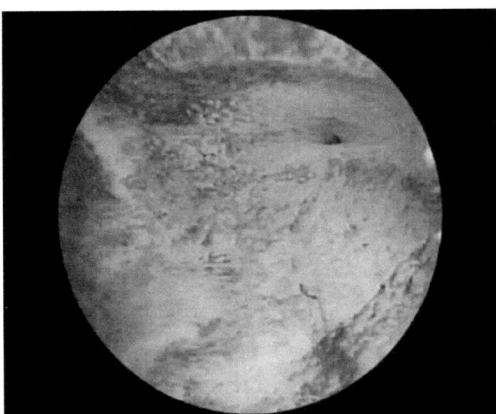

Fig. 18.1 Hysteroscopic endometrial ablation
(For color version, see Plate 4)

Hysterectomy

Definitive Treatment of AUB

Indications of hysterectomy:
- Age ≥ 40
- Failed medical treatment and minor surgical treatment like dilatation and curettage in young women with complete family.

Note: Never for very young patient.

Other Surgeries

Myomectomy and polypectomy, when these are responsible for AUB.

Suppose Mrs Faria's MBL is not excessive, but duration is prolonged almost 16–17 days. Hb is 9.8 gm%. Organic pathology has been ruled out. TVS shows thin endometrium of about 3.5 mm. She is nonsmoker and nondiabetic.

How will you treat her?

The aim of treatment is:
- To stop bleeding
- To restore synchrony to the endometrium
- To replenish iron store.

For this, patient outpatient therapy with short-term follow-up is adequate. Prolonged asynchronous breakage and shedding results in a thinned endometrium (measurable by ultrasound) and will require higher doses of estrogen to rebuild tissue and replace progesterone receptor sites.

Progestin therapy alone will not generally stop the bleeding in this case.

A cascade of oral contraceptives is to be started as soon as possible, as she has no contraindications to the use of estrogen. This should be a 30 or 35 μg ethinyl estradiol monophasic pill, to be given at high doses with a slow decline. An easy formula is one pill qid for 4 days, then one pill tid for 4 days, then one pill bid for 4 days, then one pill daily. Nausea may need to be taken care of.

Once the cascade regimen is completed, the severity of the bleeding and the degree of anemia will dictate how long oral contraceptive use is recommended at regular dosing intervals. Antifibrinolytic agent such as tranexamic acid (1 g four times daily) reduces the amount of blood loss by 50%. Its use is usually well-tolerated by the patients.

If she does not have an active bleeding *oral contraceptives are treatment of choice* and a 30–35 μg preparation is usually adequate. Supplemental iron should be encouraged. Re-evaluation in 3–6 months is recommended.

Progestins alone are also an effective treatment for anovulatory bleeding. Medroxyprogesterone acetate may be prescribed in a dose of 5–10 mg per day or micronized progesterone 100–200 mg per day for 10–14 days, starting on day 16 of the cycle, to induce stromal stability, which is then followed by a withdrawal flow.

Case scenario: *Miss Marium, an 18-year-old girl has complaints of excessive bleeding during menstruation. From menarche (at 13 years) her cycle is irregular. Bleeding occurs 2–3 months apart. Every time bleeding is heavy but for which she did not receive any medication as it was tolerable. This time bleeding occurs after 2½ months of amenorrhea. Bleeding is so heavy that she has to change the regular sanitary pad every 1–2 hours. Her body mass index (BMI) is 32 and she has abnormal hair growth over the arms, legs, abdomen and face. Ultrasonography (USG) shows normal uterus with polycystic ovaries. Her thyroid-stimulating hormone (TSH) and prolactin level is normal.*

How will you treat this case?

This is a case of *metropathia hemorrhagica* in polycystic ovarian syndrome (PCOS) patient.

Aim of the Rx

- To stop the bleeding as soon as possible (ASAP)
- To restore subsequent normal menstrual cycles.

To stop bleeding ASAP combined PSI/antifibrinolytics and high-dose progesterone is to be given
- Antifibrinolytics 500 mg qds or if needed 1 g qds for 5 days
- Norethisterone or medroxyprogesterone 30-40 mg daily in divided doses till stoppage of bleeding; usually bleeding arrested within 2-3 days
- Followed by same tablet 10-15 mg in divided doses for 3 weeks.

In subsequent cycles:
- Antifibrinolytics 500 mg qds from day 1 to 5
- Norethisterone or medroxy progesterone 5 mg tds from day 5 to 25 in each cycle can be given.

This regimen should be continued for three to four cycles. Afterwards patient can keep on oral contraceptives (OCPs) for 6-12 months.

She will be advised for weight reduction, which can resume her normal menstrual cycles.

> Suppose her bleeding is not stopped with progesterone. What other measure can be taken for immediate stoppage of bleeding?

Estrogen in high doses can stop bleeding. Conjugated estrogen 25 mg IV every 4-6 hours till bleeding ceases or for 24 hours, then OCP is started (Anderson, 1990).

RELATED INFORMATION

In PCOS or in other anovulatory condition, there is absence of active corpus luteum in the ovary. A group of follicle begins to ripe, but no one gets maturity. So there is production of estrogen from multiple growing follicles. There is no ovulation. Follicles become cystic and continues to release estrogen. So there is unopposed action of estrogen on endometrium. Endometrium becomes hyperplastic usually cystic type (Swiss cheese), but occasionally adenomatous. At a time endometrium becomes so thick that estrogen cannot support, it anymore and estrogen withdrawal bleeding takes place. Usually, it is preceded by a short period of amenorrhea and sometimes bleeding may continue 2-8 weeks and it is so heavy to threated life. This sort of bleeding was designated as metropathia hemorrhagica. As bleeding takes place after a period of amenorrhea it may confuse with ectopic pregnancy or abortion. But the bleeding of metropathia hemorrhagica is painless, which is the differentiating point between the other two situations where pain is invariable. Those who want pregnancy, ovulation induction can make the woman ovulatory and restores menstruation.

> **Case scenario:** Mrs Halima, mother of two children aged 32 years complaints of irregular pervaginal (PV) bleeding for 3 months. Her menstrual cycle is irregular ranging from 35-55 days. Her LMP was 3 months back, which was a bit heavy and was associated with pain. Since then she bleeds off and on, which is altered and fresh mixed. USG shows nothing abnormality in pelvic organs. Her built is average and she has no other medical or endocrinological disorder. She received progesterone, antifibrinolytics but bleeding did not stop completely.
> What do you want to do for this patient?

This may be a case of incomplete abortion of early pregnancy. Though, USG reveals nothing abnormality yet it might be incomplete abortion. As attachment of fine membranes cannot be detected by all machines or sonologist:
- She must have to do a β-hCH to exclude or identify pregnancy status
- Oral antibiotic is to be started
- Dilatation and curettage is to be done even in case of negative β-hCH
- Curettage material is to be sent for histopathology.

> **Case scenario:** Mrs Banu, aged 42 years, mother of three children, age of last child is (ALC)11 years, has been suffering from frequent menstruation at 15-30 days interval with heavy bleeding persisting for 5-10 days. She has been suffering from this problem for last 2 years and took different medicines from time-to-time, but the symptoms are deteriorating day by day.
> What treatment options can be offered to this patient?

She should be offered surgical treatment. This age group patient usually does not response to medical treatment. So surgical treatment is ideal for this patient. Before that she should be screened to exclude malignant status.

The options are:
- Dilatation and curettage can be done for once. May be cured after dilatation and curettage. If complaint recurs there is no further indication for dilatation and curettage. One should go for:
  - Endometrial ablation or
  - Hysterectomy

BIBLIOGRAPHY

Albers JR, Hull SK, Wesley RM. Abnormal Uterine Bleeding. Americal Family Physician. 2004;69: 1915-26.

Andersson JK, Rybo G. Levonorgesterol-releasing intrauterine device in the treatment of menorrhagia. Br J Obstet Gynaecol. 1990;97:690-4.

Bayer SR, Decuherny AH. Clinical manifestation and treatment of dysfunctional uterine bleeding. JAMA. 1993;269:1823-8.

Cameron IT, Norman JE. Endometrial biochemistry in menorrhagia. In: Asch R, Studd J (Eds). Progress in Reproductive Medicine, Vol II, New York: Partheness Publishing; 1995.pp.267-79.

Coulter A, McPherson K, Vessey M. Do British women under go too many or too few hysterectomies? Soc Sci Med. 1988;27:987-94.

DeVore GR, Owens O, Kase N. Use of intravenous Premarin in the treatment of dysfunctional uterine bleeding: a double randomized control study. Obstet Gynecol. 1982;59(3):285-91.

Dewhurst's Textbook of Obstetrics and Gynaecology for post-graduates, 6th edn. Blackwell Science Ltd; 1999.

Dockery CG, Shappard BL, Daly L, et al. The fibrinolytic enzyme system in normal menstruation and excessive uterine bleeding and effect of tranexamic acid. Euo J Obstet Gynaecol Reprod Biol. 1987;24:309-18.

Fraser IS, Critchley HO, Munro MG, et al. A process designed to lead to international agreement on terminologies and definitions used to describe abnormalities of menstrual bleeding. Fertil Steril. 2007;87(3):466-76.

Fraser IS, Critchley HO, Munro MG. Abnormal uterine bleeding: getting our terminology straight. Curr Opin Obstet Gynecol. 2007;19(6):591-5.

Hallberg L, Hogdahl A, Nilsson L, et al. Menstrual blood loss: a population study. Variation at different ages and attempts to define normality. Acta Obstet Gynecol Scand. 1996;45:320-51.

Jaideep Malhotra, Narendra Malhotra, Joseph Kuvan, et al. Approach to abnormal bleeding. In: Pankaj Desai, Varenha Malhotra, Uvru Shui (Eds). Principles of Practice of Obstetrics and Gynaecology. 3rd edn, Jaypee Brothers Medical Publishers, India, 2008.

Jeffcoate's Principles of Gynaecology, 7 edn. Kumar Pratap, Malhotra Narendra. Publishers: Jaypee Brothers Medical Publishers, New Delhi. 2008. p. 977.

MORI. Women's health in 1990. Market Opinion and Research International Clinical Endocrinology (Oxford). 1990;53:359-66.

Munro MG, Mainor N, Basu R, et al. Oral medroxyprogesterone acetate and combination oral contraceptives for acute uterine bleeding: a randomized controlled trial. Obstet Gynecol. 2006;108(4):924-9.

Munro MG. Abnormal Uterine Bleeding. Cambridge: Cambridge University Press; 2010.

Munro MG, Critchley HO, Broder MS et al. FIGO classification system (PALM-COEIN) for causes of abnormal uterine bleeding in nongravid women of reproductive age. FIGO Working Group on Menstrual Disorder. Int J Gynaecol Obstet. 2011;113:3-13.

Phillips G, Chien PF, Garry R. Risk of hysterectomy after 1000 consecutive endometrial laser ablation. Br J Obstet Gynecol. 1998;105:897-903.

Prentice A. Medical management of menorrhagia. BMJ. 1999;319(7221):1343-45.

Somen Bhattacharjee. Abnormal bleeding in adolescents. In: Roza Olyai, Dilip Kumar Dutta (Eds). Recent Advances in Adolescent Health India. Jaypee Brothers Medical Publishers; 2011.

Vercellini P, Cortesi I, Oldani. The role of transvaginal ultrasonography and outpatient diagnostic hysteroscopy in the evaluation of patients with menorrhagia. Hum Reprod. 1997;12:1768-71.

Vessey MP, Villard-Macintosh L, Mc Pherson K, et al. The epidemiology of hysterectomy: finding in a large cohort study. Br J Obstet Gynaecol. 1992;99:402-7.

CHAPTER 19

Postmenopausal Bleeding

Saria Tasnim, Farhat Hossain

INTRODUCTION

Bleeding from the genital tract occurring after the menopause has been established, i.e. after 1 year of cessation of menstruation is called postmenopausal bleeding (PMB). It is likely to be caused by pathologic disease, and it must always be investigated. It is considered as cancer until proved otherwise (Karlsson et al. 1995). Significant pathology is found in women with PMB in 10–20% cases.

The PMB is a common clinical problem representing 5% of all gynecology outpatient attendances (Moodley and Roberts, 2004). A good percentage of patents with PMB are accounted for by malignant disease of the cervix or of the body of uterus. As such PMB demands prompt evaluation. Since, many of the elderly patients are unable to determine the site of bleeding nongynecological causes such as disease of the bladder, urethra and rectum should also be excluded in PMB.

> **Case scenario:** Mrs Kohinoor Begum a 60-year-old menopausal lady has come to you with the complaints of pervaginal bleeding for 3 days.
> How will you evaluate the patient?

Detail history is to be taken from the patient in regards to:
- Age of menopause
- Parity: Multiparous women are candidates for cervical cancer while nulliparous or women with low parity are more likely to develop endometrial carcinoma.
- Details of bleeding:
  - *Nature of bleeding:* Irregular bleeding or bleeding ON and OFF is associated with genital tract malignancy. On the other hand, regular cyclical bleeding is indicative of dysfunctional uterine bleeding (DUB).
  - *Duration of bleeding with episodes:* Patients having one episode of PMB are seen not to find any abnormality. The bleeding results due to break in endometrial blood vessels secondary to sudden emotional shock or upset more likely in hypertensive patients. 70–80% of these patients do not bleed again afterwards.
  - *Postcoital bleeding:* Patients of cancer cervix reports postcoital bleeding as the earliest symptom particularly those having exophytic growth in the cervix.
  - *Association of foul smelling vaginal discharge:* This symptom is present in patients having cervical cancer.
  - *Association of burning vagina or introitus:* This symptom is present in senile vaginitis.
  - *Presence of medical disorder such as diabetics mellitus (DM) and hypertension:* DM and hypertension are common association in endometrial cancer.
  - *Any history of hormone replacement therapy (HRT) intake:* If so, its duration and whether HRT has been withdrawn or not.
  - Any history of tamoxifen intake for breast cancer.
  - History of tuberculosis or contact.
  - History of bleeding disorder, i.e. epistaxis, bruising, etc.
  - Any bleeding from bladder, urethra, rectum present or not.

Thorough physical examination including breast examination.

> What will be your stepwise approach for Mrs Kohinoor?

- Detailed history.
- General examination including breast examination.
- Local examination of vulva, urethra for caruncles and anal region for fissures and piles in order to rule out non-gynecological causes of bleeding. Bleeding from these sites can be mistaken for vaginal bleeding.
- Pap smear before pelvic examination
- Speculum examination is done to exclude growth in the cervix and senile vaginitis.
- Bimanual examination to exclude uterine and adnexal pathology.
- Transvaginal sonography: It is an established first step in the evaluation of PMB. A thickened or asymmetric endometrial lining or an obvious intrauterine lesion is an indication for more thorough evaluation.
- Endometrial sampling: It is the most accurate screening method available for PMB to exclude endometrial polyp, endometrial hyperplasia or endometrial cancer. It is done as an office procedure and is just as accurate as dilation and curettage.
- Hysteroscopy: It has greatly improved the diagnostic accuracy in the evaluation of endometrium. It allows visual inspection of endometrial cavity and gives the opportunity to perform directed biopsies. It must be used where it is available instead of doing direct endometrial sampling.

RELATED INFORMATION

Causes of Postmenopausal Bleeding

- Indiscriminate use of estrogen for HRT. Thirty percent (30%) of patients with PMB report using exogenous estrogen.
- Senile vaginitis or senile endometritis:
    - It is responsible for 30% cases of PMB.
- Genital tract malignancy.
    i. *Endometrial cancer:* About 15% patients of PMB on evaluation are found to have the disease.
    ii. Cervical cancer
- Endometrial hyperplasia: About 5% of PMB is due to this condition.
- Endometrial polyp, cervical polyp: About 10% of patients on evaluation are found to have the condition.
- Estrogen producing tumor of the ovary.
- Large ovarian tumor affecting the vascularity of uterus—Misfit tumor.
- Genital tuberculosis.
- Dysfunctional uterine bleeding.
- Genital prolapse with decubitus ulcer.
- Disease of blood and capillaries.
- Bleeding from urethra, bladder and rectum.

Clinical Features of Diseases Strongly Related to PMB

- *Endometrial cancer*: PMB is the predominant symptomology. Two-thirds of the patients are obese and hypertensive. Combination of obesity, hypertension and DM with endometrial cancer is called *corpus cancer syndrome*. Risk of endometrial cancer increases with age.
  Speculum examination shows cervix without any growth or ulcer. *Bimanual examination* reveals bulky uterus in some cases, but in early stages uterus may be atrophied.
- *Cervical cancer*: The patient complaints of postmenopausal bleeding and excessive vaginal discharge, which may be foul smelling. In some patients, there is history of postcoital bleeding.
    - *Speculum examination reveals:* Exophytic growth replacing the cervix or there is ulceration in the cervix.
    - *Bimanual examination* shows changes depending on the stage of the disease. Uterus may normal or bulky, fornices may be free or involved. Usually cervix is hard, friable, fix and bleeds on touch.
    - *Rectovaginal examination* shows bilateral parametrium is free or fixed.
- *Senile vaginitis*: The patient complaints of:
    - Postmenopausal yellowish discharge or PMB
    - Excoriation and soreness of vulva
    - Dysuria, if urethra is involved
    - Fullness of vagina.

- On speculum examination, the vagina appears as multiple reddened areas in the vault and around the urethral orifice. This is called speckled red vagina.
- Bimanual examination reveals atrophied uterus.

Investigation for Postmenopausal Bleeding

Transvaginal Sonography

Transvaginal sonography (TVS) is the most popular noninvasive investigation for assessing endometrium in women with PMB. TVS has a high sensitivity for detecting endometrial cancer and other endometrial disease (Smith et al. 1998). The threshold value for endometrial thickness is 4 or 5 mm below which endometrial pathology is unlikely. This has been established after numerous trials in women with PMB. In general, endometrial thickness greater than 4 or 5 mm is used as USG criteria for determining whether or not endometrial sampling is indicated in PMB (Dreisler et al. 2009; Gupta et al. 2002). Since, HRT increases endometrial thickness, the specificity of USG criteria is low. TVS also gives information about irregular or heterogeneous echotexture of endometrium in endometrial cancer in addition to the increased thickness of endometrium.

Saline Infusion Sonography

Saline infusion sonography infuses saline into the uterine cavity during ultrasound to improve the image. The saline separates the two walls of endometrium, allowing better measurement of endometrial thickness. Fibroids or polyps appear as filling defect in the cavity of uterus in saline infusion sonography. The sensitivity and specificity of saline infusion sonography for endometrial cancer are comparable with the high sensitivity and specificity of diagnostic hysteroscopy (Clark et al. 2002). It is more accurate than hysteroscopy in diagnosing endometrial hyperplasia (Widrich et al. 1996) and is more accurate than transvaginal ultrasonography in diagnosing intracavitary lesions (De Varies et al. 2000; Krample et al. 2001).

Endometrial Sampling

If results of pelvic ultrasound show endometrial thickness of 5 mm or more, it is advisable to perform an endometrial biopsy. Sampling of endometrium can be done using pipette device or Vabra device. Endometrial aspirator samples greater endometrial surface but less well-tolerated. In low economic setting, Karman's cannula is used for endometrial sampling. It is done as an office procedure to exclude endometrial polyp, endometrial hyperplasia or endometrial cancer in PMB. It is just as accurate as dilatation and curettage, but obviates the need of general anesthesia.

Hysteroscopy

Hysteroscopy allows direct visualization of endometrium and intrauterine cavity using flexible fiberoptic cable with carbon dioxide as the distending medium. It has the advantage that directed biopsy can be obtained, endometrial polyps and submucosal leiomyoma can be removed. It can be used as an office procedure and is particularly useful in patients having persistent abnormal bleeding. For women with PMB, hysteroscopy is the basic tool for precise diagnosis of various endouterine pathologies with sensitivity and specificity 97% and 98.66% respectively (Tandulwadkar et al. 2009).

> *After completion of history taking, physical examination and investigation it is found that Mrs Kohinoor's endometrium is hyperplastic in ultrasonography and after biopsy it shows hyperplasia without atypia. No other problem is detected at any point.*
>
> How will you treat her?

This case should be considered as a case of DUB. Endometrial hyperplasia in patients without cytologic atypia responds well to progestin therapy, with an expected response rate of 80%.

- In treating endometrial hyperplasia without atypia, it is reasonable to start with 20 mg of medroxyprogesterone twice a day for 3-6 months.
- Then an endometrial biopsy should be repeated. If hyperplasia is still present, a

hysteroscopy should be performed for a definitive diagnosis.
- If hysteroscopy confirms the presence of hyperplasia, one of the following two options can be adopted:
  1. An additional 3 months of progesterone therapy can be given followed by another endometrial biopsy.
  2. Hysterectomy.

If there is hyperplasia with atypia, then how will you manage her?

Hyperplasia with atypia responds less well to progesterone treatment. So treatment should be as follows:
- Definitive treatment: In the postmenopausal woman definitive treatment should be hysterectomy with or without oophorectomy because of the risk of concomitant and future malignancy.
- Those patients medically unfit for surgery can be treated with high-dose progesterone, but need to be reassessed frequently with endometrial sampling to ensure reversal of changes as pathology may progress to malignancy in time.

What are the different types of endometrium that we receive following endometrial sampling in PMB?

The endometrium is:
- Normal in 50%
- Atropic in 20%
- Endometrial hyperplasia in 15%
- Endometrial polyp in 3%
- Endometrial cancer in 2%.

Case scenario: Mrs Gaitri, a 60-year-old lady complaints of PMB. On evaluation, the cervix is healthy looking, but the vagina is speckled red. TVS reveals endometrial thickness of 3 mm. What is the possible diagnosis?
What are the bases of diagnosis?

Senile vaginitis is the possible diagnosis.

Diagnosis is made by exclusion of all other possible causes of PMB. TVS, cervical smear or biopsy, and endometrial sampling are essential in all cases before senile vaginitis is assumed to be the cause of PMB.

RELATED INFORMATION

Cause of Senile Vaginitis

Senile vaginitis occurs due to loss of vaginal resistance secondary to estrogen deficiency. As a result common pyogenic organisms invade the vaginal tissue. Most common of postmenopausal bleeding is atrophic senile vaginitis (Iatrakis et al. 1997).

Treatment of Senile Vaginitis

Estrogen preparation either orally or locally is given for 3 weeks. The patient is examined after 1 week, and if features of vaginitis persist estrogen can be repeated again.

Is there any role of antibiotic in the treatment of senile vaginitis?

Antibiotic is not necessary. Vaginal resistance is quickly restored by giving estrogen preparation and infection is eradicated. When the estrogen therapy is suspended, then there is minimum chance of relapse of disease.

Note: By any route estrogen may induce uterine bleeding and the patient should be warned of this.

Case scenario: Mrs Nazma, a 55-year-old multiparous woman complaints of PMB. Her TVS reveals endometrial thickness of 3 mm and endometrial sampling shows scanty endometrium. Pap smear yielded atypical cells, for which colposcopy guided cervical biopsy was done. The histopathology report was squamous cell carcinoma, grade II.
What will be the treatment option in this patient?

This patient now has to be clinically staged for cancer cervix. Since, there was no growth in the cervix, obviously this is a case of early stage disease. The ideal treatment for this patient would be modified radical hysterectomy with pelvic lymphadenectomy followed by external beam radiotherapy (EBRT) depending upon the histopathology report.

Case scenario: Mrs Hasina, a 70-year-old lady who reported for postmenopausal bleeding. On evaluation, no cause could be identified in the genital tract, but there is recurrence or persistence of bleeding per vagina.
What will be the treatment option?

In postmenopausal bleeding, in spite of negative result of investigations, if pervaginal bleeding recurs or persists it strongly recommends *Total Abdominal Hysterectomy with bilateral salpingo-oophorectomy*. There are evidences showing detection of early cancer of uterus, fallopian tube or ovary in such circumstances. Evidence suggests that 10% patients develop pathology in 2 years.

BIBLIOGRAPHY

Clark TJ, Voit D, Gupta JK, et al. Accuracy of hysteroscopy in the diagnosis of endometrial cancer and hyperplasia: a systematic quantitative review. JAMA. 2002;288(13):1610-21.

de Vries LD, Dijkhuizen FP, Mol BW, et al. Comparison of transvaginal sonography, saline infusion sonography, and hysteroscopy in premenopausal women with abnormal uterine bleeding. J Clin Ultrasound. 2000;28:217-23.

Dreisler E, Sorensen SS, Ibsen PH, et al. Value of endometrial thickness measurement for diagnosing focal intrauterine pathology in women without abnormal uterine bleeding. Ultrasound Obstet Gynecol. 2009;33(3):344-8.

Gupta JK, Chien PF, Voit D, et al. Ultrasonographic endometrial thickness for diagnosing endometrial pathology in women with postmenopausal bleeding: a meta-analysis. Acta Obstet Gynecol Scand. 2002;81(9):799-816.

Iatrakis G, Diakakis I, Kourounis G, et al. Postmenopausal uterine bleeding. Clin Exp Obstet Gynecol. 1997;24:157.

Karlsson B, Granbergs, Wikland M, et al. Transvaginal ultrasonography of the endometrium in women with postmenopausal bleeding: a Nordic multicentre study. Am J Obstet Gynecol. 1995;172(5):1488-94.

Krampl E, Bourne T, Hurlen-Solbakken H, et al. Transvaginal ultrasonography sonohysterography and operative hysteroscopy for the evaluation of abnormal uterine bleeding. Acta Obstet Gynecol Scand. 2001;80(7):616-22.

Moodley M, Roberts C. Clinical pathway for the evaluation of postmenopausal bleeding with an emphasis on endometrial cancer detection. J Obstet Gynaecol. 2004;24(7):736-41.

Smith-Bindman R, Kerlikowske K, Feldstein VA, et al. Endovaginal ultrasound to exclude endometrial cancer and other endometrial abnormalities. JAMA. 1998;280(17):1510-7.

Tandulwadkar S, Deshmukh P, Lodha P, et al. Hysteroscopy in postmenopausal bleeding. J Gynaecol Endosc Surg. 2009;1(2):89-93.

Widrich T, Bradley LD, Mitchinson AR, et al. Comparison of saline infusion sonography with office hysteroscopy for the evaluation of the endometrium. Am J Obstet Gynecol. 1996;174(4):1327-34.

CHAPTER 20

Recurrent Pregnancy Loss

Rashida Begum, Firoza Begum

INTRODUCTION

According to World Health Organization (WHO), miscarriage is expulsion or extraction of embryo or fetus weighing 500 g or less—a stage that corresponds to a gestational age of up to 20 weeks (WHO, 1977). More acceptable definition is spontaneous expulsion before viability. Recurrent pregnancy loss (RPL) is a heterogeneous condition characterized by three or more consecutive pregnancy loss before the age of viability. Prevalence of RPL is 0.6–2.3% shown by different studies (Warburton, 1987; Stray-Pederson, 1979; Fertility and Employment, 1979). According to ESHRE early pregnancy guideline development group two consecutive losses can be considered as recurrent pregnancy loss [ESHRE 2017].

> **Case scenario:** *Rabeya, married for 2 years has come to you with amenorrhea for 6 weeks. She has history of three previous spontaneous abortions. She is very much anxious about this pregnancy outcome.*
>
> *How will you approach for managing this patient?*

Detailed History is to be Taken

- *Maternal age:* Advancing maternal age is associated with a decline in both the number and quality of the remaining oocytes. Miscarriage is inversely proportional to age of the mother. The risk of miscarriage is highest where the woman is ≥ 35 years of age.
- *Paternal age:* Advanced paternal age has also been identified as a risk factor for miscarriage. Risk involved when age of the man is ≥ 40 years.
- *Environmental risk factors:* Maternal cigarette smoking and caffeine consumption have been associated with an increased risk of spontaneous miscarriage in a dose-dependent manner. However, current evidence is insufficient to confirm this association.
- *Heavy alcohol consumption:* It is toxic to the embryo and the fetus. Even moderate consumption of five or more units per week may increase the risk of sporadic miscarriage.

Menstrual History

Menstrual cycle: History of oligomenorrhea/amenorrhea/menorrhagia before the current pregnancy may signify the underlying endocrinological disorders responsible for recurrent pregnancy loss (RPL) like thyroid disorder, hyperprolactinemia and polycystic ovary syndrome (PCOS).

Last menstrual period (LMP): To assess gestational age.

About Signs and Symptoms of Pregnancy

- Vomiting
- Morning sickness.

Obstetric History

Detail of Previous Abortions

Age of gestation during previous abortion to identify whether it is in first or second trimester? As causes are different in different trimester:
- Pattern of onset of abortion
- Started with pain in the abdomen followed by expulsion
- Started with pervaginal (PV) bleeding followed by pain and expulsion
- Started with rupture of the membrane followed by pain and sudden expulsion; possibility of cervical incompetence

- Only altered PV bleeding and no pain or expulsion, evacuation needed for expulsion; possibility of missed abortion
- No complain; diagnosed ultrasonographically that fetus was dead; missed abortion
- If it is after attainment of quickening complain of loss of fetal movement and diagnosed dead fetus by USG; missed abortion
- Requirement of dilatation, evacuation or curettage
- Whether there was any precipitating factors such as history of fall, blow in the abdomen, heavy work, rough journey, history of coitus, etc.
- History of febrile illness, possibility of viral infections
- Whether she knows about blood grouping
- If Rh-ve whether she received any Rh anti-D antibody or not.

History of any Medical Diseases

- Diabetes
- Hypothyroidism/Hyperthyroidism
- Hyperprolactinemia
- Hypertension
- History of PIH
- Family history of diabetes and hypertension.

Patient should be Examined Thoroughly

- Pulse
- Blood pressure
- Anemia
- Thyroid gland
- Abdominal examination
- Bimanual examination.

> On enquiry and after examination, you elicited that she is 35 years old, normotensive, having no thyroid problem. Her mother is diabetic. Her 2 hours postprandial blood sugar was normal in previous pregnancies. Her menstrual cycle is regular and LMP was 6 weeks back. Her previous abortions were first at 10 weeks, second and third at 8 weeks. On every occasion she started PV bleeding then pain and ended with expulsion. First time it was complete abortion, but last two occasions needed curettage. Her blood group is A+ve.
> On the basis of above findings, what investigations do you like to do for this patient?

- First of all, an ultrasonogram is to be done to confirm the intrauterine pregnancy, gestational age and cardiac activity. As well as to rule out any uterine abnormality particularly developmental anomaly and myomas close to the cavity.
- Routine tests such as Hb%, VDRL, HBsAg, urine routine examination (R/E) and microscopic examination (M/E).
- Glucose tolerance test (GTT) as her mother is diabetic, she is a high-risk patient for developing gestational diabetes mellitus (GDM).
- Thyroid-stimulating hormone (TSH), prolactin are to be done.
- Antiphospholipid antibodies: All women with recurrent miscarriage should be screened for antiphospholipid antibodies.
- Karyotyping of both partner.

RELATED INFORMATION

Approaches of investigation in recurrent pregnancy loss (RPL) depend upon mode, number and time of previous miscarriages. Investigations for first trimester abortions are not same as investigations for second trimester abortion. A particular woman does not need all investigations for diagnosis the cause of her abortions. Different protocols are prepared by different societies, which are evidence based. Investigation also based on predicted causes of RPL.

Following are the causes of RPL:
- Genetic causes:
  – Chromosomal rearrangements (trisomy, monosomy X, triploidy)
  – Translocation, inversion or deletion in the parents
  – Lethal genes.
- Hormonal causes:
  – Corpus luteum insufficiency
  – Severe thyroid disease
  – Diabetes mellitus
  – Polycystic ovaries with inappropriate luteinizing hormone (LH) secretion.
- Anatomic causes:
  – Cervical incompetence
  – Uterine septa
  – Bicornuate, unicornuate uterus

- Diethylstilbestrol exposure
- Uterine fibroids
- Adenomyoma
- Intrauterine adhesion (Asherman's syndrome).
• Infectious causes:
- Toxoplasmosis
- Urea/*Mycoplasma*
- *Chlamydia*.
• Immunologic causes:
- Antiphospholipid syndrome
- Alloimmune mechanisms.
• Thrombophilias:
- Antithrombin, protein C, protein S, factor V Leiden deficiencies
- Factor XII, Factor XIII and fibrinogen deficiencies
- Hyperhomocysteinemia.
• Metabolic and toxic factors:
- Wilson's disease
- Heavy metal poisoning.
• Psychologic causes.
• Endometriosis.
• Environmental teratogens.
• Male factors.
• Unexplained.

Possible causes of first trimester miscarriages: Antiphospholipid antibodies, chromosomal abnormalities, endocrine and metabolic factors, infection, inherited thrombophilia, immunological factors and unexplained.

Possible causes of second trimester miscarriages include: Anatomical abnormalities such as cervical incompetence, septate uterus, unicornuate uterus, bicornuate uterus, didelphic uterus, uterine fibroids, adenomyoma, uterine septum, endometrial polyps and Asherman's syndrome.

Pattern of abortion: Repeated mid-trimester abortion without apparent cause starting with escape of liquor followed by painless expulsion of the product of conception is very much suggestive of RPL due to cervical incompetence.

Aborters are classified into three groups (Carp et al. 1997):
• *Primary RPL group:* Women with three or more consecutive miscarriages with no pregnancy progressing beyond 20 weeks.
• *Secondary RPL group:* Women who have had three or more miscarriages after a pregnancy that having gone beyond 20 weeks gestation, may have ended in live birth, still birth or neonatal death.
• *Tertiary RPL group*: Women who have had at least three miscarriages that are not consecutive. These are patients with miscarriages, followed by a live birth, then a further string of miscarriages.

Approaches of Investigations

According to recommendation of RCOG, ACOG and ESHRE following investigations can be done. Though all are not equally recommended by three groups:
• *Parental karyotyping (Recommended by RCOG, ACOG, ESHRE)*. Peripheral blood karyotyping of both partners should be performed in couples with recurrent miscarriage where testing of products of conception reports an unbalanced structural chromosomal abnormality. Parental karyotyping is not routinely recommended in couples with RPL by ESHRE. It could be carried out after individual assessment of risk [ESHRE 2017]. In approximately 2–5% of couples with recurrent miscarriage, one of the partners carries a balanced structural chromosomal anomaly; most commonly a balanced reciprocal or Robertsonian translocation.

Risk of miscarriage in couples with:
- Reciprocal translocation—50%
- Robertsonian translocation—25%
   The risk of miscarriage is influenced by the size and the genetic content of the rearranged chromosomal segments.
• *APS assessment (recommended by RCOG, ACOG, ESHRE):* Anticardiolipid antibody (aCL), antiphospholipid antibody (aPL) and lupus anticoagulants (LA) are done. For the diagnosis of antiphospholipid syndrome there must be two positive tests for either lupus anticoagulant or anticardiolipin antibodies of immunoglobulin G and/or immunoglobulin M class, at least 12 weeks apart present in a medium or high titer over 40 g/L, or above the

99th percentile. Screening for β2 glycoprotein I antibodies (a β2 GPI) can be considered after two pregnancy losses [ESHRE 2017].

The mechanisms by which antiphospholipid antibodies cause pregnancy morbidity include inhibition of trophoblastic function and differentiation, activation of complement pathways at the maternal-fetal interface resulting in a local inflammatory response and, in later pregnancy, thrombosis of the uteroplacental vasculature causing placental insufficiency.

Antiphospholipid antibodies are present in 15% of women with recurrent miscarriage. By comparison, the prevalence of antiphospholipid antibodies in women with a low-risk obstetric history is less than 2%. In women with recurrent miscarriage associated with antiphospholipid antibodies, the live birth rate in pregnancies with no pharmacological intervention has been reported to be as low as 10%.

- *Fetal karyotyping* (recommended by RCOG, but not routine) *ACOG, insufficient evidence.* No less than 50% of clinically recognized pregnancy losses show a chromosomal abnormality (Boue, 1975; Hassold, 1980; Simpson, 1987). If chorionic villus sampling (CVS) is performed after ultrasound diagnosis of fetal demise, the frequency is 75–90% (Sorokin, 1991; Strom, 1992). The risk of miscarriage resulting from chromosomal abnormalities of the embryo increases with advancing maternal age. It is important to note that as the number of miscarriages increases, the risk of euploid pregnancy loss increases. Genetic analysis of pregnancy tissue is not routinely recommended by ESHRE but it could be performed for explanatory purposes [ESHRE 2017].
- *Uterine cavity assessment* (recommended by RCOG, ESHRE) *ACOG insufficient evidence.* Distortion of the uterine cavity may be found in approximately 10–15% of women with RPL. All women with recurrent miscarriage should have a pelvic ultrasound to assess uterine anatomy. Hysterosalpingography can be used to assess uterine cavity, but it cannot distinguish between a septate and bicornuate uterus. So recently hysteroscopy has tended to replace the uncomfortable X-ray. Hysteroscopy is associated with much less discomfort, but also cannot distinguish between a septate and bicornuate uterus. However, it is the best procedure for diagnosing polyp, fibroid, etc. Three-dimensional (3D) ultrasonogram is the best procedure for distinguishing between a septate and bicornuate uterus. Combined hysteroscopy, laparoscopy and if possible three-dimensional ultrasound scanning should be used for definitive diagnosis.
- *Thyroid function testing* (recommended by ESHRE only). Thyroid screening by doing thyroid stimulating hormone [TSH] and thyroid peroxidase [TPO]-antibodies) is recommended by ESHRE in women with RPL. It is recommended to follow up abnormal TSH and TPO levels by testing thyroxine (T4) level [ESHRE 2017].
- *Plasma Glucose:* Fasting insulin and fasting glucose is not recommended by ESHRE, in women with RPL to improve next pregnancy prognosis [ESHRE 2017].
- *Tests for hereditary thrombophilia* (recommended by ESHRE as advanced investigation only). Hereditary thrombophilia screening is recommended by ESHRE only for research purpose or in women with additional risk factors for thrombophilia [ESHRE 2017].
- *Prolactin testing:* Prolactin testing is not recommended in women with RPL in the absence of clinical symptoms of hyperprolactinemia (oligo/amenorrhea) [ESHRE, 2017].
- *Antinuclear antibodies (ANA) testing:* ANA testing could be considered for explanatory purposes [ESHRE, 2017].

Other tests like TORCH testing is not recommended. Alloimmune testing is not recommended. Test for LPD like serum progesterone and hCG testing, measurement of homocysteine plasma levels are not recommended by ESHRE [ESHRE, 2017].

> *After doing tests you found that antiphospholipid antibodies are positive. All other test reports are normal.*
> *How will you manage her?*

She is a case of antiphospholipid syndrome. She should be treated by low-dose aspirin at a dose of 81 mg/day plus heparin, preferably low-molecular weight heparin (LMWH) at a dose of 40 mg sc daily to prevent further miscarriage and it should be continued till 34–35 weeks of pregnancy when extra-uterine survivability of fetus is possible. Alternative to LMWH unfractionated heparin at a dose of 5,000 IU sc twice daily can be given.

> How do they prevent miscarriage?

By preventing formation of microthrombus it increases placental circulation and prevent death of the fetus.

> What is the advantage of low-molecular weight heparin?

The risk of heparin therapy such as hemorrhage, osteoporosis, and heparin-induced thrombocytopenia is substantially less frequent with LMWH. The increased bioavailability and longer therapeutic half-life of LMWH also allows less frequent injections. In addition, there is no overlap between the anticoagulant effect and the antithrombotic effect, hence there is no bleeding and little need for monitoring. So emergency cesarean section or delivery can be managed without fear of hemorrhage. On the other hand unfractionated heparin should be omitted at least 48 hours before delivery.

RELATED INFORMATION

Appropriate management can greatly reduce the fetal and maternal morbidity in antiphospholipid syndrome (APS). A meta-analysis reported that treatment with aspirin or aspirin plus unfractionated heparin leads to a significant increase in the live birth rate among women with antiphospholipid syndrome. An 80% live birth rate was seen after heparin and aspirin, compared with 44% after aspirin alone (Kutteh 1996). Combined aspirin and heparin significantly reduces the miscarriage rate by 54%.

After the diagnosis of APS is made, women should be advised to start aspirin and heparin treatment after confirmation cardiac pulsation in their next pregnancy. No evidence suggests that preconceptional treatment of APS improves pregnancy outcome.

Low dose aspirin (81 mg/day) should be initiated as soon as the patient has a positive urinary pregnancy test result. Subcutaneous low-dose heparin therapy in the form of low molecular weight heparin (enoxaparin/clexane) 1 mg/kg/day or unfractionated heparin (Calciparine) 5,000 IU twice daily should be initiated when intrauterine pregnancy and cardiac pulsation is confirmed by USG and treatment should be continued up to 34 completed weeks of pregnancy. Dose of LMWH depends on duration of gestation at which previous losses took place:

- Patients with three or more prior early pregnancy losses should be treated by 1 mg/kg/day. It is a prophylactic dose for thrombosis. The RPL that occurs prior to the 10th weeks of gestation is frequently due other causes than APS and is less specific for APS than pregnancy loss that occurs after 10 weeks (Branch, 2003; Derksen, 2004).
- Patients who have at least one fetal loss after the 10th week of pregnancy are at increased risk of thrombosis during pregnancy and puerperium and should be treated by full therapeutic dose of heparin (e.g. enoxaparin 1 mg/kg body weight every 12 hours) (Tincani 2003).

During the first 3 weeks of heparin treatment, women should have a weekly platelet count to detect heparin-induced thrombocytopenia. Although aspirin plus heparin treatment substantially improves the live birth rate of women with recurrent miscarriage associated with antiphospholipid antibodies, these pregnancies remain at high risk of complications during all three trimesters, including repeated miscarriage, preeclampsia, placental insufficiency, fetal growth restriction, preterm birth (Branch, 1992; Lima, 1996) and necessitates careful antenatal surveillance.

There are no adverse fetal outcomes of low dose aspirin reported in the meta-analysis of randomized controlled trials. Heparin does not cross the placenta and hence there is no risk of fetal hemorrhage or teratogenicity. Heparin can, however, be associated with maternal complications including bleeding, hypersensitivity reactions, heparin-induced thrombocytopenia, and when used for long, osteopenia and vertebral fractures may occur. The loss of bone mineral density at the lumbar spine associated with low-dose long-term heparin therapy is similar to that which occurs physiologically during normal pregnancy.

Monitoring

Full dose UH therapy requires monitoring of partial thromboplastin time (PTT) or factor Xa level. Patients in whom baseline PTT is prolonged due to presence of lupus anticoagulant in APS should be monitored by Xa level. Prophylactic dose of LMWH does not need monitoring as it does not prolong the PTT. However, full anti-coagulation with LMWH may require monitoring by Xa.

What are the antiphospholipid antibodies?

Antiphospholipid antibodies (aPL) are a heterogeneous group of autoantibodies directed against different antigens predominantly anionic phospholipids. They are anticardiolipin (aCL), antiphosphatidylethanolamine (aPE), antiphosphatidylserine (aPS), antiphosphatidylcholine (aPC), antiphosphatidylglycerol (aPG), antiphosphatidylinositol (aPI), antiphosphatidic acid (aPA) and lupus anticoagulant (LA).

What are the obstetric complications of APS?

Pregnancy-induced hypertension (PIH), intra-uterine growth retardation (IUGR), premature labor, gestational diabetes mellitus (GDM) and still birth.

Rabeya responded the treatment and she completed 37 weeks. Fetal condition is absolutely fine. She has no complaints.
How long will you continue the pregnancy?

As this is a very high-risk pregnancy and Rabeya is elderly and fetus attained the gestational age of maturity pregnancy is to be terminated by elective cesarean section or can be induced with intensive fetal monitoring.

Case scenario: *Mrs Aklima, a nulliparous woman, has come to you for consultation about pregnancy as she had four consecutive miscarriages. Three were first trimester and one was second trimester miscarriage. Every time she was on antenatal care and received progesterone in the oral form from second pregnancy. All were missed abortions at 8, 13, 15 and 18 weeks of pregnancy. She has some recent relevant investigations including paternal karyotyping, APS and hereditary thrombophilia testing. All are normal. No test of abortuses were done. Patient does not want to do any invasive investigations.*
What will be your suggestion for her next pregnancy?

As all are missed abortions these may be due to fetal abnormality or defective placental circulation. As fetal test was not done in previous pregnancies so to exclude chromosomal defect chorionic villus biopsy is indicated. But patient does not want to do any invasive investigation. So considering defective placental circulation for hypercoagulation status of pregnancy, anticoagulant treatment such as aspirin and heparin can be started once she will get pregnant. It may be helpful in recurrent missed abortion. Empirical use of heparin and aspirin improves placental circulation and prevent death of the fetus. It is recommended to give therapeutic dose of heparin if previous abortion was beyond 10th weeks, but for empirical use prophylactic dose is appropriate as antiphospholipid antibody is negative in this case. Missed abortion may also occur in thrombophilia. Thrombotic mechanisms due either to APS or to hereditary thrombophilias are more likely to cause fetal demise in first trimester miscarriage (Preston, 1996; Grandone, 1997). If either of these is found in the presence of recurrent second trimester fetal death, treatment by anticoagulant is warranted. New thrombophilias are constantly being identified. Microparticles and protein Z deficiency are two such examples. These thrombophilias are not usually excluded in any investigation protocol. Hence, there is a place for using anticoagulants on an empirical basis in the absence of APS or hereditary thrombophilia. However, no trial has assessed anticoagulants in unexplained recurrent second trimester losses.

What is thrombophilia?

Thrombophilia is a condition where there are defects in coagulation factors.

> How thrombophilias cause RPL?

Thrombophilia causes microthrombus in the placenta resulting in abortion and other adverse obstetric outcome. It causes decidual thrombosis, fetal thrombotic vasculopathy, fetal stem vessel thrombosis, infarcts, hypoplasia, spiral artery thrombosis and previllous fibrin deposition. By this way it reduces placental circulation and causes fetal demise.

RELATED INFORMATION

Thrombophilias, whether hereditary or acquired have been found in a significant number of women with recurrent abortions without apparent cause. The most common acquired thrombophilia is antiphospholipid syndrome. Hereditary thrombophilias that have been reported to be associated with RPL include antithrombin, protein C, and protein S deficiencies, factor V Leiden (FVL), mutation of factor II, homozygosity of methylenetetrahydrofolate reductase (MTHFR), which leads to hyperhomocysteinemia. Deficiencies of factor VIII and fibrinogen, all are associated with pregnancy loss. FVL is the most common cause of hereditary thrombophilia (Seligsohn and Lubetsky, 2001).

Mechanism of abortion is same as APS. So treatment remains the same thromboprophylaxis. Aspirin 81 mg and low molecular heparin 40–80 mg daily till 35 weeks of pregnancy can prevent RPL associated with thrombophilias (Brenner et al. 2005).

> What is the newer concept of using intravenous immunoglobulin and corticosteroids in RPL with APS?

Neither corticosteroids nor intravenous immunoglobulin therapy improve the live birth rate of women with recurrent miscarriage associated with antiphospholipid antibodies compared with other treatment modalities; rather their use may provoke significant maternal and fetal morbidity. Well known prednisolone toxicities such as GDM, hypertension, preeclampsia, infections and osteoporosis contributed to the abandonment of prednisolone therapy for APS pregnancy (Lassere and Empson, 2004; Empson et al. 2002; ACOG, 1998). However, prednisolone therapy does have a place in treating the APS that is secondary to SLE.

> **Case scenario:** Mrs Nasima is carrying for 8 weeks. She had two previous blighted ovum and one 8 weeks live fetus expelled spontaneously. After thorough investigation you found nothing abnormality.
> How will you manage her?

Here the case may be unexplained. So 'tender loving care' will be enough for this type of patient. As live birth rates of 35–85% are reported in couples with unexplained RPL without any treatment (ACOG practice bulletin). Meta-analysis of randomized prospective studies suggests that 60–70% women with unexplained RPL will have a successful next pregnancy (Jeng, 1995). If patient is anxious empirical progesterone can be given till 12 weeks of pregnancy. Though the available data suggest that the use of empirical treatment in women with unexplained recurrent miscarriage is unnecessary and should be resisted. So counseling and supportive care holds the mainstay in management as available evidences suggest that unexplained recurrent miscarriage have an excellent prognosis for future pregnancy outcome without pharmacological intervention if supportive care alone is offered in the setting of a dedicated early pregnancy assessment unit. Though repeated missed abortion can be treated empirically by aspirin and heparin to prevent thrombotic defect of placenta.

RELATED INFORMATION

Role of Progesterone in RPL

Role of progesterone in RPL is debatable. The difficulty in determining the role of progesterone in preventing recurrent pregnancy loss is due to difficulty in determining who has progesterone deficiency and in establishing the diagnosis. There is no question that low-serum progesterone levels are associated with poor pregnancy outcome. Luteal phase defect (LPD) is an important aspect of progesterone deficiency. One study found that 70% of women with serum progesterone below 15 ng/mL successfully completed the first trimester with aggressive progesterone therapy strongly implies that low serum progesterone can be a correctable cause of miscarriage (Check, 1990). Even if it is used empirically miscarriage can be prevented. In a trial with unexplained RPL a significant reduction in the miscarriage rate was observed in women receiving dydrogesterone 10 mg orally daily in early pregnancy compared with those who remained untreated (El-Zibdeh, 2005).

Role of hCG in RPL

A Cochrane review (Scott, 2000) suggested that evidence for the use of hCG treatment in the prevention of RPL remains inconclusive and there is insufficient support for its routine use. So hCG therapy is not for all cases of RPL. It can be used in the following situations:
- Those with repeated early loss prior to a positive fetal heart beat.
- Those with an irregular cycle, would appear to be more likely to benefit. Sowing these criteria around 30% of cases of recurrent miscarriage could be offered hormonal support, with a success rate of around 85% (El-Zibdeh, 2005). Progesterone can be used for the same reason, but hCG has the advantage of being more 'natural' with similar effect as it works through releasing progesterone, from corpus luteum. Moreover, it is responsible for efficient corpus luteal function, which not only releases progesterone, but also other peptides, which might have some role for preventing abortions.

Despite inconsistent evidence reported in the literature, treatment with progesterone supplements and human chorionic gonadotropin hormones is often employed as a method of attempting to prevent miscarriage. In addition, some clinical studies support the administration of 17-alpha-hydroxyprogesterone in preventing preterm delivery.

> **Case scenario:** Mrs Tahera, 30-year-old woman presented with the history of three previous abortions at 18, 22 and 24 weeks of pregnancy.
>
> What investigations you will suggest her before planning the next pregnancy?

As all the cases are midtrimester abortions, the possible causes of midtrimester abortions are anatomical factors such as hypoplastic uterus, septate uterus and cervical incompetence or any space occupying lesion of uterus such as myoma, adenomyoma or uterine synechiae. Thrombophilias and antiphospholipid syndrome should be kept in mind. The information about the previous pregnancies is very important like:
- *Process of abortion:* Painless expulsion of the product of conception with sudden uterine contraction (suggestive of *cervical incompetence*).
- Hypoplastic uterus may be a factor in this case as the gestational age has progressively increased. In each pregnancy, uterus gained the capacity to accommodate the fetus.
- Arcuate uterus has a greater proportion of second trimester loss (in both arcuate and subseptate uterus, the length of the remaining cavity is shorter and there may be fundal distortion).
- There may be distortion of the shape of uterus due to multiple fibroids or short cervical length < 2.5 cm, which predispose to preterm labor.
- Presence of medical disorders such as antiphospholipid syndrome, uncontrolled DM.

The following investigations should be done for Mrs Tahera:
- *Ultrasonogram of the uterus and adenexae:* (preferably three dimensional):
  - To detect uterine malformations such as hypoplastic uterus, septate or arcuate uterus
  - To detect myoma and adenomyoma, and polyp of the uterus.
- Hysterosalpingography (HSG) to evaluate the contour of the uterine cavity, cervical canal and fallopian tubes.
  Or
  Hysteroscopy to evaluate uterine cavity.
- Laparoscopy to diagnose congenital and acquired anomalies.
- Endocrine assessments, TSH, FT4, prolactin, LH, blood sugar.

RELATED INFORMATION

Investigation of Uterine Integrity

Many different investigative tools are available to see the uterine integrity:

Ultrasonography

In patients with RPL particularly in repeated second trimester abortions imaging studies are important during initial work-up in order to assess the integrity of the uterus. Ultrasonography is currently the most readily available and least invasive mode of imaging in case of suspected uterine abnormalities.

a. *Transvaginal Sonography*
   Transvaginal sonography (TVS) is usually the initial step, but is now enhanced using 3D mode ultrasound. TVS allows accurate and rapid characterization of the uterus including its size and position as well as the presence of anomalies such as a duplicated cervix, duplicated uterus, uterine septum or unicornuate uterus. TVS is also useful in determining the size and location of the fibroid uterus as well as the presence of adenomyoma, intrauterine polyp and endometrial irregularities that might suggest adhesions. In pregnant state transvaginal USG a non-invasive procedure can be done to assess cervical length, shape and predict miscarriage and preterm birth in high-risk pregnancies. Ultrasound signs suggesting cervical incompetence are shortening of endocervical canal, funneling of internal os and sacculation or prolapse of the membrane into the cervix. A short cervix < 2.5 cm, is the best independent predictor of preterm birth before 34 weeks.

b. *Three-dimensional Ultrasound*
   Three-dimensional (3D) is now accepted as an accurate and reproducible means for the diagnosis of congenital anomalies. It has clear advantage over HSG, hysteroscopy and laparoscopy for the diagnosis of congenital uterine anomaly, since it is a non-invasive method. It has been suggested that the ability to visualize both the uterine cavity and the myometrium on a 3D scan facilitates the diagnosis of uterine anomalies and enables easy differentiation between subseptate and bicornuate uteri.

c. *Color Doppler Ultrasound*
   Color Doppler ultrasound may also allow visualization of intraseptal vascularity and may help in distinguishing the avascular from vascular septum.

Hysterosalpingography

Hysterosalpingography has long been used to evaluate the contour of the uterine cavity, cervical canal and fallopian tubes. Though radiopaque medium allows the accurate identification of filling defects, scarring and septum, it alone cannot differentiate between a septate uterus and bicornuate uterus. Furthermore, it cannot determine the myometrial extension or the size of intrauterine lesions. Therefore, HSG is primarily used to assess tubal patency, and has a limited role in the imaging of uterine malformation.

HSG provides information about the diameter and the shape of the cervical canal. A funnel-shaped isthmus is taken to be diagnostic for cervical insufficiency. Not applicable during pregnancy. If HSG shows funneling of the canal Hegar test to measure the diameter of the endocervical canal can be done. A cut-off of 6-8 mm is usually taken as to make the diagnosis of cervical insufficiency (Page 1958; Toaff et al. 1977). But recent advances of ultrasonographic assessment of cervical canal length replaced the use of both HSG funneling assessment and Hegars dilator test.

Intravenous Pyelography

Intravenous pyelography is recommended during the work-up of congenital anomalies. Defects in the urinary tract are commonly seen when a uterine anomaly is diagnosed.

Sonohysterography

Sonohysterography (SHG) was carried out by the intrauterine injection of an isotonic saline solution by Valenzano et al (Valenzano et al. 2006). The sensitivity and specificity of SHG was the same as for hysteroscopy. He, therefore, concluded that transvaginal SHG with saline solution is a low-cost, easy and helpful examination method for uterine malformations. If it can be done with 3D it allows precise recognition of lesions. It was further suggested that if 2D and 3D SHG are normal, invasive diagnostic procedure such as hysteroscopy can be avoided.

Magnetic Resonance Imaging

Magnetic resonance imaging (MRI) is an accurate non-invasive technique for the evaluation of uterine anomalies. HSG and SHG have replaced its use so MRI is justified only in special cases where its high accuracy and detailed elaboration of uterovaginal anatomy is needed for planning the most appropriate corrective surgery (Pui, 2004). However, the utility of MRI remains limited due to its cost.

Diagnostic Hysteroscopy

Hysteroscopy offers the best and most direct assessment of the uterine cavity. During the procedure the intracavitary structures can be directly visualized and directed biopsies can be obtained when indicated. This simple outpatient procedure remains the method of choice for assessment of the presence and extent of intrauterine adhesions. It is also the optimal method to evaluate the size and extension of polyps and submucous myoma. However, hysteroscopy alone cannot fully differentiate between a septate and a bicornuate uterus; laparoscopy or SHG is required to complete the evaluation.

Diagnostic Laparoscopy

Laparoscopy allows the surgeon to assess the outer surface of the uterus and other pelvic structures. It is used to establish the precise diagnosis of the various congenital and acquired anomalies. Currently laparoscopy is rarely used just to clarify uterine anomaly, and is generally reserved for women in whom interventional therapy is likely to be undertaken.

> What is cervical incompetence or cervical insufficiency?

It is a clinical diagnosis characterized by recurrent painless cervical dilatation **(Fig. 20.1B)** and spontaneous mid-trimester loss, generally in the absence of obvious predisposing conditions such as spontaneous membrane rupture, bleeding or infection. The pathophysiology of cervical insufficiency is still poorly understood. The cervix of a woman with cervical incompetence contains a higher proportion of smooth muscle cells compared with the cervix of a pregnant woman with cervical competency **(Fig. 20.1A)** (Bucking, 1965; Roddick, 1961). Deficiencies of cervical collagens (Rechberger, 1988; Petersen, 1996) cervical elastin (Leppert, 1987) or other structural, mechanical components of cervical connective tissue have been postulated as etiological factors. These factors normally resist softening, effacement and dilatation caused by the gravitational effect of the fetus and amniotic fluid.

> What are the other causes of cervical weakness?

Other causes of cervical weakness are:
Trauma to the cervix from:
a. Surgical procedures such as conization
b. Dilatation and curettage
c. Traumatic delivery
d. Traumatic instrumental delivery with cervical tearing
e. Forceful expulsion of the fetus before full dilatation of cervix leading to cervical tear.

> Among TAS and TVS, which is better to detect funneling of cervical canal and why?

Both transabdominal and transvaginal USG can diagnose cervical insufficiency. But TVS is better predictor for cervical insufficiency. Limitation of transabdominal USG is it requires full bladder in order to visualize the cervix, which can cause false-negative result. Because full bladder can press on the dilated cervix and can cause lengthening of the canal (Andersen, 1991; Confino, 1986). This problem can be overcome if a vaginal probe is used. Funneling and shortening can be identified. Ultrasound can detect dilatation of internal os before external os is affected.

> Tahera conceived again. Now she is 10 weeks pregnant. What measure do you like to take for cervical insufficiency?

Cervical cerclage operation by McDonald technique or Shirodkar technique is to be done after 12 weeks of pregnancy before dilatation of cervical canal. The success rate is reasonably high in properly selected cases at 14 weeks before dilatation of the cervix.

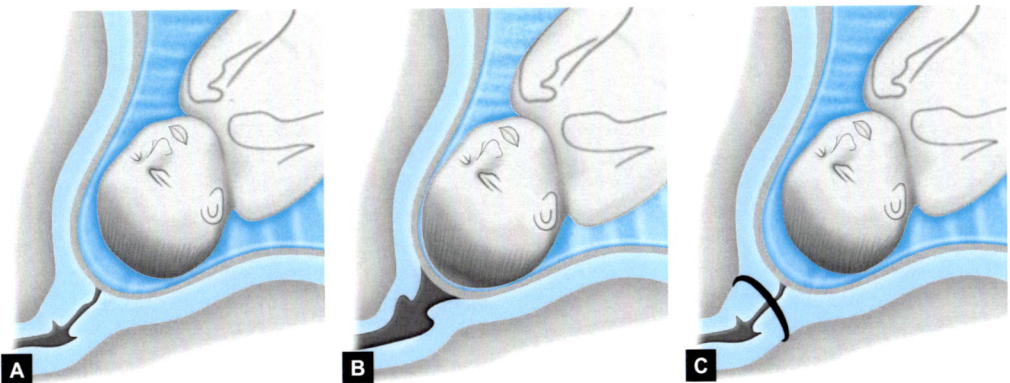

Figs 20.1A to C (A) Competent cervix; (B) Incompetent cervix; (C) McDonald suture

RELATED INFORMATION

Techniques of Cerclage

McDonald Technique

It is the simplest procedure to perform (Fig. 20.1C). The procedure consists of suturing of the cervix as high as possible by a purse-string suture in five or six bites. The knot is positioned on the anterior aspect of the cervix at 10–11 O'clock and the free end of the threads are tied leave a loop in order to facilitate early removal. Advantage of this technique is that it can be performed by relatively junior staff. However, the disadvantage of the McDonald technique is that in cases of high cervical tears it may not be possible to place the suture high enough. Ideally, the suture should be placed at the level of the internal os.

The Shirodkar Technique

A transverse incision is made on the anterior side of the cervix and the bladder is pushed up above the internal os. A vertical incision is then made in the posterior vaginal wall. The stitch is placed in two bites, penetrating the cervical tissue laterally. The mucosal incisions are then closed. Advantage of this technique is that suture can be given up to 3 cm higher than the McDonald technique.

Abdominal Approach

If the suture needs to be placed still higher or in case of severe cervical scarring after multiple failures of vaginal cerclage an abdominal approach can be used (Davis, 2000). It can be performed by laparotomy or laparoscopy (Scibetta, 1998). In the technique of Anthony, et al. the bladder is mobilized, the uterine arteries are identified and tunnels are created medial to the uterine arteries, a 5 mm Mersilene tape is then passed through the tunnels and the stitch is tied anteriorly.

Though cervical cerclage is a recognized treatment option for cervical incompetence, but it is associated with potential hazards related to the surgery and the risk of stimulating uterine contractions and hence should be considered only in women who are likely to benefit. As evidences suggest that if a woman had history of 2 or 3 miscarriages without bleeding or clear sign of labor preceding the miscarriage may benefit from prophylactic cerclage at 13–14 weeks.

> Is there any role of cervical cerclage in prevention of preterm birth?

The role of cervical cerclage in the prevention of preterm birth has been examined in a recently published RCOG Green-top Guideline Cochrane review of four randomized controlled trials found no conclusive evidence that prophylactic cerclage reduces the risk of pregnancy loss and preterm delivery in women at risk of preterm birth or midtrimester loss owing to cervical factors. A meta-analysis of individual patient-level data from four controlled trials reported that women with singleton pregnancies, a short cervix (less than 25 mm) and previous second trimester miscarriage, cerclage may reduce the incidence of preterm birth before 35 weeks of gestation (RR 0.57, 95% CI 0.33–99) (Berghella, 2005).

> **Case scenario:** Mrs Rehana has history of four consecutive pregnancy losses. By two-dimensional ultrasonography her uterus found septate.
> What will be your decision for her next pregnancy?

After exclusion of other causes if it is found that septum might be responsible for RPL then hysteroscopic metroplasty (septoplasty/septal resection) is to be done before next pregnancy.

RELATED INFORMATION

Although there are no randomized controlled studies, observational studies have reported impressive results following incision of a septum in patients with RPL. Following hysteroscopic metroplasty the cumulative birth rates at 36 weeks were 75% in septate and 67% in subseptate uterus (Fedele et al. 1993). A meta-analysis of published retrospective data of observational studies comparing pregnancy outcome before and after hysteroscopic metroplasty indicated a marked improvement after surgery (Homer, 2000). Author suggested that septate uterus *per se* is not an indication for surgical intervention as it is not always associated with poor obstetric outcome. Even in women with one miscarriage it is not indicated as after a single miscarriage 80–90% will have live birth in the next pregnancy.

Another nonrandomized trial shown 85% live birth rate after hysteroscopic septum resection (Grimbizis et al. 2001). Due to low morbidity associated with hysteroscopic resection of septum, abdominal surgery is rarely indicated. Hysteroscopic metroplasty is associated with increased risk of uterine rupture in subsequent pregnancy in comparison to uncomplicated hysteroscopic resection of submucous myoma and polyp (Sentilhes et al. 2005). However, a more liberalized approach to treatment is advocated by most authorities in light of the simplicity, minimal postoperative sequelae, and improved reproductive outcome associated with hysteroscopic metroplasty (Homer, 2000; Grimbizis et al. 2001).

Role of Surgery in Other Situations

It is generally agreed that adhesions, polyps and protruding submucous myomas should be hysteroscopically resected. Other intramural myomas, which compress the cavity or distort the cavity should be removed. Due to significant morbidity and lack of controlled data abdominal metroplasty for bicornuate uterus is reserved for only those patients with recurrent and severe second and third trimester problems.

> **Case scenario:** Mrs Farida, 23 years old had two pregnancy losses at 16 and 18 weeks of pregnancy. She is now 10 weeks pregnant and on investigation she was found to have bacterial vaginosis.
> What will be your suggestions for her?

The presence of bacterial vaginosis in the first trimester of pregnancy has been reported as a risk factor for second-trimester miscarriage and preterm delivery, though the evidence for an association with first trimester miscarriage is inconsistent. A randomized placebo-controlled trial reported that treatment of bacterial vaginosis early in the second trimester with oral clindamycin significantly reduces the incidence of second-trimester miscarriage and preterm birth in the general population. So she should be treated by Clindamycin for the bacterial vaginosis.

> **Case scenario:** Mrs Laila, aged 26 years, para- 0 + 3 first trimester abortions and known case of hypothyroidism. Now her thyroid function is normal, but antithyroid antibody (ATA) is positive.
> What is your comment regarding this report and her repeated pregnancy loss?

Systemic maternal endocrine disorders like thyroid disease have been associated with miscarriage. However, in treated cases thyroid dysfunction is not a risk factor for recurrent miscarriage. With normal thyroid function ATA have no impact on pregnancy outcome (Rushworth, 2000). One possibility is that positive ATAs coincide with other autoimmune disorders suggesting an immunoregulatory dysfunction as the underlying cause of the reproductive losses. Up to 45.5% of patients with active systemic lupus erythematosus have positive ATAs. So patient should be counseled accordingly and other causes of RPL should be evaluated.

> *Why TORCH is not recommended for routine investigation of RPL?*

Any severe infection that leads to bacteremia or viremia can cause sporadic miscarriage. But for an infective agent to appear as an etiologic factor of repeated pregnancy loss, it must be capable of persisting in the genital tract, and avoiding detection, or must cause symptoms to disturb the woman. Toxoplasmosis, rubella, cytomegalovirus, herpes and listeria infections do not fulfill these criteria. They may cause sporadic miscarriage, but not responsible for recurrent miscarriage. That is why TORCH is not recommended as routine investigation for RPL.

> *What is the immunological basis of RPL?*

- Immune-mediated abortions are known to be characterized by either autoimmune or alloimmune disturbances
- In autoimmune abortions the development of placenta and the embryo is affected by maternal autoantibodies
- In alloimmune abortions, the maternal immune system reacts against the embryo and damages trophoblast through allogeneic, rejection-type reactions
- Approximately 30% of women with unexplained RSA have increased serum levels of autoantibodies; autoimmune abortions are associated with APA, ANA, LA, AssDNA, AdsDNA
- Alloimmune abortions are associated with different cytokines such as TH1, TH2, NK cells
- For prevention of autoimmune abortions thromboprophylaxis is needed.

To prevent alloimmune abortions:
- Active immunization of women using paternal or third party lymphocytes are needed.
- Passive immunization in the form of intravenous administration of immunoglobulin G (IVIG).

> **Case scenario:** *Marufa, a known case of PCOS with history of recurrent miscarriage.*
> *Will you suggest metformin in prevention of recurrent miscarriage in her present pregnancy?*

Yes. Patients with PCOS have an increased rate of pregnancy loss (> 50%), predominantly during early gestation (Glueck et al. 2002). The underlying causes include obesity, hyperinsulinemia, hyperandrogenemia, insulin resistance, poor endometrial receptivity and elevated LH. There are several studies confirming the findings of LH hypersecretion in RPL (Glueck et al. 2001). Hyperinsulinemia and insulin resistance have been claimed to be a potential cause of the high rate of RPL in patients with PCOS and have been linked to many of the metabolic and endocrine abnormalities potentially associated with the physiopathology of RPL. Metformin has been the main treatment advocated to reduce RPL in PCOS patients. It is a category B drug and clinical practice is always ahead of evidence-based practice. Different small trials shows reduced incidence of abortion in PCOS on metformin (Glueck et al. 2001; Begum et al. 2004). Some investigators consider that the potential benefit of metformin out-weight its risks and advocate its use to reduce miscarriage (Stadtmauer, 2002). *So she can be given metformin or continue it if she is on metformin.* However, there are no randomized controlled trials to assess the role of metformin in women with recurrent miscarriage and this should be explored.

The increased risk of miscarriage in women with PCOS has been attributed to insulin resistance and hyperinsulinemia. There is a relation of increased abortion with high LH level. Though mechanism is not known.

> *If chromosomal analysis of any one of partner shows abnormality, what will be your suggestions for them?*

The couple should be offered genetic counseling and if available should be referred to clinical geneticist.

Options of treatment are:
- Preimplantation genetic diagnosis (PGD) and transfer of good embryos through ART
- ART with donor egg.

> **How male factor contributes to RPL?**

Role of sperm factors (oxidative stress, mitochondrial mutations and DNA damage) in spontaneous abortion has been focused now a days. Role of sperm DNA integrity is now believed to be a critical limiting factor that affects both fertility and embryogenesis. Sperm DNA damage may lead to impaired fertilization, pre- or post- implantation failure, disrupted embryonic development and early pregnancy loss. One of the most important factors leading to DNA damage in sperm is oxidative stress. Seminal ROS levels are significantly more among the males of RPL.

BIBLIOGRAPHY

American College of Obstetricians and Gynecologists. Anticoagulation with low-molecular-weight heparin during pregnancy. ACOG Committee opinion 211. Washington DC:ACOG; 1998.

Andersen HF. Transvaginal and transabdominal ultrasonography of the uterine cervix during pregnancy. J clin Ultrasound. 1991;19:77-83.

Begum MR, Khanom N, Quadir E, Ferdous J, Begum MS, Khan F, Begum A. Prevention of GDM by Continuing Metformin Therapy Throughout Pregnancy in Women with Polycystic Ovary Syndrome (PCOS). J Obstet. Gynaecol Res. 2009;35(2):282-6.

Berghella V, Odibo OA, To MS, et al. Cervix on ultrasonography meta-analysis of trials using individual patient-level data. Obstet Gynecol. 2005;106:181-9.

Boue J, Boue A, Lazar P. Retrospective and prospective epidemiological studies of 1500 karyotyped spontaneous human abortions. Teratology. 1975;12:11-26.

Branch WD, Khamashta MA. Antiphospholipid syndrome: obstetric diagnosis, management, and controversies. Obstet Gynecol. 2003;101:1333-44.

Branch WD, Silver RM, Blackwell JL, et al. Outcome of treated pregnancies in women with antiphospholipid syndrome: an update of the Utah experience. Obstet Gynecol. 1992;80:614-20.

Brenner B, Hoffman R, Carp HJA, et al. The LIVE-ENOX investigators. Efficacy and safety of two dose of enoxaparin in women with thrombophilia and recurrent pregnancy loss: The LIVE-ENOX study. J Thromb Haemost. 2005;3:227-9.

Buckingham JC, Buethe RA, Danforth DN. Collagen-muscle ratio in clinically normal and clinically incompetent services. Am J Obstet Gynecol. 1965;92:232-7.

Carp HJ A, Torchinsky A, Portuguese S, et al. The Recurrent Miscarriage Immunotherapy Trialists Group. Paternal leukocyte immunization after five or more miscarriages. Hum. Reprod.1997; 12:250-5.

Check JH, Winkel CA, Check ML. Abortion rate in progesterone treated women presenting initially with low first trimester serum progesterone levels. Am J Gynecol Health. 1990;4:33-4.

Confino E, Mayden KL, Giglia RV, et al. Pitfalls in sonographic imaging of the incompetent uterine cervix. Acta Obstet Gynecol Scand. 1986;65:593-7.

Davis G, Berghella V, Talucci M, et al. Patients with a prior failed transvaginal cerclage: a comparison of obstetric outcomes with a either transabdominal or transvaginal cerclage. Am J Obstet Gynecol. 2000; 183:836-9.

Derksen RH, Khamashta MA, Branch DW. Management of obstetric antiphospholipid syndrome. Arthritis Rheum. 2004;50:1028-39.

El-Zibdeh MY. Dydrogesterone in the reduction of recurrent spontaneous abortion. J Steroid Biochem Mol Biol. 2005;97:431-4.

Empson M, Lassere M, Craig JC, et al. Recurrent pregnancy loss with antiphospholipid antibody: a systematic review of randomized therapeutic trials. Obstet gynecol. 2002;99:135-44.

ESHRE early pregnancy guideline development group. Guideline of the European Society of Human Reproduction and Embryology for Recurrent Pregnancy Loss; 2017.

Fedele L, Arcaina L, Parazzini F, et al. Reproductive prognosis after hysteroscopic metroplasty in 102 women: life-table analysis. Fertil Steril. 1993;59: 768-72.

Fertility and Employment 1979. The Danish Data Archives No. 0363, Odense University.

Glueck CJ, Philips H, Cameron D, et al. Continuing metformin throughout pregnancy in women with polycystic ovary syndrome appears to safely reduce first-trimester spontaneous abortion; a pilot study. Fertil Steril. 2001;75:46-52.

Glueck CJ, Wang P, Fontaine RN, et al. Pregnancy outcome among women with polycystic ovary syndrome treated with metformin. Hum Reprod. 2002;17:2858-64.

Grandone E, Margagline M, Colaizzo D, et al. Factor V Leiden is associated with repeated and recurrent unexplained fetal losses. Thromb Haemost. 1997;77:822-4.

Grimbizis GF, Gamus M, Tarlatzis BC, et al. Clinical implications of uterine malformations and hysteroscopic treatment results. Hum Reprod update. 2001; 7:161-74.

Hassold TJ. A cytogenetic study of repeated spontaneous abortions. Am J Hum Genet. 1980;32:723-30.

Homer HA, Li TC, Cooke ID. The septate uterus: a review of management and reproductive outcome. Fertil Steril. 2000;73:1-14.

Jeng GT, Scott JR, Burmeister LF. A comparison of meta-analytic results using literature vs individual patient data. Paternal cell immunization for recurrent miscarriage. JAMA. 1995;274:830-6.

Kuttech WH. Antiphospholipid antibody-associated recurrent pregnancy loss: treatment with heparin and low-dose aspirin is superior to low-dose aspirin alone. Am J Obstet gynecol. 1996;174:1584-9.

Lassere M, Empson M. Treatment of antiphospholipid syndrome in pregnancy—a systematic review of randomized therapeutic trials. Thromb Res. 2004; 114:419-26.

Leppert PC, Yu SY, Keller S, et al. Decreased elastic fibers and desmosine content in incompetent cervix. Am J Obstet Gynecol. 1987;157:1134-9.

Lima F, Khamashta MA, Buchanan NM, et al. A study of sixty pregnancies in patients with the antiphospholipid syndrome. Clin Exp Rheumatol. 1996; 14:131-6.

Page EW. Incompetent internal os of the cervix causing late abortion and premature labor. Technique for surgical repair. Obstet Gyecol. 1958;12:509-15.

Petersen LK, Uldbjerg N. Cervical collagen in non-pregnant women with previous cervical incompetence. Eur J Obstet Gynecol Reprod Biol. 1996;67:41-5.

Preston FE, Rosendaal FR, Walker ID, et al. Increased fetal loss in women with heritable thrombophilia. Lancet. 1996;348:913-16.

Pui MH. Imaging diagnosis of congenital uterine malformation. Comput Med Imaging Graph. 2004;28:425-33.

Rechberger T, Uldbjerg N, Oxlund H. Connective tissue changes in the cervix during normal pregnancy and pregnancy complications by cervical incompetence. Obstet Gynecol. 1988;71:563-7.

Roddick JW, Buckingham JC, Danforth DN. The muscular cervix-a cause of incompetency in pregnancy. Obstet Gynecol. 1961;17:562-5.

Rushworth FH, Backos M, Rai R, et al. Prospective pregnancy out-come in untreated recurrent miscarries with thyroid autoantibodies. Hum Reprod. 2000;15:1637-9.

Scibetta JJ, Sanko SR, Phipps WR. Laparoscopic transabdominal cervicoisthmic cerclage. Fertil Steril. 1998;69:161-3.

Scott JR, Pattison N. Human Chorionic gonadotrophin for recurrent miscarriage. Coehrane Database Syst Rev. 2000;(2):CD000101.

Seligsohn U, Lubetsky A. Genetic susceptibility to venous thrombosis. N Engl J Med. 2001;344:1222-31.

Sentilhes L, Sergent F, Roman H, et al. Late complications of operative hysteroscopy: predicting patients at risk of uterine rupture during subsequent pregnancy. Eur J Obstet Gynecol Reprod Biol. 2005;120: 134-8.

Simpson JL, Bombard AT. Chromosomal abnormalities in spontaneous abortion: frequency, pathology and genetic counseling. In: Edmonds KB, (Ed). Spontaneous Abortion. Oxford: Blackwell; 1987. pp.51-76.

Sorokin Y, Johnson MP, Uhlmann WR, et al. Postmortem chorionic villus sampling: correlation of cytogenetic and ultrasound findings. Am J Med Genet. 1991;39:314-16.

Stadtmauer LA, Wong BC, Oehninger S. Should Patients with polycystic ovary syndrome be treated with metformin? Benefits of insulin sensitizing drugs in polycystic ovary syndrome- beyond ovulation induction. Hum Reprod. 2002;17:3016-26.

Stray-Pedersen B, Lorentzen-Styr AM. The prevalence of toxoplasma antibodies among 11,736 pregnant women in Norway. Scand J Infect Dis. 1979;11: 159-65.

Strom CM, Ginsberg N, Applebaum M, et al. Analyses of 95 first trimester spontaneous abortions by chorionic villus sampling and karyotype. J Assist Reprod Genet. 1992;9:458-61.

Tincani A, Branch W, Levy RA, et al. Treatment of pregnant patients with antiphospholipid syndrome. Lupus. 2003;12:524-9.

Toaff R, Toaff ME, Ballas S, et al. Cervical incompetence: diagnostic and therapeutic aspects. Isr J Med Sci. 1997;13:39-49.

Valenzano MM, Mistrangelo E, Lijoi D, Fortunato T, Lantieri PB, et al. Transvaginal sonohysterographic evaluation of uterine malformations. Eur. J Obstet. Gynecol. Reprod. Biol., 2006;124:246-9.

Warburton D, Strobino B. Recurrent spontaneous abortion. In Bennet MJ, Edmonds DK, (Eds). Spontaneous Recurrent abortion. Oxford: Blackwell Scientific; 1987.p.193.

World Health Organization. Recommended definitions; terminology and format for statistical tables related to perinatal period. Acta Obstet Gynecol Scand. 1977;56:247-53.

CHAPTER 21

Genitourinary Fistula

Muna Shalima Jahan, Rashida Begum, Sayeba Akhter

INTRODUCTION

Genitourinary fistula is a condition where an abnormal communication develops between female genital organs with the urinary tract and/or rectum. The women with fistulae suffer from constant leaking of urine, stool or both. In developing world, genitourinary fistulae are mostly of obstetric origin, whereas in developed countries the causative factors are nonobstetric, primarily occurs as complication of surgeries or malignancies.

> **Case scenario:** Mrs Nargis Akhter, 19-year-old, Para 1 (dead), comes to gynecology outpatient clinic of your hospital with complaints of continuous dribbling of urine for last 2 years.
> How will you proceed to diagnose the case?

Detailed History

History of Dribbling of Urine

- Since, when she has started dribbling?
- Does she have any urge for urination?
- Was there any precipitating factor such as delivery, surgery, etc?
- If any history of surgery, then what type of surgery, it was?
- If it was pregnancy related, then following questions need to be asked:
  - Was she a booked case?
  - Was there any antenatal visit?
  - Was it a term pregnancy?
  - How long was the duration of labor?
  - Where did the delivery occur?
  - What was the mode of delivery?
  - Who conducted the delivery?
  - Whether she had suffered from fever or any offensive vaginal discharge following delivery?
  - What was the time interval of delivery and dribbling of urine?
  - Did the child survive?
  - Whether any operative intervention was needed for delivering the baby?
- Is she menstruating regularly?
- If not, in the absence of menstruation, is there any cyclical lower abdominal pain?

Other Complaints

- Does she suffer from dyspareunia/apareunia?
- Can she hold stool/loose stool/flatus?
- Does she have any neurological problem?
- Social history?

Treatment History

Did she receive any treatment for this? Particularly any surgical treatment?

Examination

Physical examination is to be done thoroughly.

> On enquiry, you elicited that it was her first pregnancy and she never took any antenatal care (ANC). She went to labor spontaneously at term and had labor pain for 5 days. Finally, she delivered a dead male baby at home and the delivery was conducted by traditional dai. After delivery, she had risen of temperature. She started dribbling 6 days after delivery. Dribbling is continuous and there is no urge of micturition. She has no complaints about defecation. Her menstrual cycle has not established, since delivery and she has no history of lower abdominal pain. Her husband left her and got married again, so there is no complaints about coitus.
>
> *Contd...*

Contd...

> Uriniferous smell is present all around. On physical examination, she is moderately anemic, underweight, height 138 cm. Abdomen is soft and not tender. On inspection, her vulva is excoriated and urine is continuously dribbling from vagina. After introduction of speculum into the vagina a small hole is seen at midvagina through which bladder mucosa is protruding and urine is continuously draining out. On bimanual examination an opening felt in the midvagina, which admitted tip of the finger. Rest of the vagina is healthy. Cervix is almost flushed. Uterus normal size. Nothing abnormality is detected after per rectal (PR) examination. She did not receive any treatment.
>
> What is your diagnosis?

The clinical diagnosis is vesicovaginal fistula (VVF) with secondary amenorrhea.

RELATED INFORMATION

Obstetric fistula results from prolonged neglected obstructed labor. Exact prevalence of fistula cases is not known and as often estimates are based on women, who seek treatment, so may be grossly underestimated. Estimates are up to two million in Africa alone (Brain and Andrew, 2009). Women of South-East Asia and some Arab countries also suffer from obstetric fistulae. Situation Analysis of Obstetric Fistula in Bangladesh, done in 2003, showed that an estimated total number of about 71,000 women are living with obstetric fistulae and newer cases are being added every day.

A woman with obstetric fistulae suffers not only from urinary or fecal incontinence, but also from extensive physical and psychosocial morbidities. Researchers put this broad range of injuries under the heading of 'Obstructed Labor Injury Complex' (Arrowsmith, 1996). The typical scenario of an obstetric fistula patient is a small, innocent, poor village girl, illiterate and ignorant, lives in an unhygienic condition, thriving malnourished, smelly, physically disabled, psychologically broken hearted, socially outcast, who remains jobless, childless, helpless and lives without any hope. The fistula patients has three life, *first* is the life of a common village girl, which she had before developing the fistula, *second* the most miserable, neglected, uncivilized life, when she was living with fistula and the *third* when she is cured from fistula and seems to be born second time with a new life.

Genitourinary fistula is developed between ureters/bladder and/or urethra with uterus/cervix/vagina, which results in continuous dribbling of urine.

Types of Fistula

There are different types of fistula:
1. Vesicovaginal fistula (VVF): An abnormal communication between urinary bladder and vagina. This is the most common type of genitourinary fistula **(Fig. 21.1)**.
2. Urethrovaginal fistula.
3. Ureterovaginal fistula.

A combination of vesicoureterovaginal and other less common types are also reported.

Genitourinary fistula can be classified in different ways.

Mostly it is classified on the basis of certain factors:
- Size
- Site.

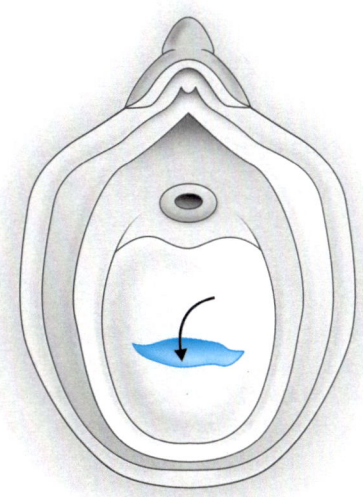

Fig. 21.1 Vesicovaginal fistula

According to Size

- Tiny admit only a small probe
- Small (0.5–1.5 cm)
- Medium (1.5–3 cm)
- Large (>3 cm) including circumferential loss of urethrovesical junction
- Extensive, major loss of bladder and urethra, with a large gap between the two.

According to Location

- *Juxta-urethral:* Most common fistula developed at the urethrovesical junction usually with some loss of urethra.
- *Vesicovaginal or mid-vaginal:* The fistula usually develops at the base of bladder and remains away from urethral orifice.
- *Juxtracervical:* Fistula that formed near the cervix, usually following cesarean section.
- *Vesicouterine and vesicocervical fistule* are rare and almost always develop following cesarean section.
- *Ureterovaginal fistula:* An abnormal communication between ureter and vagina. This is less common and usually develop following surgical trauma and rarely developmental/congenital.

There is no universal standardized classification of fistula. Two recent attempts have been made to standardized classification system, one of them is by Kees Waaldijk and the most experienced fistula surgeon. Waaldijk classification is mostly used by African surgeons.

Waaldijk Classification (Waaldijk, 1994)

- *Type I:* Fistula 5 cm or more away from external urethral orifice (EUO) and not involving the closing mechanism.
- *Type II:* Fistula that involves the closing mechanism (<5 cm away from EUO):
  - Without (sub) total involvement of the urethra:
    - Without circumferential defect
    - With circumferential defect.
  - With (sub) total involvement of urethra:
    - Without circumferential defect
    - With circumferential defect.
- *Type III:* Miscellaneous fistula, ureterovaginal and other exceptional fistula.

Genitourinary fistula may be congenital or acquired. Congenital variety is rare and often associated with other urogenital anomaly. According to the social development and healthcare status of a country etiology of acquired genitourinary fistula differs. In low resource countries, i.e. Bangladesh, most of the genitourinary fistulas are of obstetric origin, developed as a sequel of prolonged neglected labor though fistula following pelvic, especially gynecologic surgeries are increasing in number. Whereas in developed countries, nonobstetric causes like radiation or surgery are frequently responsible for fistula formation.

Mechanism of Development of Obstetric Fistula

Obstetric fistula develops as a sequel of prolonged obstructed labor, resulting from pressure necrosis of both bladder and vaginal wall, but may result from direct injury during operative delivery.

Pressure Necrosis

When labor is prolonged and becomes obstructed, vaginal wall and the bladder and/or rectum are compressed between pubic bone and fetal head. Persistent compression for at least three hours, compromises the blood supply and this wide spread ischemic vascular injury leads to pressure necrosis (Arrowsmith, 1996). When the pressure is relieved, the necrosed tissue begins to slough out within 3–5 days resulting in fistula formation. Site and extent of fistula depend on the level and duration of obstruction.

Direct Injury

Caused by:

- Instruments used in destructive procedures to deliver stillborn infants or in criminal abortion
- Inappropriate application of forceps
- Symphysiotomy
- Cesarean section
- Cesarean hysterectomy.

Direct injury results in leakage of urine immediately after the procedure except tying or the inclusion of bladder tissue or ureter within the knot.

Factors for Making the Woman Vulnerable for Developing Obstetric Fistula

- Many physical and socioeconomic factors are involved in the development of obstetric genitourinary fistula.
- Early marriage and child bearing at young age.
- Malnutrition and short stature leading to cephalopelvic disproportion in first pregnancy.
- Long duration of obstruction and/or delivery of a still birth.
- Less access to obstetric care services directly play role in developing obstetric fistula.
- Lack of education, poverty, cultural and religious practices and above all United Nations Population Fund (UNFPA) outlined 3 classic delays in receiving health care, all these issues indirectly make the woman vulnerable to development of obstetric fistula (Muleta et al. 2010; Meyer et al. 2007).

Nonobstetric Causes of Fistula

- Injury at the time of gynecologic or urological surgery.
- Extension of malignant or granulomatous diseases.
- Foreign body, e.g. forgotten vaginal pessary.

Surgical Trauma

Because of close anatomical relation between the female reproductive tract and the ureter/bladder, the risk of the development of fistula increases after pelvic surgery (Demirci et al. 2012). Among gynecological operations, hysterectomy is particularly related to the causation. Emergency cesarean hysterectomy, hysterectomy for malignant or large tumors, or for pelvic inflammatory disease or severe endometriosis, all increase the risk of damage. Anatomical conditions, such as adiposity and narrow space in the lesser pelvis also pose risk of injury during dissection. Mechanism of fistula development following hysterectomy or other pelvic surgeries are tissue devascularization, and denervation and the location of the injury on the bladder and its proximity to the vaginal cuff is also important (Demirci et al. 2012; Duong et al. 2009).

Radiation

Radiation therapy induces an endarteritis, which leads to tissue necrosis, and subsequent potential fistula formation. Usually this type of fistula occurs months to years after radiation therapy.

Trauma and Foreign Body

Trauma sustained during sexual activity or sexual assault, accidental trauma of genital tract rarely can be responsible for fistula formation. Foreign bodies such as a neglected pessary, an aerosol cap, and vesical calculi are also documented agents.

Corrosive Agents

Use of corrosive agents used as a treatment of prolapsed uterus or dyspareunia are also found during clinical practice.

Other Rare Causes

Include chronic diseases such as urinary tuberculosis, lymphogranuloma venereum, inflammatory bowel disease and autoimmune diseases.

> Suppose you could not find the fistula easily, but urine is coming out through the vagina.
> How will you proceed further for the diagnosis?

In such a case examination under anesthesia (EUA) and dye test need to be done.

RELATED INFORMATION

During evaluation, it is mandatory to differentiate urinary leakage through a VVF or ureterovaginal fistula (extra-urethral leakage) from stress/urge/urinary incontinence (transurethral leakage).

Physical Examinations

Proper physical examination is facilitated by:
- Use of a speculum
- Good lighting
- Positioning (lithotomy/Trendelenburg/left-lateral/knee-chest as appropriate).

In the case of a large VVF, urine is encountered immediately after introduction of speculum; in most cases, the fistula can be visualized easily and the diagnosis is confirmed. In certain situation confusion may arise and special tests need to be done.

Simple Dye Test

It is done when fistula could not be seen or palpated and to exclude more than one fistula. The patient with lithotomy position, a speculum is inserted into the vagina to facilitate inspection. If the fistula is not easily visualized, the vaginal apex is sponged dry, and 60 mL of dilute solution of methylene blue is instilled in the bladder via a catheter. After 1 minute, patient has to be asked to cough. If VVF is present, dye will be seen coming out through the fistulous opening into vagina.

Three Swab Test

This is a special dye test, which helps in delineating the site of fistula and to differentiate uretero vaginal, vesicovaginal and urethro-vaginal fistula. Three cotton swabs are placed in the vagina one at the upper vagina, one at the middle, and one in the lower vagina. Diluted methylene blue is instilled into bladder through a catheter and wait for 1 minute. Swab need to be removed one after another. If the upper swab is soaked with urine, but unstained with dye and the lower two remain dry, it is ureterovaginal fistula. If the middle swab is stained with dye and upper and lower swabs remain dry, it is vesicovaginal fistula. If the upper two swabs remain dry and lower swab stained with dye, it is urethrovaginal fistula.

If none of the swabs is stained, there could still be a fistula. The test has to be repeated using 200 mL of dye. The patient should be allowed to walk for 20 minutes and then the swabs again have to be removed one by one and inspect. Sometimes tiny fistula needed careful search as there is a chance of missing it. If still there is doubt double dye test may be done.

Examination Under Anesthesia

Sometimes *examination under anesthesia* may be needed for proper evaluation of fistula. This is useful:
- In examination of patients with vaginal stenosis, tenderness and with small fistula.
- In planning surgery, especially in difficult and residual cases.
- Usually EUA is done/planned just before proceeding to surgery.
- Routine careful per rectal examination is mandatory. Otherwise there is a chance of missing rectovaginal fistula (RVF). Sometimes small RVF is hidden behind the fibrous band in posterior vagina.

> Suppose during proper physical examination, a fistula of about 2 × 1.5 cm found in the bladder base through which bladder mucosa is protruding. A metal catheter introduced through urethra came out through the fistula indicating integrity of urethra. There is no scarring of vaginal mucosa.
> Do you think this patient needs dye test?

No, dye test is not always necessary to delineate the fistula. If the fistula is not obvious or there is doubt of associated smaller additional fistula, then dye test might help. But, here fistula is obvious and be felt and seen.

> This patient has no urge for micturition. Suppose, she is having continuous dribbling and urge as well, what could be the possibility?

She might have ureterovaginal fistula.

Ureterovaginal fistula usually involves one ureter and traumatic in origin. So, accumulation of urine into the bladder through other ureter is responsible for desire to pass urine along with incontinence due to communication of opposite ureter with the vagina. In a very big vesicovaginal fistula, following a too long labor, one of the ureter may open in the vagina directly due to involvement of the ureterovesical junction in the ischemic process. More often, they are caused by operative injury during cesarean section or an emergency hysterectomy for a ruptured uterus.

> Why Nargis Akhter is not having her regular menses?

She might be suffering from secondary amenorrhea of *hypothalamocortical origin* due to strong desire to stop leaking anything through vagina or due to ischemic damage of endometrium following prolonged labor or due to obstruction in the outflow of menstrual blood, e.g. cervical stenosis.

RELATED INFORMATION

Often VVF is not the only consequence of prolonged obstructed labor rather may be associated with some other physical and social morbidities.

These injuries may include, total urethral loss, stress incontinence, hydroureteronephrosis, renal failure, bladder calculi formation, rectovaginal fistula, rectal atresia, anal sphincter incompetence, urine dermatitis, amenorrhea, cervical destruction, vaginal stenosis, pelvic inflammatory disease, secondary infertility, osteitis pubis and foot-drop. Among the serious social problems are divorce, separation from their families, exclusion from religious and social activities, worsening poverty, malnutrition, and almost unendurable sufferings (Arrowsmith et al. 1996).

Urine Dermatitis

Excoriation of vulva and inner thigh from the irritation of continuous leakage of urine, especially if concentrated. There may be superimposed secondary infection.

Vaginal Stenosis

Vaginal size may be significantly reduced from extensive scarring and fibrosis of vaginal mucosa. A ring-like stenosis usually occurs at the level of mid-vagina. In some cases even tip of the finger cannot be negotiated.

Secondary Amenorrhea

May be due to ischemic destruction of endometrium, or of *hypothalamocortical* origin. In some women due to vaginal or cervical stenosis, cryptomenorrhea may be present. Those patients will also have cyclical lower abdominal pain.

Foot Drop

It is a manifestation of compression damage to the lumbosacral plexus. About 90% patients with foot drop slowly recover, but may take up to 2 years. There may also be saddle anesthesia with loss of anal reflex and the risk of pressure sores (Brian et al. 2009).

Musculofascial and Bone Damage

The levator ani and the pelvic fascial supports are subject to ischemic damage. Pelvic X-ray reveals damage to the region of symphysis pubis in about 30% cases of obstetric fistula.

Complete Perineal Tear or Rectovaginal Fistula

Sometime patients do not complain about fecal incontinence and routine per-rectal examination is therefore needed to exclude coexistent rectovaginal fistula. The incidence of combined fistula ranges from 5% to 10%. Isolated RVFs are rare.

Depression and Suicidal Tendency

It is common among fistula patients. Study in Ethiopia found 100% of patient had positive psychological disorder test (Brian et al. 2009).

> In this case your diagnosis is VVF, associated with secondary amenorrhea.
> What will be your next task in managing this patient?

Definitive treatment is local repair by flap splitting method and before that a meticulous preoperative work-up is mandatory. Before proceeding to repair, a thorough examination should be done to delineate the condition of uterus, cervix and upper vagina. After a comprehensive work-up, she should be counseled adequately regarding the surgical procedure and the anticipated outcome. After successful repair, in some cases, menstruation may resolve spontaneously.

RELATED INFORMATION

Before going for definitive surgery, it is necessary to assess the general condition of the patient and the status of the fistula. The patient should be physically fit for anesthesia and surgery. If any problem can be identified that need to be addressed first:
- Anemia should be corrected and any comorbidity should be treated before surgery.
- General health to be improved with nutritious diet and required supplementation.

- Vulval and perineal dermatitis should be treated with zinc oxide ointment or a cream containing lanolin.
- In addition to routine preoperative investigations, following important relevant investigations are often required:
  - *Urinalysis and urine culture* may identify the presence of a concomitant infection, which should be treated with appropriate antibiotic. This is needed, when there is sacculation in the upper vagina with some stagnation of urine, but usually due to continuous drainage of urine bladder remain empty and cystitis does not occur (Sayeba, 2006).
  - *Preoperative cystourethroscopy* may be necessary in some cases to evaluate the anatomic relationship of the fistula. The exact location of the fistula in relation to the ureteric orifices, its size and status of bladder and neck should be determined. Additional fistulous communications need to be excluded to reduce the risk of surgical failure. Practically, the role of cystourethroscopy is doubtful to many fistula surgeons and therefore, limited.
  - *Intravenous urography* may help in assessing ureteral anatomy.
  - *Plain X-ray abdomen* to delineate bladder stone.

Note: Good ultrasonographic evaluation can supplement IVU and X-ray.

Immediate Preoperative Preparation

- Adequate hydration by advising to drink plenty of water
- Bowel should be kept empty preferably by using glycerine suppository:

> The patient is now prepared for surgical repair.
> What will be the preferred route of repair?

Transvaginal repair.

RELATED INFORMATION

Female genitourinary fistula can be repaired through different approaches.
- Transvaginal
- Transabdominal
- Transvesical
- Combined route.

Whenever possible transvaginal repair is the preferred method of repair for both vesicovaginal and urethrovaginal fistula but depends on the familiarity of the surgeon. Gynecologists always prefer vaginal route, but urologists often prefer abdominal route. Vaginal route can avoid abdominal incision, more acceptable to the women, postoperative discomfort is less and vaginal stenosis can be corrected simultaneously.

The location of the fistula and the degree of tissue loss will dictate the approach to repair. The abdominal approach should be reserved for situations in which access to the fistula is limited. Involvement of the ureter may also require an abdominal approach to facilitate ureteral reimplantation.

In certain circumstances, a combined vaginal and abdominal approach may be helpful.

> What are the points in favor of successful repair of VVF in this patient?

This patient is having a single fistula, small in size, located at bladder base, not involving ureteral orifices or urethra or bladder neck. She also has no vaginal stenosis/scarring and this is the first approach of surgical repair. All these features go in favor of successful repair.

RELATED INFORMATION

Success of Repair Depends On

A. Factors Related to Fistula

- *Number and site of fistula:* Single fistula at the bladder base away from bony attachment or cervix heals well after repair.
- *Size of fistula(s):* The smaller the fistula, higher the success of repair.
- *Adherence to pubic symphysis/pubic bone:* Difficult to separate and less mobilization, which may increase tension on suture line.
- *Presence of inflammation, infection and fibrosis around fistula:* Should resolve first before attempting local repair.

- *Scarring/Fibrosis of bladder or vaginal mucosa:* All the fibrous tissue from fistula margin to be removed before placing sutures. So, prospect of healing is more following repair if less scarring and less fibrous tissue.
- *Relationship of ureteric orifices to the edge of fistula:* Involvement of one or both ureteric orifices indicate large fistula size and complex one. Before repair identifying and protecting both ureteric orifices is mandatory.
- *Involvement of urethra:* Increases chance of postrepair incontinence, may not be through fistula, but due to nonfunctioning or incomplete functioning of sphincter mechanism.
- *Presence of bladder calculi:* To be identified by passing a metallic catheter into bladder and if any, should be removed first. Presence of calculi increases chance of infection and break up of suture line.
- *Bladder capacity:* If bladder capacity is less chance of failure is more.

B. Factors Related to Surgery

- *Timing of surgery:* After 3-6 months from occurrence (depends as well on surgeon's judgment)
- *Expertise of the surgeon*, more than average manual dexterity of the surgeon in suturing
- *Experienced assistants*
- *Adequate dissection and mobilization* of the vaginal wall from the bladder wall around fistula
- *Tension free, watertight closure of the fistula*
- *Proper hemostasis*
- *Catheter care:* Continuous postoperative bladder drainage and quality of other postoperative care.

C. Case Complexity

The best chance at closure of the fistula is the primary attempt.

The complexity of cases vary widely, 25% are reasonably simple, 50% are technically challenging and remaining 25% can be extremely challenging. Every fistula surgery has a chance of success and failure. Even experts cannot cure every case. Successful closure of the fistula cannot make the patient always dry. Even after successful repair of fistula, some 15-20% will have severe stress incontinence due to damage of urethral sphincteric mechanism. An expert surgeon who repairs all cases can at best probably make 65-75% really dry (Wall et al. 2005; Zheng and Anderson, 2009).

Patient should be informed about the anticipated outcome of repair before surgery. In addition, she should also be counseled about postoperative management, length of hospital stay and cost.

> *After local repair, how are you going to take postoperative care of this patient?*

Postoperative care is very important for the success of the repair:
- Continuous urinary drainage is the key issue. So, transurethral catheter should be kept for 14-21 days (as per surgeon's preference).
- Vaginal pack if inserted, should be removed after 24 hours postoperatively.
- Adequate hydration will ensure irrigation of the bladder and help to remove clots and debris that could obstruct the catheter. Patient should be instructed to drink large amount of water daily, so that urine will be as clear as drinking water.
- To move bowel regularly, the patient should be encouraged to take large amount of vegetables and fresh fruits. If necessary laxatives to be given.
- According to hospital protocol, prophylactic antibiotic is to be given. Regarding antibiotic use and its continuation, postoperatively much controversy is there as infection plays no role in the causation of fistula, and if infection occurs it is due to contamination during surgery.
- Strenuous activity should be avoided for at least 3 months.
- Resumption of sexual activity should also be after 3 months following repair.

> *Suppose, this patient has come to you with this problem 10 days after delivery. Would you like to perform the repair right now? If not, give your reasons.*

No, an interval of at least 3 months from injury to repair in obstetric fistula is generally recommended. This delay allows for the tissues to become free from infection or edema, and tissue reaction to get subside. Some surgeons do repair, when wound became clean, even before 3 months.

Delay of closure has a significant negative impact on a patient's quality of life and social isolation.

> Do you think conservative treatment plays any role in the healing of fistula in this type of patient?

If size of the fistula is small and patient comes just after the development of fistula, it would have been possible to treat her conservatively with continuous catheterization with the aim of spontaneous healing.

RELATED INFORMATION

When the genitourinary fistula is small, sometimes continuous bladder drainage using an indwelling urinary catheter immediately after its development, leads to spontaneous closure. Fistulae <2 cm in greatest dimension has the prospect of spontaneous healing in 20-40% cases, when catheter is kept for 4-6 weeks, even in case of large fistula, size becomes smaller with continuous bladder drainage, which facilitates future successful repair.

If the fistula has not closed within 4 weeks, it is unlikely to do so, probably due to collagen deposition and epithelialization of the fistulous tract.

In the event of leakage of urine after removal of the catheter following repair, recatheterization is advocated for further duration with the hope of spontaneous healing of residual fistula.

After a cesarean section for prolonged obstructed labor, the catheter should be retained for at least 10 days. If there is urinary leakage after removal of the catheter, it should be reinserted immediately and kept for another 2-3 weeks.

Early repair: Some surgeons showed very good results in repairing selected fistula before 3 months (Waaldijk, 2004).

> Suppose in this patient, local repair is successful and now you are going to discharge her from hospital.
> What instructions do you like to give her?

The patient should be instructed:
- To avoid over distension of bladder by frequent voiding
- To avoid sexual intercourse and strenuous activity for at least 3 months
- To avoid pregnancy for 6 months
- During pregnancy to have regular antenatal care
- To have mandatory hospital delivery by elective cesarean section
- To perform Kegel's pelvic floor exercise, if there is any urethral incontinence.

> Suppose the fistula is a large one involving bladder neck and adherent to pubic bones.
> What measure during local repair may improve the chance of success of repair?

Interposition of graft can be done to improve the chance of healing.

RELATED INFORMATION

Labial fat graft (Martius graft) has been using by many fistula surgeons for long. The idea of Martius graft is to bring good tissue with its blood supply into the area of repair. The vascular supply to the graft inferiorly from the internal pudendal artery and superiorly from the external pudendal artery. In mobilizing a labial fat pad pedicle, the surgeon must preserve one of these vascular bundles.

Recently, a lot of controversy arises about the use of this graft. Many expert surgeons are now restricting its use only in selected cases.

Martius grafts may be used in recurrent fistula, where there is lack of vaginal skin to cover the repair site, to support urethral repair or where water tight closure is not possible (Brian et al. 2009).

To prevent the postrepair incontinence, certain measures could be taken such as lengthening of urethra, repair of pubocervical fascia, if possible and urethral support with a fibromuscular sling (Browning, 2004; Browning, 2006).

> After successful repair, Mrs Nargis again developed dribbling though small in amount.
> How will you manage her?

She will be managed either by pelvic floor exercise or sling procedure, or by using urethral plug.

She will be counseled that after successful closure of fistula at least 20% may develop some incontinence. She will be assessed properly and then will be managed conservatively by pelvic floor exercise for at least 6 months. If still there is significant stress incontinence, some surgical procedures such as lengthening of urethra and fibro-muscular sling or rectus fascia sling can be done (Browning, 2006). She will be counseled and informed that complete cure may not be possible that can minimize her frustration. Before proceeding to surgical procedure, dye test must have to be done to exclude minute fistula. In the hand of experts, only 50% can be made dry. Urethral plug can be used in severe cases to stop the urine draining out through the urethra (Brian et al. 2009).

> Suppose local repair fails in this patient. What are you going to do for her?

The patient has to be counseled and advised to come back after 3 months to take the second attempt of repair. If the first attempt of local repair fails, second attempt should be taken after 3 months to allow the tissue reaction get subside and infection get clear. Several attempts can be taken to repair the fistula, so long surrounding tissues are available for repair.

> Case scenario: Mrs Rahela had an operation for VVF 4 years ago. It was failed. After that she underwent 3 more surgeries, but still she is suffering from dribbling. Now fistula becomes smaller, but there is no tissue available for repairing. Margins are bounded by bones.
> How will you manage this patient?

This patient needs urinary diversion as last resort of treatment.
Types of operation need to be individualized based on the type of fistula and choice of patient.

RELATED INFORMATION

Urinary diversion is the last resort to achieve a socially acceptable solution for the unfortunate patients of genitourinary fistula. This should be restricted only for inoperable fistula, e.g. failed repair with damaged urethra, very small bladder and severe fibrosis or severe vaginal stenosis obstructing visualization and access to fistula.

Urinary diversion is indicated when the bladder can no longer safely function as a reservoir for urine storage.

Indications

- Bladder cancer requiring cystectomy
- Neurogenic bladder conditions that threaten renal function
- Severe radiation injury to the bladder
- Intractable incontinence in females
- Chronic pelvic pain syndromes.

Types of Diversion

Noncontinent or Conduit Urinary Diversion

Diversion into a noncontinent conduit is considered less technically demanding and is associated with the fewest postoperative complications; therefore, this technique is the criterion standard. Noncontinent urinary diversion is performed by any of the two ways. It needs lifelong use of urostomy bags:
1. Directly anastomosing the ureters to the anterior body wall: Cutaneous ureterostomy. Direct ureter anastomosis with the skin is the only form of diversion that does not require use of the gastrointestinal tract. In adults, cutaneous ureterostomy is currently rarely performed.
2. Using a segment of bowel to anastomose in a similar manner to the anterior wall for ostomy bag drainage.
   The bowels most commonly used for noncontinent conduit diversion are:
   - 15–25 cm of ileum (most commonly used) called ileal conduit
   - Colon
   - Jejunum bowel segments (least commonly used).

Continent Urinary Diversion

The most commonly used bowel segments for continent urinary diversion are either:
- Ileum or a combination of terminal ileum
- Ascending colon.

Pressure for storage and emptying of the urine needs to be low as high storage and voiding pressures ultimately cause high-pressure reflux nephropathy and may result in renal failure. Except ureterosigmoidostomy, other bowel segments used for continent diversion need initial detubularization. The bowel segments are then refashioned in a more spherical shape, which increases capacity and decreases luminal pressure by a magnitude of 3–4 times lower than the original segmental pressure.

Continent diversion may be further categorized into three types:

1. *Orthotopic or neobladder diversion:* Orthotopic diversion or neobladder is the reconstructed pouch anastomosed to the native urethra. The continence mechanism in an orthotopic diversion is the native urethral rhabdosphincter.
2. *Continent catheterizable diversion:* Patients with a continent catheterizable stoma have a one-way valve mechanism fashioned at the insertion site that leads into the urinary storage system.
3. *Ureterosigmoidostomy:* It consists of anastomosing the ureters to the sigmoid colon in a non-refluxing manner. This diversion method relies on the anal sphincter for continence. For reasons listed in complications, ureterosigmoidostomy is becoming a less popular method of continent diversion.

Contraindications

- The major contraindications to urinary diversion are bowel-type specific. Because of refractory metabolic abnormalities, jejunal segments should be used only in the absence of another acceptable type of bowel segment.
- Bowel injured by radiation should not be used for diversion.
- Patients with poor renal function, severe metabolic abnormalities, significant proteinuria should not undergo diversion with continent reservoirs.
- Lack of motivation is unable to catheterize a continent reservoir should not undergo diversion in this manner.
- Spinal cord injuries associated with poor hand coordination are absolute contraindications for continent urinary diversion (including neobladder) because of the need for intermittent catheterization and the potential for catastrophic complications if these individuals fail to do so.
- Bowel abnormalities such as Crohn disease, severe irritable bowel syndrome, fat malabsorption and potentially, ulcerative colitis preclude the surgeon from taking long segments of bowel.
- Patients with a preoperative creatinine clearance of less than 60 mL/minute should not undergo continent urinary diversion.
- Those with a prior history of high-dose radiotherapy to the abdomen and/or pelvis should not have long lengths of small bowel used.

Preoperative Evaluation

Prior to urinary diversion, following need to do:

a. *Renal function assessment*: Assessment of the patient's *renal function* is important. A minimum creatinine clearance of 60 mL/min necessary prior to performing continent diversion. A minimum of renal function is necessary because of the increased renal demand created by continent urinary diversion. Because of the increased contact time of urine with bowel segments, previously eliminated renal products are reabsorbed and must again be re-excreted.
b. *Sphincter function test*: Before continent diversion anal sphincteric function must be tested. It must be competent.
c. *Laboratory studies*: To exclude infection and assessing metabolic status, specifically metabolic acidosis. Following tests are to be done:
    - Arterial blood gas (if significant metabolic acidosis is expected)
    - Acid-base disturbance graph
    - Complete blood cell count
    - Urinalysis and urine culture (if indicated)
    - Electrolytes, blood urea nitrogen (BUN) and creatinine.
d. *Imaging studies*:
    - *Ultrasonography*: It is a desirable method for imaging the upper urinary tracts.
    - *Intravenous pyelography*: Most urologists are comfortable with the anatomical information obtained from an intravenous pyelography (IVP). Depending on the evaluating physician's preference, IVP

is an excellent method of imaging the integrity and drainage of the upper urinary system.
- CT scanning: Non-contrast CT scanning is most useful for demonstrating the presence of urinary calculi; if absent, performing a contrast-enhanced study alone or after non-contrast images is probably more useful for assessing drainage, function and integrity.

Preoperative Care

- Preoperatively a full mechanical and antibiotic bowel preparation is to be given. If large-bowel segments are to be used, an air-contrast barium enema is recommended to rule out significant diverticulosis or other conditions that may exclude large bowel for use in urinary diversion.
- It needs to be discussed about several options of urinary diversion with each patient preoperatively.

Peroperative Care

- The surgeon should be very familiar with the intended procedure as decision may be changed according to patient's need. Thoroughly irrigate the bowel contents after isolating the limb that will be used for diversion. The bowel reanastomosis should be widely patent and should be performed along the antimesenteric segments.
- The Wallace anastomosis allows for widely patent ureteral orifices, which are less likely to become obstructed. This procedure also allows for reflux of urine, which theoretically may predispose patients to long-term reflux nephropathy.
- A nonrefluxing anastomosis though significantly diminishes the risk of reflux nephropathy, it is also more prone to stricture and obstruction, which ultimately may lead to reoperation and repair.
- So to reduce urinary reflux, Wallace type of anastomosis with a properistaltic segment of nondetubularized ileum is recommended.
- Detubularizing continent reservoirs and reconstructing them in a more spherical shape is of paramount importance. This procedure allows for greater capacity and most importantly for reduced storage pressure.
- In the case of neobladder construction, isolated bowel loop should be tested to see mesenteric mobility prior to disrupting bowel continuity.
- Stents are recommended to bridge the ureteral anastomosis.
- When a neobladder is constructed, a urethral Foley catheter and suprapubic tube are left in place.
- When a continent catheterizable reservoir is constructed, a stenting catheter is left in place, in the efferent limb and a suprapubic tube is placed through a separate portion of the reservoir, and brought out through a stab incision in the skin. Noncontinent diversion is drained by ureteral stents only.

Postoperative Care

The length of time drainage tubes should stay in place varies according to individual practice:
- Stent the ureteral anastomosis for 2 weeks.
- The urethral Foley catheter is left in place for 2 weeks before removal.
- The suprapubic tube is then clamped and the reservoir, cycled with post-void residuals, is to be checked.
- At the third postoperative week, the suprapubic tube is removed.

Postoperative Monitoring

- *History:* In case of noncontinental diversion, patient needs to ask, how much urine is normally obtained with each void or catheterization.
- *Biochemical tests*
- *Ultrasonography:* Mild hydronephrosis is not unusual after continent diversion.
- *IVP* is performed at 6 weeks postoperatively.
- *CT scan:* It is extremely valuable for assessing a ruptured continent urinary reservoir or for determining the presence of fistulous communication of the urinary tract with the gastrointestinal or genital tracts.
- *Cystography:*
  - Distension of the continent reservoir with contrast is indicated, when the patient is

thought to have a ruptured segment. The reservoir must be assessed in at least two views, and the conduit must be adequately distended.
- Cystography to rule out a rupture is best performed under real-time imaging, thereby allowing the reservoir to be monitored throughout the entire distension phase.

Complications

Early Complications
These include:
- Postoperative ileus or bowel obstruction: More common in continent diversions
- Ureter-bowel anastomotic leak
- Acute pyelonephritis
- Urinoma.

Late Complications
- Metabolic disturbances may result from the interaction of urine with the absorptive surface of the bowel used for the procedure
- Ischemic strictures
- Peripheral vascular disease
- Chronic obstructive pulmonary disease
- Infection.

Complications Related to Type of Diversion

Conduit diversion

Jejunal segments
Jejunal segments pose the most medically challenging metabolic abnormality with regard to urinary diversion. More water and electrolyte loss. The net effect in 27% of patients is a hyperkalemic, hyponatremic, hypochloremic metabolic acidosis, known as the jejunal conduit syndrome.

Ileal and colonic segments
- Patients in whom ileal and colonic segments were used may develop hyperchloremic metabolic acidosis, which is likely caused by increased ammonium and chloride absorption by the bowel segment from the urine.
- Because of the poor absorptive capacity of colonic segments, these patients tend to develop hypokalemia more often than those in whom small-bowel segments were used.
- Patients with sepsis or decreased hepatic functional reserve, who develop ammonia hyperabsorption by the bowel segment are at risk for hyperammonia and encephalopathy.

Continent diversion

Metabolic abnormalities
Increased bowel surface area or contact time with urine results in greater solute reabsorption and more pronounced abnormalities. Patients with continent reservoirs, which have both a greater surface area for absorption and prolonged contact times with urine, have a higher incidence of metabolic abnormalities.

Vitamin B_{12} deficiency
The terminal ileum is the exclusive site of vitamin B_{12} absorption in humans. Most urinary diversions in which ileum is used are performed in a way to compensate for the physiology of vitamin B_{12} absorption; however, more than 50 cm of resection appears to be the critical length at which abnormal B_{12} absorption may be expected. Long-term follow-up studies in patients with shorter ileal segments demonstrate a 25-28% incidence of complications from vitamin B_{12} deficiency. Patients in whom more than 50 cm ileum is resected are at increased risk for vitamin B_{12} deficiency, which usually does not become clinically apparent for at least 2 years.

Rupture of reservoir
One of the most devastating complications is rupture of the reservoir, which is most common in continent diversions. Hypercontinence of the catheterizable reservoir often leads to an elevated storage pressure and results in rupture. Bacterial peritonitis invariably results when a bowel segment used for diversion ruptures.

Other Complications

- Secretory and/or osmotic diarrhea
- Stomal stenosis, dermatitis, prolapse, retraction and parastomal hernias (incidence; 15-40%)
- Poor drainage of conduit or reservoir
- Retention in the continent reservoir

- Volvulus and retention in conduit (rare)
- Urinary lithiasis (especially in patients with secretory diarrhea and chronic dehydration)
- Recurrent symptomatic infections
- Ureterosigmoidostomy: Adenocarcinoma, urosepsis, ureteral stenosis, and/or hydronephrosis.

Treatment of Complications

Early Complications

- Most commonly, the treatment is intravenous hydration and possible nasogastric tube placement guided by abdominal radiography and laboratory studies.
- If the integrity of the ureteral-bowel anastomosis is suggested to have been compromised, consider performing further imaging studies using ultrasonography and IVP. Some degree of hydronephrosis is common, so it should not be overdiagnosed.
- One of the most catastrophic complications of continent diversion is reservoir rupture and bacterial peritonitis manifested by abdominal distension, and abdominal pain. It should be presumed to have a ruptured reservoir until proven otherwise. Contrast-enhanced CT scanning of the abdomen and pelvis is diagnostic.
- This condition is a surgical emergency that requires exploration, repair, and broad spectrum intravenous antibiotics. The risk of bacterial peritonitis and increased morbidity needs prompt consultation with an urologist early in patient care. If urinary reservoir rupture goes undiagnosed and untreated, the outcome can be fatal.
- A continent catheterizable reservoir, that is unable to catheterize via the efferent limb is a medical emergency. Ultrasound-guided percutaneous drainage may be required. Blind percutaneous drainage is discouraged because of the risk of injury to the mesenteric vascular pedicle that supplies the reservoir.
- Urinoma may be treated with percutaneous drainage and/or stenting of the appropriate urinary segment in an effort to aid in closure of the abnormal communication.

Late Complications

- Urinary obstruction is best treated in the short-term with percutaneous drainage or consultation with a urologist and retrograde drainage.
- Prevention is the most effective treatment for vitamin B_{12} deficiency. Strongly consider periodic parenteral replacement in patients with a urinary diversion in which ileum was used.
- Electrolyte abnormalities are best treated in the short-term with intravenous hydration and acidosis correction. The patient should receive lifelong supplementation with oral potassium and/or sodium citrate. Chlorpromazine or nicotinic acid may be given to patients in whom sodium loading may be dangerous.
- Administer sodium chloride and thiazide diuretics to patients with jejunal conduit syndrome.
- Diagnosing and treating concomitant pyelonephritis, obstruction, or urinary stasis is important in a patient with metabolic abnormalities; otherwise, the patient is sure to be refractory to treatment.
- Secretory diarrhea is initially treated with cholestyramine (4 g PO bid) in an attempt to decrease colonic exposure and to free bile salts. Dietary fat restrictions are recommended for patients with significant steatorrhea (i.e. >20 g/day).
- Osmotic diarrhea is treated by slowing bowel motility with oral agents (e.g. loperamide, diphenoxylate and difenoxin) to decrease transit time.

Prognosis

Using continent reservoirs as the primary means of diversion has gained popularity, since the techniques have become more refined. Patients receiving continent diversion instead of noncontinent stomas perceive themselves as having a better body image and an improved quality of life. Recent reports do not demonstrate any adverse effects on prognosis or long-term survival for patients with continent versus noncontinent diversion.

Case scenario: Mrs Alo, a 21-year-old short-statured lady developed VVF as a consequence of prolonged obstructed labor. A macerated baby delivered after 3 days of labor pain. She had history of rise of temperature and foul smelling discharge from vagina. After 10 days of delivery, she developed dribbling of urine. She was consulted by a local doctor, but continued to live with the problem. Now after 2 years she has come to your tertiary hospital seeking cure from her suffering. On examination it was found that vagina is so narrow to introduce the speculum. Digital examination explored a big fistula about ≥4 cm in diameter in the middle of posterior part of vagina with massive scarring of surrounding tissue.

How will you manage this case?

This patient is suffering from a complex obstetric fistula. As the patient gave history of foul smelling vaginal discharge, probably she suffered from vaginal and/or pelvic infection following delivery. Infection and ischemia from prolonged obstructed labor resulted in extensive vaginal wall injury leading to scarring and eventual vaginal stenosis. This fistula is a large one (probably ≥4 cm) and associated with vaginal stenosis, so falls in the category of complex fistula demanding comprehensive evaluation before surgical planning.

After adequate evaluation, if the scarring is not that extensive hindering vaginal route approach and assumption of adequate tissue availability after dissection and mobilization for repair, then attempt can be taken for vaginal repair with or without vaginoplasty. In this case, lateral relaxing incisions in the scar tissue, will provide better accessibility to the fistula.

RELATED INFORMATION

Characteristics of Complex Fistulas

Several factors define the complexity of a fistula (Genadry et al. 2007). These are:
- *Site*: In relation to the bladder neck and ureteral orifices, especially circumferential one when urethra is completely separated from bladder.
- *Size:* When it is greater than 4 cm and involves the continence mechanism, particularly if reduces the residual bladder volume.
- *Number:* If multiple or associated with presence of RVF.
- *Severity of scarring:* It determines the fistula's accessibility and mobility as well as the vagina's residual capacity and function.
- *Repeat surgery:* A simple fistula may become complex, when repair fails and with successive failed repair, becomes more complex.

Note: A VVF is even more complicated, when it is greater than 6 cm, particularly if the urethra is absent, there is severe scarring, and/or it is combined with a RVF.

Evaluation of Complex Fistulas

Comprehensive assessment of complex fistulas addresses general health of the patients like that of simple fistula with meticulous evaluation of the status of their urogenital tissues.

Urogenital tissue status includes the size of lesions, number of fistulous tracts, degree of scarring of the vagina and urethral sphincter, length of residual urethra (which determines the degree of urethral reconstruction to be performed and the patient's future continence), residual bladder capacity, and status of the ureters.

A vesicocervical or vesicouterine communication should be ruled out.

Vaginal Scarring

Often large fistula is associated with extensive vaginal wall scarring making it too short and narrow for continuing sexual activities, sometimes even total atresia occurs. Gynatresia is the term referring to a greatly foreshortened and stenotic vagina, which is more likely to occur when a large fistula is repaired. Moreover, the flaps and tissue grafts used during vaginal reconstruction to close large or persistent/recurrent fistulas may further decrease vaginal caliber and sexual function (Gutman et al. 2007). The size and status of the vagina dictate the need for vaginal, augmentation and/or reconstruction.

Management of Complex Fistulas

Every element of evaluation needs to be considered in choosing appropriate technique and route for surgical repair:
- Like managing simple fistula, most fistula surgeons in general, prefer vaginal route as

a first attempt to treat complex fistulas. This approach minimizes the risk of operative and postoperative complications, but may be associated with more vaginal scarring and further shortening.
- In case of large fistula encased in dense vaginal scarring large episiotomy or lateral relaxing incisions (either unilateral or bilateral) are needed for adequate exposure. Often vaginoplasty with removal of scar tissues is required, supplemented with amnion graft or myocutaneous flap.
- The abdominal route is more frequently preferred, when bladder augmentation or ureteral reimplantation is needed, or in the presence of associated pelvic pathology. Abdominal approaches may be extraperitoneal or intraperitoneal. With the intraperitoneal technique, an omental flap can be interpositioned to secure the separation, which also provides fresh blood supply; with the extraperitoneal technique, a bladder mucosal flap may be used to cover the large defect.
- A combined approach is indicated when the first approach chosen did not provide good exposure or did not lead to successful repair, or when a single route does not permit the complex treatment.

> **Case scenario:** Mrs Hasina, a 27-year-old lady delivered a dead baby at home by dai 6 months back. 8 days after delivery she developed dribbling of urine through vagina. Along with this, she gives history of foul-smelling vaginal discharge with periodic, uncontrolled escape of gas and also noticed that stool is passing through vagina when it becomes loose watery. On examination you found two holes, one at the upper part and other at mid-vagina. Urine is coming through the upper one, size of which is moderate. During per rectal (P/R) examination finger passed through the lower one. Her anal sphincter is competent. There is minimum scarring.
>
> Outline your plan of treatment

This patient is having combined vesicovaginal and rectovaginal fistula following prolonged obstructed labor. This also is a complex fistula.

Before planning treatment she needs to be properly evaluated. As this patient is having a moderate sized VVF with less scarring and a RVF at mid-vagina with no sphincter deficiency, local repair of both fistulas through vaginal route can be approached in one sitting after adequate bowel preparation (3-5 days).

RELATED INFORMATION

Development of combined VVF and RVF is 5-10% of surgically treated patients, though a large series reported 11-17% (Wall, 2004; Kelly and Kwast, 1993). More extensive damage caused by pressure necrosis and incur more stress and morbidities to the patient, and additional challenge to the surgeons. In addition to remaining continuously wet and smelly, these patients also experience repeated infections, malnutrition and psychological problems sometimes resulting in frank depression (Ojengbede, 2007). Resulting mostly from obstetric trauma, acquired rectovaginal fistulae may also arise as a complication of a repaired fourth-degree perineal tear. Less commonly develops as a result of direct surgical injury to the rectum or vagina, ischemia, or postoperative infection. Inflammatory bowel disease such as ulcerative colitis or Crohn disease may result in complex rectovaginal fistula. Very occasionally primary or metastatic disease in surrounding organs (rectum, cervix, uterus or vagina) may result in rectovaginal fistula. Fistula may occur several years after completion of radiation therapy, which is an infrequent cause.

Types of RVF

- *Low:* Vaginal opening near the posterior fourchette.
- *Mid*: From the level of the cervix to just superior to the posterior fourchette.
- *High:* Fistula is in the area of the posterior fornix.

Thorough and meticulous physical examination is to be done to determine site, size and number of both fistulas before any surgical plan. By passing a probe through vaginal hole and placing a finger in rectum, fistula tract can be identified. At the same time, tissues about the fistula are to be delineated and perineal body and integrity of anal sphincter need to be evaluated. A proctosigmoidoscopy examination usually done to ensure that the mucosa of the intestinal tract is normal.

Surgical Repair

- *Multiple stage:* Traditionally fistula surgeons practice multiple-stage repair with closure. First closure of VVF and performing temporary colostomy for fecal diversion, especially in cases of high and/or large RVFs. RVF closure is usually recommended following a mandatory 2–3 months interval period of VVF repair.
- *Single stage:* Repair of both VVF and RVF done in a single sitting, especially if the RVF is of low or mid-variety and less than 3 cm in diameter.

Multiple stage approach is because of fear of soiling of the surgical field by fecal matter and consequent infection and eventual breakdown of suture line. But, this multiple stage procedure increases patient's risk in terms of anesthetic hazards, operative morbidities, hospital stays and cost, and in particular colostomy associated series of morbidities such as skin irritation, recurrent hemorrhage, stoma infection, prolapse, or periosteal herniation (Ojengbede, 2007). Considering all these factors, fistula surgeons are now moving towards performing single stage closure with a commendable success rate.

For successful repair of combined fistula 3–5 days bowel preparation including mechanical cleansing and antibiotic gut sterilization is mandatory. Adequate hydration by advising 4–6 L of water daily and previous night enema need to be ensured.

> **Case scenario:** Mrs Khaleda underwent an operation (hysterectomy) for fibroid uterus. At 5th postoperative day she developed acute abdomen, which was corrected by conservative treatment. But, after 3 weeks of operation she developed passage of fluid through vagina having uriniferous smell. It was continuous, but, small in amount. She has urge of voiding and she voids normally. You examined and found nothing abnormality except escape of fluid. You did routine examination (R/E) and microscopic examination (M/E) of the fluid suspecting urine, which commented as urine sample. Then you did three swab tests which revealed that 1st swab was wet with clear fluid no dye came out and other two were not soaked.
>
> What is your diagnosis and how will you manage her?

This is a case of ureterovaginal fistula at the vaginal vault/caff. As this has developed as a complication of hysterectomy and involves one of the ureters, and diagnosed 3 weeks after the initial insult, so proper evaluation is to be done by examination, abdomino-pelvic ultrasound and intravenous urography. A preliminary cystoscopy with ureteric catheterization/assessment is to be done followed by definitive procedure.

Definitive treatment will depend on the level of damage from uterovesical junction and also on the extent of damage.

RELATED INFORMATION

Ureterovaginal fistula resulting from ureteral injuries are almost always iatrogenic, occurring after abdominal, vaginal, or laparoscopic pelvic surgery. Among the gynecological surgeries hysterectomy is the most commonly causative factor in developed world, but in low resource countries obstetric operations, e.g. cesarean section and cesarean hysterectomies are often responsible. Occurrence of both vesicovaginal and ureterovaginal fistula at the same time has also been described, but very infrequently.

Iatrogenic trauma to the ureter may be the result of laceration, suture ligation, transaction, electrocautery, a crush injury or ischemia due to the devitalization of the ureteral blood supply. Ureterovaginal fistulas from gynecologic surgery are usually close to the bladder, i.e. the lower third of the ureter is usually affected, and the vulnerable sites of injury to the lower third of the ureter include the lateral edge of the uterosacral ligament, ventral to the uterine artery and then just lateral to the cervix and fornix of the vagina (Murtaza et al. 2012).

Clinical Presentation

Patients presentation varies according to the nature of trauma. The main presentation of the ureterovaginal fistula is urinary incontinence despite the normal act of micturition. Complete ligation results in acute ureteral obstruction, causing abdominal or flank pain, low-grade fever and ileus. However, ureteral transaction often goes unrecognized, resulting in urinoma, ileus, and subsequent fistula to the vaginal cuff. Ureteral crush or cautery injury to the ureter can result in sloughing or perforation of the ureter and a delayed presentation of urinoma or ureterovaginal fistula.

Diagnosis

Diagnosis of ureterovaginal fistula by simple vaginal speculum examination is often difficult. Diagnosis requires a combination of cystoscopy, intravenous pyelography and retrograde ureteropyelography. The retrograde pyelogram may be useful to localize the level of obstruction and the fistula as well. In resource poor countries where sophisticated investigation facilities are not available there standard three swab test and simple abdominal sonogram are often help in diagnosis. Three swab test helps in differentiating from vesicovaginal fistula and stress incontinence, but fails to determine which ureter is involved (Randawa, 2009). The cystogram may be useful to exclude a coexistent vesicovaginal fistula. CT urography also has a definitive role in the diagnosis of ureterovaginal fistula.

Management

The main aim of the treatment of ureterovaginal fistula is the restoration of the urinary continence, prevention of urosepsis and preservation of renal function. Prompt diagnosis and appropriate surgical intervention has excellent results for ureterovaginal fistula with no recurrence and minimal complications.

Though timing of definitive surgery depends on time of identification, surgeon's discretion and patient's condition, early repair (as early as at 4 weeks) is now being preferred by many surgeons. If the open surgical procedure is not being considered immediately, an attempt should be made for ureteral stenting or percutaneous nephrostomy for early drainage of the affected upper urinary tract as the partial ureteral obstruction is almost always present. Recently, conservative noninvasive or minimal invasive approach including endoscopic ureteric stent insertion (for 6-8 weeks) as primary management has been recommended, as reported success rate of resolution of fistula is high (Otaibi, 2012; Ajamaheswari, 2013; Selzman, 1995). When the retrograde approach of ureteric stenting is impossible, percutaneous nephrostomy and antegrade stent insertion can be tried as second step. Primary treatment with percutaneous nephrostomy has been reported to be less effective. If stenting is not feasible or failed then surgery is the option.

Surgical Options

- *Ureteroneocystostomy:* Refers to reimplantation of the ureter into the bladder. This procedure is done to correct distal ureteral injuries in close proximity to the bladder that measure 3-5 cm.
- *Psoas hitch:* Means extending the bladder's dome and lateral wall and anchoring the bladder wall to the surface of the psoas muscle to cover distal ureteric loss up to 5-8 cm. This procedure helps in mobilization of the bladder with fixation above the iliac vessels to create a tension free ureteral anastomosis. Here, ureter is implanted into an immobilized part of bladder, which prevents kinking during filling and emptying of the bladder.
- *Boari flap ureteric reimplantation:* Boari-Ockerblad flap is a useful adjunct when the diseased or injured segment of ureter is too long or ureteral mobility is too limited to perform a primary ureteroureterostomy or when a psoas hitch is not sufficient. Boari flaps can be created to bridge a 10-15 cm defect. If needed, spiral bladder flaps can be constructed to reach the renal pelvis in some circumstances. If both ureters are diseased or injured, bilateral Boari flaps may be created, if bladder capacity permits.

The bladder flap is prepared by freeing the peritoneum off the posterolateral surface of bladder. The flap length will depend on the size of the ureteral defect, and the base should be slightly broader than the apex. The flap should be at least 4 cm wide at the base and 2-3 cm at the tip (or three times the diameter of the ureter) to avoid constriction of the ureter after tubulization. Longer the flap, the wider must be the base. If greater length is required and bladder capacity permits, an oblique or S-shaped incision can be made.

- *Transureteroureterostomy:* This technique is used in cases of an obliterated or severely injured distal ureter, such as in cases of radiation damage, ischemia or total distal ureteral loss (e.g. ureteral avulsion during ureteroscopy). The health of the distal ureter is assessed with retrograde pyelography, CT intravenous pyelography, or ureteroscopy. The recipient ureter should be of adequate caliber, free of significant vesicoureteral reflux, and without significant stricture.
- *Ureteroureterostomy:* The technique of primary anastomosis of the ureter is used to repair upper to mid-ureteral injuries when the proximal- and distal-segments on either side of the injury are healthy and when the injured segment is relatively short. This can be determined with a combination of retrograde and antegrade fluoroscopic studies. The injuries commonly described that are appropriate for ureteroureterostomy include congenital anomalies of the ureter such as retrocaval ureter, penetrating injuries to the ureter from gunshot, e.g. iatrogenic injuries usually incurred during surgical mis-steps, i.e. complete ligation. The latter may either be identified at the time of surgery or delayed, in which case the presentation is often of a urinoma and/or ureteral stricture.

Complications Associated with Ureterovaginal Fistula Repair

- Urinary extravasation at the ureteral hiatus is usually minimal when the ureter is stented and usually ceases when urinary drainage is adequate.
- Bladder spasms are amenable to long-acting anticholinergics and are often related to larger more rigid stents.
- Stenosis at the anastomosis is usually due to attenuated ureteral blood supply, tension on the anastomosis, kinking of the ureter in a psoas hitch or compression of the intramural ureter in a tunneled reimplant. This is often amenable to ureteral balloon dilation and stenting. If unsuccessful or recurrent stenosis occur, then ureteral reconstruction using a more advanced technique may be necessary.

> Do you think obstetric fistula can be prevented? If so, how?

Yes, obstetric fistula is a completely preventable maternal morbidity. Basically prevention can be primary prevention, secondary prevention and tertiary prevention.

Primary Prevention

Delaying age at marriage and first childbirth by restricting and implementing law of marriage, increasing female education and access to family planning.

Secondary Prevention

Providing quality maternal health services (antenatal care including birth planning, safe delivery care and postnatal care) easily accessible, acceptable and affordable to women.

Tertiary Prevention

Early recognition of prolonged or obstructed labor through use of partograph, early referral to comprehensive emergency obstetric service center (CEmOC), timely cesarean section and catheterization at least for 10 days in prolonged obstructed labor. In addition, proper care should be taken during cesarean section, instrumental delivery or hysterectomy and if any injury is suspected, need immediate identification, repair and appropriate postoperative care.

BIBLIOGRAPHY

Ajamaheswari, et al. Management of ureterovaginal fistulae: an audit. Int Urogynecol J. 2013;24(6):959-62.

Arrowsmith S, Hamlin EC, Wall L. Obstructed labor injury complex: obstetric fistula formation and the multifaceted morbidity of maternal birth trauma in the developing world. 1996;51(9):568-74.

Brian Hancock, Andrew Browning. Practical Obstetric Fistula Surgery. London: The Royal Society of Medicine Press Limited; 2009.

Browning A. A new technique for the surgical management of urinary incontinence after obstetric fistula repair. Br J Obstet Gynecol. 2006;113(4):475-8.

Browning A. Prevention of residual urinary incontinence following successful repair of obstetric vesicovaginal fistulae using a fibro-muscular sling. BJOG. 2004;111(4):357-61.

Demirci U, Fall M, Gothe S, et al. Urovaginal fistula formation after gynaecological and obstetric surgical procedures: Clinical experiences in a Scandinavian series. Scand J Urol. 2013;47(2):140-4.

Duong TH, Gellasch TL, Adam RA. Risk factors for the development of vesicovaginal fistula after incidental cystostomy at the time of a benign hysterectomy. Am J Obstet Gynecol. 2009;201(5):512.

Genadry RR, Creanga AA, Roenneburg ML, et al. Complex obstetric fistulas. Int J Gynaecol Obstet. 2007;99:S51-6.

Gutman RE, Dodson JL, Mostwin JL. Complications of treatment of obstetric fistula in the developing world: gynatresia, urinary incontinence, and urinary diversion. Int J Gynaecol Obstet. 2007;99:S57-64.

Kelly J, Kwast BE. Epidemiologic study of vesico-vaginal fistula in Ethiopia. Int Urogynecol J. 1993;4:278-81.

KM Al-Otaibi Ureterovaginal fistulas: The role of endoscopy and a percutaneous approach. Urol Ann. 2012;4(2):102-5.

Meyer L, Ascher-Walsh CJ, Norman R, et al. Commonalities among women who developed vesicovaginal fistulae as a result of obstetric trauma in Niger: results from a survey given at the National Hospital Fistula Center, Niamey, Niger. Am J Obstet Gynecol. 2007;197(1):90.

Muleta M, Rasmussen S, Kiserud T. Obstetric fistula in 14,928 Ethiopian women. Acta Obstet Gynecol Scand. 2010;89(7):945-51.

Murtaza B, Mahmood A, Niaz WA, et al. Ureterovaginal fistula—etiological factors and outcome. J Pak Med Assoc. 2012;62(10):999-1003.

Ojengbede OA, Morhason-Bello IO, Shittu O. One-stage repair for combined fistulas: myth or reality? Int J Gynecol Obstet. 2007;99:S90-3.

Randawa A, Khalid L, Abbas A. Diagnosis and management of ureterovaginal fistula in a resource-constrained setting: experience at a district hospital in northern nigeria. Libyan J Med. 2009;4(1):41-3.

Sayeba Akhter. Principle and Practices in Management of Female Genital Tract Fistula, 1st edition. Dhaka: Terracotta press; 2006.

Selzman AA, Spirnak JP, Kursh ED. The changing management of ureterovaginal fistulas. J Urol. 1995;153(3 Pt 1):626-8.

Waaldijk K. Step by Step of Vesicovaginal Fistulas. Edinburgh: Campion Press; 1994.

Waaldijk K. The immediate management of fresh obstetric fistulas. Am J Obstet Gynecol. 2004;191: 795-9.

Wall LL, Arrowsmith SD, Briggs ND, et al. The obstetric vesico-vaginal fistula in the developing world. Obstet Gynecol surv. 2005;60(7 Suppl 1):S3-S51.

Wall LL. The obstetric vesicovaginal fistula: characteristics of 899 patients from Jos, Nigeria. Am Obstet Gynecol. 2004;190(4):1011-9.

Zheng AX, Anderson FW. Obstetric fistula in low-income countries. Int J Gynaecol Obstet. 2009;104(2):85-9.

INDEX

Page numbers followed by *f* refer to figure and *t* refer to table.

A

Abdomen
　plain X-ray 324
　swelling of 177
Abdominal cramps 213
Abdominal examination 1, 181, 304
Abdominal hysterectomy 302
　total 159, 195, 247
Abdominal pain 176
　lower 53, 56, 144
　severe 136
Abdominal pregnancy 138
　fates of 138
Abdominal sonogram, simple 335
Abdominal trauma 97, 140
Abortion 253
　alloimmune 315
　immune-mediated 315
　mechanism of 309
　midtrimester 310
　missed 135
　multiple induced 4
　previous 303
　process of 310
　related bleeding 202
　risk of 219
Abruptio placenta 2, 2*t*, 14, 15, 21, 30, 58, 59, 97
　cause of 16
　cesarean section in 19
　history of previous 17
　management of 22
　risk in 17
Abscess, appendicular 183
Accessory gland infection, history of male 274
Acetic acid 227, 230
Acetowhite lesion 227
Acidosis 72
Acne 293
Actinomycin 150, 151, 155, 156
Add-back therapy 246
Adenexae, ultrasonogram of 310
Adenocarcinoma 202, 204, 331
Adenofibroma 168, 181
Adenoid cystic carcinoma 203
Adenoma malignum 203
Adenomyoma 272, 311
Adenomyomectomy, indications of 272
Adenomyosis 163, 169, 239
　dysmenorrhea 238
　presence of 294

Adenosine triphosphate 72
Adjuvant therapy 259
　postoperative 211
Administer sodium chloride 331
Adnexal cyst, types of 172, 174
Adnexal mass 175, 182
Advanced cancer, symptoms related to 203
Aerobic coliforms 218
Afterload technique 212
Alcohol consumption, heavy 303
Alloimmune disturbances 315
Allopurinol 274
Alopecia 155
Alpha-fetoprotein 54
Amenorrhea 72, 136, 151, 323
American Cancer Society 178, 229, 232
American Diabetes Association 79
American Society for Clinical Pathology 232
American Society for Reproductive Medicine 243, 258
Amniocentesis 97
　complications of 94
Amnionitis
　cases of 45
　prolongation, signs of 45
　signs of 45
Amniotic band syndrome 51, 59
Amniotic fluid 55, 93
　bilirubin concentration 92
　collection of 55
　embolism 30
Amniotomy 70
　risk of 70
Amnisure assay 55
Ampicillin
　combination of both 56
　injection 56
Amreich's operation 210
Anal sphincter incompetence 323
Analgesics 244
Anastrozole 246
Anatomic abnormalities of placenta 41
Anatomic causes 304
Anemia 61, 90, 203, 304, 323
　congenital 98
Anemic women, placenta of 5
Anesthesia
　examination under 322
　general 27, 32, 147
Angiotensin sensitivity test 116

Angiotensin-converting enzyme inhibitor 113
Anomaly, developmental 59
Anorexia nervosa 256
Anovulation 258
　cause of 256
　chronic 259
　hypothalamic 266
Anovulatory causes 256
Anoxemia 98
Anoxia, intrapartum 19
Antecedent pregnancy, history of 152
Antenatal care 62
Antenatal check up 115
Antenatal precautions 33
Antibiotics 43
Antibody testing 91
Anticardiolipin 308
Anticonvulsant therapy 113
Antidiabetic agent 84
Antiestrogenic actions 261
Antiestrogens 259
Antifibrinolytics 291, 292, 296
Antihypertensive drugs 111, 113
Antihypertensive medications 113
Anti-Müllerian hormone 258
Antinuclear antibodies testing 306
Antiphosphatidic acid 308
Antiphosphatidylcholine 308
Antiphosphatidylethanolamine 308
Antiphosphatidylglycerol 308
Antiphosphatidylinositol 308
Antiphosphatidylserine 308
Antiphospholipid antibodies 304, 305, 307, 308
Antiphospholipid syndrome 307
Antiprogestational agents 293
Anti-rhesus antibody titers 91
Antral follicle 259
Anuria 7
Anxiety 112
Apgar score 73
Appendicitis 136
Arcuate uterus 310
Aromatase inhibitors 246, 261
Arrhythmia 121
Artificial insemination
　by donor 278
　by husband 278
Ascites 168
　pericardial effusion 98
　malignant 181
Asherman's syndrome 72, 272, 273, 305

Aspermia 256
Asphyxia 12, 72
Aspiration curettage 289
Aspirin 244, 307
    low dose 115, 272, 307
Assisted reproductive
            technique 130, 279
    complications of 282
    indications of 280
    types of 279
Asthenospermia 255, 280
    severe 278, 281
Asthma, contraindicated in 25
Asymptomatic cyst, aspiration of 172
Atonicity, causes of 28
Autologous transfusion 7
Azoospermia 256, 274, 276, 280
    nonobstructive 256, 277

B

Bacterial toxins 29
Bactericidals, negative 71
Balloon tamponade 139
    types of 26
Bandl's ring 68, 69, 69t
Basal body temperature 257
Bathroom privileges, bed rest with 56
Beta blocker 113
Beta-adrenergic agents 44
Betamethasone, injection 43, 102
Bicornual uterus 46
Bimanual examination 162,
            182, 299
Biopsy
    result, interpretation of 232
    samples for 186
    types of 232
Birth
    asphyxia 86
    injury 86
    passage, defect in 63, 64
    premature 39
    preterm 39
    prevention of preterm 313
Bishop's score 8t
Bladder 243
    calculi
        formation 323
        presence of 325
    flap 335
    small 327
    spasms 336
Blastocyst 4
Bleeding
    amount of 201
    from bowel 213
    management
        of mild 7
        of moderate 7

    nature of 201
    severe 6
    type of 201
    with episodes, duration of 298
Bleomycin 157
Blood 26
    collection of 32
    complications of 7
    group of husband 90
    semen 54
    sugar 254
    supply, ureteral 334
    volume loss 28
    with stool 177
Blood glucose 85
    control 81
        treatment of 81
    level
        increased 79
        measuring 84
    reduction of 264
    self-monitoring of 81
Blood loss 5
    fluid, amount of 12
    increased 36
    prevent further 290
Blood pressure 61, 90, 110, 113, 304
Blood product 26
    transfusion, complications of 7
Blood transfusion 5
Blood-stained discharge per vagina 56
Bloodstream spread 207
Boari flap ureteric reimplantation 335
Bone damage 323
Borderline tumors 165
Bowel abnormalities 328
Brachial plexus injuries 86
Brachytherapy 211-213, 215
Brain 151, 243
    complains 148
    metastases 191
Breast ovarian cancer, hereditary 179
Breastfeeding 85, 180
Breathlessness 148
Brenner tumor 181
Bromocriptine 259
Burning vagina, association of 298

C

Calcium
    creatinine ratio 116
    gluconate 7
Canadian diabetes association 79
Cancer 158
    cells 160
    cervix 210
Carbohydrate
    laser ablation 236
    metabolism 78

Carboplatin 189, 191, 193
Carcinoma 289
    type of 197
Cardiac disease 44
Cardiac failure, congestive 113
Cardinal ligament, medial half of 209
Catastrophic complications 328
Catheterizable diversion, continent 328
Cauliflower growth 204f
Ceftriaxone 71, 75
Cell
    carcinoma, small 203
    non-keratinizing, large 202
Cell type
    histologic 214
    unfavorable 198
Cell-mediated gamete injury 249
Cellulitis 288
Central nervous system 44, 98
Central placenta previa 4
Central precocious puberty 266
Cephalopelvic disproportion 71
Cerclage 50
    history indicated 47
    indications of 47
    operation
        after 49
        contraindications of 49
        potential risk of 49
        types of 48
    suture, removal of 50
    techniques of 313
    timing of 49
Cerebral
    artery, middle 90
    edema 118
    malaria 116, 118
    metastasis 160
    palsy 51
Cerebrospinal fluid 154
Cerebrovascular accident 111, 113
Cervarix 222
Cervical
    adenocarcinoma in situ 235
    biopsy 205
    canal 47
    cancer 201, 221, 287, 299
        cause of 204
        invasive 215
        primary prevention of 221
        recurrent 217
        secondary prevention of 223
        staging of 205
    carcinogenesis, steps in 223f
    cerclage 47, 51
        operation 46, 312
        role of 11
    conization 43
    curettage 139
    cytological test 225

cytology 224
destruction 323
dilatation 63, 110
　painless 312
dystocia 63, 68
ectopic pregnancy 139
effacement 53, 57
epithelial cells 222
epithelium
　regenerating 227
　thickness of 234
incompetency 46
insufficiency 46, 47, 312
　pathophysiology of 46, 312
intraepithelial neoplasia 204, 226, 233, 237
　grades of 234t
length measurement 45
lesions, precancerous 221
motion tenderness 162
mucus test 258
neoplasia 231
polyp 287
pregnancy 139
shortening, basis of 46
stenosis 322
tear 29
weakness, causes of 312
Cervicitis 225
Cervicovaginal cause, local 2
Cervix 319
　and pregnancy, carcinoma of 219
　barrel-shaped 215
　carcinoma 208
　carries, stump carcinoma of 218
　competent 48f, 313f
　constitutes 46
　duplicated 311
　incompetent 48f, 313f
　inflamed 227
　injury to 32, 72
　invasive cancer of 219
　laceration to 32
　mobility of 162
　precancerous disease of 221
　under colposcope 230, 231
　vagina, injury to 32
Cesarean section 19
　history of previous 3, 15
　indications of 20
CHAMOCA 156
Chemoradiation 211, 213
Chemotherapy 189, 255
　advancement of 159
　combination 156, 189
　drugs 160
　indications of 150
　monitoring during 190
　multiagent 157, 158
　neoadjuvant 191, 215

regime of 213
second-line 192, 193
single agent 189
types of 157, 189
Chest pain 177
Chlamydia 55
　trachomatis, co-infection with 205
Chlorambucil 156
Chocolate cyst 162, 164, 165, 241, 248, 250f
Cholestyramine 331
Chondroma 168
Chorioadenoma destruens 142, 151
Chorioamnionitis 29, 44, 57-59
　acute 59
　sign of 57, 58
Choriocarcinoma 142, 149, 196
Choriodecidual interface, bleeding in 42
Chorionic tissue, pathological changes in 145
Chorionic villi 147
　sampling 97
　scalloping of 146
　swelling 146
Chromopertubation 270
Cimetidine 274
Circumvallate placenta 16
Cisplatin 157, 159, 189, 213
Cisplatinum 189
Cisplatinum-etoposide 151
Classical Meigs' radical hysterectomy 209
Clear cell
　adenocarcinoma 165
　carcinoma 180
　of ovary 181
　tumors 165
Clexane 307
Clomiphene 179
　citrate 259, 260
　acts 260
　dose 260
　use of 179
　failure 261
Clonic stage 118
Clubfoot 51, 59
Coagulation defect 30
Coagulation failure 149
Coagulation profile 107, 117
Cocaine abuse 17
Coital disorder 275
Coitus interruptus 254
Collagen structure, abnormal 42
Colonic cancer 183
Colonic segments 330
Color Doppler ultrasound 311
Colpopuncture 129
Colposcope, parts of 230

Colposcopy 205, 229, 233
　directed biopsy 229
　indications of 229
　instruments for 230
　objective of 229
　supplies for 230
Columnar cells, single layer of 230
Coma, stage of 118
Complete blood count 32, 40, 106, 133, 288
Complex fistula
　category of 332
　characteristics of 332
　evaluation of 332
Conception failure 261
Condom tamponade 27
Conduit urinary diversion 327
Cone biopsy 232
Congenital anomaly 71, 144
Conization, diagnostic 232
Connective tissue tumor 168
Consciousness, level of 122
Conservative surgery 247
Constriction ring 68, 69, 69t
Contraceptive pill, combined 293
Convulsion
　causes of 118
　mechanism of 118
Cord traction, controlled 34
Cordocentesis 94, 97
Cornual pregnancy 137
　treatment of 137
Corpus cancer syndrome 299
Corpus luteum
　cyst 174
　insufficiency 304
Corrosive agents 321
Corticosteroid 56, 58, 191, 259, 309
Corticotropin releasing hormone 42
Cough 148
Counseling of patient 81
Couvelaire uterus 18, 20, 29
　port wine colored 18f
Craniotomy 73
　complications of 73
C-reactive protein 40, 56
Cryoprecipitate 26
Cryosurgery 235
　equipment of 235
　principles of 235
Cryptorchidism 255
Culdocentesis 129
Cyclo-oxygenase in platelets 115
Cyclophosphamide 156, 189, 191
Cyproterone 274
Cyst 163
　adenoma 183
　aspiration of 247, 250
　benign 164, 167
　dermoid 165-167

fall groups 162
follicular 162
functional 183
hemorrhagic 163, 191
in woman, type of 164
inflammatory 162, 165
kissing ovaries
  with 240*f*
  without 240*f*
larger theca-lutein 149
luteal 165, 172
lutein 150
malignant 163
neoplastic 162, 164
peritoneal 164, 183
physiologic 183
regression of 248
retention 162, 165
role of aspiration of 172
rupture of 167
Cystadenoma 165
Cystectomy 251
  excision of 247
  three-stage technique 251
  with vasopressin 251
Cystic hygroma 71
Cystic ovaries 247
Cystic teratoma
  benign 183, 196
  mature 167
Cystoscopy 205
Cystourethroscopy, preoperative 324
Cytologic atypia 300
Cytologic reporting, terminologies for 226*t*
Cytology 288
Cytology-based screening, limitations of 227
Cytoreduction
  benefits of 188
  optimum 188
Cytoreductive surgery 188
Cytotrophoblast 145

D

Dai 71
Danazol 245, 293
  dose 245
  mechanism of action 245
  side effects 245
Deflexion 65
Dehydration, management of 68
Dehydroepiandrosterone 42
Delivery, early 102
Depression 323
Dexamethasone 43
Dextrose in normal saline 74
Diabetes mellitus 39, 79, 89, 108, 253, 298, 304

Diabetogenic stress 78
Diarrhea 213, 292
Diathermy coagulation 247
Diazepam 120
Diazoxide 45
  side effects 45
Diclofenac 292
Dienogest 245
  side effects 245
Difenoxin 331
Diphenoxylate 331
Dipstick test, correlation of 106
Discharge
  amount of 53
  color of 53
  type of 53
Disseminated intravascular coagulation 18, 22, 30
Diuretics 113
Diverticular disease 164
Dizziness 111, 292
Docetaxel 193
Doppler ultrasonography 163
Doppler ultrasound 92
Drug
  history of 274
  side effects of 160
Ductal obstruction 275
Ductus arteriosus 44
Duhrssen's incision 29, 69
Dye test, simple 322
Dysgerminoma 194-196
Dysmenorrhea 238, 257
Dyspareunia 162, 238, 239
Dysplasia 232
Dyspnea 177, 181
Dystocia 61, 64

E

Eclampsia 16, 44, 105, 113, 117, 123, 125
  antepartum 117, 123
  case of 117
  development of 113
  impending 106
  intrapartum 117
  management of 118
  postpartum 114, 117, 123
  treatment for 119
  types of 117
Eclamptic convulsion 117, 118*f*
Ectocervix 225
Ectopic adnexal mass, chronic 135
Ectopic endometrium develop 241
Ectopic implantation 130
  tube for 131
Ectopic pregnancy 97, 100, 128, 130, 132, 137, 162, 183, 253
  causes of 130
  chronic 136

  diagnosis of 136
  resolute 134
  risk factors of 130
  sites of 130, 131*f*
Edema 61
Egg retrieval 280
Ehlers-Danlos syndrome 46
Ejaculatory dysfunction 275
Electrolyte abnormalities 331
Elevated intravascular pressure 108
EMACO therapy 156, 159
Embryo 128
  eight cell grade 1 281*f*
  transfer 279, 281
Embryonal carcinoma 180
Embryonic cells, differentiation of 241
Embryonic tissue 146
Empiric antibiotics 276
Encephalitis 116, 118
Encephalocele 71
End organ damage 271
Endocervical
  canal 225, 230
  curettage 205
  mucus plug 47
  swab 55
Endodermal sinus tumor 165, 196
Endometrial ablation 294
  indications for 294
  techniques 294
Endometrial adenocarcinoma 181
Endometrial biopsy during luteal phase 258
Endometrial cancer 287, 299
Endometrial hyperplasia 289
Endometrial implants 249
Endometrial injury 272
Endometrial sampling 289, 299, 300
Endometrioid
  adenocarcinoma 165
  borderline tumor 165
  tumors 165
Endometrioma 174, 163, 183, 241
  development of 242
  primary 242
  secondary 242
  size of 250
Endometriosis 163, 169, 179, 181, 238, 239, 241, 243, 246, 248
  associated infertility 249
  classification of 243
  development of 243
  diagnostic features of 239
  management of 249
  mild 249
  minimal 249
  pain 238
  stages of 243*t*
  surgical treatment of 250
  treatment for 244

Endometriotic lesions, inflammation of 244
Endometriotic tissue, bleeding of 244
Endometriotic women 238
Endometrium
  destruction of 294
  transcervical resection of 294
  treatment of thin 272
Endometroid adenocarcinoma 181
Endomyometritis 29
Endophytic growth 204
Endothelial damage, results of 108
Endothelial injury 108
Enoxaparin 307
Epididymis 275
Epigastric pain 104, 111, 112
Epilepsy 118
Episiotomy wound hematoma 32
Epithelioid trophoblastic tumors 151
Epsilon-aminocaproic acid 292
Ergometrine 25
Erythroblast 98
Erythroblastosis fetalis 98
Erythromycin 56
Espinosa-Flores operation 49
Estrogen 272
  resistant to 271
Etamsylate 292
Etoposide 151, 157, 159
Euglycemia 86
Exhaustion, sign of 61
Exogenous gonadal steroids 288
Exophytic growth 204, 204f
Exploratory laparotomy 195
Extraperitoneal rupture 135
Extrauterine pelvic tissues 151

F

Facial flushing 112
Fallacy-contaminated substances 54
Fallopian tubes 209, 243
Familial ovarian cancer syndrome, developing 180
Fasting glucose, impaired 79
Fasting plasma glucose 79
Febrile convulsion 116
Female infertility, causes of 256
Female partner, preparation of 278
Fenretinide 180
Fertility
  alternate treatment for 199
  drugs
    risk of 179
    use of 179
  effect of chemotherapy in 198
  preserving surgery 209, 219
  sparing surgery 198
  treatment 269
    advanced 278
    proceed for 248

Fertilization, impairs 249
Fetal
  anemia
    detect 90
    diagnosis of 92
  blood sampling 94, 102
  cause 63
  complications 12, 123
  condition 90
  death 95, 97
  distress 21
  factors 71
  fibronectin
    immunoenzyme testing 54
    test 40
  genotype, detect 92
  goiter 71
  heart rate 21, 53, 110
  heart sound 73
  hemolytic process 95
  hypoxia 113
  infection 95
  karyotyping 306
  lie, abnormal 61
  lung maturity, assessment of 55
  macrosomia 81
  membrane in vagina 48
  movement 56
  pulmonary maturity 95
  stress 42
  testing, nonreassuring 58
Feto reduction 97
Fetomaternal hemorrhage 89, 96
Fetomaternal transfusion 98
Fetus 143
  and neonate 85
  effects on 72
  invariably dies 72
  management of 92
Fever 53
Fibroid 163, 176, 239, 300
Fibroma 168
Fibronectin 108, 116
Fibrosis, severe 327
FIGO anatomic staging 154t
FIGO staging of cervical cancer 205t
Fistula 319
  edge of 325
  factors related to 324
  fibrosis around 324
  formation 320
  management of complex 332
  nonobstetric causes of 321
  number of 324
  obstetric 319, 320
  prevention of 73
  site of 324
  subsequent 334
  types of 319
Folic acid deficiency, role of 17

Folinic acid 155
Follicular cyst, simple 174
Follicular predominant phase, early normal 266
Follicular rupture 178
Foot drop 72, 323
Foreign body 321
Fornices region 152
Fornixes, lump felt through 162
Fresh frozen plasma 7, 26
Fulguration 247
Future pregnancy, chemotherapy in 157

G

Galactorrhea 151
Gamete intrafallopian transfer 279
Gamma rays act 211
Gardasil 222
Gastric
  cancer 183
  discomfort 292
Gastroenteritis 136
Gastrointestinal complications 213
Gastrointestinal toxicity 190
Gemcitabine 193
Genetic
  causes 304
  factors 43, 178
  predisposition 242
  testing 154
Genital organs, female 318
Genital sepsis 72
Genital tract 2, 39, 298
  infection 41
  injury to 29
  lower 33, 55
  malignancy 299
  trauma 32
    management of 32
Genitalia, evaluation of external 287
Genitourinary
  fistula 318, 319, 320, 326
  female 324
  tract infection 39
Gentamycin 71, 75
Germ cell tumor 165, 167, 174, 180, 195
Gestational age 5, 8, 39, 104, 303
Gestational choriocarcinoma 196
Gestational diabetes mellitus 78, 86, 308
  complications of 85, 86
  development of 80
  high-risk 80
  management of 84
  perinatal complications in 86
  risk factors for 80
  treatment of 85

Gestational hypertension 105
Gestational sac in right tube 129f
Gestational trophoblastic
　disease 142, 143
　neoplasia 142
　tumor 142
Gestations, multiple 16
Gestrinone 245, 293
Glandular cell 227
Glasgow coma scale 116, 122, 122t
Glibenclamide 82, 83
Glisson's capsule 108
Glomerular endothelial damage 108
Glucocorticoids 84, 102
Glucose
　intolerance 86
　testing 78
　tolerance
　　impaired 79, 81
　　normal 79, 81
　test 304
Glyburide 82, 83
Glycemic
　control, poor 84
　fluctuations 84
Gonadal dysgenesis 196
Gonadotropin 179, 259
　low dose 259, 262
　releasing hormone 179, 251, 260
Gonadotropin-releasing hormone
　agonist 246
　protocol 280
　treatment of 172
Gonorrhoea 55
Graft, interposition of 326
Granulocytopenia 155
Granulosa tumors 165
Gross residual disease 216
Gunshot 241

H

Haemorrhage, management of
　postpartum 24
Haultain procedure 36
Head, descent of 110
Headache 44, 111, 112, 293
Heart
　damage to 160
　failure, congestive 98
HELLP syndrome 30, 106, 115, 124, 125
Hemangioma 168
Hematogenous 186
Hematoma
　broad ligament 30, 135
　formation 17, 28
　retroperitoneal 15
　retroplacental 16
　unmanageable 28

Hematuria 203, 240
Hemoglobin
　estimation 6
　percentage 62
Hemolysis 106
　produces heme 98
　signs of 124
Hemolytic anemia 292
　in infants 54
Hemoptysis 148, 203
Hemorrhage 15, 31, 149
　accidental 14
　antepartum 1, 2, 39, 89
　arresting of 26
　blood transfusion 151
　intracranial 72
　intracystic 167
　intraperitoneal 136
　major 218
　minor 218
　obstetric 28t
　pontine 116
　postpartum 18, 24, 28, 72
　severe 25
　sign of internal 15
Hemostasis, defective 290
Hepatic edema 108
Hepatic function test parameters 190
Hepatic resection 159
Hepatotoxicity 155
Hereditary thrombophilia,
　tests for 306
Hernia, diaphragmatic 51, 59
Herpes simplex virus 205
Heterotopic pregnancy 134
Heterozygous 89
Hip dislocation 51, 59
Hirsutism 293
Homozygous 89
　rhesus positive 99
Hormonal causes 304
Hormonal therapy 244
Hormone 244
　assay 257
　replacement therapy 179, 298
Horseback riding 140
HPV
　testing 228
　vaccination 222
HPV-DNA testing 228, 229
Human blood group 89
Human carcinogens 221
Human chorionic gonadotropin 142, 179, 265
Human immunodeficiency virus
　infection 233
Human insulin 83
Human papillomavirus 204, 221, 223
Humoral immune 242
Hyaluronic acid 46

Hydatid cyst of morgagni 172, 173
Hydatidiform mole 142-144, 151
　development of 144
　diagnosis of 145
　invasive 151
　management of 146
Hydralazine 112
Hydramnios, acute 15
Hydrocele 255
Hydrocephalus 61, 71, 144
Hydronephrosis 164
Hydrops fetalis 71, 98
Hydrosalpings 183
Hydrosalpinx 164
Hydrothorax, right-sided 168
Hydroureteronephrosis 323
Hydroxyurea 156
Hyoscine butylbromide, injection 31
Hyperandrogenism 258
　causes 263
　sign of 286
Hyperbilirubinemia, causes 54
Hyperglycemia 45
Hyperhomocysteinemia 309
Hyperinsulinemia 263, 315
Hyperkeratosis 231
Hyperprolactinemia 151, 253, 256, 266, 303
Hyperproliferative trophoblastic cells 143
Hypersensitivity reaction 191
Hyperspermia 256
Hypertension 39, 108, 202
　in pregnancy, classification of 105
　management of 111
　pregnancy-induced 39, 104, 105, 308
Hypertensive encephalopathy 113
Hyperthyroidism 44, 253, 256
Hypertonic
　dysfunction 66
　uterine
　　action 67
　　inertia 66
Hypofibrinogenemia 18
Hypogastric artery ligation,
　bilateral 145
Hypoglycemia, treatment of 81
Hypogonadotropic
　hypogonadism 256
Hypomenorrhea 287
Hypo-osmotic swelling test 275
Hypoplasia 309
Hypoplastic uterus 310
Hypoproteinemia 98
Hypospermia 256
Hypotension 45, 121
Hypothalamic pituitary failure 256
Hypothalamocortical origin 322, 323
Hypothermia 44

Hypothyroidism 256
Hypotonic dysfunction 66
Hypotonic uterine action 67
Hypovolemic shock 17, 137
Hypoxia 108
   evidence of 125
   to hypoperfusion 29
Hysterectomy 145, 187, 295
Hysteria 118
Hysterosalpingogram 270
Hysterosalpingography 311
Hysteroscopic endometrial
       ablation 295*f*
Hysteroscopic metroplasty 314
Hysteroscopy 288, 289, 299, 300
   confirms 301
   diagnostic 312
   disadvantages 289
   indications 289
Hysterotomy 145

I

Iatrogenic absence 273
Iatrogenic preterm delivery 43
Ibuprofen 292
Icterus gravis neonatorum 98
Ifosfamide 157, 191
Ileal segments 330
Ileus 334
Immature teratoma 196
Immotile cilia syndrome 255
Immunoassay test 55
Immunologic causes 305
Immunoprophylaxis 99
In vitro fertilization 248, 279
   indications of 280
   steps of 280
Inco-ordinate uterine action 29, 67
Indigo carmine, dye test by 54
Indomethacin 44
   dose and duration 44
   side effects 44
Infants worldwide, death of 39
Infarcts 309
Infection 31, 42, 89, 167, 171, 272, 324
   intra-amniotic 47
   intrauterine 11, 58, 72
   natural 222
   transmission of 7
Infectious causes 305
Infectious status, diagnose 55
Infertility 72, 253
   primary 253
   secondary 253
Infiltrating lesions, deeply 241
Inflammation, presence of 324
Inflammatory cells, infiltration of 46
Infracolic omentectomy 186, 187, 195
Infracolic omentum 186

Insomnia 104, 111
Insulin 86
   analog 83
   doses of regular 85
   rapid-acting 83
   resistance
      diagnosis of 263*t*
      in ovulation, effect of 263
   resistant 264
   secretion 82
   sensitizer 259
   sensitizing agents 263
   therapy 84
Insulin-dependent diabetes,
       uncontrolled 44
Intense modulating radiation
       technique 212
Interleukin-1 107
Intermenstrual bleeding 203, 290
International Federation of
       Gynecology and Obstetrics
       207, 287
International Ovarian Tumor
       Analysis 169
Interstitial pregnancy
   development of 137
   risk factors for 137
Intestinal obstruction 51, 59, 167
Intestine 243
Intra-amniotic infection,
       diagnosis of 57
Intracardiac injection 135
Intracavitary radiation 216
Intracavitary radiotherapy 212
Intracellular proteins 227
Intracytoplasmic sperm injection 279,
       281, 281*f*
Intramyometrial injection 10
Intranatal precautions 33
Intraperitoneal chemotherapy,
       role of 189
Intraperitoneal rupture 135
Intrauterine
   blood transfusions 95
   contraceptive device 292, 239
   death 22, 98
   device 128, 288, 291
   fetal death 30, 59
   growth
      restriction 12, 144
      retardation 308
   insemination 278
   negative blood group, incidence
       of 96
   polyp 311
   pressure, increased 43
   progestogens 292
   transfusion 95, 102
      indications 95
      risk of 95
      types of 95

Intravascular fluid 109
Intravascular status, assessment of 7
Intravenous
   antibiotics 58
   bolus 112
   continuous drip 112
   fluid, administration of 7
   immunoglobulin 309
   pyelography 311, 328
   urography 205, 324
Introitus 298
Invasive cancer, preclinical 232
Ipsilateral pelvic 195
Iron deficiency anemia, treatment
       of 291
Irradiation, local 191
Irregular bleeding, pregnancy-
       related 201
Ischemic damage 323
Itching per vagina 53

J

Jejunal segments 330
Johnson maneuver 36

K

Kallmann's syndrome 256
Karman's cannula 300
Kartagener syndrome 255
Karyotype 146
Karyotypic abnormality 196
Ketoacidosis, management of 68
Ketones 72
Kidney
   damage to 160
   function tests 106
Klinefelter syndrome 255
Krukenberg's tumor 197, 197*f*

L

Labetalol 111
Labial fat graft 326
Labor
   active management of 70
   cervical dilatation, normal 63
   dystocia 61, 64, 65, 70, 76
      amniotomy 69
      role of amniotomy in 69
      role of oxytocin in 70
   first stage of 63
   management
      during 85
      of third stage of 33
   pain
      clinical indicators of 57
      exclusion of false 61
      suspected 57

precautions of 114
precipitate 66
predicting preterm 45
premature 308
preterm 40, 95
risk factors for preterm 46
second stage of 15, 63, 64
spontaneous preterm 84
stages of 63
Lactic acid, accumulation of 72
Laparoscopic cystectomy 248
Laparoscopic dye test 270f
Laparoscopic ovarian drilling 266
    indications of 266
    over gonadotropin,
        advantages of 267
Laparoscopic procedure, second 251
Laparoscopic surgery, poor 249
Laparoscopy 129, 134, 139, 210, 258, 270
    advantages of 270
    diagnosis by 241
    disadvantages of 270
    disease 248
    role of 193
Laparotomy 129, 134
Lecithin, tested for 55
Leiomyoma 168, 183
Leopold maneuvers 65
Lesion
    excision of 247
    subtle 241
    variety of 241
Letrozole 259
Leukocyte count 58
Leukoplakia 231
Levonorgestrel
    intrauterine system 292
    releasing intrauterine 245
Lifestyle modification 259
Ligaments, round 242
Lignocaine 274
Liley curve, limitation of 94
Liley's curve 93f
Lipoma 168
Lipoprotein, high-density 293
Liposomal doxorubicin 193
Liquid-based cytology 226
    advantages of 226
    disadvantages of 226
Liquor amni 143
Liquor, color of 110
Listeria infections 315
Lithotomy 32
Liver function tests 106, 107, 114, 117
Loading plus maintenance dose 119
Lomiphene 261
Loop electrocautery excision
        procedure 43, 236
    advantages 236

complications 237
equipment 236
principles of 236
success 237
Low birth weight 12
    cause of 39
Low motility, causes of 255
Lower uterine, development of 11
Low-molecular weight heparin 307
Lumbar puncture 154
Lumbosacral plexus 323
Luminal pressure 328
Lump, origin of 162
Lungs 151, 243
Lupus anticoagulant 308
Luteal phase defect 265, 309
    causes 265
    diagnosis 265
    frequency 265
    treatment 265
Luteinized unrupture follicle syndrome 249, 256, 260, 264
    causes 265
    diagnosis 265
    frequency 265
    treatment 265
Luteinizing hormone 304
Lymph node 151, 210
    bearing tissue 209
    para-aortic 186
    regional 206
    status 214
Lymphadenectomy 186, 187
Lymphangioma 168
Lymphatic and vascular
        embolism 242
Lymphatic dissemination 185
Lymphatic spread 206
Lymphovascular space invasion 214

M

Macrosomia 84-86
    evidence of 84
    incidence of 85
Magnesium
    action of 112
    sulfate 36, 44, 85, 113, 119, 120
Magnetic resonance imaging 11, 17, 241, 290, 312
Malaria 255
Male infertility, causes of 275
Male partner, evaluation of 274
Malformations, congenital 85
Malignancy index, risk of 168
Malposition 64
    causes 64
    diagnosis 64
Marfan's syndrome 46
Marriage, age of 202

Massive postpartum hemorrhage,
        complications of 37
Maternal
    age 303
    blood, contamination of 54, 94
    complications 12
    death, cause of 123
    endothelial cells, function of 108
    hyperglycemia 85
    pre-eclampsia 108
    pulse rate 57
    pyrexia 49
    weight gain 80
Maternal-specific factors 107
McBurney's point 169
McDonald suture 48, 48f, 313f
McDonald technique 313
Meconium causes 94
Medical disease 39
Medical disorder, history of 274
Medical nutrition therapy 82
Medroxyprogesterone 291, 296
Mefanamic acid 291
Meigs' syndrome 168
Membrane
    artificial rupture of 5, 8, 19, 62
    prelabor rupture of 53
    premature
        activation of 42
        rupture of 53
    rupture of 95
Menarche, age of 176
Meningitis 116, 118
Menopausal
    state 244
    status 169
    symptoms 213, 268
Menopause 176
Menorrhagia 238-240, 287, 292
Menses, regular 322
Menstrual bleeding 287, 322
Menstrual blood loss, reduction of 292
Menstrual calendar 291
Menstrual cycle 201, 303
    irregular 268
    previous 128
Menstrual history 104, 303
Menstrual period, last 303
Menstrual regulation 253
Menstrual status 225
Menstruation
    painful 257
    regular cyclical 257
Mesenteric thrombosis 136
Mesonephroid adenocarcinoma 181
Metabolic
    abnormalities 330
    acidosis 72
    control, inadequate 80
    derangement 264, 267
    factor 305

Index

Metalloproteinases, several matrix 42
Metaplastic epithelium 223
Metaplastic squamous
    epithelium 230
Metastasis 153
Metastatic disease 188
Metformin 83, 264
Methotrexate 133, 150, 151, 155, 156
    contraindications of 134
    injection 11
    side effects of 156
    therapy, monitoring of 134*t*
    toxic effect of 155
    treatment
        advantages of 134
        disadvantages of 134
Methyldopa 111, 113
Methylenetetrahydrofolate
    reductase 309
Meticulous surgery 187
Metronidazole 71, 75
Metropathia hemorrhagica 295, 296
Metrorrhagia 287
Microinvasive carcinoma, surgery
    for 209
Midcycle pain 257
Middle-cerebral artery, advantages
    of 92
Mifepristone 293
Miscarriage 100, 307
    cause of 310
    threatened 100
Misoprostol 25, 34, 58
Mittelschmerz pain 257
Molar pregnancy 97, 100, 143, 150, 253
    causes of 144
    complications of 149
    diagnosis of 142
    evacuation of 146
    previous history of 149
    snowstorm appearance 143*f*
    types of 144
Molar tissue, sign of dissemination
    of 143
Mole
    complete 144, 147, 145, 146*t*
    invasive 142, 151
    partial 144, 145, 146*t*
Monofollicular development 262
Monsel's solution 231
Morgagni's cysts 173
Mother, affection of 99
Mother's blood glucose 85
Motility
    non-progressive 254
    progressive 254
M-rules (malignant) 169
Mucinous adenocarcinoma 165
Mucinous borderline tumor 165
Mucinous cystadenocarcinoma 180

Mucinous cystadenoma 166, 174
Mucinous ovarian cancer 185
Mucinous tumors 165, 181
Müllerian agenesis 241
Müllerian tumors 165
Multicystic ovaries 266
Multifollicular ovaries 266
Multiovular multiple pregnancy 5
Multiparity 15, 70
Multiparous 74
    with epidural 64
    without epidural 64
    women 73, 75, 164
Multiple pregnancy, hyperplacentosis
    in 108
Mumps 255
Musculofascial 323
Myeloid leukemia, acute 158
Myocardial infarction, acute 113
Myoma 271
    treatment of 272
Myomatous polyp 287
Myomectomy 295
Myometrial gap junctions,
    increment of 42
Myometrium
    activation of 41
    premature activation of 41

N

Naproxen 292
National Diabetes Data Group 79
Nausea 44, 104, 111, 112, 121, 213, 292
Necrospermia 255
Neodymium-doped yttrium
    aluminum garnet 294
Neonatal
    hypoglycemia 86
    infection 58
    intensive care unit 71
    management 85
    respiratory distress syndrome 43
Neoplasia 227
    type of 151
Neoplasm 255
Nephrotoxicity 189
Neuroendocrine carcinoma 203
Neuromuscular toxicity 44
Neurotoxicity 189, 191
Neutropenia 190
Nicotine 274
Nifedipine 85, 111, 112, 274
Nitrazine paper test 54
Nitrofurantoin 274
Nitroglycerine 36, 44
Nitrous oxide 31
Noncorrectable factors, treatment
    of 273
Nondiabetic pregnant woman 82

Nongestational choriocarcinoma 180
Nonpolyposis colorectal cancer,
    hereditary 179
Nonresponding endometrium 273
Nonsteroidal anti-inflammatory
    drugs 244, 265
Nonstress test 57
    abnormal 57
Norethindrone 246
Norethisterone 296
    acetate 245
Normal saline, application of 230
Nucleus 279
Nulliparous
    cause in 63
    lady 160
    spontaneous labor in 70
    with epidural 64
    without epidural 64
    women 178
        cystectomy 164
Nutritious diet 323

O

O negative blood 26
Oblique arrest 65
Obstetric
    complications 85
    conditions 22
    fistula
        developing 321
        development of 320
    history 104, 303
    management 71
    origin 318
    practice, modern 3
Obstetrical complications 41
Obstetrical disease 39
Obstetrical management 119
Obstructed labor 70
    in mother and fetus 72
    injury complex 319
Obstructive azoospermia 277
Occipitosacral arrest 65
Odor of discharge 53
Oligoasthenoteratospermia 280
Oligohydramnios 111
Oligomenorrhea 268, 287
Oligo-ovulation 258
Oligospermia 255, 276, 280
Oliguria 7, 104, 111
Oocyte depletion during
    chemotherapy 199
Operative delivery, increased 72
Oral contraceptive 244
    combined 291
    history of 177
    pill 39, 180, 244, 291
    use, long-term 204

Oral glucose tolerance test 79t
Oral hypoglycemic agent 82, 83
Oral medroxyprogesterone 245
Oral tocolysis 43
Osteitis pubis 72
Osteoma 168
Ototoxicity 189
Ovarian abscess 183
Ovarian artery ligation 27
Ovarian blood vessels 185
Ovarian cancer 176, 187
   advanced 188
   CT scan in 184
   early 187
     stage 190
   etiology of 178
   higher risk of 179
   risk of 176, 179
   role of
     MRI in 184
     PET scan in 184
     tumor markers in 184
   stages of 192t
   syndrome 166
   treatment of 189
Ovarian carcinoma 188
Ovarian chocolate cystectomy, bilateral 248
Ovarian complex cyst, bilateral 172
Ovarian cyst 160
   aspiration of 172
   benign 163, 164, 168
   complications of 167
   etiology of 164
Ovarian dysgerminoma 195
Ovarian endometrioma 240
Ovarian epithelial cancer, recurrent 192
Ovarian failure 256
Ovarian germ cell tumors 196
Ovarian hyperstimulation
   controlled 248
   cycles, controlled 282
   syndrome 150, 261, 263, 282
Ovarian malignancy 176, 191
   primary 164, 181
   staging of 186
Ovarian mass 162
   inflammatory 183
Ovarian neoplasia 162
Ovarian neoplasm 163
Ovarian pregnancy 139
Ovarian reserve 249, 258
   loss of 251
   reduced 171
   test 258
Ovarian stimulation 259
   with monitoring 280

Ovarian torsion 15, 170, 183
   complications of 171
   fate of 171
   predisposing factors for 170
Ovarian tumor 163
   benign 163, 167, 182
   cause of 178
   classification for 165
   malignant 181, 183, 198
   nature of 163
   pathogenesis of 166
   role of laparoscopy in 168
   secondary malignant 197
   stages of 192
   treatment of malignant 187
   types of malignant 180
Ovary
   mucinous adenocarcinoma of 185
   sudden rupture of 140
   wedge resection of 266
Ovulation
   cascade 257
   diagnosis of 257
   failure 261
   inducing agents 259
   induction of 259
Ovulatory cycles 178
Ovulatory dysfunction 256
Oxaliplatin 193
Oxygen species, reactive 55
Oxytocin 8, 25, 58, 70, 146, 147
   augmentation 70
   doses of 19
   drip 19, 36
   infusion 25, 69
   injection 30
   role of 67, 68

P

Packed red cell 7
Paclitaxel 193
Pain
   character of 61
   chronic 171
   control 218
   killer, management of 68
   pattern of 238
Painful defecation 240
Palliative treatment 217
Palpable liver 203
Pap smear 221, 288, 299
   procedure of 225
   role of 202
Pap test 221
   abnormal 229
   abnormalities in 228
   repeat 229
Papillary serous cystadenoma 166

Para-aortic lymphadenectomy, bilateral 195
Paraovarian cyst 164, 172, 173, 183
Parental karyotyping 305
Parenteral antibiotics, management of 68
Parenteral medroxyprogesterone acetate 245
Partial thromboplastin time, activated 19
Paternal age 303
Paternal genotype 99
Paternal-specific factors 107
Pathologic disease 298
Peak systolic velocity, advantages of 92
Pedicle, torsion of 167
Pedunculated leiomyoma 164
Pelvic
   abscess 183
   adhesions 128
   exenteration 217
   exenteration, total 217
   infection 163
   inflammatory disease 130, 183, 253, 323
   kidney 164, 183
   lymph node 186, 211
   lymphadenectomy 208, 209, 210
   lymphocele 164
   pain 203
   peritoneum 242
   radiation 211
   sidewall involvement 217
   walls 64, 249
   washing 195
Pelvis
   adequacy of 8
   contracted 76
Peptic ulcer, perforated 136
Per vaginal
   bleeding 176
   discharge 203
   examination 1, 40, 61, 128
Perabdomen examination 287
Perimenopausal bleeding 203
Perinatal death 86, 95
Perineal dermatitis 324
Perineal tear, repair of complete 32
Periosteal herniation 334
Peritoneal biopsies 195
Peritonitis 171
Persistent amenorrhea, causes 294
Pervaginal bleeding, irregular 201
Pervaginal examination 287
Physical stress, excessive 140
Pill amenorrhea 39
Pioglitazone 263

Placenta 15, 16, 31, 143
　accreta 11
　　diagnosis of 11
　　enlargement of 5
　previa 1, 2, 2t, 3-5, 9, 10, 97
　　anterior 10
　　cesarean section in 10
　　diagnosis of 3, 4
　　enlargement of 5
　　in multiple pregnancy 5
　　management of 7
　　risk of 5
　　types of 3f
　　with labor pain 15
Placental abruption 16, 17
Placental alpha-microglobulin-1 test 55
Placental hematoma 18
Placental implantation 29
Placental infraction, causes 16
Placental location, diagnosis of 17
Placental oxygenation 107
Placental separation, severe degree of 12
Placental site trophoblastic tumor 142, 151
Plasma glucose 78, 80, 306
Plasmapheresis 103
Plasminogen activator-1 108
Platelet 26
Pleura 243
Polycystic ovarian syndrome 80, 254, 286, 295, 303
Polyembryoma 180
Polyhydramnios 84
　development of 80
Polymenorrhagia 287
Polymenorrhea 287
Polymerase chain reaction 228
Polyp 300
　treatment of 272
Polypectomy 295
Postcoital bleeding 203, 298
Posterolateral fornix 182
Postinsulin hypoglycemia 84
Postmenopausal bleeding 203, 298
　causes of 299
　investigation for 300
Postmenopausal women 172
Postnatal manifestations 98
Postnatal prophylaxis 100, 101
Postpartum hemorrhage, causes of 28
Post-trachelectomy stenosis 219
Pouch of Douglas 242, 243
Powder-burn lesions 241
Precancers, prevention of 221
Pre-eclampsia 84, 105, 106, 115, 149, 307
　cause of 107

　complications of 115
　developing 107
　etiology of 107
　in woman, risk of 116
　pathology of 107
　prediction of 116
　risk factors for 107
　severe 44, 106, 111, 115
　sign of 104
　symptoms of 104
Pregestational diabetic women 83
Pregnancy 128, 164
　causes during 118
　facilitate 278
　first affected 101
　high-risk 84
　hypertension in 16, 105
　loss, recurrent 303
　metformin in 83
　multiple 97
　signs of 128, 303
　symptoms of 128, 303
　termination of 100, 110, 114
　test 288
Pregnancy-associated factors 107
Preimplantation genetic diagnosis 279
Prelabor rupture of membranes, risk factors of 55
Premature birth, causes of 41
Premature ovarian failure 268
Premature preterm rupture membrane 51
Premenstrual mastalgia 257
Prepregnancy techniques 47
Preterm birth, complications of 51
Preterm labor, advanced stage of 45
Procaine 274
Proctoscopy 205
Progesterone 291
　administration of 51
　midluteal phase 257
Progestins 244, 245
Progestogens 292
Progressive disease 190
Prolactin testing 306
Prophylactic
　antibiotics 56
　chemotherapy 150
　oophorectomy 180
　salpingectomy 180
Prophylaxis, antenatal 100
Propranolol 113
Prostacyclin, production of 108
Prostaglandin 55, 146
　synthetase inhibitor 291, 292
Protein
　rich platelet 272
　S deficiencies 309
Proteinuria 15, 108, 111

Psammoma bodies 166
Pseudogestational sac 129
Pseudo-Meigs' syndrome 168
Pseudomyxoma peritonei 166
Psoas abscess 164
Psoas hitch 335
Puberty, delayed normal 266
Pubic bone, adherence to 324
Pubic symphysis bone, adherence to 324
Puerperal cerebral thrombosis 118
Pulmonary
　arterial occlusion 153
　congestion 44
　edema 113, 294
　hypoplasia 51, 59
　insufficiency, acute 149
　maturity 58
Pulse 61, 304
Pyosalpings 183

R

Radical hysterectomy 208, 209
　complications of 210
　with lymphadenectomy 208
Radical trachelectomy 219
Radiotherapy 255
　complications of 213
Rashes 293
Rectal atresia 323
Rectal bleeding 203
Rectal cancer 183
Rectovaginal examination 178, 182, 203, 299
Rectovaginal fistula 72, 322, 323
　types of 333
Rectovaginal septum 242
Rectum and pelvic colon 243
Recurrent disease 192
　therapeutic options for 216
　treatment of 216
Recurrent pregnancy loss, role of progesterone in 309
Red blood cells 95
Renal failure 323
Renal function 328
　assessment of 7, 328
　impairment 121
　preservation of 335
Renal insulinage 79
Renal shutdown 25
Renal toxicity 191
Reproductive organs, damage to 160
Rescue cerclage 47, 48
Reserpine 274
Reservoir, rupture of 330
Residual disease, volume of 192
Resistant ovary syndrome 269

Resistant recurrent cancer,
    treatment 193
Respiratory depression 44
Respiratory distress syndrome 56
Resuscitation 25
    component of 25
    management for 19
Retordine 44
Retroperitoneal hematomas, large 33
Retroperitoneum 151
Retroplacental hematoma,
    formation of 18
Rhesus
    antibody 91
    antigen 89
    blood group 89
    D gene 101
    incompatibility 96
    isoimmunization 89, 92, 96, 97
    negative 89
        mothers 96
        pregnant women 101
        women, monitoring of 91
    positive 89
        fetus 91, 96
Ringer's lactate 7, 67
Rollover test 116
Rosiglitazone 263
Rupture membrane 57
Rupture of uterus, causes of 76

S

Sacral backache 240
Sacrococcygeal teratoma 61
Sacroiliac joint 64
Saline infusion sonography 289, 300
Saline sonosalpingogram 270
Salpingitis 128
    isthmica nodosa 130
Salpingo-oophorectomy 194, 196
Salpingo-oophoritis 288
Salvage therapy 156, 217
Sayeba's condom tamponade 27f
Scalp alopecia 190
Scarring, severity of 332
Schiller test 229, 231
Schroeder's ring 68
Sclerotherapy 247
Scoliosis 51, 59
Semen analysis 254
Semen parameter
    abnormal 255, 275, 278
    normal 254, 255t
Seminoma 255
Senile endometritis 299
Senile vaginitis 299, 301
Sepsis 149, 155, 171
Septicemia 29

Septum, treatment of 273
Serosal cell metaplasia 241
Serous
    adenocarcinoma 165
    adenofibroma 166
    borderline tumor 165
    cystadenocarcinoma 180
    cystadenoma 166, 174
    tumors 165, 166
Sertoli cell tumors 165
Serum
    estradiol 257
    progesterone 132
    uric acid 106
Severity of bleeding, classification
    of 6t
Sex cord-stromal tumors 165
Sex hormone binding globulin 245
Sexually transmitted
    disease 55, 128, 255
    infection 286
Sheehan's syndrome 256
Shirodkar suture 48
Shirodkar technique 313
Shock 31, 149
    hemorrhagic 15
Shoulder dystocia 86
Sickle-cell disease 44
Sildenafil (viagra) 272
Silver nitrate 231
Skeletal compression
    deformities 51, 59
Skin toxicities 190
Slurred speech 121
Smelling vaginal discharge 298
Soft tissue obstruction 71
Sonographic diagnosis 47
Sonohysterography 311
Speculum
    examination 203, 299
    use of 321
Sperm
    cervical mucus contact test 275
    concentration 254
    cryopreserved 278
    factors, role of 316
    function, special tests for 275
    motility 254
Sphincter function test 328
Sphingomyelin, tested for 55
Spiral artery thrombosis 309
Spironolactone 274
Squamocolumnar junction 227, 230
Squamous cell 227
    atypical 226, 228
    carcinoma 202, 204, 205
        advanced 218
        antigen 202
Squamous intraepithelial lesion 226

Squamous metaplasia 231
    immature 227
Stable disease 190
Status eclampticus, case of 122
Stenosis 336
Steroid 43, 46, 274
    hormones 286
    labor, doses of 45
Streptococcus, group B 55
Stress
    fetal 41
    history of 274
    incontinence 323
    maternal 41, 42
Submucosal leiomyoma 300
Submucosal myoma 290
    resection of 314
Subseptum, treatment of 273
Suburethral region 152
Subzonal injection 279
Suicidal tendency 323
Sulfonylurea 83
Sulphasalazine 274
Supracervical hysterectomy 10
Suprapubic subcutaneous fibrosis 213
Supraventricular rhythm 111
Syncytiotrophoblast 145
Syndactyly 144
Systematic peritoneal biopsies 186
Systemic maternal endocrine
    disorders 314
Systemic methotrexate 137
    multidose 137

T

Tachycardia 45
Tamoxifen 259, 261, 298
Teletherapy 211
Tensile strength, causes of
    decreased 42
Teratoma 181
    immature malignant 180
    mature 174
Teratospermia 255, 280
Terbutaline 36, 44, 69
    side effects 44
Terminal ileum 330
Testicular feminizing syndrome 196
Testicular sperm extraction 275
Theca lutein cysts 174
Therapeutic tocolysis, role of 57
Thiazide diuretics 331
Three swab test 322
Thrombocytopenia 108, 155, 292
    mild 125
    moderate 125
    severe 125
Thrombophilia 305, 308, 309

Thrombophlebitis 31
Thromboplastin 18
Thromboxane, formation of 115
Thyroid
　disease, severe 304
　disorder 303
　function test 288, 306
　gland 304
　storm 149
Thyroid-stimulating hormone 304
Thyrotoxicosis 144
Thyroxin 259
Tissue 29
　anoxemia 98
Tocodynamometer 65, 67
Tocolysis 45, 57, 84
　high-dose 45
　use of 43
Tocolytic agent 44, 69
Tonic stage 118
Toxic factors 305
Toxicity 156, 190
　evaluation of 156
　monitoring of 190
　risk of 134
Tranexamic acid 291, 292
Transabdominal
　cerclage 49
　sonography 3
　ultrasonogram 163
Transitional cell tumors 165
Transplacental hemorrhage,
　　　volume of 97
Transureteroureterostomy 336
Transvaginal
　repair 324
　sonography 288, 289, 299, 300,
　　311
　ultrasonogram 258
　ultrasonography 3, 128, 163
　ultrasound 40
Triage test 228
Troglitazone 263
Trophoblast
　implantation site 146
　neoplasm of 145
Trophoblastic disease 148
Trophoblastic fragments 108
Trophoblastic hyperplasia 146
Trophoblastic stromal
　　　inclusions 146
Trophoblastic tissue 147
　dies 150
　embolization of 147
　proliferation of 144
Tubal abortion 135
Tubal block, bilateral 269
Tubal disease 164

Tubal ectopic pregnancy 129f
Tubal mole 135
Tubal pregnancy 135
　rupture 135
　unruptured 129f
Tubal surgery 130
Tuberculosis 253
Tubo-ovarian abscess 164
Tumor marker 163
　alpha-fetoprotein 194
Tumor masses, large 188
Tumor stage 192
Tumor volume 214
Tumor-necrosing factors 107
Turner's syndrome 179
Twisted ovarian tumor 171

U

Ulcerative growth 204f
Umbilical cord, short 17
United Nations Population Fund 321
Ureteric orifices 325
Ureteric tunnel 209
Ureteroneocystostomy 335
Ureterosigmoidostomy 328, 331
Ureteroureterostomy 336
Ureterovaginal fistula 72, 320, 322, 334
Ureters 243
Urethra
　damaged 327
　involvement of 325
Urethral loss, total 323
Urethral plug 326
Urethrovaginal fistula 322, 324
Uric acid 106
Urinary diversion 328
Urinary extravasation 336
Urinary obstruction 331
Urinary problem 53
Urinary protein 110
Urinary tract, infection in 39
Urine
　culture 324
　dermatitis 323
　history of dribbling of 318
Uriniferous smell 319
Urinoma 334
Urogenital tissue 332
Uterine
　abnormalities 42
　anomaly 183
　artery 208, 209
　　Doppler 116
　bleeding
　　abnormal 286, 287, 294
　　dysfunctional 287, 298
　cavity assessment 306
　contractility 147

　contraction 57, 66, 67, 110
　counter traction 30
　defect 41
　factor infertility 271
　fatigability 29
　fibroid 16
　horn, noncommunicating 183
　inertia 63, 67
　infection 95
　integrity, investigation of 310
　inversion 30, 36, 37
　malformation 16
　muscle relaxation 36
　myometrium 151
　perforation 149
　rigidity 21
　septum 311
　structural abnormality 29
　synechiae 273
　tenderness 57
　tetany 69
Uteroplacental apoplexy 18
Uterosacral ligaments 207, 242
Uterovesical junction 334
Uterovesical pouch 242
Uterus 16, 129, 209
　abnormalities of 46
　atonicity of 28
　bicornuate 137
　capacity of 29
　duplicated 311
　empty 129f
　hardening of 61
　injury to 31
　outer coat of 242
　overdistension of 16, 42, 55
　palpation of 25
　previous scar in 4
　rupture 15, 30, 72, 75
　septate 46, 310
　size of 162
　subseptate 29
　ultrasonogram of 310
　unicornuate 137, 311

V

Vaccination
　age for 222
　types of 222
Vaccine, schedule of 223
Vagina 243, 319
　laceration to 32
　upper one-third of 209
Vaginal bleeding 17, 53
Vaginal cornification 261
Vaginal delivery 9, 59
Vaginal examination 177
Vaginal margin, close 214

Vaginal metastasis 153
Vaginal mucosa 325
Vaginal progesterone 51
Vaginal route 210
Vaginal scarring 332
Vaginal sidewall hematoma 32
Vaginal smear test 257
Vaginal stenosis 72, 323
Vaginal swab, high 55
Vaginal tissue fistula, ischemic change of 73
Vaginal wall 25
Vaginitis 225
Valval hematoma 30
Varicocele 255, 276
Vas deference 275
Vasopressin 251
Venous thrombosis, deep 218
Ventouse 61
Verrucous carcinoma 203
Vesicles, grape-like 144f
Vesicovaginal fistula 72, 213, 319, 319f, 322, 334, 335
    development of 72
Vigorous sexual intercourse 140
Vincristine 156
Virus-like particles 222
Visual disorders, develops 125
Visual disturbances 111
Visual inspection with acetic acid 227
Vitamin B_{12} deficiency 330, 331
Vomiting 44, 104, 111, 112, 121, 292
von Willebrand disease 288
Vulva 243
Vulval hematoma 32, 33
Vulval pad, inspection of 57

W

Waaldijk classification 320
Wertheim's original operation 208
Wurm operation 49

Y

Yolk sac tumor 165, 196

Z

Zona dissection, partial 279
Zona drilling 279
Zygote intrafallopian transfer 279